# Multi-Modal EEG Monitoring of Severely Neurologically Ill Patients

Xuefeng Wang • Feng Li • Suyue Pan
Editors

# Multi-Modal EEG Monitoring of Severely Neurologically Ill Patients

Springer

*Editors*
Xuefeng Wang
Department of Neurology
The First Affiliated Hospital of
Chongqing Medical University
Chongqing
China

Feng Li
Department of Neurology
The First Affiliated Hospital of
Chongqing Medical University
Chongqing
China

Suyue Pan
Department of Neurology
Nanfang Hospital of Southern Medical
University
Guangzhou
Guangdong
China

ISBN 978-981-16-4492-4 ISBN 978-981-16-4493-1 (eBook)
https://doi.org/10.1007/978-981-16-4493-1



This Springer imprint is published by the registered company Springer Nature Singapore Pte Ltd.
The registered company address is: 152 Beach Road, #21-01/04 Gateway East, Singapore 189721, Singapore

# Contents

# Contributors[1]

[1]The names on the list are in alphabetical order.

**Feng Li** Department of Neurology, The First Affiliated Hospital of Chongqing Medical University, Chongqing, China

**Guoxing Zhu** Department of Neurology, Huashan Hospital, Fudan University, Shanghai, China

**Jiyuan Li** Department of Neurology, The First Hospital of Shanxi Medical University, Taiyuan, Shanxi, China

**Li Kuang** Department of Psychiatry, The First Affiliated Hospital of Chongqing Medical University, Chongqing, China

**Lihong Huang** Department of Neurology, The First Affiliated Hospital of Chongqing Medical University, Chongqing, China

**Qun Wang** Department of Neurology, Beijing Tiantan Hospital, Capital Medical University, Beijing, China

**Shengnian Zhou** Department of Neurology, Qilu Hospital of Shandong University and Brain Science Research Institute, Shandong University, Jinan, Shandong, China

**Suyue Pan** Department of Neurology, Nanfang Hospital of Southern Medical University, Guangzhou, Guangdong, China

**Wei Dan** Department of Neurosurgery, The First Affiliated Hospital of Chongqing Medical University, Chongqing, China

**Wei Jing** Department of Neurology, Shanxi Bethune Hospital Affiliated to Shanxi Medical University, Taiyuan, Shanxi, China

**Weina Chai** Department of Neurosurgery, The First Affiliated Hospital of Chongqing Medical University, Chongqing, China

**Xiaojiang Jiang** Department of Neurology, The Third Affiliated Hospital of Army Medical University, Chongqing, China

**Xiaoyi Li** Department of Neurophysiology, Guizhou Provincial People's Hospital, Guiyang, Guizhou, China

**Xin Tian** Department of Neurology, The First Affiliated Hospital of Chongqing Medical University, Chongqing, China

**Xuefeng Wang** Department of Neurology, The First Affiliated Hospital of Chongqing Medical University, Chongqing, China

**Yao Wang** Department of Neurology, Nanfang Hospital of Southern Medical University, Guangzhou, Guangdong, China

**Yicong Lin** Department of Neurology, Xuanwu Hospital, Capital Medical University, Beijing, China

**Yin Yan** Department of Neurology, Chongqing University Central Hospital, Chongqing Emergency Medical Center, Chongqing, China

**Ying Zhang** Department of Neurology, Xi'an International Medical Center Hospital, Xian, Shaanxi, China

**Yongming Wu** Department of Neurology, Nanfang Hospital of Southern Medical University, Guangzhou, Guangdong, China

**Yuanfeng Zhou** Department of Neurology, Children's Hospital of Fudan University, Shanghai, China

**Yuangui Huang** Department of Neurology, Xijing Hospital, The Fourth Military Medical University, Xi'an, Shaanxi, China

**Yuping Wang** Department of Neurology, Xuanwu Hospital, Capital Medical University, Beijing, China

**Zhongming Huang** Phecda (China) Limited, Guangzhou, China

# List of Abbreviations

| | |
|---|---|
| ABP | Absolute band power |
| AC | Alternating current |
| AC-ECoG | Alternating current electrocorticography |
| ACC | Anterior cingulate cortex |
| ACNS | American Clinical Neurophysiology Society |
| ADHD | Attention-deficit hyperactivity disorder |
| ADR | $\alpha/\delta$ Power ratio |
| AE | Autoimmune encephalitis |
| AED | Antiepileptic drug |
| AHI | Apnea–hypopnea index |
| AMPAR | α-Amino-3-hydroxy-5-methyl-1-4-isoxazolepropionic acid receptor |
| AP | Action potential |
| APACHEII | Acute Physiology and Chronic Health Evaluation II |
| ATP | Adenosine triphosphate |
| AUC | Area under the curve |
| aEEG | Amplitude-integrated electroencephalogram |
| aSAH | Acute subarachnoid hemorrhage |
| BAEP | Brainstem auditory evoked potential |
| BDNF | Brain-derived neurotrophic factor |
| BERD | Brief electroencephalogram rhythmic discharge |
| BIPD | Bilateral independent periodic discharge |
| BIPLED | Bilateral independent periodic epileptiform discharge |
| BIS | Bispectral index |
| B(I)RD | Brief (potentially) ictal rhythmic discharge |
| BRD | Brief rhythmic discharge |
| BS | Burst suppression |
| BSI | Brain symmetry index |
| CANTB | Cambridge Automated Neuropsychological Test Battery |
| CAP | Cranial artery pressure |
| Caspr2 | Contactin-associated protein-like 2 |
| CBF | Cerebral blood flow |
| CDSA | Color density spectral array |
| CHD | Congenital heart disease |
| CLV | Continuous low voltage |
| CNS | Central nervous system |
| CNV | Continuous normal voltage |

| | |
|---|---|
| COSBID | Cooperative Studies on Brain Injury Depolarizations |
| CPAP | Continuous positive airway pressure |
| CPC | Cerebral Performance Category |
| CPCR | Cardiopulmonary cerebral resuscitation |
| CPOT | Critical Care Pain Observation Tool |
| CPR | Cardiopulmonary resuscitation |
| CRRT | Continuous renal replacement therapy |
| CRS-R | Coma Recovery Scale-Revised |
| CSD | Cortical spreading depolarization/cortical spreading depression |
| CSE | Convulsive status epilepticus |
| CSF | Cerebrospinal fluid |
| CSI | Cerebral state index |
| CT | Computed tomography |
| CTA | Computed tomography angiography |
| CTP | Computed tomography perfusion |
| cEEG | Continuous electroencephalogram |
| c/s | Cycles per second |
| DAI | Diffuse axonal injury |
| DC-ECoG | Direct current electrocorticography |
| DFT | Discrete Fourier transform |
| DNV | Discontinuous normal voltage |
| DPFC | Dorsal prefrontal cortex |
| DRS | Disability Rating Scale |
| DTABR | $\delta+\theta/\alpha+\beta$ Ratio |
| DWI | Diffusion-weighted imaging |
| EBA | Excessive $\beta$ activity |
| ECG | Electrocardiogram |
| ECI | Electrocerebral inactivity |
| ECMO | Extracorporeal membrane oxygenation |
| ECoG | Electrocorticography |
| ECS | Electrical silence |
| EDB | Extreme $\delta$ brush |
| EEG | Electroencephalogram |
| EEG-R | EEG reactivity |
| EGDS | Early goal-directed sedation |
| EIEE | Early infantile epileptic encephalopathy |
| EME | Early myoclonic encephalopathy |
| EMG | Electromyography |
| EP | Evoked potential |
| EPSP | Excitatory postsynaptic potential |
| ERP | Event-related potential |
| ET | Envelope trend |
| FBDS | Faciobrachial dystonic seizure |
| FDG | F-deoxyglucose |
| FDG-PET | F-deoxyglucose positron emission tomography |
| FFT | Fast Fourier transform |
| FIRDA | Frontal intermittent rhythmic $\delta$ activity |

| | |
|---|---|
| FIRES | Febrile infection-related epilepsy syndrome |
| FT | Flat trace |
| fMRI | Functional magnetic resonance imaging |
| G1 | First grid |
| G2 | Second grid |
| GABA | γ-Aminobutyric acid |
| GC | Glasgow coma score |
| GED | Generalized epileptiform discharge |
| Gly | Glycine |
| GPD | Generalized periodic discharge |
| GPED | Generalized periodic epileptiform discharge |
| GPI | Glycosylphosphatidylinositol |
| GRDA | Generalized rhythmic δ activity |
| GTCS | Generalized tonic-clonic seizure |
| HIE | Hypoxic ischemic encephalopathy |
| HREZ | Isoniazid, rifampicin, ethambutol and pyrazinamide |
| ICP | Intracranial pressure |
| ICU | Intensive care unit |
| IEE | Ictal epileptiform event |
| IEFP | Ictal epileptic field potential |
| IFSECN | International Federation of Societies for electroencephalography and Clinical Neurophysiology |
| IIC | Ictal–interictal continuum |
| ILAE | International League Against Epilepsy |
| IPSP | Inhibitory postsynaptic potential |
| IRDA | Intermittent rhythmic δ activity |
| LGI1 | Leucine-rich glioma inactivated 1 |
| LPD | Lateralized periodic discharge |
| LPDs+ | Lateralized periodic discharges plus |
| LPR | Lactic acid-to-pyruvate ratio |
| LRDA | Lateralized rhythmic δ activity |
| MAP | Mean arterial pressure |
| MCD | Malformation of cortical development |
| MCS | Minimally conscious state |
| MDD | Major depression disorder |
| MIDT | Monetary incentive delay task |
| MMPSI | Malignant migrating partial seizures of infancy |
| MPFC | Medial prefrontal cortex |
| MRF | Midline-and-right-frontal |
| MRI | Magnetic resonance imaging |
| mRS | Modified Rankin Scale |
| mV | Millivolt |
| mm | Millimeter |
| ms | Millisecond |
| NCS | Nonconvulsive seizure |
| NCSE | Nonconvulsive status epilepticus |
| NICU | Neurocritical care unit |
| NIHSS | National Institutes of Health Stroke Scale |

| | |
|---|---|
| NIRS | Near-infrared spectroscopy |
| NIV | Noninvasive ventilation |
| NMDA | N-methyl-D-aspartate |
| NMDAR | N-methy1-D-aspartate receptor |
| N-PASS | Neonatal Pain, Agitation and Sedation Scale |
| NREM | nonrapid eye movement |
| NSAb | Neuron surface antibody |
| NSE | Neuron-specific enolase |
| OAA/S | Observer's Assessment of Alertness/Sedation |
| OAE | Otoacoustic emission |
| OCT | Optical coherence tomography |
| OFC | Orbitofrontal cortex |
| OIRDA | Occipital intermittent rhythmic δ activity |
| ONSD | Optic nerve sheath diameter |
| OS | Ohtahara syndrome |
| OSAS | Obstructive sleep apnea syndrome |
| $PaCO_2$ | Arterial partial pressure of carbon dioxide |
| $PaO_2$ | Arterial partial pressure of oxygen |
| $PbtO_2$ | Partial brain tissue oxygen tension |
| PD | Periodic discharge |
| PET-CT | Positron emission tomography-computed tomography |
| PHDA | Paroxysmal high-amplitude δ activity |
| PICU | Pediatric intensive care unit |
| PLED | Periodic lateralized epileptiform discharge |
| PLEDs+ | Periodic lateralized epileptiform discharges plus |
| PLIDD | Periodic long-interval discharge |
| PNDA | Persistent nonrhythmic δ activity |
| PSG | Polysomnography |
| PSIDD | Periodic short-interval discharge |
| PSP | Postsynaptic potential |
| PTSD | Posttraumatic stress disorder |
| PWI | Perfusion-weighted imaging |
| qEEG | Quantitative electroencephalogram |
| RASS | Richmond Agitation and Sedation Scale |
| RAV | Relative α variation |
| RAWOD | Regional attenuation without δ |
| RBP | Relative band power |
| RDA | Rhythmic δ activity |
| RdoC | Research Domain Criteria |
| REM | Rapid eye movement |
| ROC | Receiver operating characteristic |
| RPFC | Right prefrontal cortex |
| RSE | Refractory status epilepticus |
| SAH | Subarachnoid hemorrhage |
| SAS | Riker Sedation-agitation Scale |
| SBP | Systolic blood pressure |
| SC | Spreading convulsion |
| SD | Spreading depression |

| | |
|---|---|
| SE | Status epilepticus |
| SEF | Spectral edge frequency |
| SEP | Somatosensory evoked potential |
| SIRPID | Stimulus-induced rhythmic, periodic or ictal discharge |
| SLSEP | Short-latency somatosensory evoked potential |
| SPECT | Single-photon emission computed tomography |
| SQI | Signal quality index |
| SSRI | Selective serotonin reuptake inhibitor |
| STDS | Standard traditional directed sedation |
| $StcO_2$ | Cerebral tissue oxygen saturation |
| TBI | Traumatic brain injury |
| TCA | Transcranial acoustic |
| TCD | Transcranial Doppler ultrasonography |
| TIRDA | Temporal intermittent rhythmic δ activity |
| TMD | Tympanic membrane displacement |
| TNF-α | Tumor necrosis factor-α |
| TOAST | Trial of ORG 10172 in Acute Stroke Treatment |
| TTM | Targeted temperature management |
| TW | Triphasic wave |
| UWS | Unresponsive wakefulness syndrome |
| μV | Microvolt |
| VEP | Visual evoked potential |
| VGKC | Voltage-gated potassium channel |
| VLPFC | Ventrolateral prefrontal cortex |
| VPFC | Ventral prefrontal cortex |
| VS | Vegetative state |
| WHO | World Health Organization |

# Part I

# Electroencephalogram (EEG) Basis and Quantitative Electroencephalogram (qEEG) Technology

# Basic Theory of EEG

1

Guoxing Zhu, Yuangui Huang, and Xuefeng Wang

## Contents




G. Zhu
Department of Neurology, Huashan Hospital, Fudan University, Shanghai, China

Y. Huang
Department of Neurology, Xijing Hospital, The Fourth Military Medical University, Xi'an, Shaanxi, China

X. Wang (✉)
Department of Neurology, The First Affiliated Hospital of Chongqing Medical University, Chongqing, China



**Abstract**

EEG is the most sensitive method to reflect the functional state of the brain. In neurocritical care units (NICUs), most patients often cannot express their feelings because of consciousness disorders, clinical physical examination and imaging examination cannot achieve continuous evaluation, and routine electrocardiogram (ECG)-blood pressure-cerebral oxygen





X. Wang et al. (eds.), *Multi-Modal EEG Monitoring of Severely Neurologically Ill Patients*, https://doi.org/10.1007/978-981-16-4493-1_1

saturation monitoring has difficulty reflecting the changes in patients' brain function sensitively, which easily leads to a delay in treatment and the deterioration of the patient's condition; therefore, continuous and sensitive (EEG) monitoring is important for neurocritical patients. On the other hand, the EEG waveform is complex because different patterns may represent different stages of a disease, and even different sleep-wake states in the same stage of a disease may also lead to deviation in the EEG interpretation. In the NICU, many monitoring instruments and clinical operations can easily lead to various EEG artifacts. How to explain the significance of changes in EEGs reasonably and distinguish artifact interference accurately will have an important impact on the decisions of clinicians. This chapter briefly introduces the basic concepts of EEG, normal EEG waves, and key points in EEG interpretation and emphasizes the common artifact recognition techniques in the NICU. Throughout the chapter, we put forward our own views, and we hope to provide a solid foundation for the contents described in the following chapters in this book.

**Keywords**

EEG · Mechanism of the formation · Basic concepts · Recording methods · Severely ill patients · Recognition of artifacts

EEG is a method to record and trace the bioelectrical activity of brain neurons. Since the German neuropsychiatrist Hans Berger began to study human EEG in 1924, EEG has been developed all over the world and began to serve clinical and scientific services. The International Society of EEG and Clinical Physiology was established in 1947, and the first International EEG Conference was held in the United Kingdom. In China, in the early 1980s, Beijing took the lead in establishing the epilepsy and EEG group, followed by the establishment of corresponding organizations in various provinces and regions across the country. On this basis, the National Society of EEG and Epilepsy was born, and its meeting was held every 2 years. Currently, EEG examination has been popularized in hospitals throughout the world as a mature technology, serving the majority of patients. After the 1970s, with the development of electronic technology, dynamic cassette EEG, EEG video monitoring systems, digital EEG, and stereotactic EEG came into being, providing more opportunities for research in the fields of epilepsy, epileptic seizure-type diagnosis, and sleep physiology and pathology.

## 1.1 Formation of EEG

The human brain, similar to other parts of the body, such as the heart and muscles, can generate bioelectricity. The recording of brain bioelectrical activity by placing electrodes on the scalp is called EEG. However, the current generated by the human brain is very weak; therefore, it must be amplified one million times, and through electromagnetic induction, the pulsed direct current traced from the scalp electrodes is converted to alternating current (AC), and then by multipole amplification, recorded on record paper. Therefore, the commonly seen EEG is an indirect image of brain electrical activity.

## 1.2 Mechanism of the Formation of an EEG

The human brain includes four parts: cerebrum, diencephalon, cerebellum, and brain stem. The brain is divided into two cerebral hemispheres, which are connected together by the corpus callosum and the anterior and posterior commissures of the brain. The outermost surface of the cerebral hemisphere is gray matter, which is mainly composed of nerve cells, and it is called the cerebral cortex. The deep part of the cerebral hemisphere is composed of fibers of nerve cells called white matter. The cerebral hemisphere is divided into four lobes: the frontal, parietal, occipital, and temporal lobes. The diencephalon is located between the two cerebral hemispheres above the midbrain, including the thalamus, hypothalamus, and third ventricle; and the brainstem is divided into the midbrain, pons, and medulla oblongata.

The cerebral cortex is the highest center of human advanced neural activity and the main anatomical basis of brain-wave activity. The human cerebral cortex is composed of approximately 14 billion neurons and countless synapses that form a large and complex information transmission network. The cerebral cortex is divided into six layers, from the outside to the inside: (a) molecular layer: there are horizontal cells inside, and the axons within this layer run horizontally on the surface of the cortex with lateral conduction function; (b) outer granular layer (small pyramidal cell layer); (c) pyramidal cell layer: the apical dendrites are as long as the cortical surface; (d) inner granular layer (astrocytic layer); (e) ganglion cell layer; (f) fusiform or polymorphic cell layer: the axons of this layer extend to adjacent white matter. The central nervous system (CNS) is basically composed of nerve cells (neurons), glial cells, and nerve fibers. Nerve cells are composed of cell bodies and protrusions extending from the cell bodies. The latter are divided into two types, dendrites and axons, according to their functions. Each neuron has multiple dendrites, and each dendrite branches repeatedly to form a branch shape. Dendrites are the most active part of nerve excitement transmission, and they receive external impulses. Dendrites are divided into short dendrites and apical dendrites; the former connect with neurons, and the latter extend to the surface of the cortex. Each neuron has only one axon, whose function is to transmit nerve impulses from the cell body. Nerve impulses are not directly transmitted from one neuron to the next but must pass through a contact point, called a synapse. The terminus of a neuron is divided into many small branches, and the end of each small branch expands into a spherical shape, called a synaptosome, which is attached to the cell body or dendritic surface of the next neuron. At the contacts of the synapses, each is separated by a membrane. The axon membrane at the end of the axon is called the presynaptic membrane, the cell body membrane or dendritic membrane opposite to it is called the postsynaptic membrane, and the gap between the two membranes is called the synaptic cleft. There are dense protrusions on the inner side of the presynaptic membrane that form a vesicle fence. The synaptic corpuscle contains a large number of synaptic vesicles containing neurotransmitters. Synaptic vesicles release transmitters through the vesicle barrier. In some parts of the postsynaptic membrane, there is a special substance that can bind to neurotransmitters called receptors.

Brain electrical activity originates from the cerebral cortex, and brain electrical activity is generated by the postsynaptic potential (PSP) of pyramidal neurons and their vertical apical dendrites.

In the static state, if a microelectrode is inserted into a cell, there will be a potential difference between the inside and the outside of the membrane. The potential inside the cell membrane is low, 60–90 mV negative relative to the outside of the membrane. If no stimulation is given to neurons, this potential difference remains constant. This potential difference between the inside and the outside of the membrane is called the resting potential or membrane potential. The formation of membrane potential is related to the concentration of various ions in the fluid inside and outside the cell. Under normal circumstances, the main positive ion in the intracellular fluid is $K^+$, and the main negative ion is organic acid. In the extracellular fluid, the main positive ion is $Na^+$, and the main negative ion is $Cl^-$. The cell membrane has certain selectivity for ion permeability. In the static state, the permeability to $K^+$ is the largest, followed by $Cl^-$; the permeability to $Na^+$ is very small, only 1/50 that of $K^+$, and the cell membrane is completely impermeable to organic matter. Ions always diffuse from places with high concentrations to places with low concentrations; therefore, $K^+$ diffuses out of the cell through the cell membrane, while the organic anions inside the cell stay inside the cell. It is difficult for $Na^+$ outside the cell to diffuse into the cell through the cell membrane. Therefore, there are many positive ions outside the cell membrane, and the potential is high; there are many negative ions inside the cell membrane, and the potential is low. This phenomenon of polarity is called the polarization state. Because the positive and negative charges inside and outside the membrane attract each other, the positive and negative ions are arranged outside and inside the cell membrane, so a potential difference is formed inside and outside the membrane, which is the static potential mentioned above.

When a neuron is excited, the permeability of the cell membrane to ions is changed, and the permeability of the cell membrane to $Na^+$ is selectively increased. Therefore, $Na^+$ diffuses from the outside of the cell to the inside of the cell, increasing the positive ions in the membrane and canceling the original membrane potential, which is called depolarization. Finally, the potential inside the cell is even higher than that outside the cell. The potential change generated at this time is called the action potential (AP). When the AP reaches the peak, the permeability of the membrane to $Na^+$ decreases, and the permeability to $K^+$ increases significantly, so $K^+$ diffuses out of the membrane and returns to a positive polarization state outside the membrane and a negative polarization state inside the membrane, which is called repolarization. In the process of repolarization, with the help of the Na-K pump of the cell membrane, the excess $Na^+$ that has diffused into the cell is transported to the outside of the cell, and the extra $K^+$ is transported to the cell. Since the solutions on both sides of the cell membrane are conductive, a circular current loop is formed between the nerve segments in the excitatory and resting parts. This circular current loop depolarizes the previously dormant nerve membrane in the adjacent region, forming a new excitation region. A local circuit is formed between the new excitement area and the next adjacent part. Repeatedly, the excitement spreads along the nerve fiber.

Nerve impulses are not directly transmitted from one neuron to the next but are connected in the form of synapses. When the nerve impulse is transmitted from the presynaptic neuron to the postsynaptic neuron to the synapse, transfer mediators (such as acetylcholine and γ-aminobutyric acid (GABA) stored in the synaptic corpus are released and act on the postsynaptic membrane through the synaptic cleft. The transmitter binds to receptors in the postsynaptic membrane, which temporarily changes the permeability of the postsynaptic membrane to ions, changing the membrane potential and generating a local current. When the local current reaches certain intensity, the excitement is transmitted to the next neuron, and this potential is called the PSP. If the chemical transmitter released from the synaptic corpuscle is acetylcholine, it will increase the permeability of the postsynaptic membrane to $Na^+$, $K^+$, and $Cl^-$, but the permeability to $Na^+$ is the greatest, causing a depolarizing PSP, namely, an excitatory postsynaptic potential (EPSP); an EPSP is a temporary partial reduction of membrane potential. If synaptic vesicles release GABA, the permeability of the postsynaptic membrane to $K^+$ increases, causing excessive polarization of the postsynaptic membrane, which is called an inhibitory postsynaptic potential (IPSP). An IPSP is a temporary increase in membrane potential. The potentials generated by the synapses in different parts of the cell are summed up in the membrane potential of the cell body.

The total potential of the cerebral cortex mainly occurs in the large pyramidal cells arranged in the vertical direction in the cortex. Most of the current is limited to the cortex, and a small part of it passes through the meninges, cerebrospinal fluid (CSF), and the head to the scalp, causing different potential levels in different parts of the scalp. The amplitude of these potential differences is 10–100 μV, which can be recorded between two electrodes. This is the basis of EEG [1].

## 1.3 EEG Distribution, Waveform, and Amplitude

Since EEG waves represent the synchronous potential difference of a group of nerve cells in a certain area of the cerebral cortex, EEG analysis should be conducted from seven aspects, namely, frequency, amplitude, waveform, phase relation, the mode of occurrence of abnormal waves, the breadth of distribution, and responsiveness to various stimuli.

### 1.3.1 Frequency

Frequency refers to the number of times a certain wave repeats in 1 s. It is usually expressed in cycles per second (c/s) or Hz. The wavelength of the scattered slow wave can be measured and expressed by the time it occupies. The frequency of brain waves is divided into four frequency bands: δ frequency band: 3/s or less; θ frequency band: 4–7/s; α frequency band: 8–13/s; and β frequency band: 14/s or more (usually 14–40/s). The frequency band of EEG is one of the important criteria for evaluating abnormalities in clinical practice. Waves below 8/s are called slow waves, and waves above 13/s are called fast waves.

### 1.3.2 Amplitude

Amplitude represents the height of a wave, expressed in μV. It is determined by comparing the distance of a wave from its peak to the intersection of the two-point line of the wave and the height of the standard signal recorded under the same gain and filtering conditions. For example, if the height of a wave in an EEG is 10 mm, and the calibration signal of 50 μV is measured to be 5 mm, then the amplitude of this wave is 100 μV. The amplitudes of the corresponding parts on the two sides should be symmetrical. The asymmetry of the amplitudes is often caused by extracerebral factors. In particular, the difference in the amplitude of the recording electrodes can be caused by different spatial distances or impedances. Therefore, the placement and resistance of the electrodes should be verified during the inspection.

### 1.3.3 Waveform

- *Sinusoidal wave*: The ascending and descending branches of a sinusoidal wave are clear and smooth.
- *Monophasic and diphasic waves*: A monophasic wave is a single-direction deflection upward or downward from the baseline, while a diphasic wave includes two components above and below the baseline.
- *Spike wave*: A spike wave looks like a spike, and a spike waves takes 20–70 ms.
- *Sharp wave*: A sharp wave is sharp-like and differs from a spike wave in that it takes more than 70 ms (between 70 and 200 ms), the upward branch is usually steeper, and the downward branch is sloping.
- *Complex wave*: A complex wave is composed of two or more continuous waves. For example, a spike-slow complex wave consists of a spike wave and a slow wave, such as a 3/s spike-slow complex wave and a 4~5/s spike-slow complex wave. Different complex waves have different clinical meanings.

### 1.3.4 Phase Relation

Phase relation refers to the synchronization and polarity relation of brain waves in one or more leads. In different leads, if the peaks and troughs of waves occur at the same time, these waves are said to be in phase; if their peaks and troughs do not occur at the same time, they are said to be out of phase. If the two wave crests are in completely opposite directions and are 180 degrees out of phase, these waves are said to be phase reversed. Phase reversed waves are a sign of the origin of brain-wave potential during bipolar tracing, and they have positioning significance.

### 1.3.5 Mode of Occurrence of Abnormal Waves

Long-range: appear continuously for 5–10 s. Short-range: appear continuously for 1–2 s. Rhythmicity: reoccur regularly. Irregularity: highly rhythmic disorder; irregular waveforms, amplitudes, and frequencies; scattered or appear occasionally. Migratory: a wave that occurs at a certain time in a certain area but occurs in another area at another time.

### 1.3.6 Distribution and Breadth

- *Universal or diffuse distribution* Electrical activity that occurs in various areas or most areas of the brain at the same time. It may be that the amplitude is higher in some regions of its distribution.

- *Lateral distribution* Appears on one side of the cerebral hemisphere or mainly on one side. This distribution is abnormal. The abnormality of the brain is located on the side of the abnormal activity or with a lack of normal activity.
- *Focal distribution* Electrical activity occurs only in a certain area of the head. The electrodes in the neighboring area may be affected and have the same electrical activity, but the amplitude of the electrical activity in the affected area is relatively low. The focal distribution should be distinguished from the predominance of a certain area accompanied by the universal distribution. For abnormal slow waves and sharp waves, this distinction is very important.

### 1.3.7 Reactivity

The normal and abnormal EEG changes induced by various methods are called reactivity. These methods include open and closed eye tests, hyperventilation, flashes or other sensory stimuli, and changes in alertness levels.

## 1.4 Common EEG Recording Methods

EEG records and traces the bioelectrical activity of brain neuron cells. The brain electrical activity recorded by scalp electrodes is usually 1–60 Hz, and the voltage is between 5 and 300/μV. The conductors placed on the scalp to export brain electrical activity are called electrodes. There are many types of electrodes. Commonly used scalp electrodes include needle electrodes, tubular electrodes, and disc electrodes; and special electrodes include sphenoid electrodes, nasopharyngeal electrodes, and intracranial electrodes.

For conventional electrode placement, the International Federation of Societies for electroencephalography and Clinical Neurophysiology (IFSECN) recommended the International 10–20 system. Electrodes are generally placed on the left and right forehead (Fp), frontal area (F), central area (C) (anteroposterior to the central groove), parietal area (P), occipital area (O), anterior temporal area (T or F7, 8), middle temporal area (T or T3, 4), posterior temporal area (T or T5, 6), earlobes on both sides (A1, A2), and the middle of the head (parietal center C). Odd-numbered electrodes are placed on the left side of the head, and even-numbered electrodes are placed on the right side of the head. The electrodes are passed through an electroencephalograph composed of several amplifiers to amplify the weak electrical activity of the brain via wires and record this activity by a recording device on paper or a computer screen. The EEG examination room should not be too bright or soundproof, but it should be quiet. There should be glass windows on the shielding wall of the EEG device so that the examiner can see the patient and observe their condition. For example, if a patient has seizures or other conditions during the tracing process, the examiner can see this and give timely treatment.

At least two electrodes are required for EEG. One electrode is connected to the first grid (G1) of the EEG machine and the other is connected to the second grid (G2). The potential difference recorded between the two electrodes forms an EEG. Each amplifier has two input terminals, which are connected to the G1 and G2 to record the potential difference. According to custom, when the potential of G1 is more negative than G2, the recorded waveform is required to be upward (negative phase, negative); conversely, if G1 is more positive than G2, the waveform is downward (positive phase, positive). Therefore, G1 is the negative terminal of the amplifier, and G2 is the positive terminal.

If there is a point with a zero potential on the body connected in parallel to the G2, the potential difference with the electrodes on other parts of the G1 is equal to the absolute value of the latter's potential change. This zero-potential point theoretically refers to the point where the body is infinitely far away from the body when it is in the electrolyte solution. In fact, this kind of absolute-zero potential does not exist. The lead method (montage) of EEG can be divided into the monopolar lead method (monopolar), using irrelevant electrodes, and the bipolar lead method (bipolar), using only active electrodes without using irrelevant electrodes.

### 1.4.1 Monopolar Lead (Fig. 1.1)

The monopolar lead method involves connecting each active electrode of the scalp with an irrelevant electrode on the same side, and the EEG traced is the potential difference between each active electrode and the irrelevant electrode. The irrelevant electrode that is often used is the ear electrode, and the zero potential of the ear electrode is set to indicate the absolute value of the potential of each active electrode on the scalp. However, in fact, the ear poles do not have absolute-zero potential and may be affected by bioelectricity other than brain electricity, such as ECG and myoelectricity. Therefore, the standard monopolar lead traces only the potential difference between the active electrodes of the scalp and the ear electrodes, which is very close in value to the absolute value of the active electrode potential. It is recommended to use average monopolar leads at the same time; that is, irrelevant electrodes use the average value of each scalp electrode potential through high-resistance input (0.5~3 M) as a reference to replace the ear electrode to eliminate the influence of the ear electrode.

### 1.4.2 Bipolar Lead (Fig. 1.2)

The bipolar lead method involves tracing the two active electrodes on the scalp connected to the G1 and G2 electrodes of the EEG machine without using extraneous electrodes. What is recorded by the bipolar lead method is the potential difference between the two active electrodes. When a monopolar lead shows an abnormal wave in a certain part, it can be confirmed on the bipolar lead; that is, phase reversed (or tit-for-tat) of the abnormal wave can be seen at the location where the abnormality occurs. The advantage of the bipolar lead method is that it is less susceptible to the influence of other bioelectricity, such as ECG, than monopolar lead, and it can eliminate artifacts caused by the activation of irrelevant electrodes. Bipolar leads must be combined and used with monopolar leads. Monopolar leads are the basis for analyzing EEG. Bipolar leads should be combined with the specific analysis of monopolar

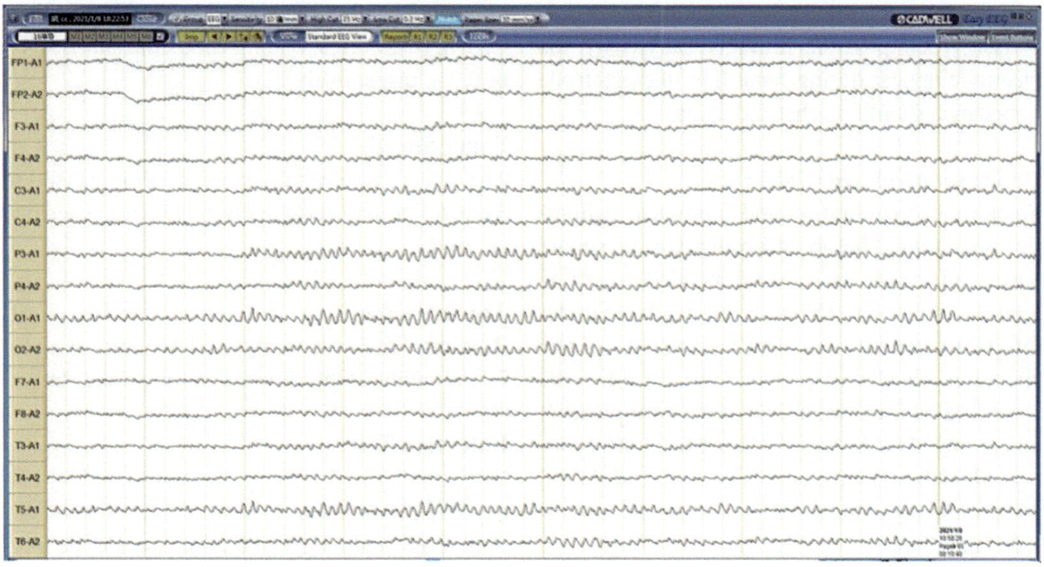


**Fig. 1.1** Monopolar lead

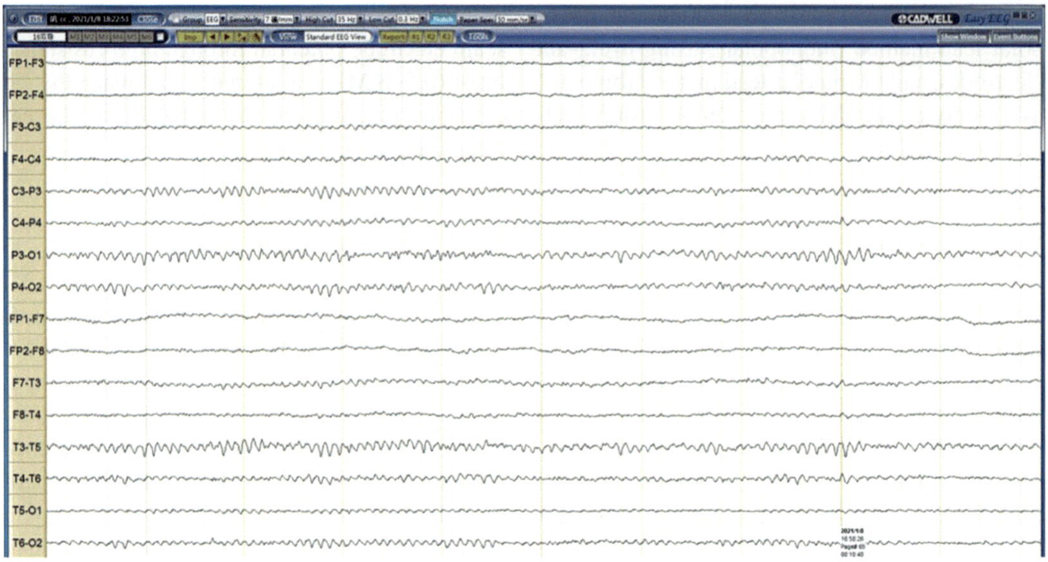


**Fig. 1.2** Bipolar lead

leads to draw correct conclusions. The bipolar lead design should be based on the principles of crisscross and triangulation [2, 3].

### 1.4.3 The Parameters to Check

**Electrode Impedance**
After the electrode is installed, the impedance between the electrode and the scalp should be measured, and it generally should not exceed 5 kΩ. When possible artifacts caused by the electrode appear during recording, the electrode impedance should be checked again.

**Calibration Voltage (Calibration)**
Square wave calibration and biological calibration are required before recording. During square wave calibration, it is recommended to try to record and measure the calibration voltage under different filter settings. The calibration voltage should be adjusted to a sensitive level, and all the recording pen tips should be at the zero position and arranged in the same straight line. After biological calibration, the curves of each lead should be completely consistent in waveform, amplitude, and phase.

**Sensitivity**
In routine recording, the sensitivity is generally set at 7 μV/mm or 10 μV/mm (adults), 10 μV/mm, or 20 μV/mm (children). The sensitivity can be adjusted in time as appropriate.

**Filtering**
In a normal recording, the high-frequency filter should not be lower than 70 Hz and should be set to 70 Hz. The low-frequency filter should not be higher than 1 Hz and should be set to 0.3 Hz or 0.5 Hz (the corresponding time constant is 0.4 s or 0.3 s, respectively).

**Paper Speed**
The speed of normal paper feeding is set to 3 cm/s. For long-term tracing, 1.5 cm/s speed can be used.

**Tracing Time**
Routine EEG recording should last at least 20 min without interference in the awake state.

**Induction Test**
Eye opening and closing, flash stimulation, and hyperventilation should be used as routine induction tests, and sleep induction should be per-

**Table 1.1** Monopolar lead combination method

| 18 Lead | | | 16 Lead | | 8 Lead | |
|---|---|---|---|---|---|---|
| Lead | Auricular lead | Average lead | Auricular lead | Average lead | Auricular lead | Average lead |
| 1 | Fp1-A1 | Fp1-AV | Fp1-A1 | Fp1-AV | Fp1-A1 | Fp1-AV |
| 2 | Fp2-A2 | Fp2-AV | Fp2-A2 | Fp2-AV | Fp2-A2 | Fp2-AV |
| 3 | F3-A1 | F3-AV | F3-A1 | F3-AV | C3-A1 | C3-AV |
| 4 | F4-A2 | F4-AV | F4-A2 | F4-AV | C4-A2 | C4-AV |
| 5 | C3-A1 | C3-AV | C3-A1 | C3-AV | O1-A1 | O1-AV |
| 6 | C4-A2 | C4-AV | C4-A2 | C4-AV | O2-A2 | O2-AV |
| 7 | P3-A1 | P3-AV | P3-A1 | P3-AV | T3-A1 | T3-AV |
| 8 | P4-A2 | P4-AV | P4-A2 | P4-AV | T4-A2 | T4-AV |
| 9 | O1-A1 | O1-AV | O1-A1 | O1-AV | | |
| 10 | O2-A2 | O2-AV | O2-A2 | O2-AV | | |
| 11 | F7-A1 | F7-AV | F7-A1 | F7-AV | | |
| 12 | F8-A2 | F8-AV | F8-A2 | F8-AV | | |
| 13 | T3-A1 | T3-AV | T3-A1 | T3-AV | | |
| 14 | T4-A2 | T4-AV | T4-A2 | T4-AV | | |
| 15 | T5-A1 | T5-AV | T5-A1 | T5-AV | | |
| 16 | T6-A2 | T6-AV | T6-A2 | T6-AV | | |
| 17 | Pz-A2 | Pz-AV | | | | |
| 18 | Cz-A2 | Cz-AV | | | | |

formed as much as possible. When conducting an induction test, it is necessary to increase the recording time accordingly.

- *Eyes open and closed test*: When the subject is awake and relaxed with eyes closed, he is asked to open his eyes for 3–5 s every 10s and to repeatedly open and close his eyes 2–3 times. The time of each eye opening and closing point is marked.
- *Flash stimulation*: The light stimulator is placed approximately 30 cm in front of the subject's eyes, and his eyes are directed to look at the center of the stimulator with his eyes closed. The brightness of the stimulator is 100,000 candles (>100 Nit), the stimulation pulse width is 0.1–10 ms, and the stimulation frequency is adjustable between 1 and 60 Hz. The duration of each frequency stimulation is 10 s, and the interval is 10s. Then, another frequency stimulation is used for 10 s. Generally, the stimulation is gradually increased from low frequency to high frequency; for example, 1 Hz → 3 Hz → 6 Hz → 9 Hz → 12 Hz → 1 5 Hz → 18 Hz → 21 Hz → 24 Hz → 27 Hz → 30 Hz.
- *Hyperventilation*: Hyperventilation recording should last at least 3 min, and the deep breathing rate should be 20–25 breaths/min. Before and after hyperventilation, recording should last for at least 1 min without changing the lead combination. Hyperventilation should not be performed on patients with severe cardiopulmonary disease, cerebrovascular disease, high intracranial pressure (ICP), sickle cell anemia, or patients with poor general conditions.
- *Sleep induction*: The process of falling asleep and the light sleep period (nonrapid eye movement (NREM) I and II), deep sleep period and rapid eye movement (REM) sleep period should be recorded.

The lead combination methods commonly used in China are shown in Tables 1.1 and 1.2.

## 1.5 Interpretation of the EEG of Healthy Adults

Whether an EEG is normal is only a statistical concept. EEG analysis has a certain degree of subjectivity and relativity, and proper training and

**Table 1.2** Bipolar lead combination method

| 18 Lead | | | | 16 Lead | | |
|---|---|---|---|---|---|---|
| Lead | Longitudinal lead | Transverse lead | Ring lead | Longitudinal lead | Transverse lead | Ring lead |
| 1 | Fp1-F7 | A1-F7 | O1-T5 | Fp1-F7 | A1-F7 | O1-T5 |
| 2 | F7-T3 | F7-F3 | T5-T3 | F7-T3 | F7-F3 | T5-T3 |
| 3 | T3-T5 | F3-Fz | T3-F7 | T3-T5 | F3-Fz | T3-F7 |
| 4 | Fp1-F3 | Fz-F4 | F7-Fp1 | Fp1-F3 | Fz-F4 | F7-Fp1 |
| 5 | F3-C3 | F4-F8 | Fp1-Fp2 | F3-C3 | F4-F8 | Fp1-Fp2 |
| 6 | C3-P3 | F8-A2 | Fp2-F8 | C3-P3 | F8-A2 | Fp2-F8 |
| 7 | P3-O1 | A1-T3 | F8-T4 | P3-O1 | A1-T3 | F8-T4 |
| 8 | Fz-Cz | T3-C3 | T4-T6 | Fz-Cz | T3-C3 | T4-T6 |
| 9 | Cz-Pz | C3-Cz | T6-O2 | Cz-Pz | C3-Cz | T6-O2 |
| 10 | Fp2-F8 | Cz-C4 | O2-O1 | Fp2-F8 | Cz-C4 | O2-O1 |
| 11 | F8-T4 | C4-T4 | Fz-F7 | F8-T4 | C4-T4 | Fz-F7 |
| 12 | T4-T6 | T4-A2 | F7-F8 | T4-T6 | T4-A2 | F7-F8 |
| 13 | Fp2-F4 | T5-P3 | F8-Fz | Fp2-F4 | T5-P3 | F8-Fz |
| 14 | F4-C4 | P3-Pz | Cz-T3 | F4-C4 | P3-Pz | Cz-T3 |
| 15 | C4-P4 | Pz-P4 | T3-T4 | C4-P4 | Pz-P4 | T3-T4 |
| 16 | P4-O2 | P4-T6 | T4-Cz | P4-O2 | P4-T6 | T4-Cz |
| 17 | O2-O1 | Fp1-Fp2 | Fz-Cz | | | |
| 18 | O1-T5 | O1-O2 | Cz-Pz | | | |

experience are very important. An EEG reflects the changes in the electrical potential of neurons. Therefore, any two diseases involving the same degree of neuron function will produce the same EEG abnormality; in contrast, an EEG abnormality can have multiple causes; therefore, the cause of a disease cannot be determined by EEG.

In the process of brain maturation, an EEG, which reflects the functional state of the brain, undergoes a developmental process from immaturity to maturity similar to that of the functional state of the brain. Therefore, individuals of different age groups have different EEG recordings; there can be multiple types of normal EEG between individuals of the same age. Moreover, the EEG described in the awake state is completely different from that described in the sleep state, and there are more inter-individual differences in awake–state EEG than in sleep-state EEG. At different stages from infancy to 19 years old, normal changes in EEG are very obvious. As age increases, EEG shifts to a more mature type. There is little change in normal EEG between 20 and 60 years old, the boundary between normal and abnormal is easy to define, and the types of abnormalities are more consistent with the basic types of encephalopathy. The EEGs of individuals older than 60 years old are similar to those of adults younger than 60 years old.

The EEG of a healthy awake adult is composed of α wave as the basic wave and a small amount of scattered fast and slow waves. Basic wave: mainly α waves or θ waves with normal distribution; symmetrical on both sides, the frequency difference of the α waves should not exceed 20% in the symmetrical part, and the amplitude difference should not exceed 50% in the occiput or 20% in the other part; the volatility should not be too high, and the average volatility of α waves is less than 100 μV. During eye opening and closing, mental activity, and stimulation sensation, α wave should have a normal response. Slow waves: These waves are scattered and of low amplitude, are mainly seen in the temporal area, and are mostly θ waves; there should be no continuous high-amplitude θ or δ waves in any part. Brain waves should be symmetrical during sleep. No abnormal electrical activity should be observed. Regardless of wakefulness or sleep, there should be no spike wave, spike-slow wave complex, etc.

The determination of an abnormal EEG is not based on a lack of normal EEG components or types but on whether the EEG contains abnormal activity or types. If an EEG contains abnormal electrical activity, no matter how many normal components it contains, it should be considered abnormal. In most abnormal EEGs, abnormal types do not completely replace normal electrical activity. They may appear intermittently or only in a certain area or areas or add to the normal background.

Abnormal EEGs are divided into four basic types: (a) epileptic activity, (b) slow wave, (c) abnormal amplitude, and (d) deviation from the normal type. Each type of abnormality may be caused by one or several types of brain diseases. Brain abnormalities are characterized by irritating or destructive lesions, which are located in the cortex, subcortex, or outside the cortex. On the other hand, many diseases cause more than one type of EEG abnormality, and for a neurological disease, not all cases have EEG abnormalities. If the brain lesions are small and long and located deep in the brain, the EEG may be normal. Although some people have abnormal EEG, they do not have any other manifestations of brain diseases. For the above reasons, EEG cannot be used alone for specific clinical diagnosis; it can only suggest a series of possible diagnoses. As with the results of other laboratory tests, EEG may be valuable in differential diagnosis and guide the choice of correct diagnosis. For example, in a patient with an unknown history of coma, the appearance of fast waves in an EEG may indicate barbiturate poisoning, the appearance of bilateral synchronous universal triphasic waves (TWs) is beneficial for the diagnosis of hepatic encephalopathy, and the appearance of focal slow waves or amplitude suppression may be beneficial for the diagnosis of subdural hematoma.

The following are the criteria for judging abnormalities in an adult EEG:

- The average amplitude of the basic rhythm is extremely high or flat and mixed in by slow waves of low amplitude.
- The basic rhythm lacks a response to various physiological stimuli on one or both sides.
- The basic rhythm wave amplitude is obviously asymmetric, >50%, or the frequency difference between the two sides of the wave is 20%.
- Slow wave activity exceeds the normal amount, especially when it is focal.
- There is a certain combination of spike waves, sharp waves, spike-slow complex waves, and sharp-slow complex waves in awake and sleep tracing.
- Slow waves and fast waves with high amplitudes erupt. More than two explosive activities occur during hyperventilation.
- The apical sharp wave, sleep spindle, and K composite wave that appear during sleep are obviously asymmetric.

## 1.6 Recognition of Common Artifacts in the EEGs of Patients in Severe Condition

An EEG is a weak bioelectric signal that needs to be magnified millions of times for the recording of this kind of electrical activity. In this process, non-EEG signals from various sources may also enter the amplifier and be mixed into EEG signals, which are called EEG artifacts. In the intensive care unit (ICU), a large number of artifacts are often produced by various instruments and equipment and the operations of staff. These artifacts are complex and diverse, and they often cause difficulties in the reading, analysis, and judgment of EEGs, thereby affecting the accuracy of EEG diagnostic results. Recognizing these artifacts is the key to improving the success of EEG diagnosis. EEG technicians often hope that the anti-interference ability of the instrument is as strong as possible, but the anti-interference ability of the instrument contradicts the fidelity of the EEG signal. Many interference signals are stronger than the EEG signal. The elimination of interfering artifacts may also cause some EEG signals to be lost, leading to the distortion of EEG waveforms. Therefore, some artifacts are inevitable, and the most important thing is to be able to identify them correctly and avoid making incorrect conclusions.

There are many artifacts in the ICU that need to be judged in real time based on the on-site

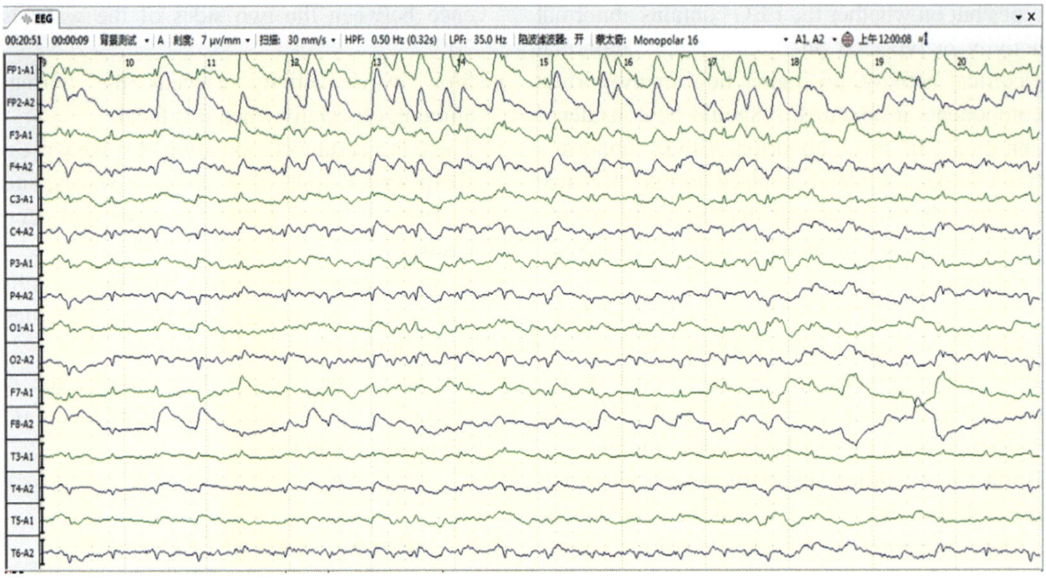

**Fig. 1.3** Eye movement artifacts

observation of the patient's condition. As time passes, it is difficult to determine the nature and source of the suspicious waveform. Therefore, in the identification of artifacts, the patient's environment and ongoing activities need to be taken into consideration as much as possible, and it is also important to be familiar with the characteristics of the instrument. To improve the identification and elimination of artifacts, reduce the false-positive detection rate of EEG, and improve the accuracy of diagnosis via EEG, researchers need to understand the scenarios in EEG recordings and patient activities in real time or through video recording to help eliminate false positives.

Common artifacts in the ICU mainly include physiological artifacts, artifacts from instrument electrodes, and artifacts from environmental electromagnetic interference. Some common artifacts that occur in the ICU are summarized as follows.

### 1.6.1 Physiological Artifacts

**Artifacts Related to Eye Movement**

In patients with emotional stress or habitual blinking, blinking artifacts of 2–4 Hz continuous high amplitude consistent with the blinking frequency may appear in the frontal and temporal region, similar to the regular "θ wave," especially in the prefrontal region (Fig. 1.3). In patients with eye movement, large slow waves can appear in the frontal and temporal regions. At this time, we can observe the patient's eye movement or make his/her eyes open to record and compare them. If the artifact is due to blinking, gently pressing the eyelid with the thumb and index finger can eliminate the artifact. Soothing the patient by advising them not to be nervous and not to move the eyes can alleviate or eliminate eye movement artifacts.

**Electromyography (EMG) Artifacts**

In patients with severe disease, abnormal mental behavior caused by disease factors or in the ICU, such as anxiety, tension, and dysphoria, can cause many EMG activity artifacts in EEG. The source can be the EMG potential, the friction potential of the clothes, the movement of the electrode wires, or the mutual contact of the wires. The graphics can be different due to the source of the artifacts, which are manifested by the baseline drift of the poor electrode contact or the single sharp pulse or continuous upper frequency sharp pulse. The waveform is indistinguishable when the upper frequency is released, and it is a thick line similar to a spicule (Figs. 1.4, 1.5 and 1.6).

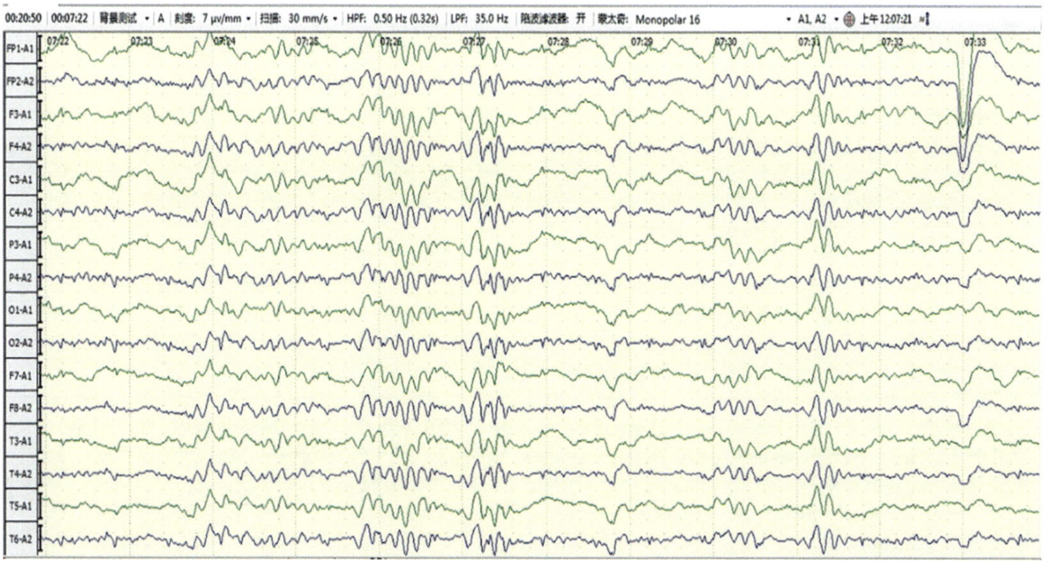

**Fig. 1.4** Artifacts caused by a patient repeatedly tapping the bed rail due to abnormal mental behavior

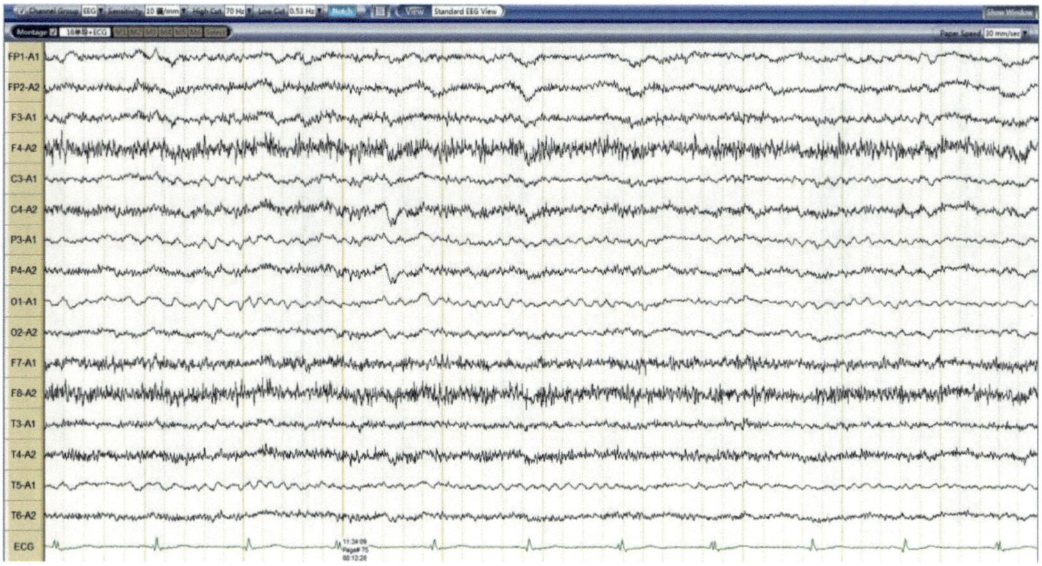

**Fig. 1.5** The patient could not relax during EEG examination, and muscle tension is seen

At this time, the operator should try not to use an upper frequency filter to eliminate the artifact but should ask the patient to relax, adjust their position, and distract their attention to reduce EMG interference.

### Masticatory-Related Artifacts

When masticatory-related artifacts occur, there are 5–10 continuous clusters of high-amplitude irregular myoelectric bursts in the bilateral anterior and middle temporal leads (F7, F8, T3, T4). There is an obvious positive deflective slow wave at the end. The slow wave can sometimes spread to a larger range or even all leads, lasting 0.2–0.5 s, with an interval of 0.5–2 s, depending on the patient's masticatory frequency while eating (Fig. 1.7). Masticatory interference is commonly observed in patients in ICU, such as those

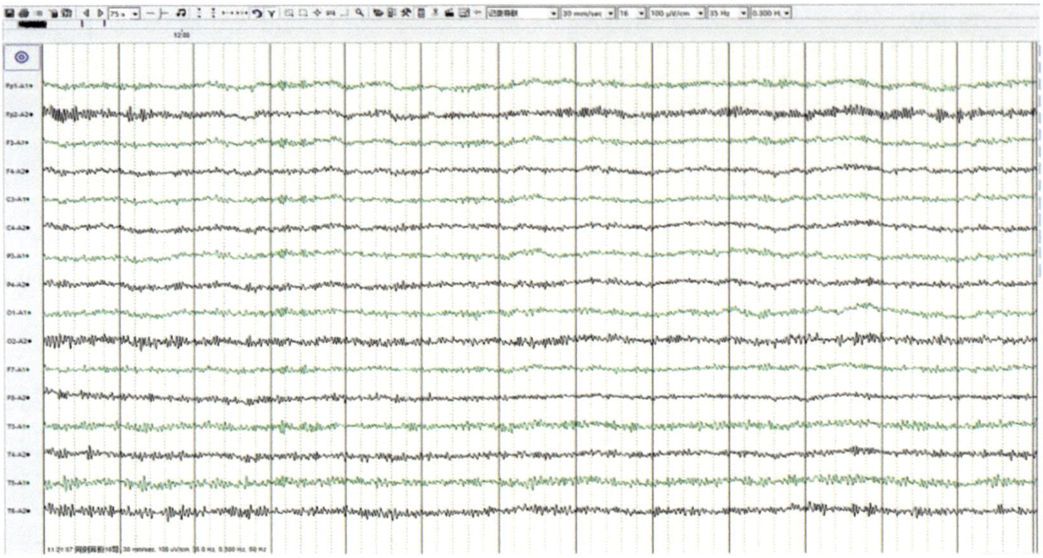

**Fig. 1.6** EEG showing EMG artifacts in a tetanus patient with whole-body muscle tension

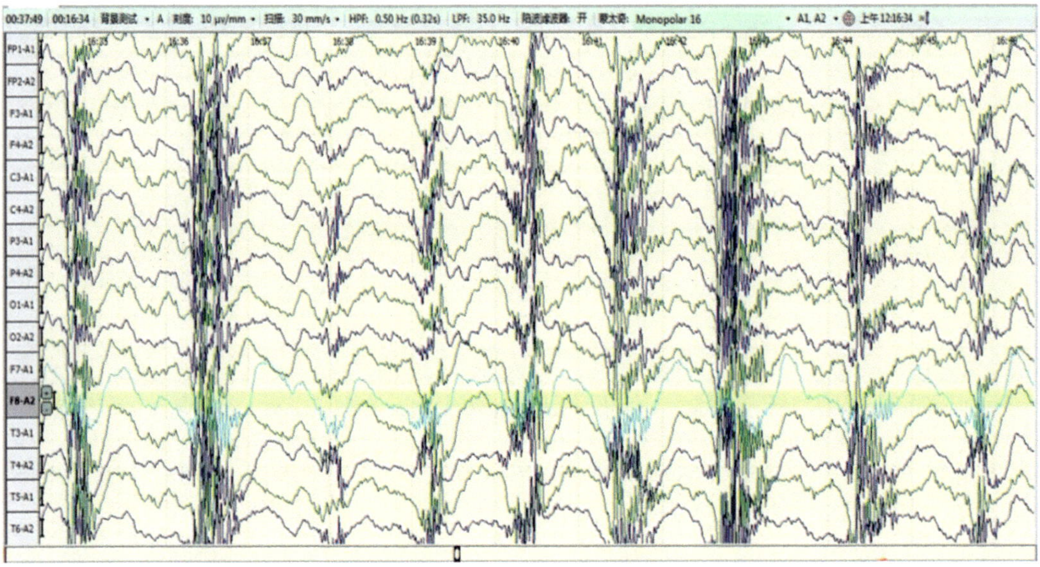

**Fig. 1.7** Artifacts caused by patient swallowing

with abnormal mental behavior or in patients with autoimmune encephalitis (AE) with involuntary oropharyngeal movements. This pattern can easily be mistaken for spiny slow waves, and it is basically impossible to analyze during mastication. Therefore, patients who can cooperate should be advised not to eat during the examination, and patients who cannot cooperate should be monitored for as long as possible to extend the recording time.

### ECG Artifacts

An artifact waveform that is consistent with the heart rate can appear in a single lead, a lead on one side and even all leads. This waveform can be a negative, positive, or two-way sharp ECG

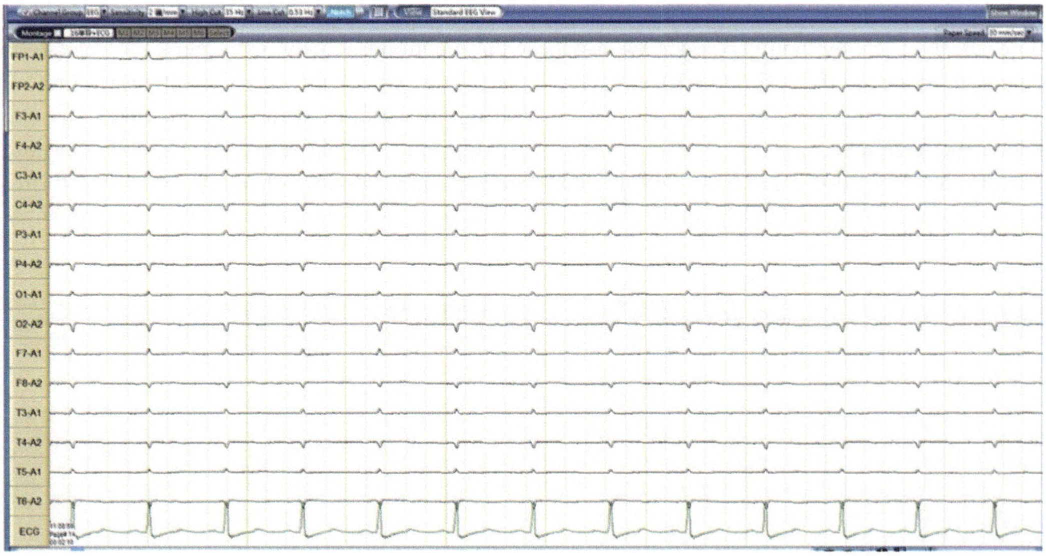


**Fig. 1.8** In the judgment of brain death, artifacts consistent with heart rate appear on all electrically silent leads

artifact, which is equivalent to the R wave of an ECG. There is no fixed relationship with background EEG activity, but the artifact is related to body position (Fig. 1.8). ECG artifacts are common in patients with short necks, obesity, and hypertension and when the ear electrodes are not properly positioned. In brain death monitoring, background brain electrical activity is almost equipotent. It is necessary to increase the sensitivity of the amplitude display (2 μv/mm), and it is difficult to eliminate the highly amplified tiny ECG artifacts. At this time, the patient's body position can be changed, trying to keep it as straight as possible to extend the distance between the neck and the heart. ECG artifacts can also be eliminated by adding dual leads or average leads; adding another lead to record the ECG can quickly determine whether an artifact is an ECG artifact.

**Perspiration-Related Artifacts**

Perspiration can cause changes in skin resistance, leading to a very slow baseline drift, but there is still brain electrical activity on an EEG (Fig. 1.9). If the baseline drifts up and down too much and exceeds the display range, the EEG cannot be analyzed. Perspiration artifacts often appear for a period of time after falling asleep. Although a patient may have no obvious perspiration, there are still changes in skin resistance and obvious baseline drift. To reduce this interference, the patient can be slightly awakened and then allowed to fall back asleep. Alternatively, a low-frequency filter can attenuate the slow baseline drift. Some patients with severe neurological illnesses perspire more, for example, in a patient with perspiration induced by stress. Resistance can be changed or electrodes can be loosened when hyperthermia causes profuse perspiration, resulting in very slow and unstable baseline movement with high amplitude, which can sometimes be masked by brain waves. At this time, the proper temperature can be maintained by physical cooling or adjusting the room temperature.

### 1.6.2 Artifacts from Instruments and Electrodes

**Artifacts Produced by a Respirator**

Patients on a respirator move passively, and the respirator causes the electrode to shift and the electrode line to swing, which can cause a large slow wave such as a slow baseline drift that is consistent with the respiratory frequency. In this situation, attempts to balance the patient's body and the removal and stabilization of the electrode wire attached to the shoulder and neck can be helpful to reduce artifacts (Figs. 1.10 and 1.11).

### Electrode Artifacts

Factors such as poor electrode fixation, long-term recording, dry conductive fluid, excessive scalp grease, and too much resistance between the electrode and the skin can cause electrode artifacts, which are intermittent or continuous irregular baseline drifts, accompanied by relatively many 50 Hz interferences, and occasionally a small number of interference waveforms, which are very similar to spike and sharp waves

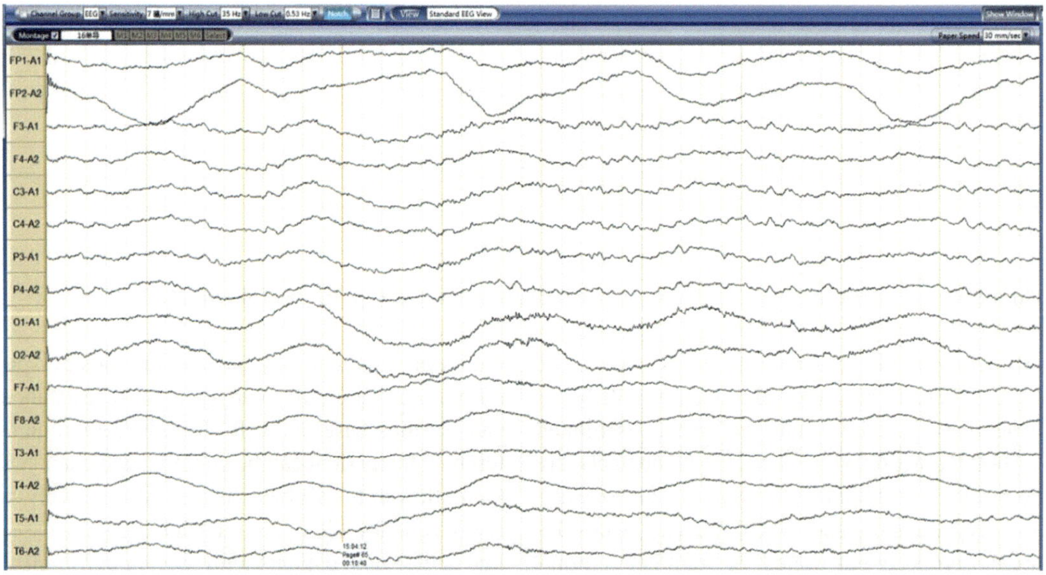


**Fig. 1.9** Skin resistance changes during perspiration, causing baseline drift

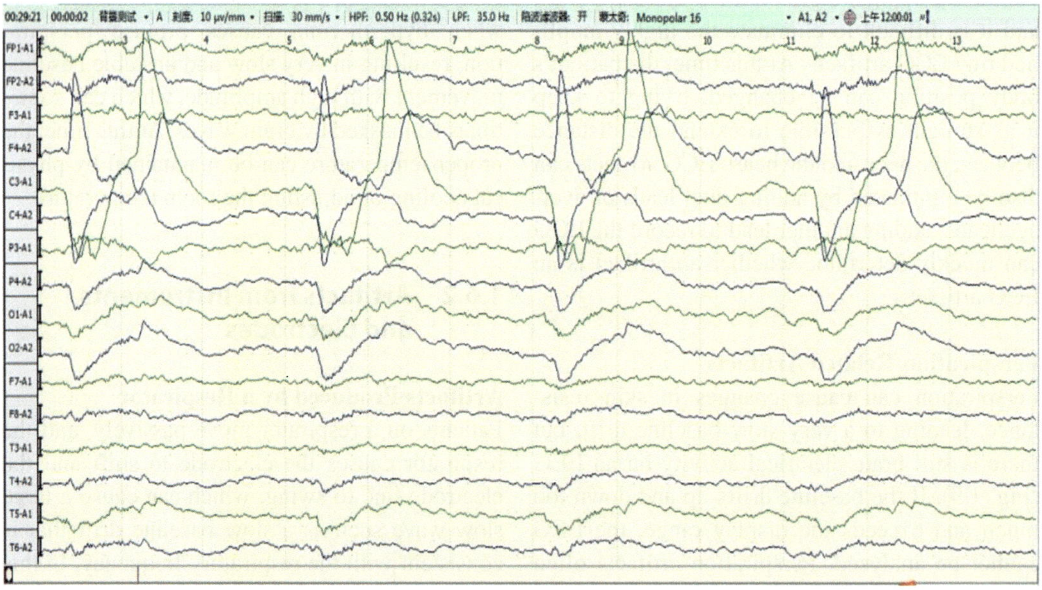


**Fig. 1.10** Respiration artifacts consistent with respiratory frequency

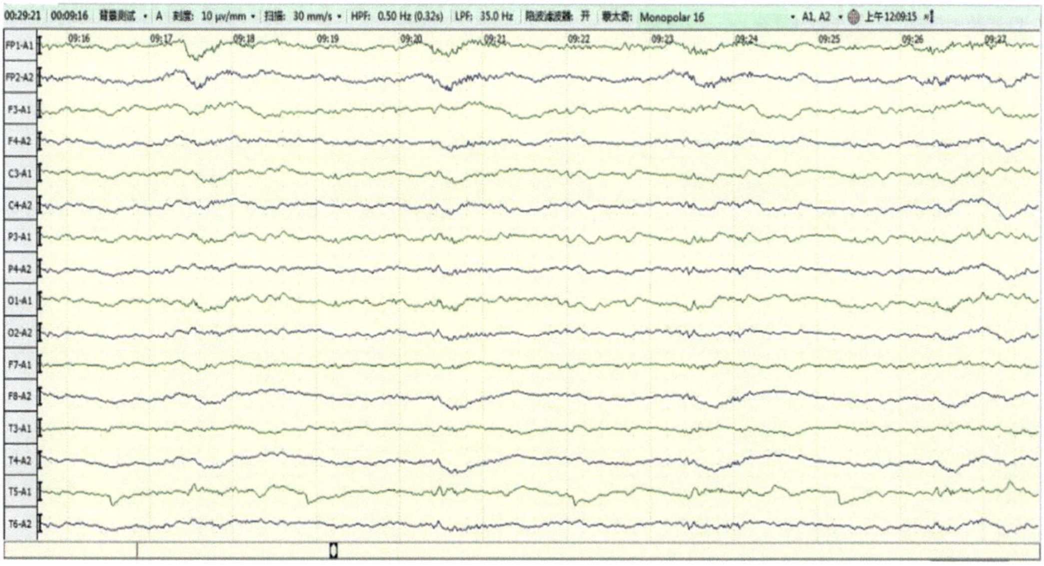

**Fig. 1.11** After adjusting the patient's position, the respirator artifacts disappeared

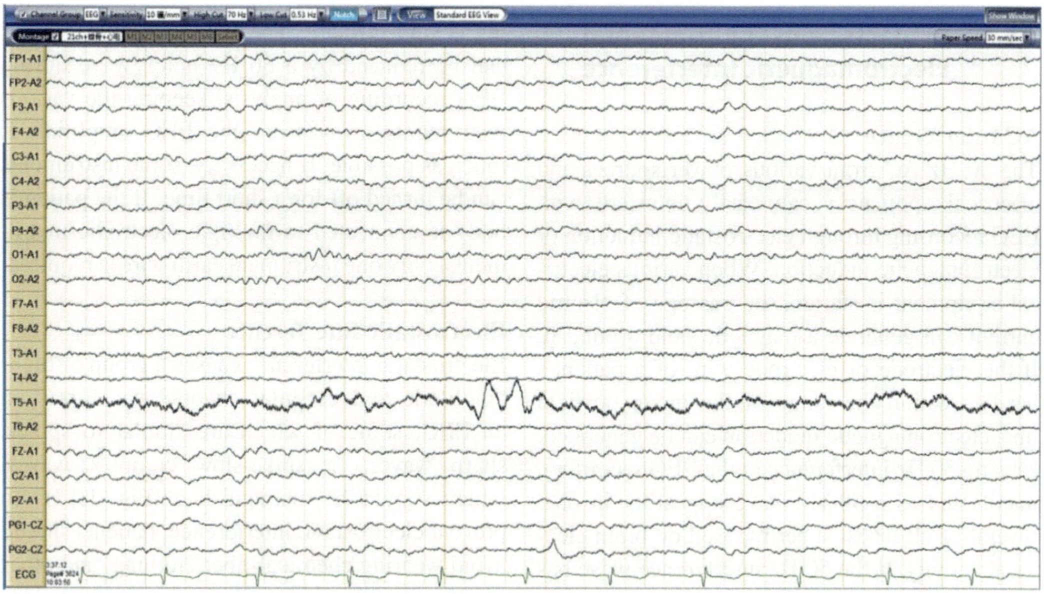

**Fig. 1.12** Artifacts caused by poor electrode fixation

(Figs. 1.12 and 1.13). Therefore, if the electrode contact of a lead is not appropriate and a large number of disorderly interference waveforms often appear, extreme caution should be used when identifying abnormal EEG waveforms in this lead, so that the interfering wave is not misinterpreted as an abnormal EEG. Because procedures are frequently performed in the ICU, electrode loosening or falling off often occurs. Therefore, it is necessary to strengthen and fix the electrode and check whether the electrode is secure in an ICU.

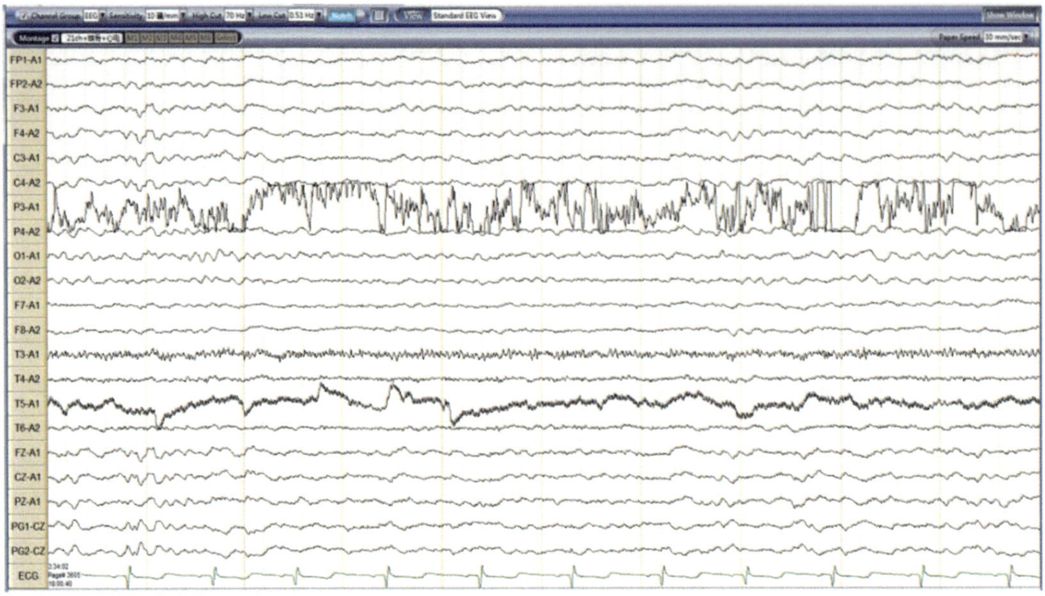


**Fig. 1.13** Artifacts caused by poor electrode contact

### 1.6.3 Artifacts from Environmental Electromagnetic Interference

**AC Interference**

The 50 Hz AC from various power sources and electrical appliances can easily interfere with EEG recording through electrostatic induction or electromagnetic induction. When various electrical equipment is started, the passage of electric current can generate a magnetic field around it. If the electrode or electrode wire of a patient's head is within the range of the magnetic field line, electromagnetic induction can be generated, causing 50 Hz interference in the EEG recording, manifested as a 50 Hz wave appearing in one, several or all leads, superimposed on brain electrical activity. If the 50 Hz interference wave has a high amplitude, brain electrical activity will be completely covered (Figs. 1.14, 1.15, and 1.16). In the ICU, various medical equipment devices, such as monitors, respirators, sputum suction devices, and infusion pumps, are present around the patients. In this environment, EEG recording is very difficult. The 50 Hz interfering wave can be reduced by a 50 Hz notch wave during EEG recording or analysis, keeping the various instruments away from the EEG amplifier as much as possible. If necessary, some instruments can be turned off for a short time. If the patient's body is connected to multiple electronic instruments, only one instrument earth wire is required.

**Electrostatic Interference**

Electrostatic interference causes a group of high-amplitude and irregular chaotic waveforms on an EEG, some of which are similar to spikes, sharp waves, or spike-slow complex waves, which should be distinguished (Fig. 1.17). To prevent electrostatic interference, patients should avoid wearing chemical-fiber clothing, and other people should avoid walking frequently beside the patient's bed during the examination. Liquid dripping from an intravenous infusion set near the electrode line of the patient's head in the ICU will also result in electrostatic interference, causing EEG artifacts (Fig. 1.18). At this

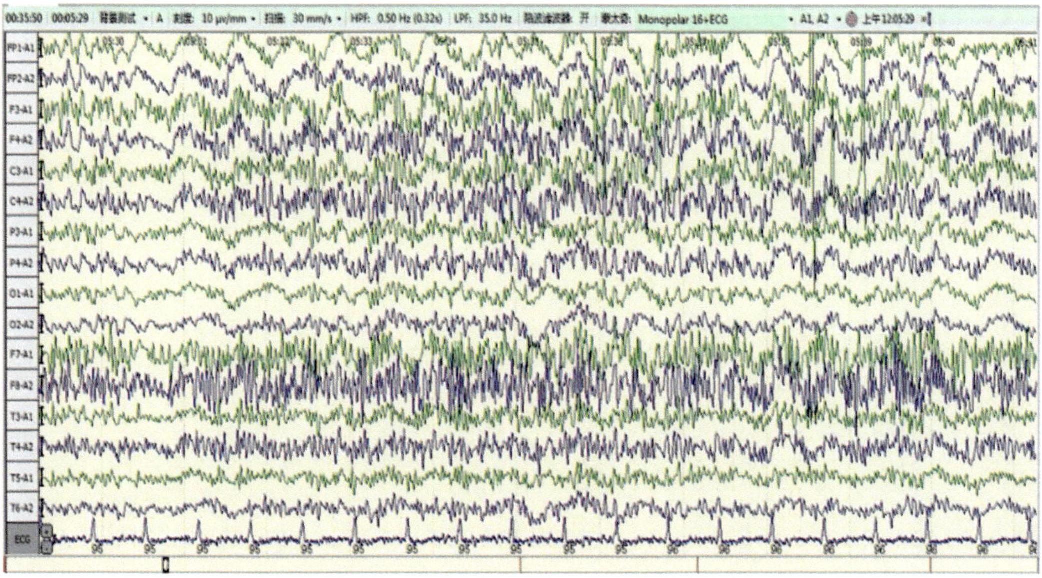


**Fig. 1.14** When using extracorporeal membrane oxygenation (ECMO), many AC artifacts will appear

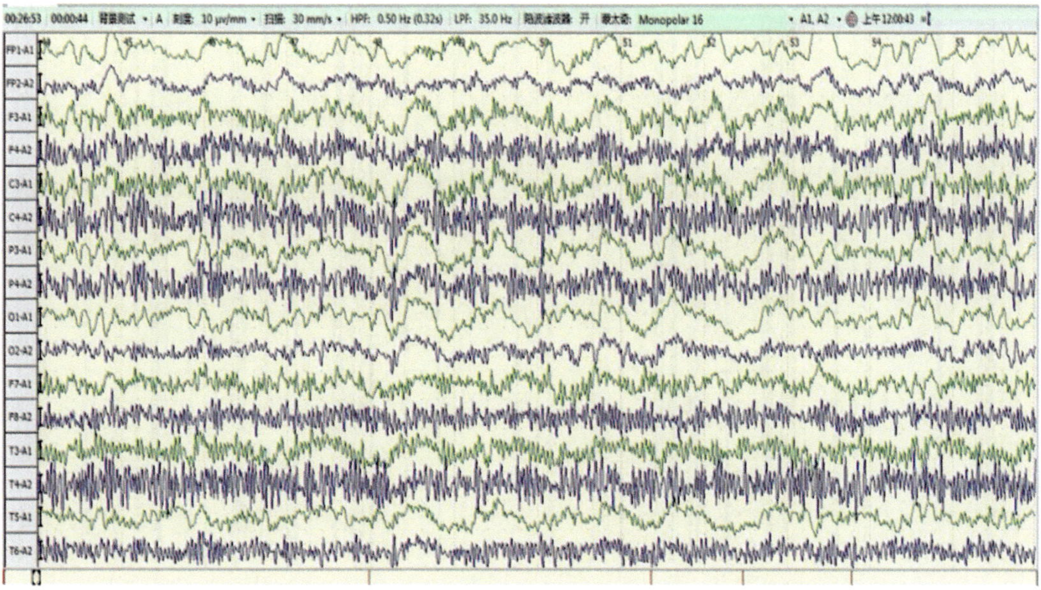


**Fig. 1.15** When using continuous renal replacement therapy (CRRT), many AC artifacts are seen

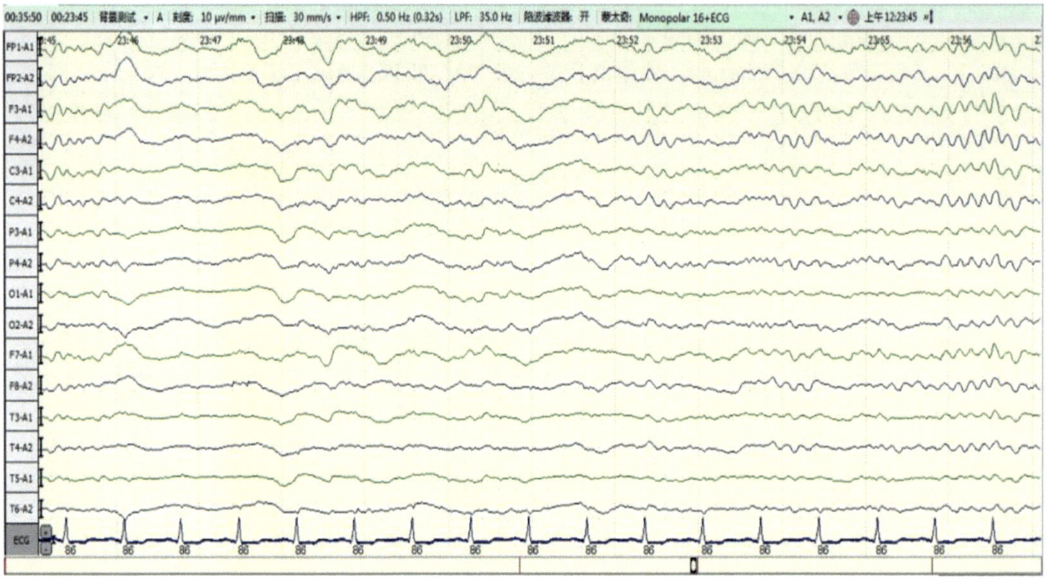


**Fig. 1.16** After stopping ECMO and CRRT, the AC artifacts disappeared

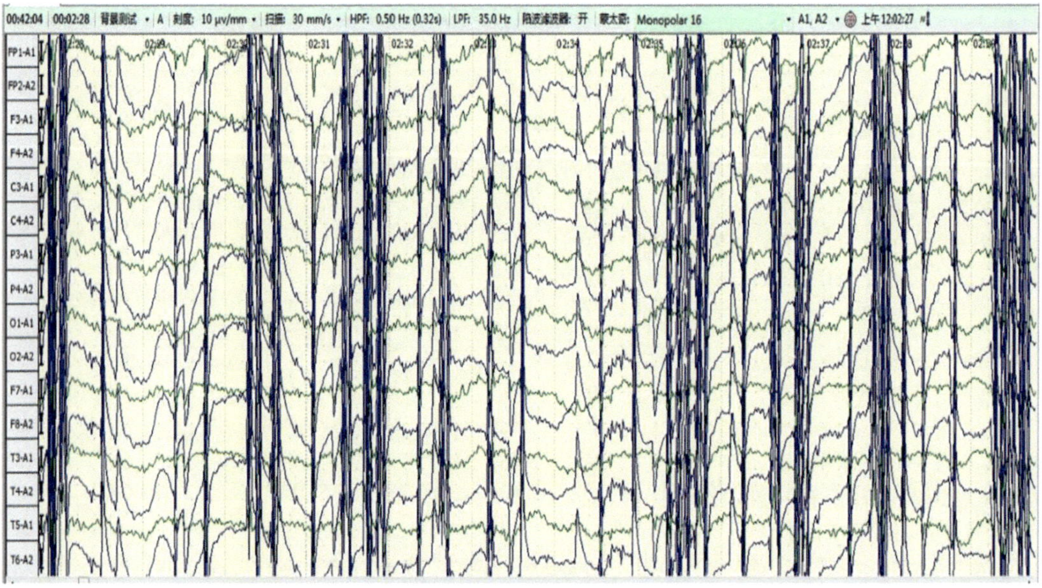


**Fig. 1.17** Electrostatic interference caused by frequent walking in the monitoring room

time, the infusion time should be marked on the EEG. When the patient's condition permits, the infusion set can be temporarily turned off, and this artifact can disappear.

**Case**

In the patient Huang, with fulminant myocarditis, after cardiopulmonary resuscitation (CPR), the EEG showed full electrical inhibition. During the examination, the patient had sudden ventricular fibrillation. The EEG showed ventricular fibrillation patterns consistent with the cardiac rhythm, which showed a slow-wave-like pattern and rhythmic distribution (Figs. 1.19, 1.20, 1.21, and 1.22).

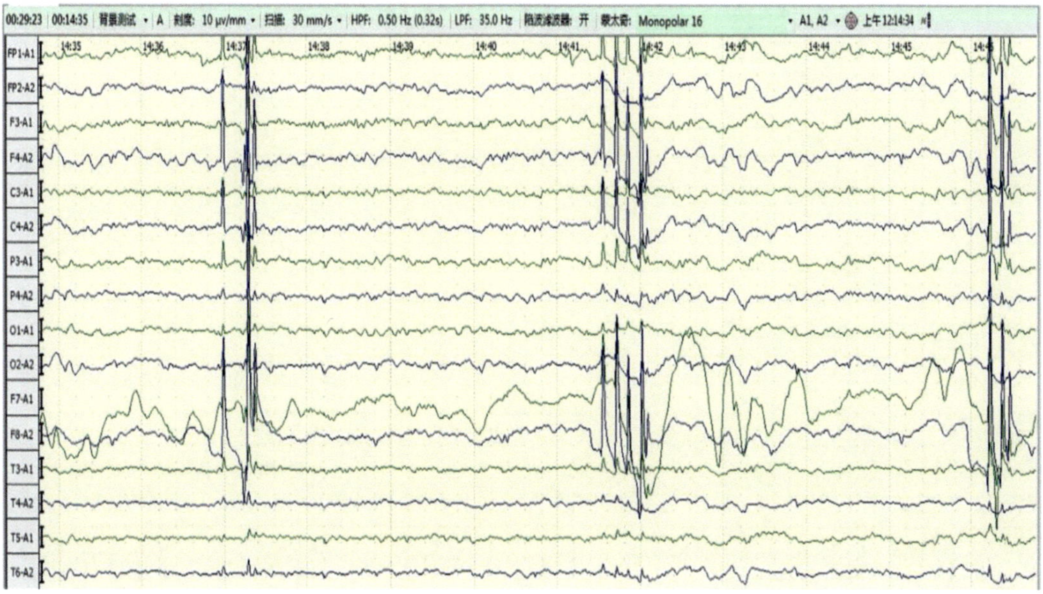


**Fig. 1.18** Because the intravenous infusion set is located near the electrode line, electrostatic pulse interference is generated when the liquid drips

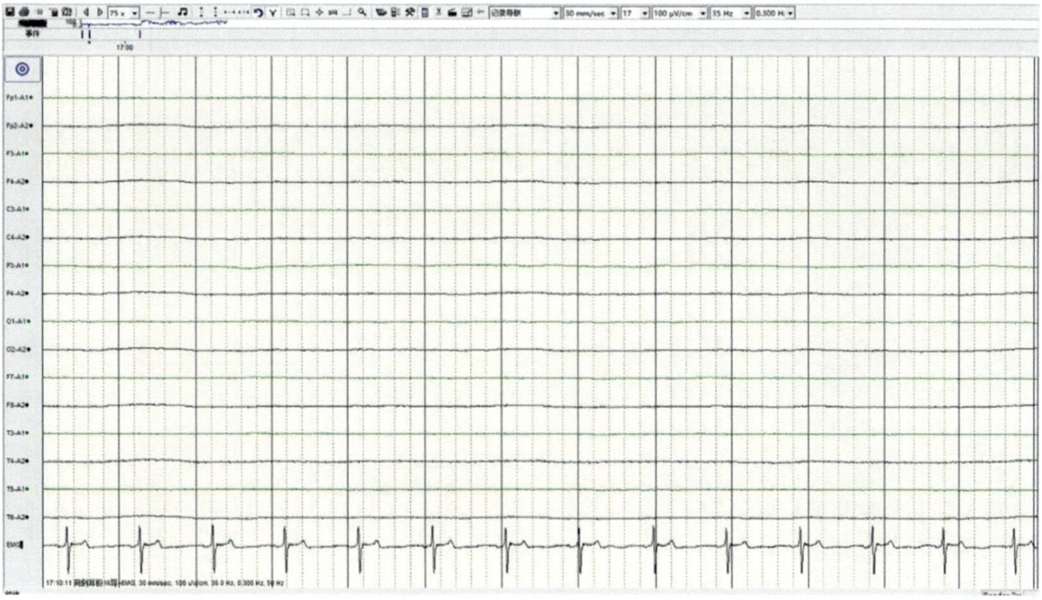

**Fig. 1.19** The EEG background is in a state of full electrical suppression

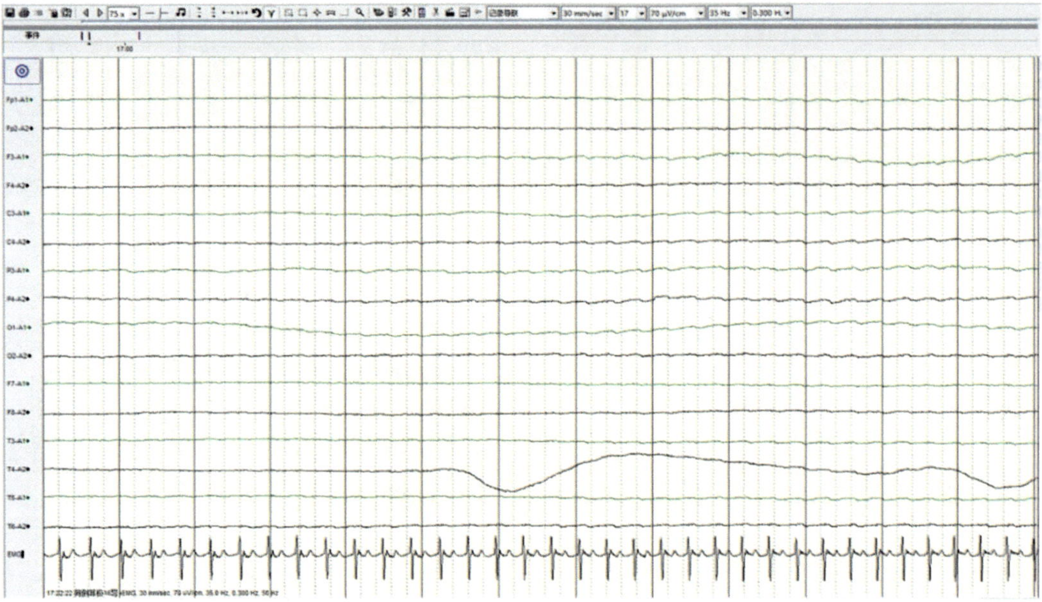

**Fig. 1.20** As the heart rate increases, the EEG gradually shows slow-wave-like artifacts consistent with the heart rate

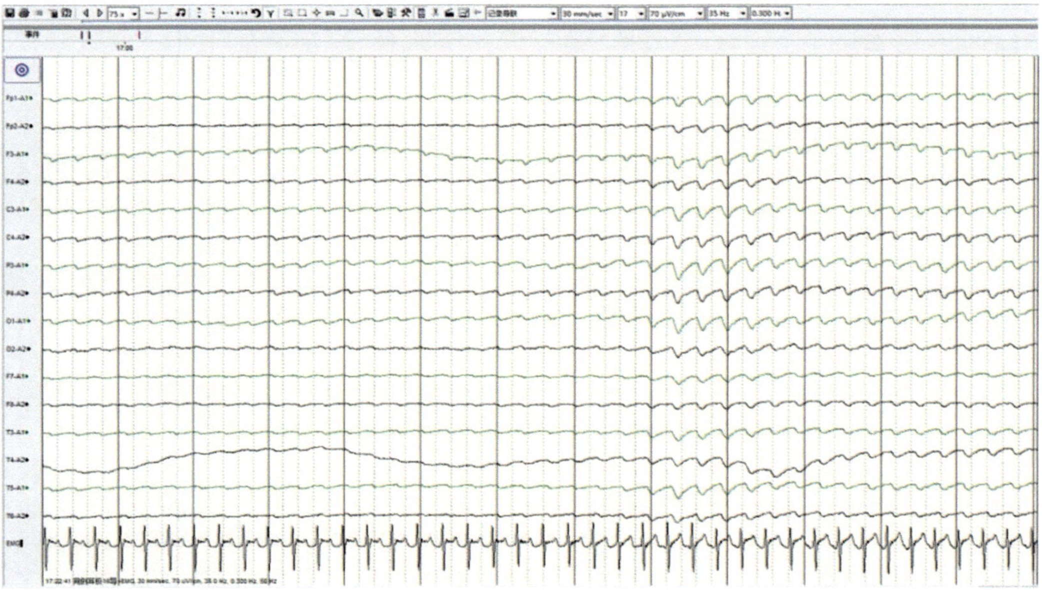

**Fig. 1.21** Slow-wave-like artifacts gradually become apparent on the EEG

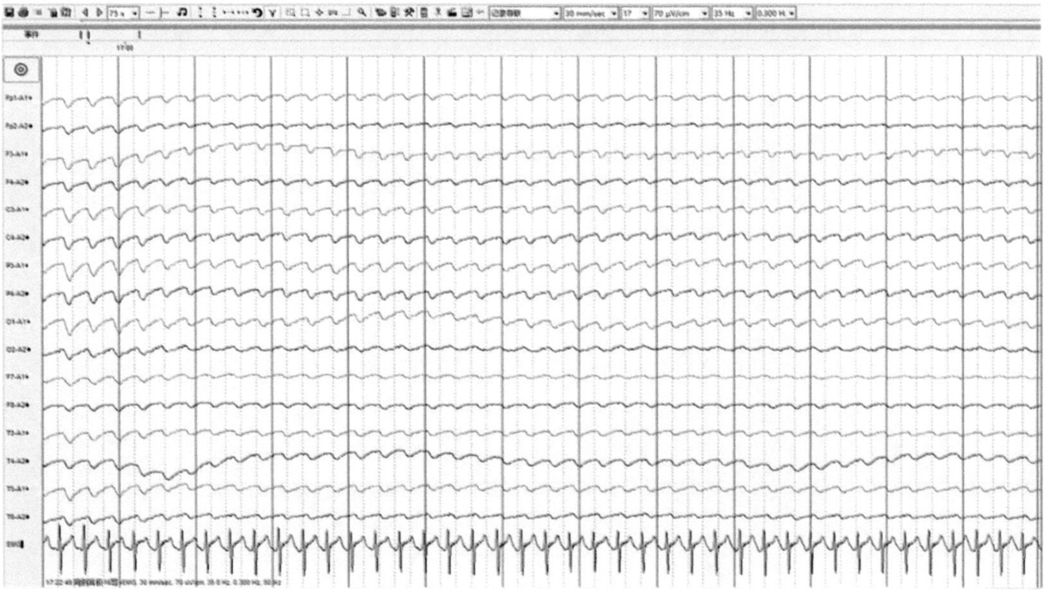

**Fig. 1.22** Slow-wave-like sample covering all leads

## References

1. Olejniczak P. Neurophysiologic basis of EEG. J Clin Neurophysiol. 2006;23(3):186–9.
2. Margitta S, Laurent K, Thomas B, et al. The standardized EEG electrode array of the IFCN. Clin Neurophysiol. 2017;128(10).
3. Kuratani J, Pearl PL, Sullivan L, et al. American clinical neurophysiology society guideline 5: minimum technical standards for pediatric electroencephalography. J Clin Neurophysiol. 2016;33(4).

# qEEG Monitoring System in Severely Ill Patients

# 2

Feng Li and Zhongming Huang

## Contents



**Abstract**

Continuous electroencephalogram (cEEG) monitoring can promptly detect abnormal brain electrical activity in critically ill patients and dynamically evaluate their brain function. However, continuous monitoring data are relatively large, the analysis time is relatively long, and the professional requirements are high, so it is difficult for nonneuroelectrophysiologists to analyze the EEG of critically ill patients at the bedside in a timely manner. qEEG compresses the original EEG signal, compressing hours or even days of data into a single screen by means of graphs and uses quantitative techniques to analyze the EEG signals in the frequency domain and time domain. qEEG intuitively reflects the patient's brain function status in the form of trend graphs, making it possible for nonneuroelectrophysiological critical care doctors to analyze and evaluate patients' brain function at the bedside. This chapter gives a detailed introduction to several qEEG analysis techniques with the greatest practical clinical value, focusing on the basic concepts, principles, interpretation points and steps, common artifacts, and identification methods of com-

F. Li (✉)
Department of Neurology, The First Affiliated Hospital of Chongqing Medical University, Chongqing, China

Z. Huang
Phecda (China) Limited, Guangzhou, China
e-mail: amin.huang@phecdachina.com



X. Wang et al. (eds.), *Multi-Modal EEG Monitoring of Severely Neurologically Ill Patients*,
https://doi.org/10.1007/978-981-16-4493-1_2

monly used trend graphs. This chapter helps clinicians quickly understand qEEG and how to use qEEG to make early predictions of a disease. This chapter lays a good foundation for subsequent chapters.

**Keywords**

qEEG · Amplitude-integrated electroencephalogram (aEEG) · Relative band power (RBP) Relative alpha variability (RAV) · Status epilepticus (SE) · Trend graph · Principle Interpretation steps · Artifacts

## 2.1 Basic Concepts of qEEG

qEEG uses mathematics and computer technology to quantify the original EEG. The amplitude and frequency of the original EEG processed by an electronic computer via analog-to-digital conversion and fast Fourier transform (FFT) form a trend map. qEEG reflects the functional state of the brain in the form of a trend map, and it is an intelligent EEG signal processing system for the noninvasive evaluation of brain function [1]. Currently, qEEG uses FFT to calculate EEG data over a period of time into parameters and then draws a graph of the relationship between the parameters and time. This graph is called the qEEG trend graph [2]. In the late 1960s, Maynard [3] developed the original aEEG predecessor, the cerebral function monitor, based on the clinical needs of continuous EEG monitoring in the adult ICU. After years of continuous attempts, qEEG has now been developed into a multichannel, multifunctional nerve function monitoring device (Fig. 2.1).

qEEG is composed of amplifiers, computers, analysis software, and acquisition components and is mainly used for brain function monitoring in critically ill patients [1, 4]. The EEG amplifier consists of signal input, analog amplification, analog-to-digital conversion, system management, and data communication. The collected EEG data are filtered, logarithmically analyzed, and FFT processed by the quantitative analysis software; and the distribution of EEG in time and space are displayed along the time axis. The quantitative analysis software analyzes EEG signals in the frequency domain and the time domain and compresses the data of several hours, or even 24 h, into a picture in the form of a trend graph, which directly reflects the brain function of the patient (Fig. 2.2).

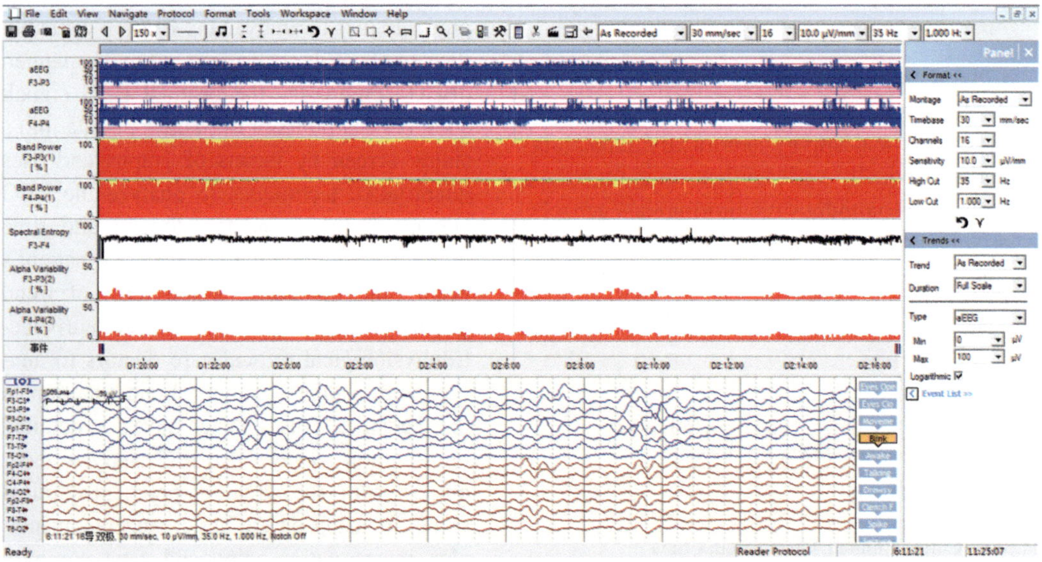


**Fig. 2.1** Sixteen-hour trend graph and the 10-s original EEG shown as the arrow. From the trend graph, the change trend of the brain function state during the whole monitoring process can be intuitively understood

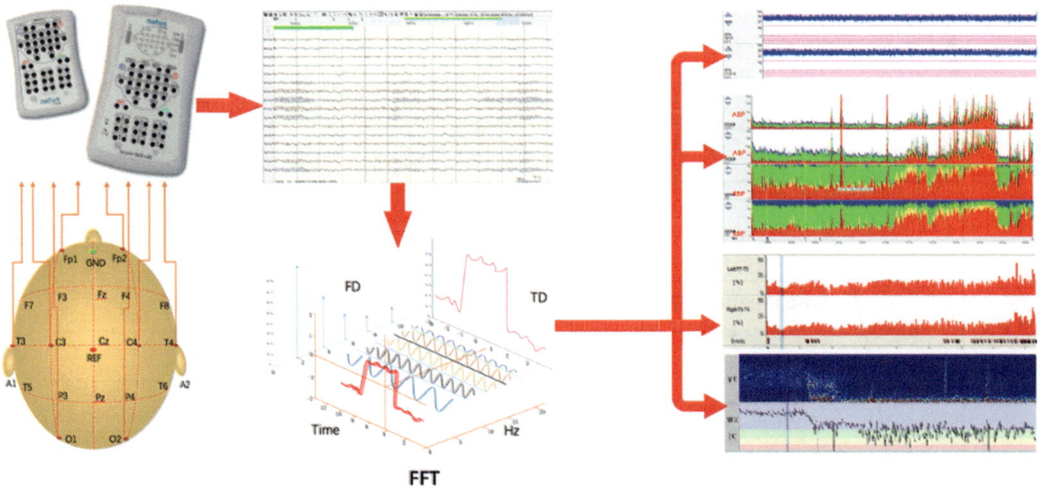


**Fig. 2.2** qEEG collects the EEG signal from the scalp, analyzes it by FFT, and displays the spectrum and power spectrum of the EEG sequence signal in the form of a trend spectrum

FFT is the basic technology used for EEG quantitative analysis. FFT folds the waveform into sine waves of different frequencies and converts the EEG waveform with nonlinear time domain characteristics into frequency domain quantities; it then calculates the amplitude and power of each frequency component, thereby presenting the energy value of the wave. The advantages of FFT are simple processing, strong applicability to the signal, and obvious physical meaning [2]. Frequency domain analysis is mainly performed through power spectrum analysis, which converts the EEG wave, the amplitude of which varies with time, into a spectrum of EEG power with a given frequency so that the α, β, θ, and δ in the EEG can be easily observed at different time nodes. Time domain analysis is mainly used to directly extract waveform features. Although a large amount of EEG information is reflected in frequency characteristics, which are easier to observe from the frequency domain, some important information is reflected more prominently in time domain characteristics, such as spikes reflecting epilepsy. qEEG uses the above analysis techniques to convert EEG signals into trend graphs. The trend graph is a compressed graph of EEG over a period of time, which can quickly show the overall situation of the patient's brain function and the trend of brain function changes over a period of time.

## 2.2 Trend Chart Commonly Used in qEEG

### 2.2.1 aEEG

#### The Principle of aEEG

aEEG passes the EEG signal through an asymmetrical bandpass filter to attenuate the electrical activity below 2 Hz and above 15 Hz, and between 2 and 15 Hz, the electrical energy of the nonrhythmic component of the EEG signal attenuates as the frequency increases (approximately 12 dB/10, that is 12 dB change for every 10-time increase), which is called filter compensation. Then, the EEG signal is amplified to minimize artifacts from ECG and current interference, sweating, exercise, and muscle activity (Fig. 2.3). The processing of aEEG also includes semilogarithmic amplitude integration. The amplified EEG waveform is processed by semilogarithmic amplitude compression (0–10 μV is a linear display, 10–100 μV is a logarithmic display), and the compressed EEG wave extracts the peak value of the EEG wave through an analog rectification module. The series of peaks are connected with smooth curves so that aEEG can reflect the maximum amplitude (the upper boundary of the aEEG waveform) and the minimum amplitude (the lower boundary of the aEEG waveform) of the original EEG. This process is called peak

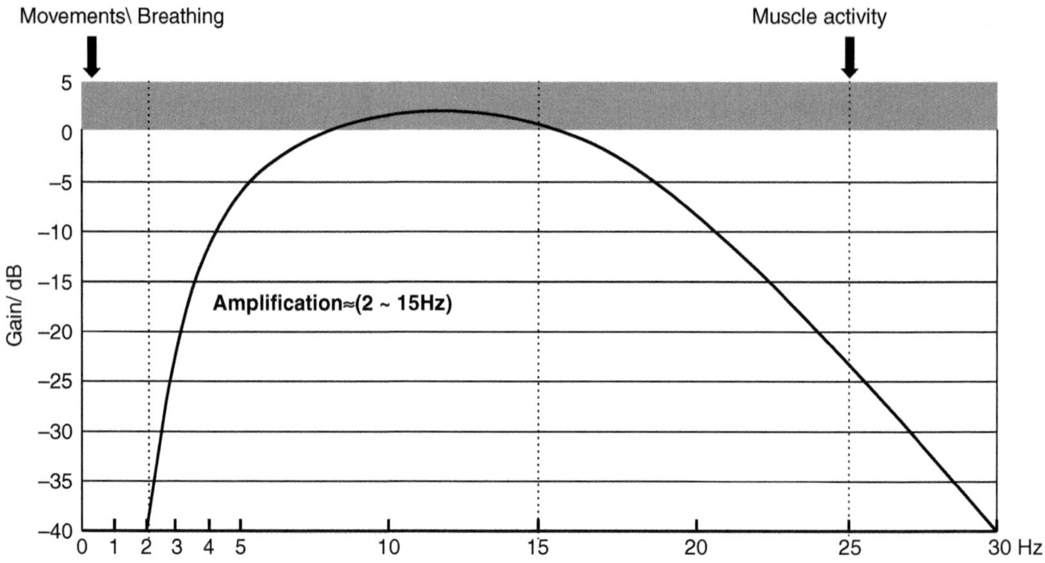


**Fig. 2.3** Asymmetric filtering can filter out noise and artifacts. Artifacts usually have a very low frequency (<1–2 Hz) (such as exercise or breathing) or a very high frequency (>25–30 Hz) (such as muscle activity), which can be reduced by using this filtering

detection and smoothing (the time constant is 0.5 s) (Fig. 2.4). In terms of time compression, in the first-generation brain function monitor, the paper speed of the EEG signal is 6 cm/h or 30 cm/h. Time compression can reflect the original EEG waveforms for up to tens of hours in a very short spectral band, which is convenient for medical staff to observe the patient's brain function status as a whole [5].

### Interpretation of aEEG

aEEG omits the complicated process of waveform and frequency analysis of the original EEG through filtering, semilogarithmic amplitude integration, correction, smoothing, and time compression. Furthermore, aEEG comprehensively evaluates the three contents of the background pattern of EEG activity, the sleep-wake cycle, and seizure, mainly based on the upper and lower boundaries and the changing trend of the bandwidth (Figs. 2.5 and 2.6). All aEEG data should be analyzed in terms of these three contents to make a complete evaluation of the patient's brain function. Long-term aEEG monitoring is compressed and compact, making it difficult to identify short-term abnormal changes. Therefore, it is suggested that the range of 2 h be used as the best display time.

To facilitate clinical analysis, a large number of researchers have classified aEEG background activities. Currently, Hellström-Westas et al. [6, 7] proposed the classification method with the most clinical applications. The interpretation method is as follows:

(1) Interpretation of background activities:
  1. Continuous normal voltage (CNV): Continuous activity, the lower boundary (minimum amplitude) is (5) 7–10 μV, the upper boundary (maximum amplitude) is 10–25 (−50) μV, the bandwidth is normal, and the prognosis is usually good (Fig. 2.7).
  2. Discontinuous normal voltage (DNV): Discontinuous activity, the upper boundary is >10 μV, the lower boundary is variable but ≤5 μV, the bandwidth is widened, there are mild aEEG abnormalities, and most of the prognoses are good (Fig. 2.8).
  3. Continuous low voltage (CLV): Continuous low-amplitude activity, the upper boundary is approximately 5 μV or

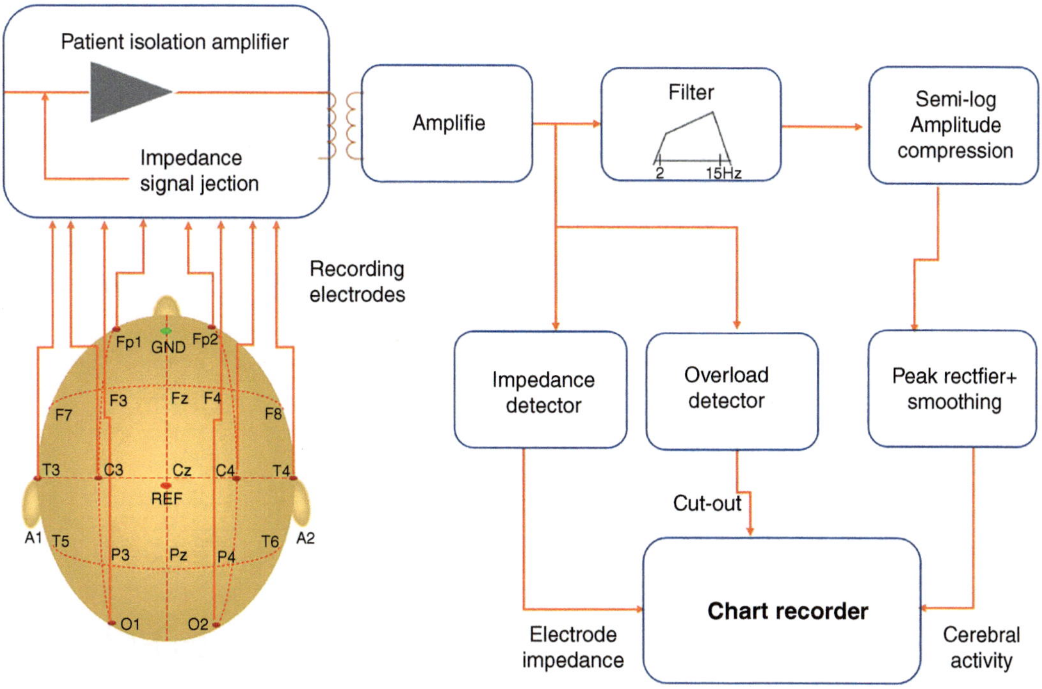


**Fig. 2.4** aEEG signal topology diagram

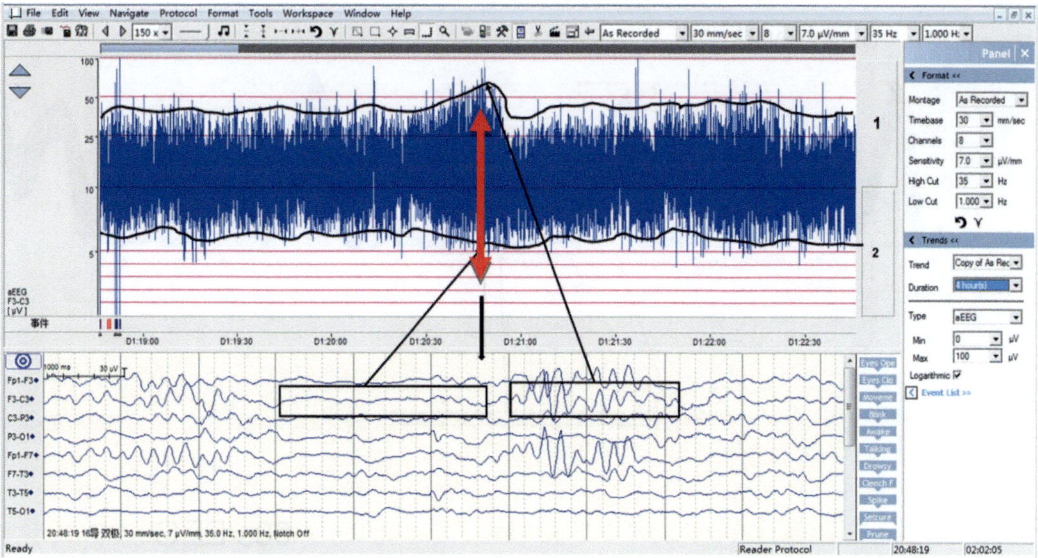

**Fig. 2.5** After compression and integration, within 10 s of the original EEG image (black arrow) corresponding to aEEG, the maximum amplitude of the original EEG constitutes the upper boundary of aEEG, the minimum amplitude constitutes the lower boundary of aEEG, and the upper and lower boundaries are called the bandwidth (red arrow)

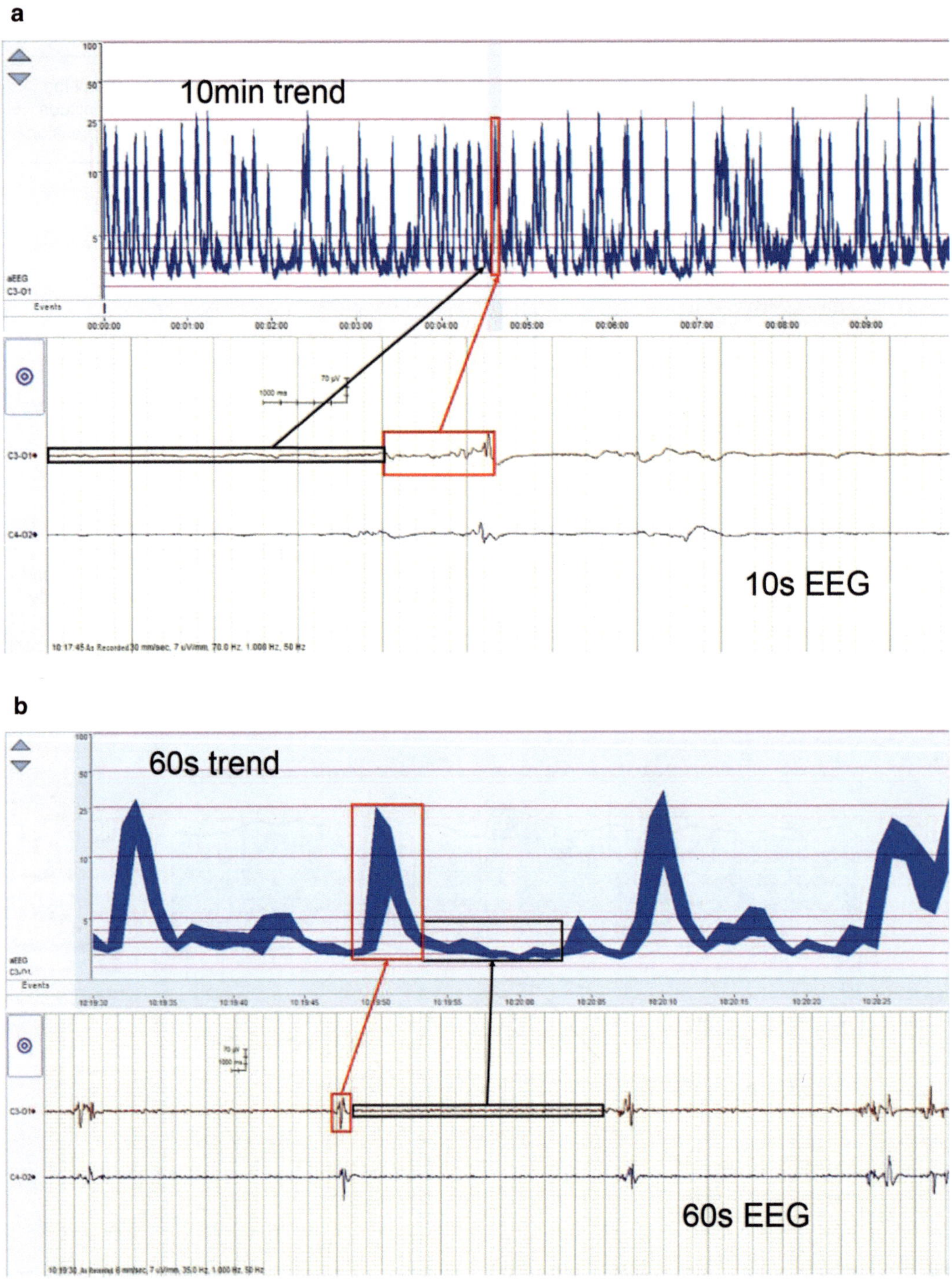


**Fig. 2.6** (**a–b**) In a patient post-CPR, EEG shows a burst suppression (BS) pattern. (**a**) A 10-min aEEG and the 10-s original EEG. (**b**) A 60-s aEEG and the 60-s corresponding original EEG. The suppressed part of the EEG corresponds to the lower boundary of aEEG, and the burst part corresponds to the upper boundary of aEEG

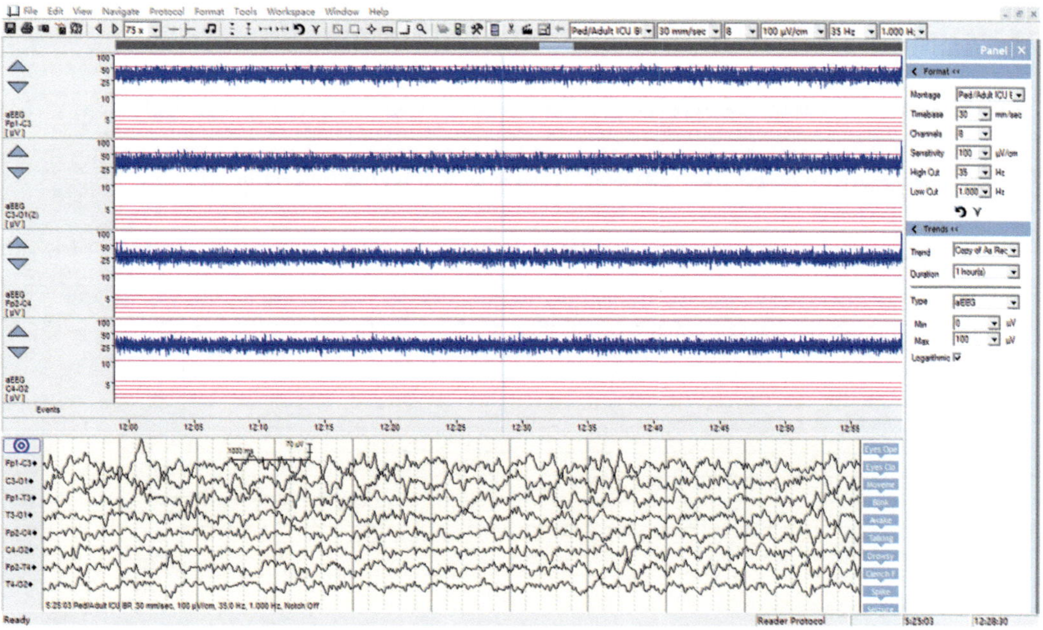

**Fig. 2.7** aEEG showing CNV; the upper boundary is 10–25 (−50) μV, and the lower boundary is (5) 7–10 μV

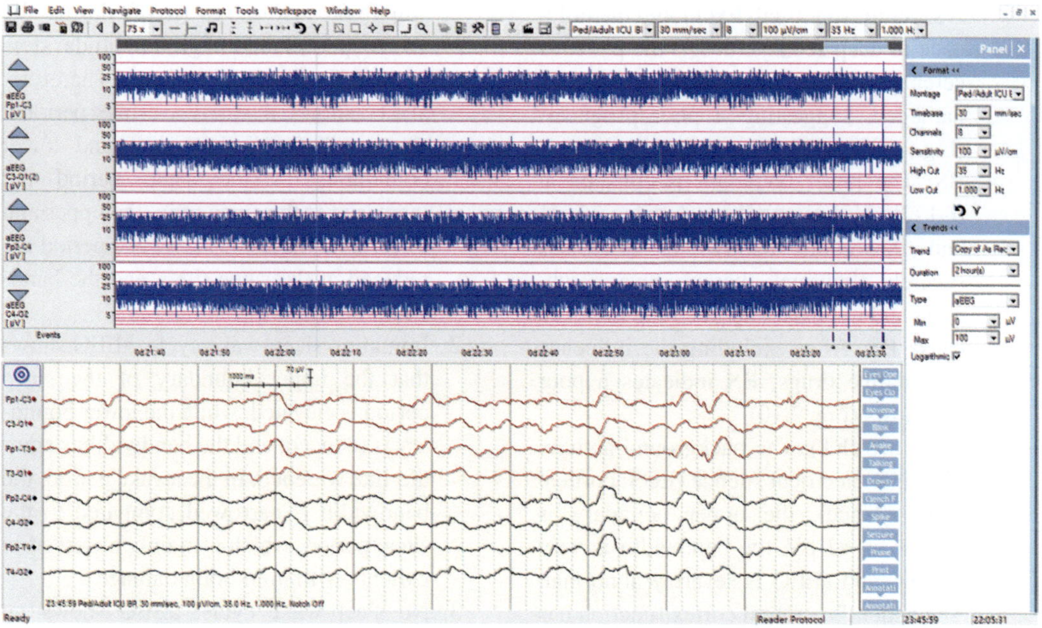

**Fig. 2.8** aEEG showing DNV; the upper boundary >10 μV, and the lower boundary ≤5 μV

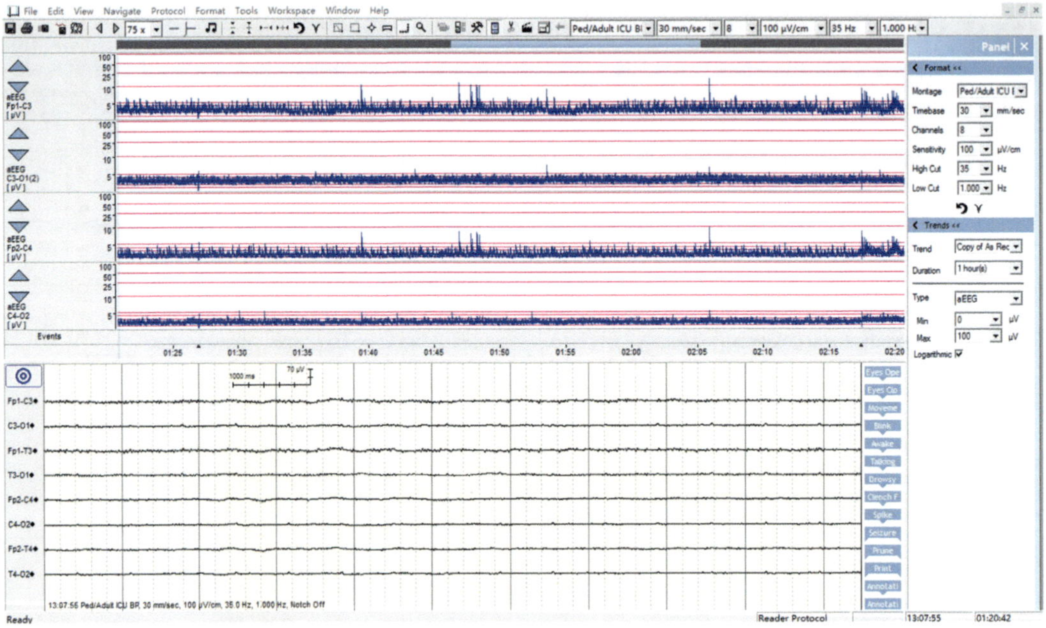

**Fig. 2.9** aEEG showing CLV; the upper boundary is approximately 5 μV or <5 μV

<5 μV, the bandwidth narrows, and aEEG is severely abnormal. Excluding the influence of deep sedative drugs, the patient's cerebral cortex function has been severely damaged, suggesting a poor prognosis (Fig. 2.9).

4. BS: The lower boundary is constant at 0–1 (2) μV, the upper boundary is >25 μV, and the comb bandwidth. aEEG is severely abnormal; there is severe ischemia and hypoxia, and deep sedation can cause BS. After excluding the influence of sedative drugs, BS indicates a poor prognosis (Fig. 2.10).
5. Flat trace (FT): The background activity is mainly electrical silence (ECS; cortical EEG silence), the upper boundary is <5 μV or <2 μV, the bandwidth is very narrow, and aEEG is severely abnormal. The patient's cerebral cortex function has been severely damaged or brain death has occurred, suggesting a very poor prognosis (Fig. 2.11).

(2) Interpretation of the sleep-wake cycle:

1. Normal sleep-wake cycle: Healthy people usually have a mature sleep-wake cycle. The original EEG is dominated by low-amplitude fast waves (α, β) during the awake period and high-amplitude slow waves (θ, δ) during sleep. Therefore, aEEG shows a sine-wave-like periodic change. That is, the upper and lower boundaries of the sleep period are increased at the same time, the upper and lower boundaries of the awake period are reduced at the same time, and the bandwidth is similar.
2. Immature sleep-wake cycle: aEEG shows that the upper boundary of the sleep period is elevated, while the lower boundary is reduced, and the bandwidth is spindle-like widened. In the awake period, the bandwidth is narrowed compared to the sleep period, which is mainly observed in patients with mild brain damage.
3. No sleep-wake cycle: aEEG shows no periodic changes in the upper and lower boundaries, which is observed in severely impaired brain function.

(3) Interpretation of epileptic seizures:

1. Single attack: aEEG shows that the upper and lower borders increase sharply at the

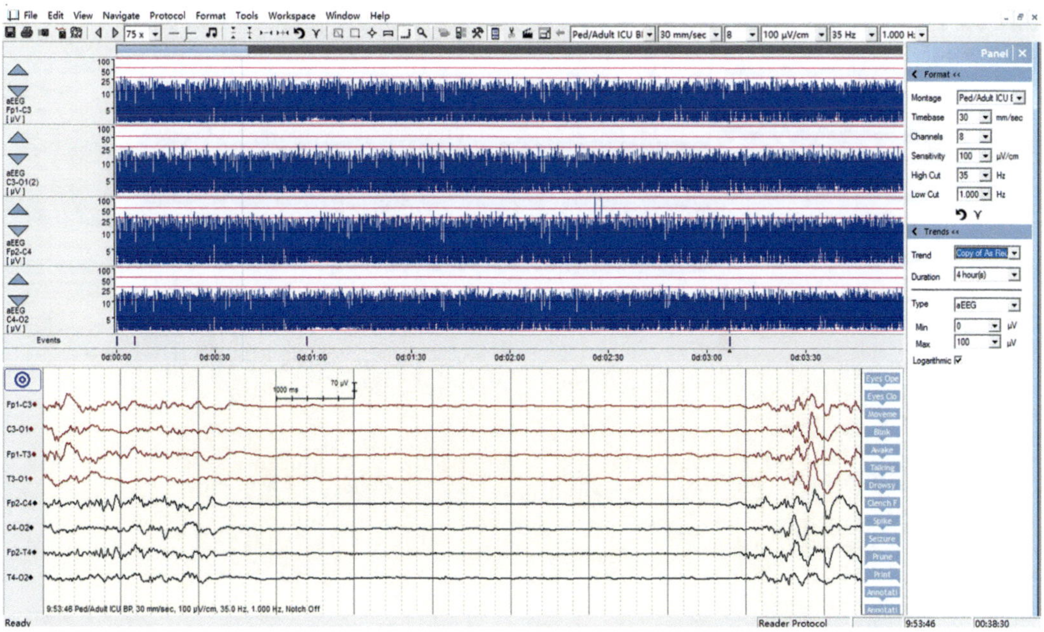

**Fig. 2.10** aEEG showing BS; the lower boundary is constant at 0–1 (2) μV, and the upper boundary is >25 μV

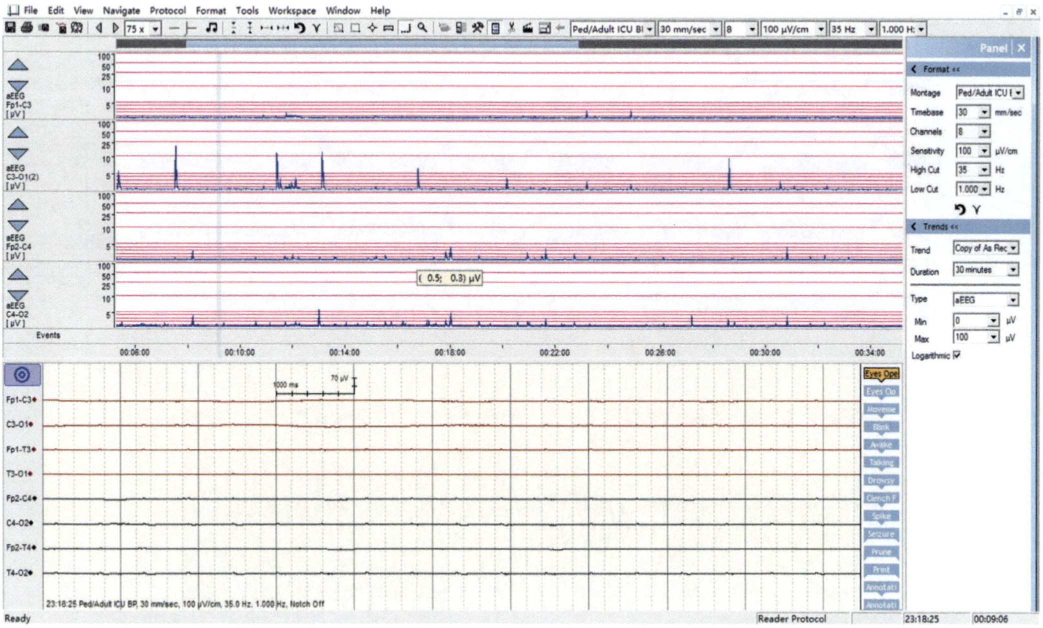

**Fig. 2.11** aEEG showing ECS; the upper boundary is <5 μV or <2 μV

same time and then decrease briefly, showing a spike shape. The cessation of seizures is manifested by the rapid decline of the upper and lower boundaries at the same time, and the whole aEEG is sharp (Fig. 2.12).

2. Single recurrent attack: A single recurrent attack within a period of time, more than three attacks within 30 min, there are multiple spikes, and there is a remission period between the two (Fig. 2.13).

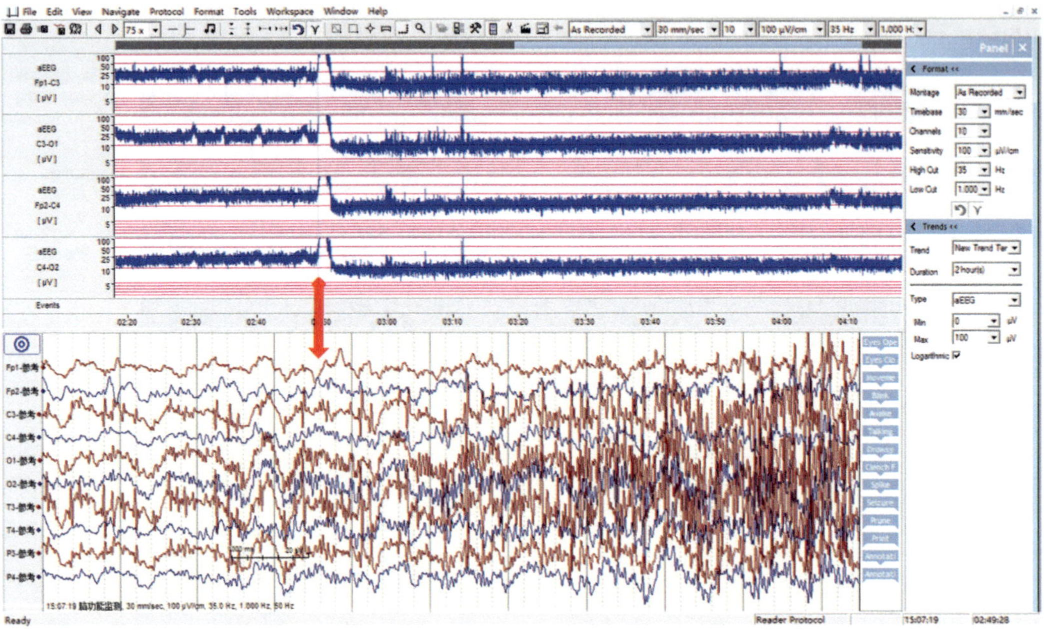

**Fig. 2.12** aEEG showing a single attack

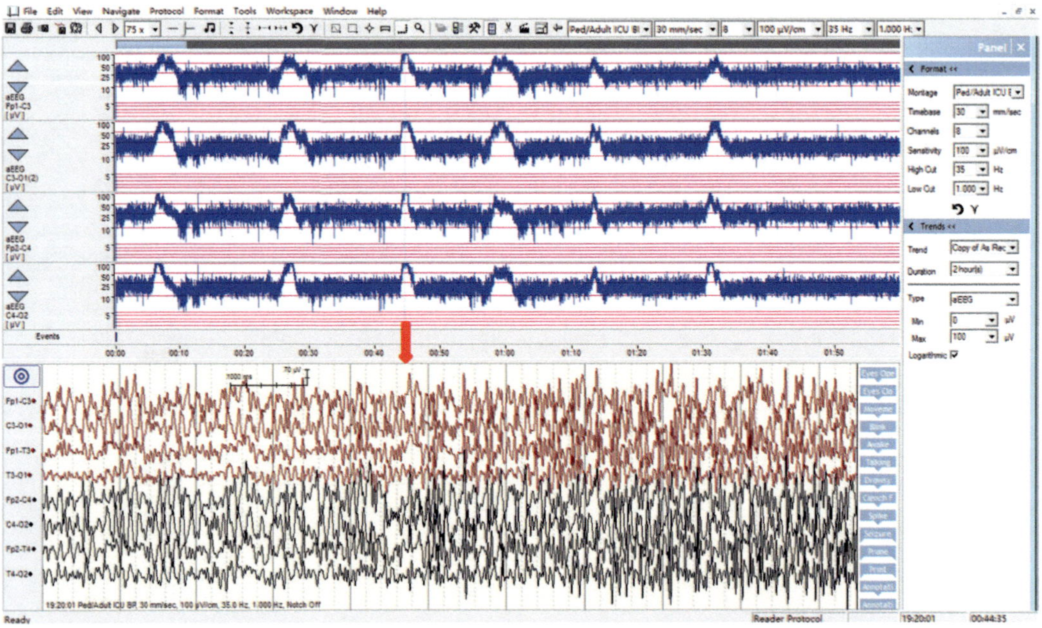

**Fig. 2.13** Single recurring seizure showing multiple "spikes"

3. SE: Discharge ≥30 min, aEEG appears as a "sawtooth pattern" (Fig. 2.14) or two forms of continuous increases in the peak and trough amplitudes (Fig. 2.15).

### 2.2.2 RBP

**The Principle of RBP**

The spectrum analysis technology has greatly helped in the analysis of the original EEG. This technology converts the EEG waveform with nonlinear changes in the time domain characteristics into a frequency domain and quantifies each frequency component. Absolute band power (ABP): band energy is the power of each band in an EEG, which is divided into ABP and RBP. ABP converts the change of the original EEG amplitude with time into the change of EEG power with frequency; that is, the absolute power value of each frequency band of α, β, θ, δ within a certain time range is obtained. Compared with RBP, ABP has difficulty distinguishing differences between different bands. RBP mainly reflects the change in EEG frequency. RBP is not the percentage of the power of each band to the total power but the ratio of the energy of one band to the total energy of all the bands, which is expressed as a percentage with different color areas (Fig. 2.16). Red represents the area under the curve (AUC) of the δ frequency band, yellow represents the AUC of the θ frequency band, green represents the AUC of the α frequency band, and blue represents the AUC of the β frequency band (Fig. 2.17).

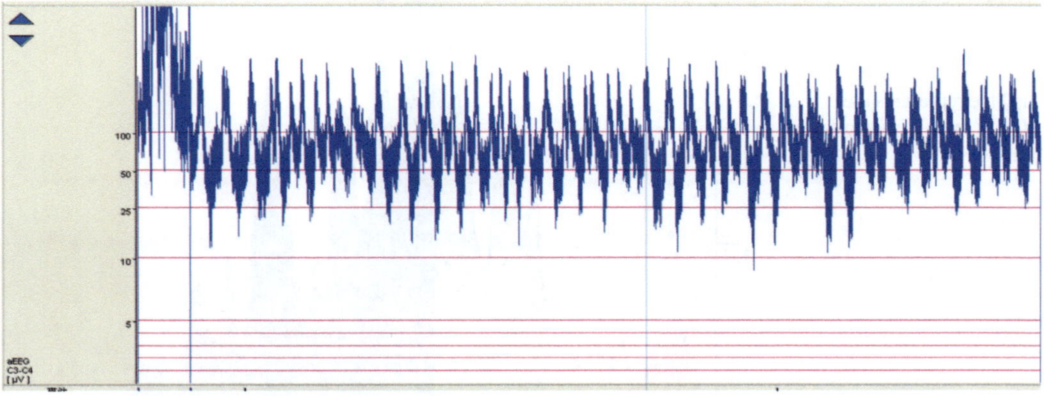


**Fig. 2.14** SE: Discharge for ≥30 min showing a "sawtooth pattern"

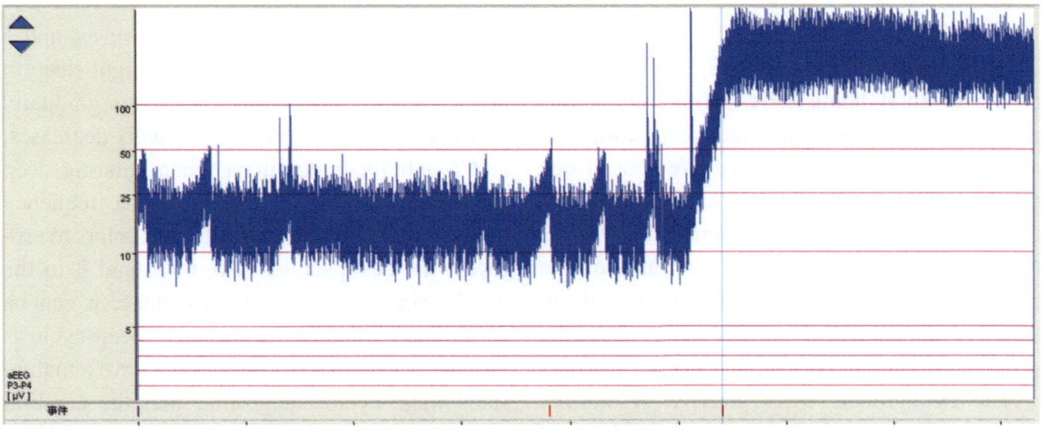


**Fig. 2.15** SE: Discharge for ≥30 min; the amplitude of the peak and valley continues to increase

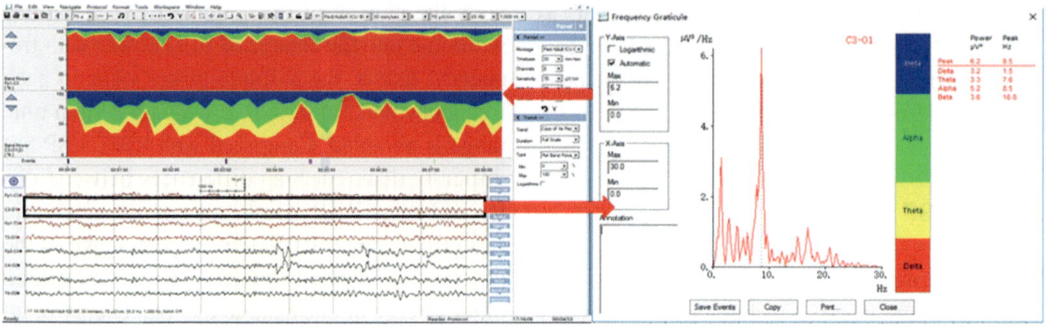


**Fig. 2.16** RBP: Through spectrum analysis of every 10 s of EEG and the display according to the relative energy arrangement of different frequency bands, different EEG frequency bands are indicated by different colors in the trend chart

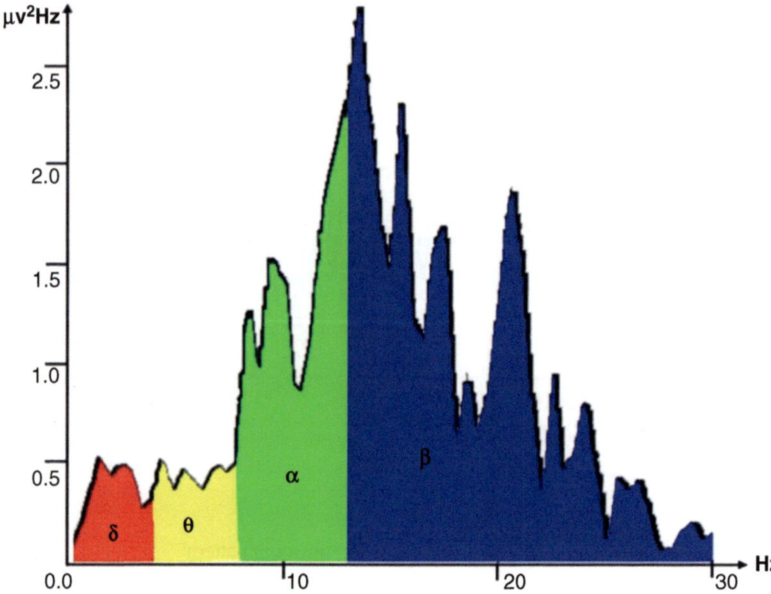


**Fig. 2.17** EEG power map: red represents the AUC of the δ frequency band, yellow represents the AUC of the θ frequency band, green represents the AUC of the α frequency band, and blue represents the AUC of the β frequency band

**The Interpretation of RBP**

The EEG activities in the corresponding regions of the cerebral hemispheres of normal adults appear synchronously and are very similar in amplitude and frequency. Once any area of one side of the brain is damaged, its EEG activity will change, and the frequency or amplitude will be inconsistent with the corresponding area on the opposite side. The difference can be visualized directly from the RBP trend graph to evaluate the symmetry of the two hemispheres (Fig. 2.18).

The background EEG activity of normal adults in the states of being quiet, awake, and with closed eyes is dominated by α rhythms. RBP shows that α waves account for more than 80%, and the proportions of β waves, θ waves, and δ waves are low. During sleep, from light sleep to deep sleep, slow-wave activity gradually increases, fast-wave activity gradually decreases, and δ activity is dominant when entering deep sleep. A trend graph expressed as the frequency domain, such as RBP, uses different colors to represent the occupancies of δ, θ, α, and β in the trend graph. From the trend change, it can be determined whether the patient's sleep cycle is normal (Fig. 2.19). Normal people have a mature sleep-wake cycle, suggesting that the cerebral cortex is functioning well. For patients with brain damage, if the sleep-wake cycle reappears, then a good prognosis is indicated.

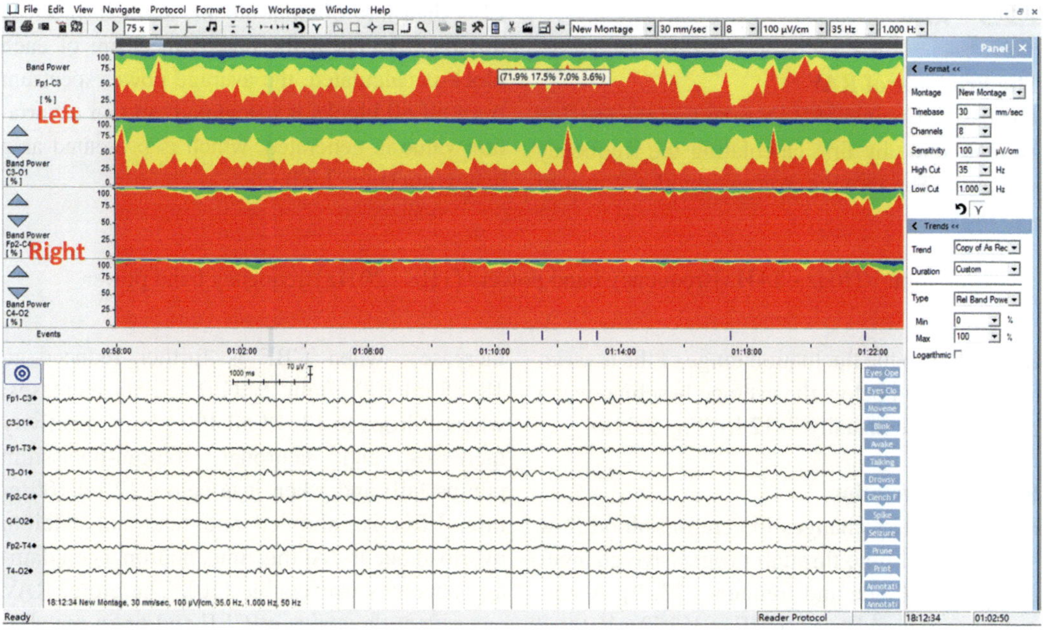


**Fig. 2.18** Patients with a right cerebral infarction. RBP shows that the right side is dominated by slow waves, and the left and right sides are obviously asymmetric

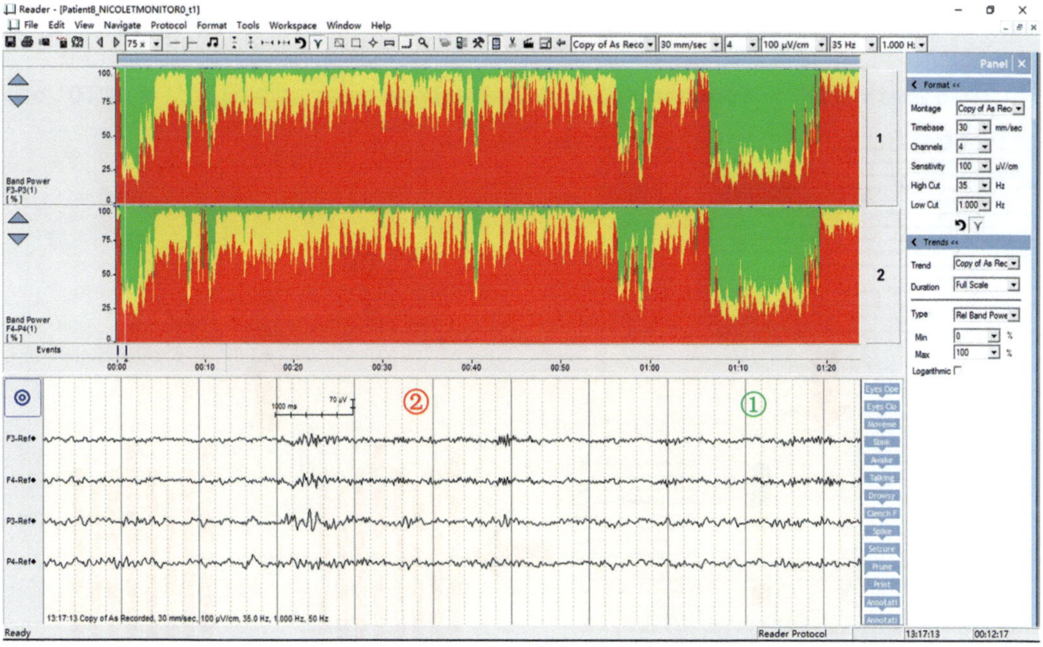


**Fig. 2.19** ① In healthy adults who are awake with eyes closed, the original EEG is dominated by alpha rhythm background activity, and RBP is dominated by the alpha band (green); ② in the sleep state, the original EEG δ rhythm background activities increase, the RBP δ band (red) is dominant, and there is a small theta wave (yellow)

### 2.2.3 RAV

**The Principle of RAV**

The basic principle of RAV is to find the moving average value by first calculating the frequency spectrum. The moving average divides 2 min of EEG data into 60 data blocks, and one block is usually 2 s. Then, the power spectrum of each block is calculated, the average power spectrum from all 60 blocks is calculated, and an α variation value is generated, which is presented as a histogram (Fig. 2.20).

$$\alpha\,\text{variation} = \left(6\,\text{Hz} - 14\,\text{Hz}\right)\text{frequency band power} / \left(1\,\text{Hz} - 20\,\text{Hz}\right)\text{frequency band power}.$$

RAV refers to the fluctuation range of the α variation above and below the average baseline over a period of time (usually 8–12 h) (Fig. 2.21a).

**RAV Interpretation**

RAV can reflect changes in cerebral blood flow (CBF) in real time through progressive changes in EEG amplitude and frequency [8, 9]. A normal person should have a CBF of 35–50 ml/100 g/min. When CBF decreases to nearly 25–35 ml/100 g/min, the EEG fast wave activity begins to decrease and anaerobic metabolism increases; when CBF is further reduced to 18–25 ml/100 g/min, EEG θ activity increases; when it drops to 13–18 ml/100 g/min, δ activity increases and neuronal sodium-potassium pumps fail; and when it is below 12 ml/100 g/min, EEG is inhibited and neuronal calcium overload occurs. At this time, neuronal cell damage becomes irreversible [10]. Therefore, RAV can reflect the status of CBF and brain metabolism, and the change trend of RAV can quickly assess the degree of neuronal ischemia, hypoxia, and cell damage.

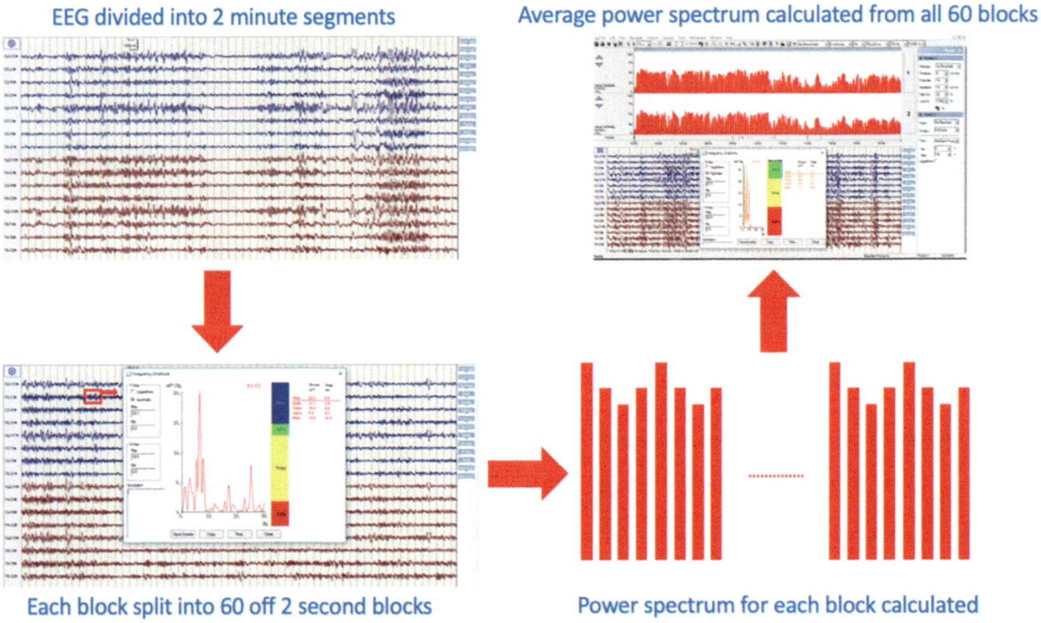


**Fig. 2.20** α variation. Divide the original 2-min EEG segment into 60 blocks of 2-s, calculate the spectrum of each block, and then average all 60 blocks of the spectrum to obtain the value of α variation, which is presented as a histogram. The change map composed of the internal histogram in a period of time is called the "RAV" trend map

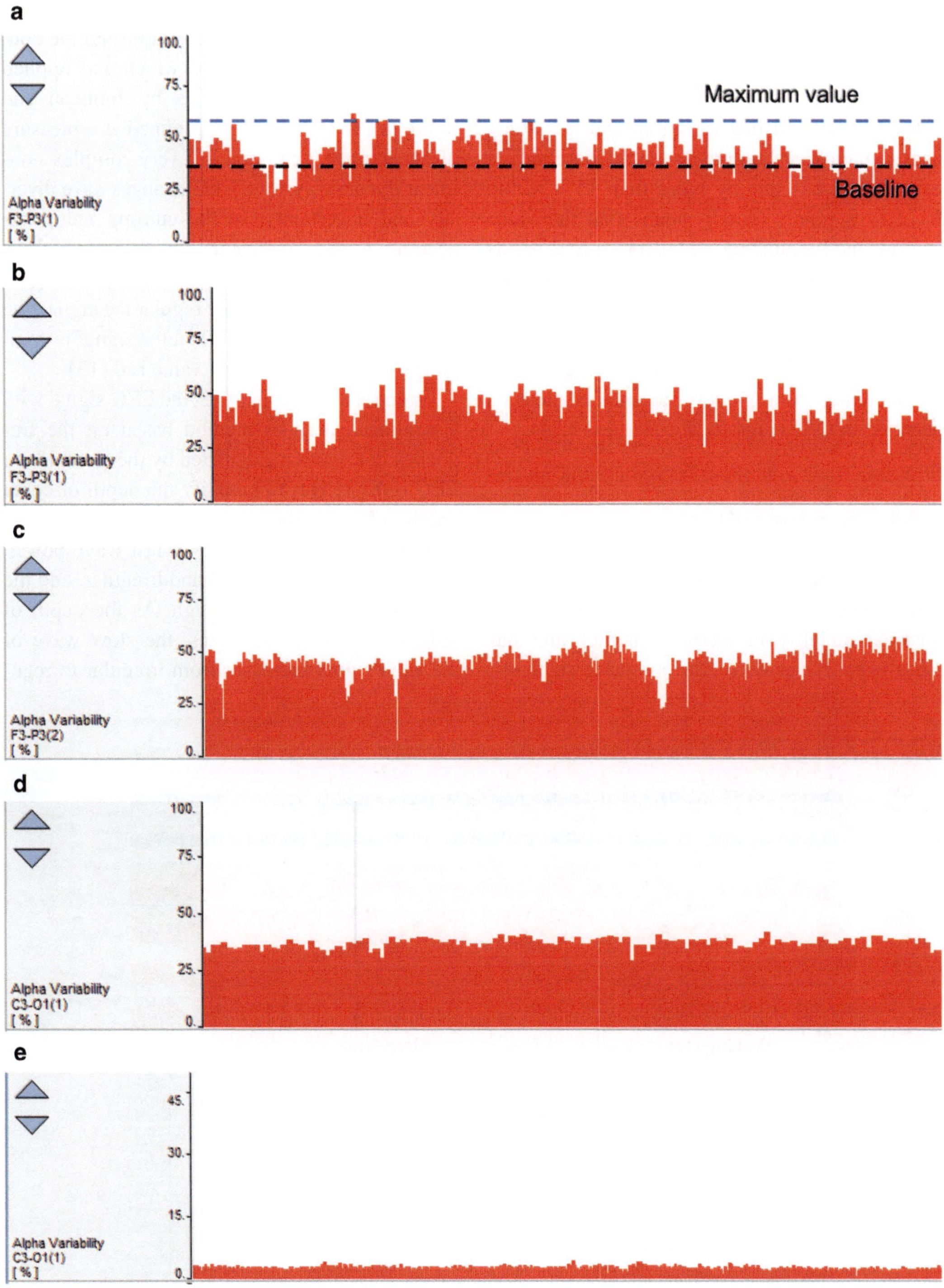


**Fig. 2.21** (**a**) When performing RAV analysis, it is necessary to select at least 8–12 h of recorded data and determine its score based on the frequency and amplitude of the relative α exceeding the baseline. (**b**) Grade 4, excellent. Excursions form baseline occurring once per hour or of greater than 15% of the median value were given a score of excellent. (**c**) Grade 3, good. Excursions of 10% at least every 4 h were given a score of good. (**d**) Grade 2, fair. Small or infrequent excursions were give a score of fair. (**e**) Grade 1, poor. No excursions greater than 2% were scored as poor

According to the research of Paul, M and Vespa [11], RAV can be divided into four levels. Four points (very good) means that every hour has a value that exceeds the baseline (the mean value of the 8–12 h α variation, and this study uses visual observation to divide the baseline) or exceeds the baseline by more than 15% within 8–12 h; 3 points (good) means that the value exceeds the baseline by 10% every 4 h; 2 points (general) means that the frequency of exceeding the baseline is rare or the amplitude is less than 10%; and 1 point (poor) means that the amplitude beyond the baseline is less than 2% (Fig. 2.21b–e). Declining from one level to another means a decrease in CBF (Figs. 2.22, 2.23, and 2.24).

### 2.2.4 Spectral Entropy

**The Principle of Spectral Entropy**

The concept of entropy was first proposed as a physical quantity in thermodynamics and has since been expanded to various research fields. Shannon introduced this concept into information theory in 1948 [12] and established the concept of information entropy, which was applied to energy spectrum analysis by Johnson and Shore in 1984 [13] and was defined as a measure of uncertainty. The brain is a very complex nonlinear dynamic system. EEG changes have diversity and uncertainty, so the entropy index has become a new indicator for analyzing these changes. The more irregular the signal, the higher the entropy value; the more regular the signal, the lower the entropy value. When the signal is completely regular, the entropy value is 0 [13].

Spectral entropy analyzes the EEG signal with a nonlinear analysis method based on the frequency distribution calculated by the frontal lobe EEG (0.8~32 Hz) to quantify the depth of coma sedation [14]. In the awake state, the frontal lobe EEG signal is dominated by a fast wave power, the EEG signal is complex and irregular, and the spectral entropy value is high. As the depth of sedation gradually increases, the slow wave of the EEG signal increases from irregular to regu-

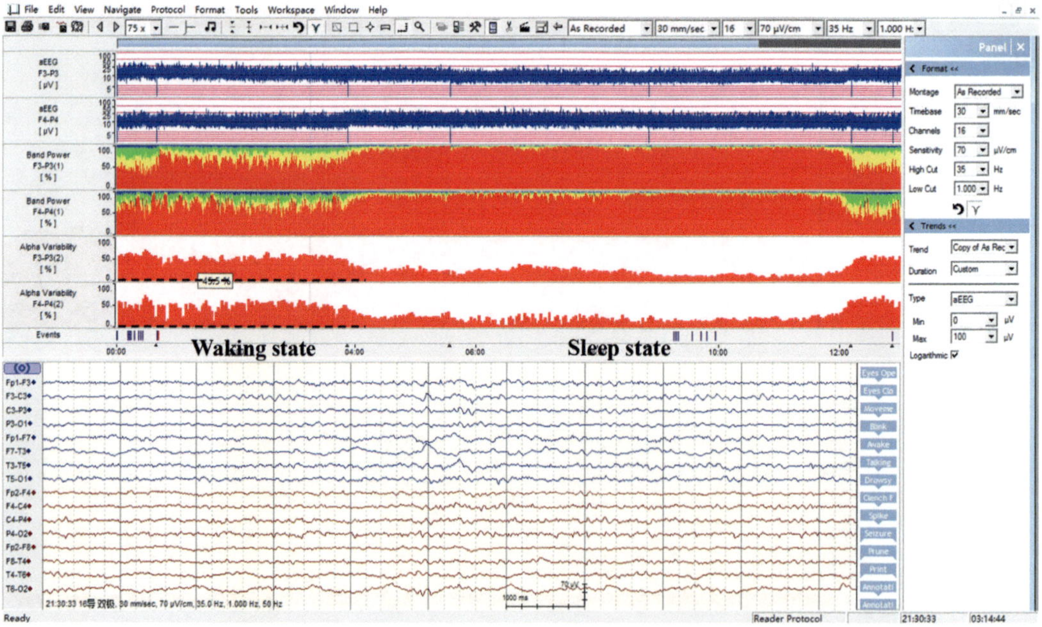


**Fig. 2.22** When the patient is awake, the α variation baseline is visually inspected (the baseline is the point at which there is no change in α variation during this time period). As shown in the figure, the patient is awake, the baseline is 45%, and the α variation range fluctuates between 45% and 70%. Thus, its RAV is 25%, which is divided into 4 points according to the level. During sleep, cerebral oxygen metabolism decreases, slow wave activity increases, and RAV decreases

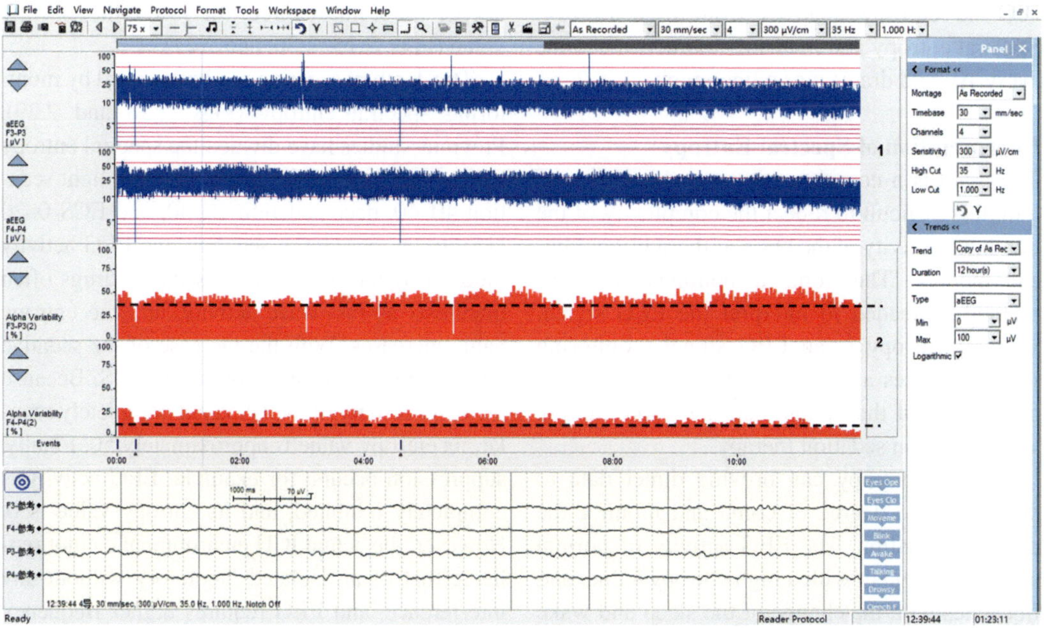

**Fig. 2.23** A 27-year-old man with a right craniocerebral injury. Through the α variation trend, it is found that the left and right hemispheres of the brain are asymmetrical. The left baseline is 40%, the α variation fluctuates between 40% and 52%, and the RAV is 12%, which is rated as 3 points; the right baseline is approximately 23%, the α variation range is between 23% and 30%, and the RAV is 7%, which is rated as 2 points

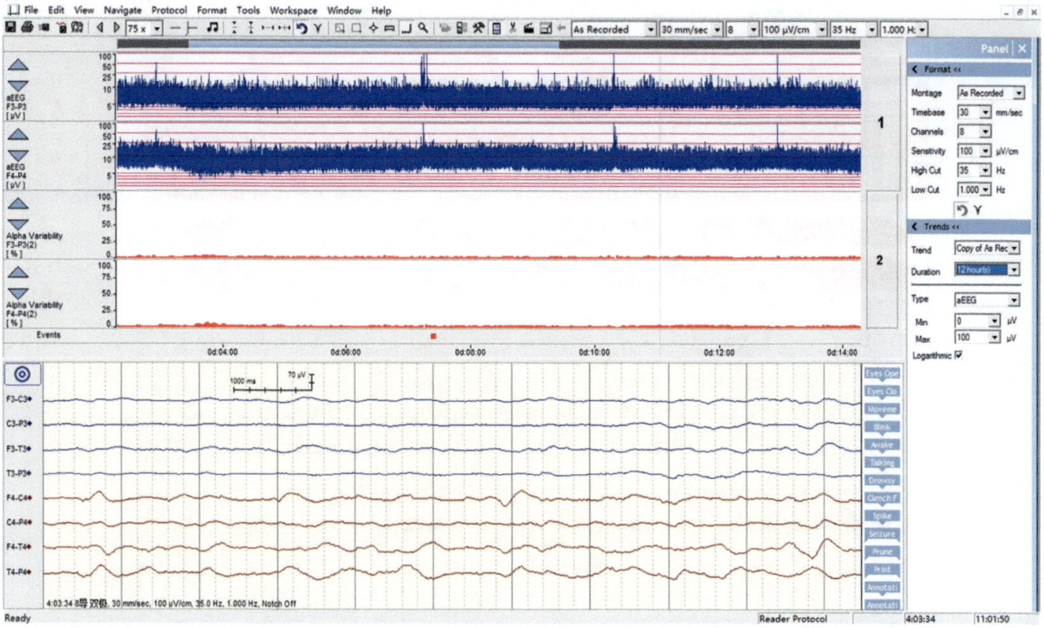

**Fig. 2.24** Hypoxic-ischemic encephalopathy (HIE) patients. aEEG showing DNV; there is no overall change in the α variation of the left and right hemispheres, the α variation between 3% and 5%, and the RAV is 2%, which is rated as 1 point

lar, and entropy changes from high to low. Spectral entropy automatically extracts the value every 10 sand draws it as a line graph.

**Interpretation of Spectral Entropy**

The brain is a complex nonlinear dynamic system. It is difficult to reflect the complexity of the nonlinear activity of the brain with traditional linear models. Therefore, a nonlinear analysis method is needed to interpret the EEG signal. Spectral entropy is an EEG signal monitoring index that uses a nonlinear model to reflect the complexity of the system and has good guiding significance in sedation therapy.

Spectral entropy can provide direct data to determine the degree of coma and monitor the depth of sedation. The EEG activity of normal adults is irregular, with a high entropy value, and fluctuates with the change of the sleep and wake cycle; the EEG activity of people in a coma caused by brain injury is mainly a slow wave that is relatively regular with low entropy, and the deeper the coma degree, the lower the entropy value (Figs. 2.25, 2.26, and 2.27).

The depth of sedation can be assessed by monitoring spectral entropy (Figs. 2.28 and 2.29). Previous studies have divided the spectral entropy values into four levels: conscious >60, light sedation 40–60, deep sedation 20–40, and ECS 0–20 [15]. In the process of sedation, the EEG activity induced by the initial use of sedative drugs often manifests as fast wave activity, and the entropy value increases. With the increase of the sedative dose, EEG activity will appear as a BS. Because the EEG activity of the BS is not completely regular, its entropy value is approximately 50. Finally, suppression occurs; for example, EEG activity is completely inhibited, and its entropy value is 0. However, the actual ICU environment cannot replicate that of an isolated laboratory without any interference, and EEG requires higher frequency sampling. Thus, EEG activity cannot be completely suppressed. Therefore, for suppressed EEG activity, the entropy value is approximately 20.

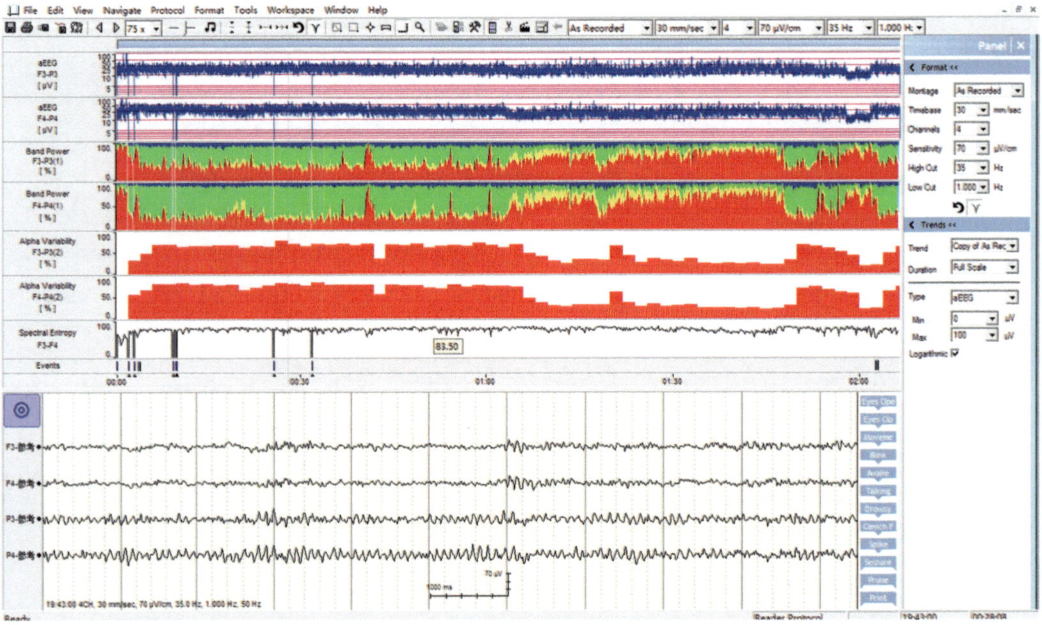

**Fig. 2.25** A healthy female. aEEG showing CNV, with a sleep-wake cycle; RBP is mainly a fast wave in the waking period and a slow wave in the sleep period. RAV is 4 points (very good); spectral entropy fluctuates between 80 and 90 in the waking period and between 70 and 80 in the sleep state

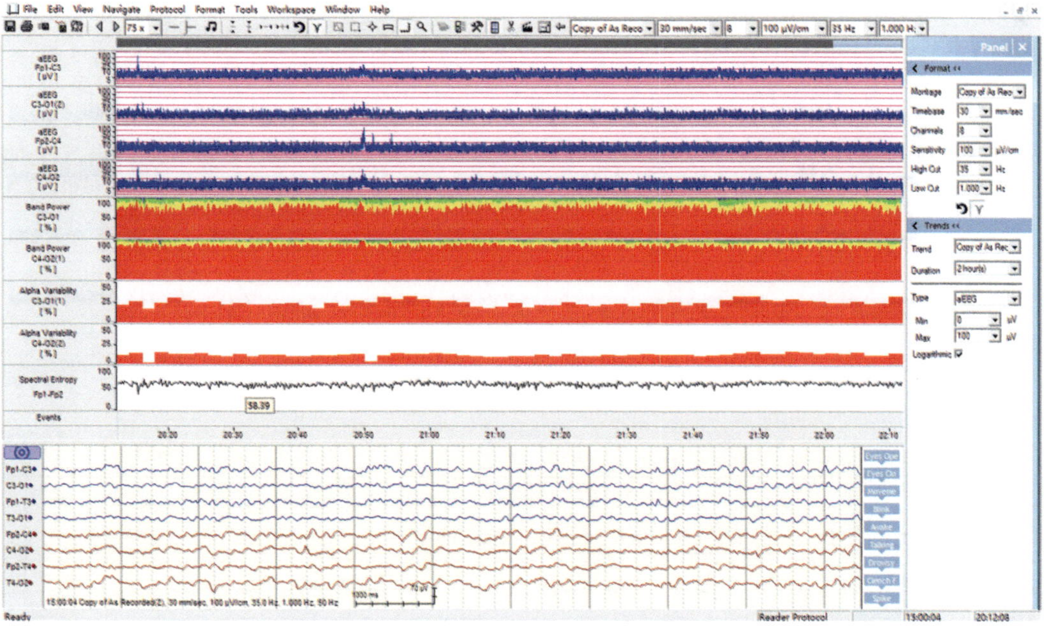

**Fig. 2.26** A 29-year-old male who presented with trauma to the right side of the brain and a superficial coma. aEEG showing that the left and right hemispheres are DNV; RBP is dominated by δ activity on both sides, the percentage of slow wave on the right is relatively large, and there is no sleep-wake cycle; the RAV of right side is poor, 1 point (poor); spectral entropy is 50–60

## 2.2.5 Other Trend Graphs

The four common trend graphs of qEEG can reflect the functional status of the cerebral cortex of patients. aEEG is used to assess the degree of brain damage in patients, monitor seizures, assist in prognostic judgment, and guide treatment plans. RBP reflects brain symmetry and the sleep-wake cycle. RAV assists in the assessment of cerebral ischemia and cerebral oxygen metabolism. Spectral entropy assesses the depth of coma and sedation to guide drug treatment [16]. Currently, these four commonly used trend maps essentially satisfy the clinical application of brain function monitoring through intuitive and simple expressions. However, through EEG analysis of the spectrum, more trend map combinations can be used to assist the clinical judgment of the patient's brain function state, including spectroscopy, ABP, envelope trend (ET), and the α/δ power ratio (ADR) (Fig. 2.30).

**Spectrogram**

A spectrogram is used to detect changes in the EEG frequency content, displaying the spectral power in color; dark blue represents low power, and dark red represents high power. In the awake state, the alpha frequency band is used as the background activity, and the corresponding spectrogram high power (dark red) is in the 8~13 Hz region; the sleep state is the δ frequency band as the background activity, and the corresponding spectrogram high power (dark red) is in the 0.5~4 Hz region (Fig. 2.31).

**ET**

ET reflects the change in EEG amplitude. To find the ET, EEG data are divided into segments with a certain length of time, the amplitude of each wave in each segment is detected, the waves are arranged according to the amplitude, and the median is used, which is the envelope value of the segment. Since the amplitude of epileptic sei-

**a**

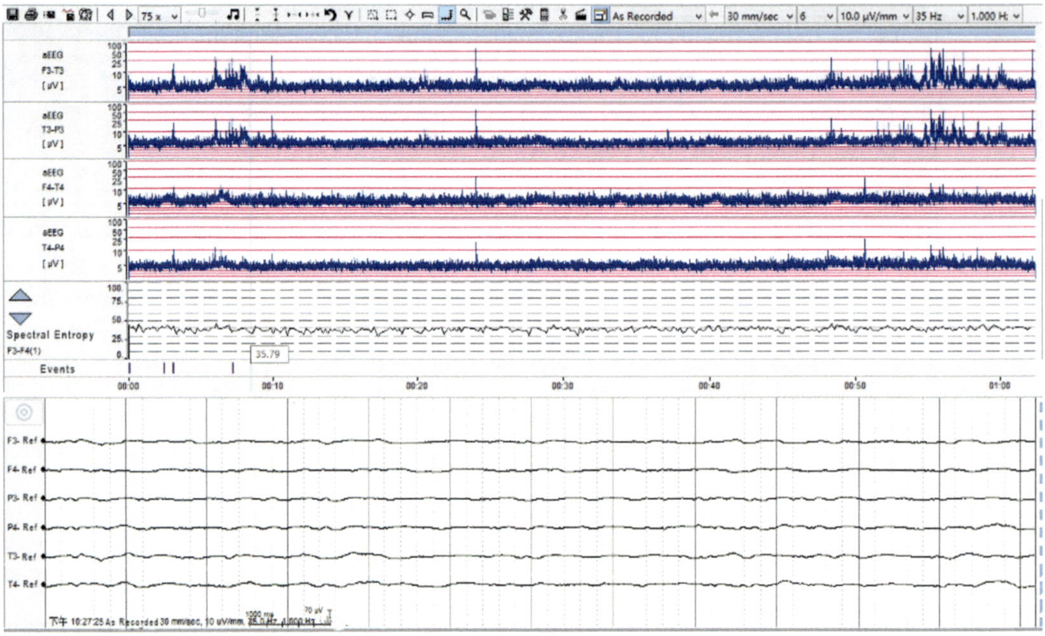


**b**

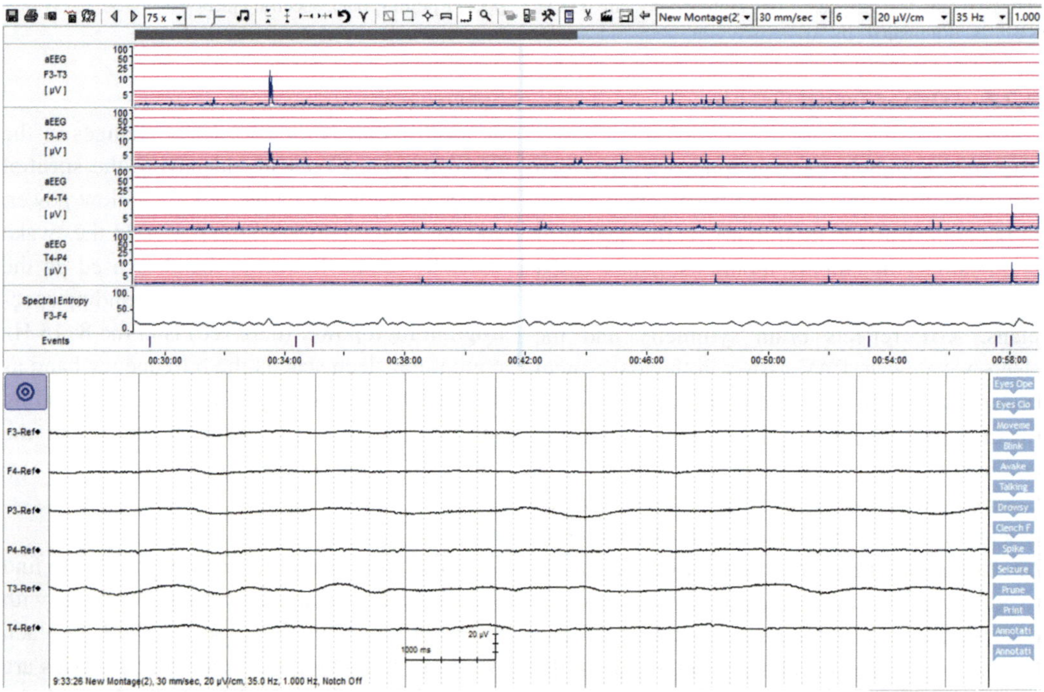


**Fig. 2.27** (**a**–**b**) A patient after receiving CPR. (**a**) aEEG monitored on day 1 after resuscitation; the upper boundary is <10 μV, the lower boundary is <5 μV, the entropy index is between 30 and 40, and the GCS (Glasgow coma scale) score is 4, deep coma. (**b**) aEEG on the 6th day; the brain function is severely abnormal, the entropy index is between 10 and 20, the deep coma is worse than on the first day, and the GCS score is 2 T. Finally, the patient died

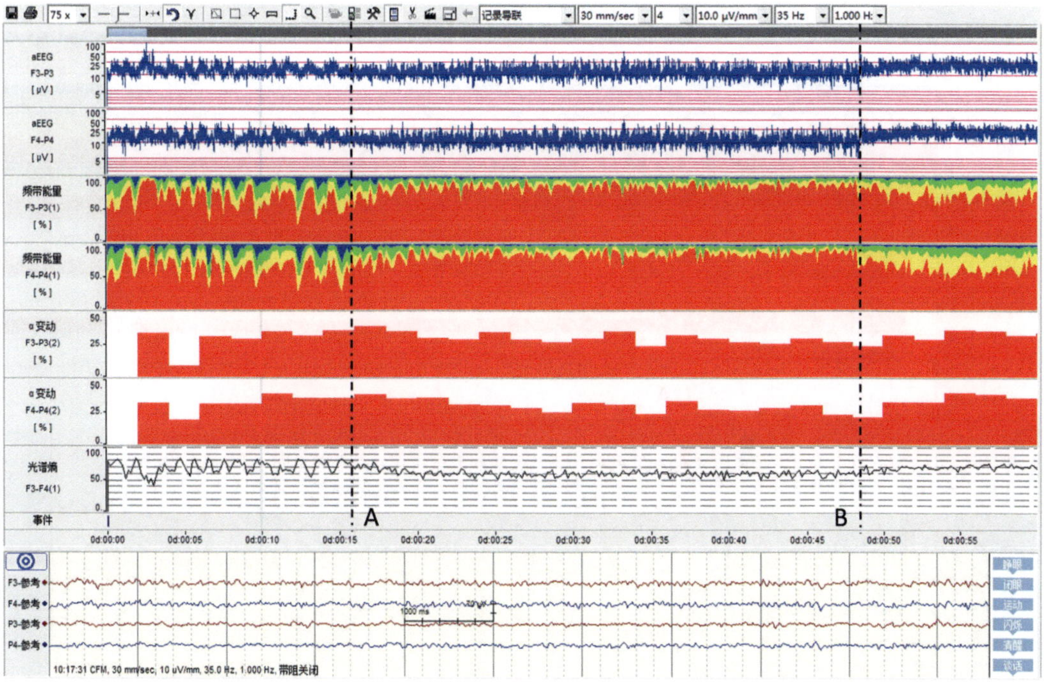


**Fig. 2.28** A patient with drowsiness after receiving CPR with clinical manifestations of limb twitching before monitoring. After the administration of propofol, qEEG monitoring indicated that the trends of EEG activity were unstable (aEEG was zigzag), and there were alternating fast and slow waves. When 5 μg/ml propofol was injected at point A, the amplitude of aEEG decreased, DNV appeared, δ activity increased, RAV decreased, and the spectral entropy value was stable between 50 and 55. After 30 min, aEEG showed a continuous background, the fast and slow waves of RBP were relatively stable, the RAV rose, and the spectral entropy was between 60 and 70

zures is usually higher than the background activity of EEG, ET is considered to be a reliable method for detecting epileptic seizures. During a seizure, aEEG shows that the upper and lower borders increase at the same time and then decrease, showing a spike shape. ET also shows a spike shape (Fig. 2.32).

### ADR

The power ratio between α (8–13 Hz) and δ (0.5–4 Hz) is ADR. ADR is related to CBF and the cerebral oxygen metabolism rate. In 2004, Claassen et al. [17] analyzed the association between the ADR of delayed cerebral ischemia after subarachnoid hemorrhage and Hunt-Hess classification (grades 4 and 5) and found that the incidence rate of delayed cerebral ischemia was 24% when ADR was moderately decreased; when the ADR increased by 3%, there was no delayed cerebral ischemia. When the ADR was lower than 10% of the baseline of six consecutive records or lower than 50% of the single record, delayed cerebral ischemia was likely to occur (Fig. 2.33).

## 2.3 Common Artifacts and Recognition of qEEG

qEEG monitoring can evaluate the patient's brain function status, cerebral ischemia, hypoxia, depth of coma, and sedation in real time and plays an important role in reasonable evaluation of prognosis; but it still has certain limitations. The complex ICU environment, various medical equipment used, and various medical and nursing operations performed can easily lead to misjudgments by personnel who lack EEG interpretation experience. This section describes the common artifacts of qEEG to help non-

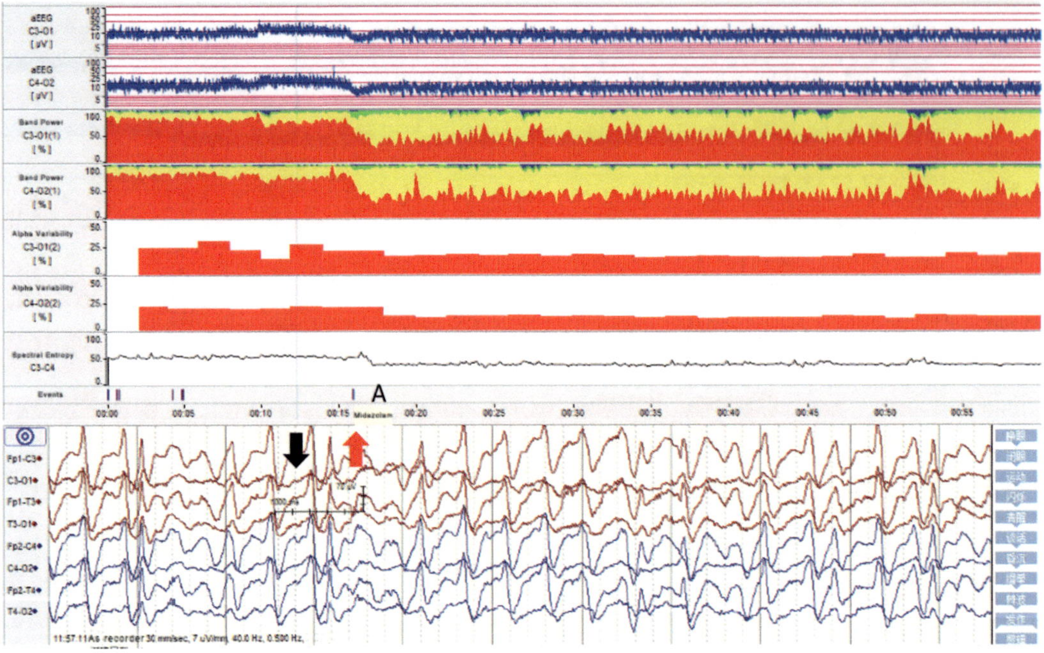


**Fig. 2.29** HIE patients. aEEG showing continuous background activity at the beginning of monitoring; the lower boundary amplitude increases after 5 min, and a high-amplitude spike is found from the original EEG (black arrow). After midazolam was administered (point A), the spike disappeared, DNV activity appeared in aEEG, RBP δ activity decreased, θ activity increased, and RAV and spectral entropy also decreased

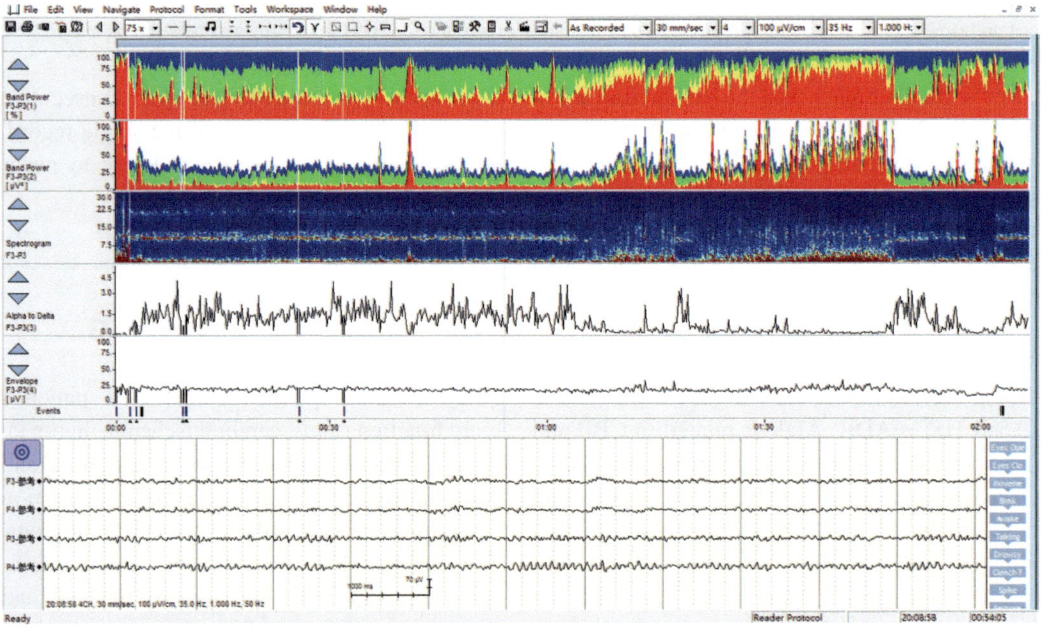


**Fig. 2.30** Combination trend map: RBP, ADR, spectrogram, ABP, 95% spectral edge frequency (95% SEF)

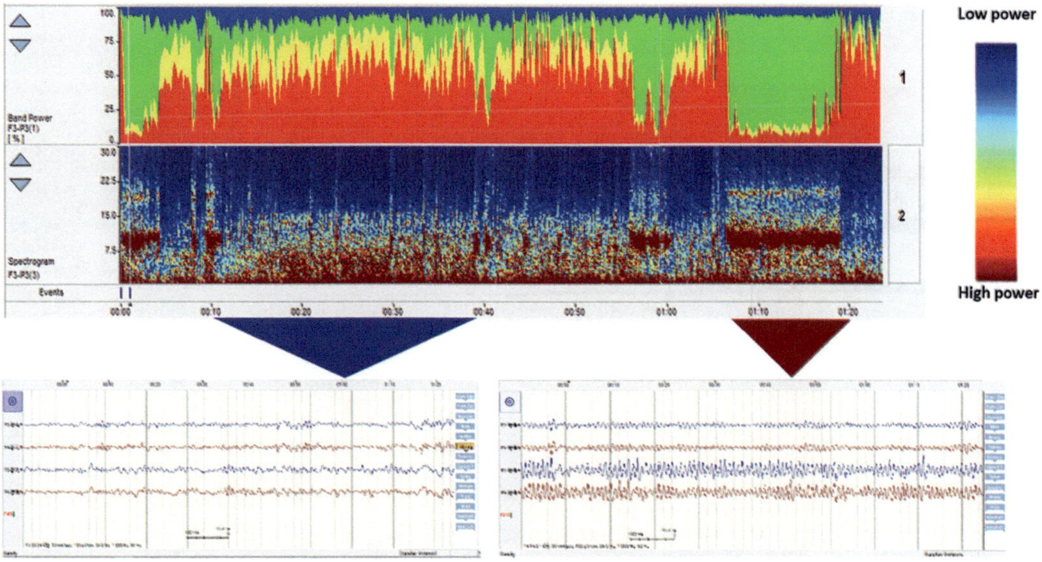


**Fig. 2.31** Spectrogram. The color represents the power level: dark blue represents low power and dark red represents high power. In the awake state, the alpha frequency band is used as the background activity, and the corresponding spectrogram high power (dark red) is in the 8~13 Hz region; the sleep state is the δ frequency band as the background activity, and the corresponding spectrogram high power (dark red) is in the 0.5~4 Hz region

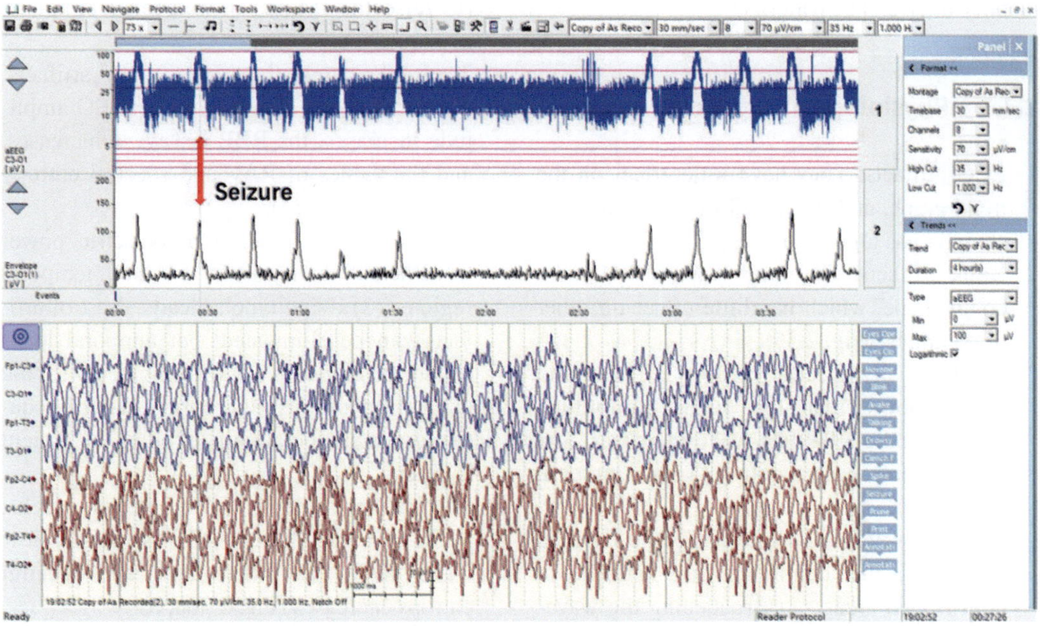


**Fig. 2.32** ET during epileptic seizures. aEEG showing that the upper and lower borders increase at the same time and then decrease, showing a spike shape. ET also shows a spike shape

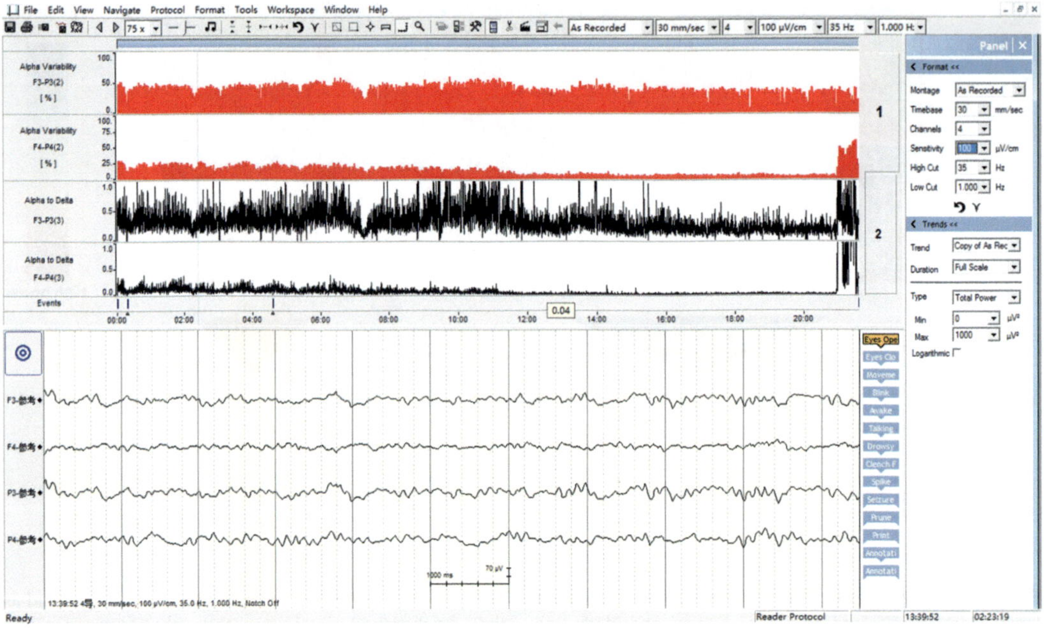

**Fig. 2.33** Comparing ADR with RAV. The left RAV is good, the right variant is bad, and the corresponding ADR also has a lower ratio on the right

neuroelectrophysiological medical staff better identify interference patterns.

### 2.3.1 Physiological Artifacts

1. ECG artifacts: They have little effect on the trend graph, and the aEEG trend graph occasionally has higher volatility (Fig. 2.34).
2. Blink artifacts: The trend graph aEEG has a comb shape, which has little effect on other trend graphs (Fig. 2.35).
3. Forehead myoelectric activity: The trend chart shows that the aEEG amplitude increases, the RBP fast wave increases, and the RAV and spectral entropy values increase (Fig. 2.36).

   Solution: (1) Adding myoelectric leads to assist with the identification of artifacts in both frontal areas. (2) Broadening the waveform to help identify myoelectric artifacts and high-frequency EEG activities by reducing the paper speed. (3) Combined with the clinical conditions, appropriate use of sedative drugs or adjustment of the patient's position (to raise the head) can relieve or eliminate most artifacts.
4. Teeth clenching (breathing tube) artifacts: The trend graph shows that the aEEG amplitude increases, the RBP fast wave increases, and the values of RAV and spectral entropy increase (Fig. 2.37).

   Solution: (1) Adding myoelectric power leads helps identify artifacts in both temporal regions. (2) Using bipolar leads, most of artifacts can be eliminated, but temporal leads cannot be eliminated. (3) Combined with the clinical conditions, appropriate use of sedative drugs can be eliminated after the patient is quiet.
5. Respiratory artifacts: In the trend graphs, aEEG is comb-shaped, RBP is mainly slow wave, RAV has little effect, and spectral entropy increases (Fig. 2.38a, b).
6. Sweating artifacts: The trend graph of the aEEG amplitude increases, RBP is dominated by slow waves, and the RAV and values of spectral entropy decrease (Fig. 2.39).

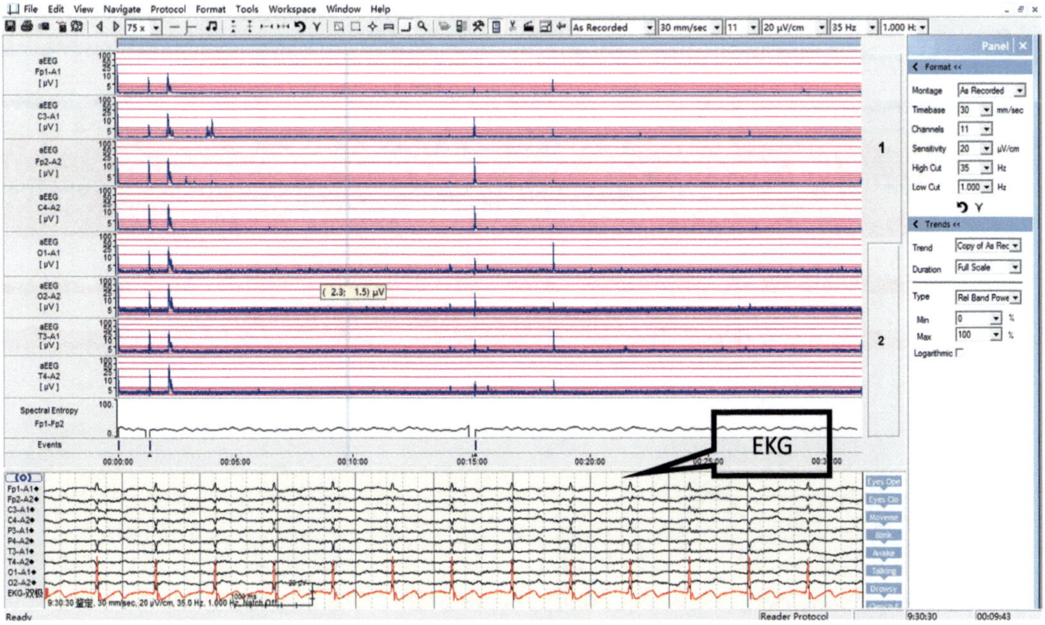


**Fig. 2.34** In patients with brain death, all EEG leads have small sharp waves. Through the ECG leads, it can be observed that the small sharp waves are synchronized with the ECG, which can help identify ECG artifacts. The aEEG trend graph also shows that some trend waves exceed 2 μV, which may be related to ECG artifacts

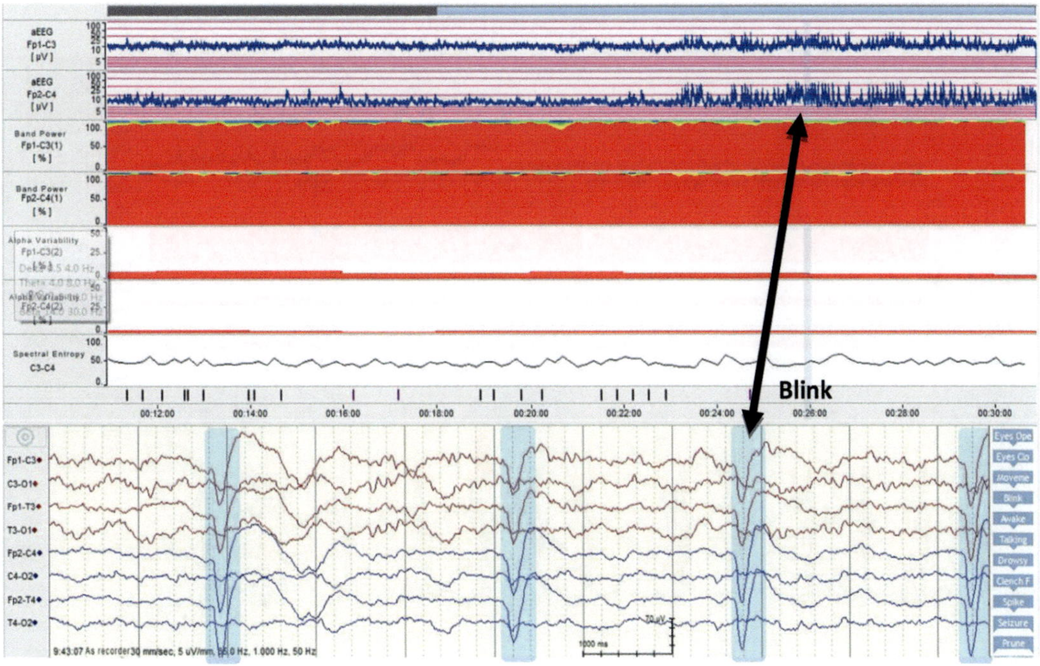


**Fig. 2.35** Blink artifacts show regular synchronous normal phase waves in all the leads in EEG and a comb shape in the aEEG trend graph

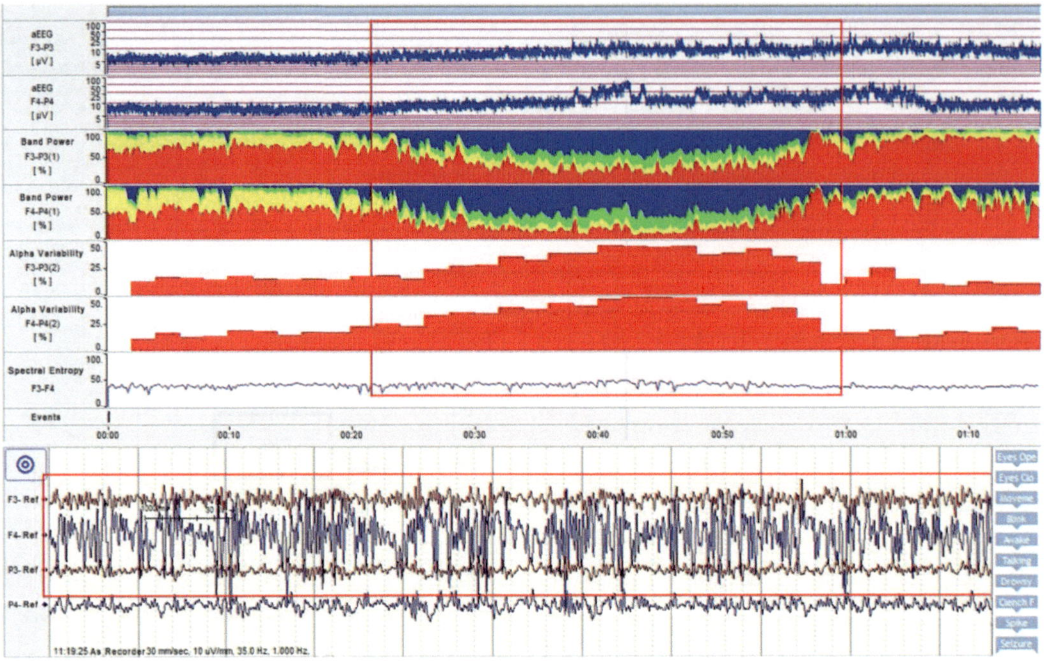

**Fig. 2.36** EEG showing continuous low-medium amplitude myoelectric activity in the bilateral frontal pole leads (in the red box), which is more obvious when frowning or looking up and disappears after being quiet. The trend chart shows that the aEEG volatility increases, RBP fast waves increase, and RAV and spectral entropy values increase

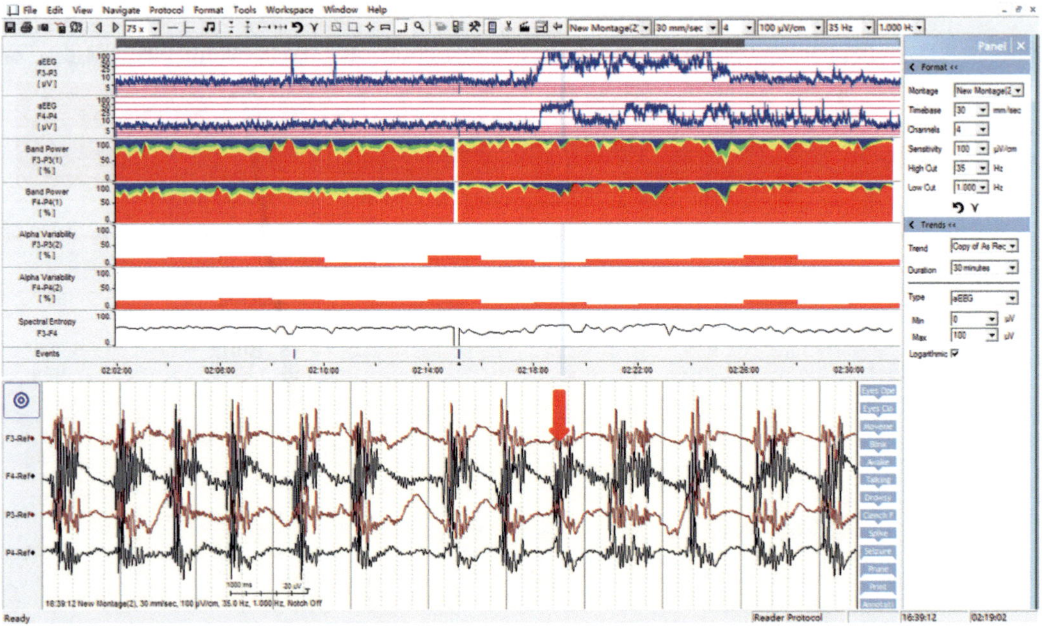

**Fig. 2.37** The masseter muscles in the temporal region show obvious movement when the patient's teeth are painfully clenched or the breathing tube is bitten, and clusters of high-amplitude irregular myoelectric bursts appear in the bilateral anterior and middle temporal leads (F7, F8, T3, T4). Sometimes EMG artifacts can spread to a larger area or even all the leads. The trend chart shows that the aEEG volatility increases, RBP fast waves increase, and the values of RAV and spectral entropy increase

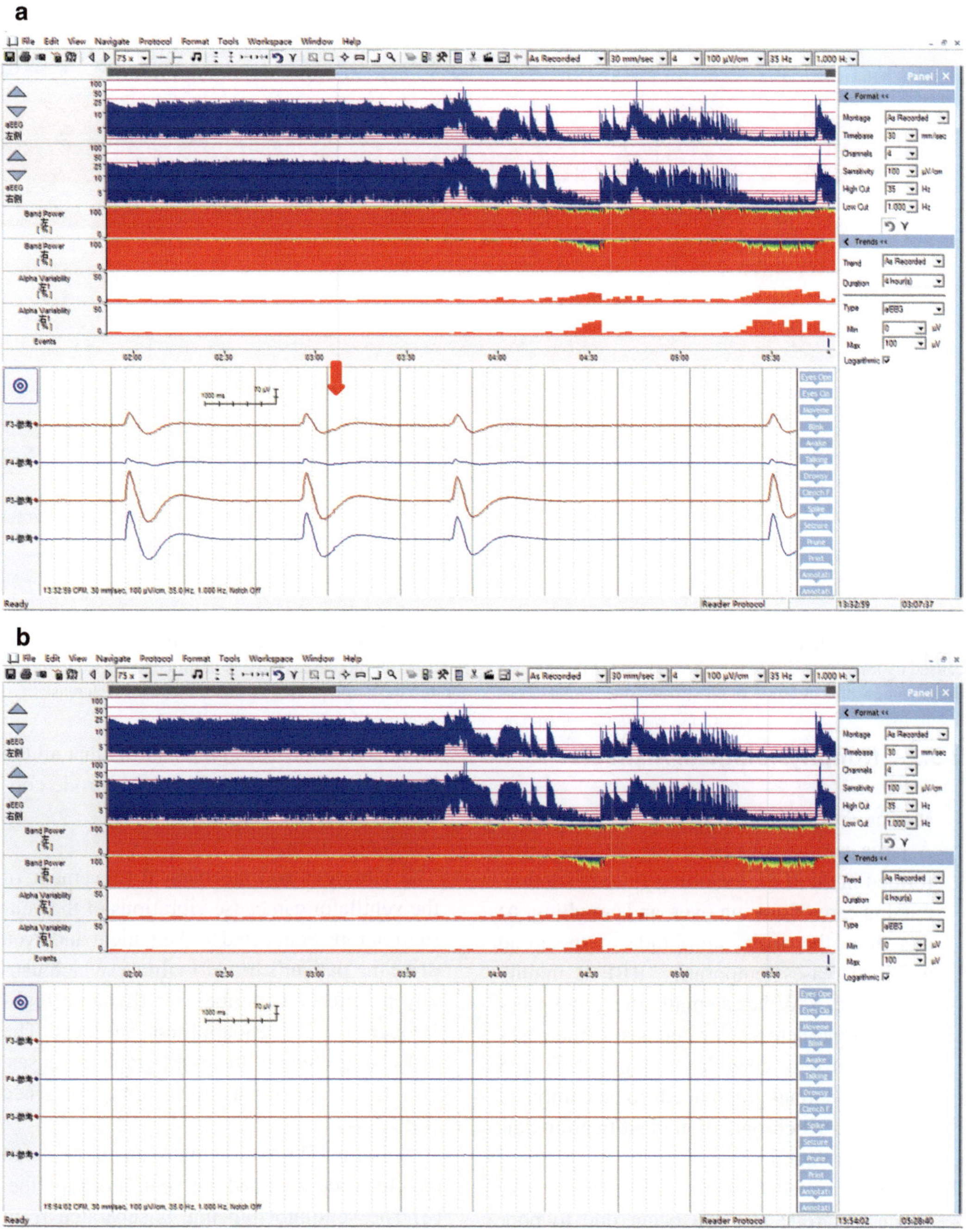


**Fig. 2.38** (**a**) The EEG of a patient's body movement caused by the patient's breathing showing a baseline drift or irregular slow waves. The trend graph of aEEG is comb-shaped, slow waves are dominant in RBP, there is less impact on RAV, and spectral entropy increases. (**b**) The interference disappears after adjusting the patient's position

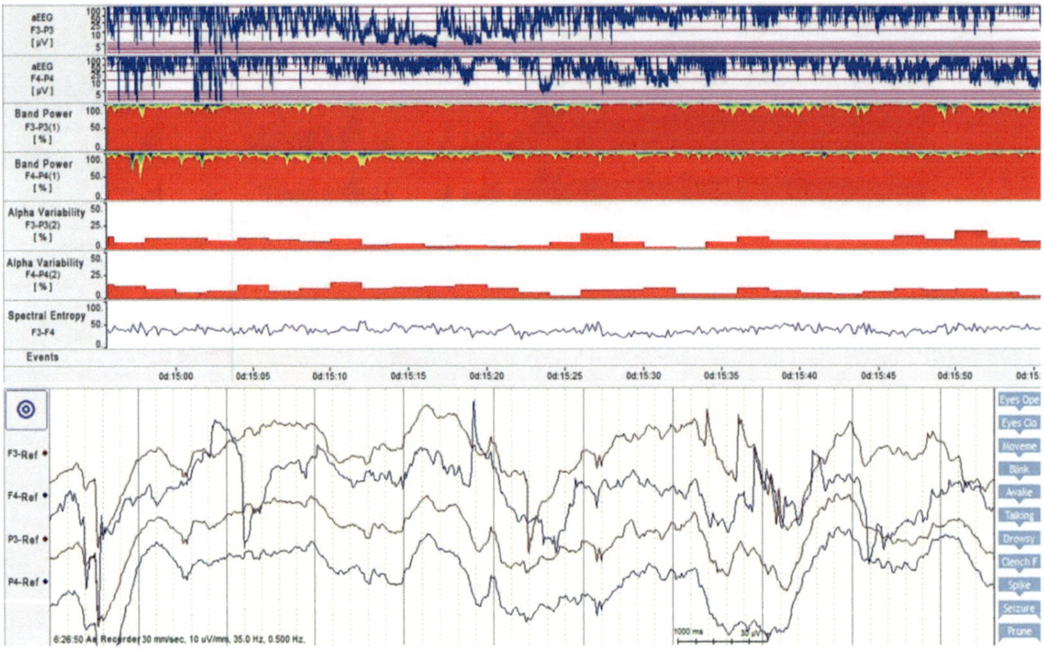

**Fig. 2.39** The artifacts of sweat gland activity potentially caused by sweating. EEG shows a wavy and slow baseline drift. When the reference electrode site sweats, the baselines of all the leads drift. The aEEG volatility of the trend graph increases, RBP is dominated by slow waves, and the RAV and values of spectral entropy decrease

## 2.3.2 Nonphysiological Artifacts

1. Motion artifact

   A large number of operations are often performed in the ICU, including sputum suction, nursing care of turning over, and coughing. At this time, the aEEG amplitude of the trend graph increases temporarily, RBP is mainly slow wave, RAV has a small effect, and spectral entropy increases or decreases (increases with persistent coughing) (Figs. 2.40 and 2.41). Thus trend graph needs to be combined with video synchronization identification during interpretation.

2. Electrode artifacts

   When electrode artifacts occur due to poor electrode solder joint contact, poor contact between the electrode and the scalp, or scalp oil or scabs, the trend graph shows that all the leads are affected by the poor electrode contact (Figs. 2.42 and 2.43).

3. Ventilator artifacts

   The vibration and mechanical movement of the ventilator can cause vibrations of the ventilation tube connected to the patient and even drive the patient's head to vibrate, which usually manifests as periodic or rhythmic high-frequency and high-amplitude artifacts. The aEEG amplitude of the trend graph increases, and the other trends have little influence (Fig. 2.44).

   Solution: (1) Avoid entanglement between the electrode wire and the ventilator pipeline. (2) The ventilator pipeline is separated from the pipeline support and fixed on the bed screen.

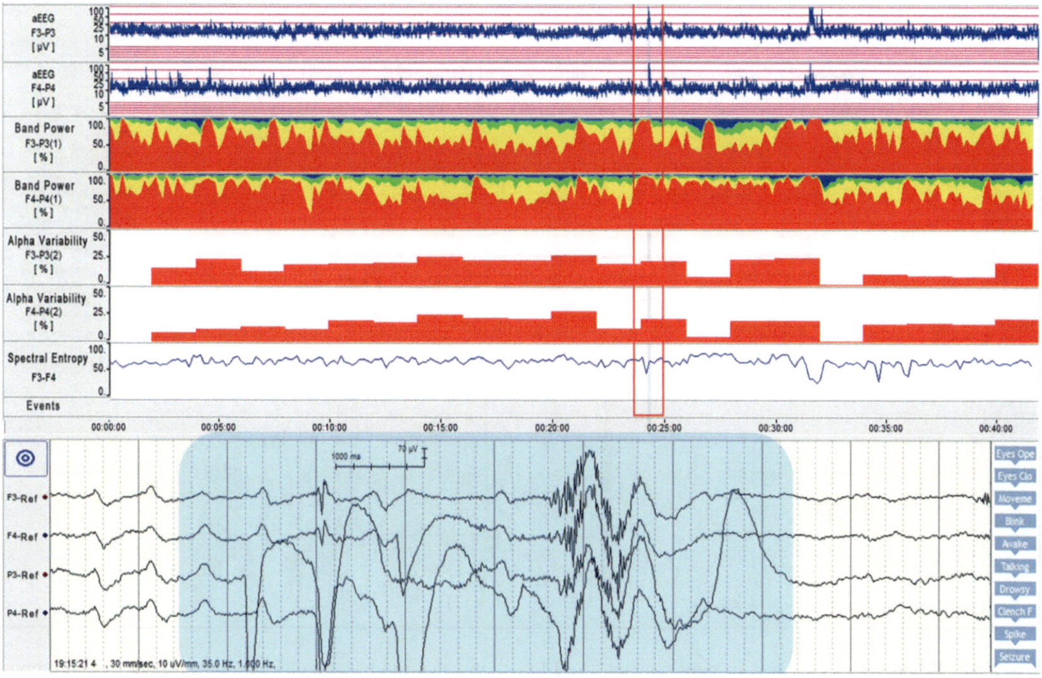


**Fig. 2.40** EEG showing rhythmic or irregular high-amplitude slow waves when the patient coughs. In the trend graphs, the aEEG amplitude transiently increases, RBP is mainly slow wave, RAV has a small effect, and spectral entropy increases or decreases (increases with persistent coughing)

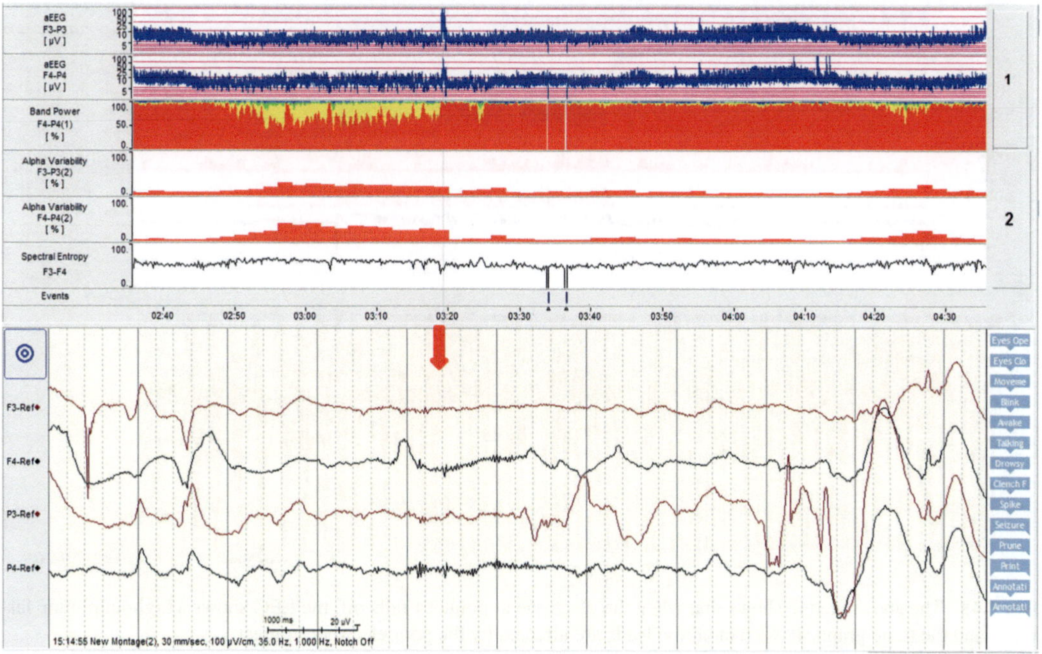


**Fig. 2.41** EEG showing rhythmic or irregular high-amplitude slow waves during sputum suction, with high-frequency myoelectric activity at the same time. In the trend graphs, the aEEG amplitude rises temporarily, RBP is mainly slow wave, RAV has little influence, and spectral entropy increases or decreases

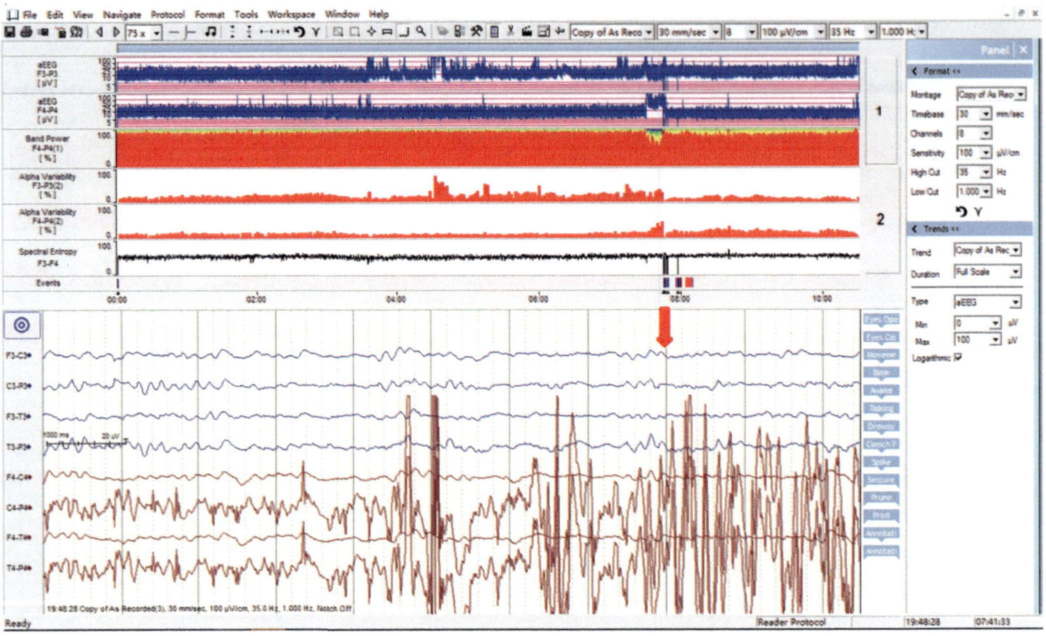

**Fig. 2.42** When the electrode is in poor contact, the EEG shows that the baseline has an intermittent or continuous irregular drift, and the trend graph shows that all the leads are affected by the poor electrode contact

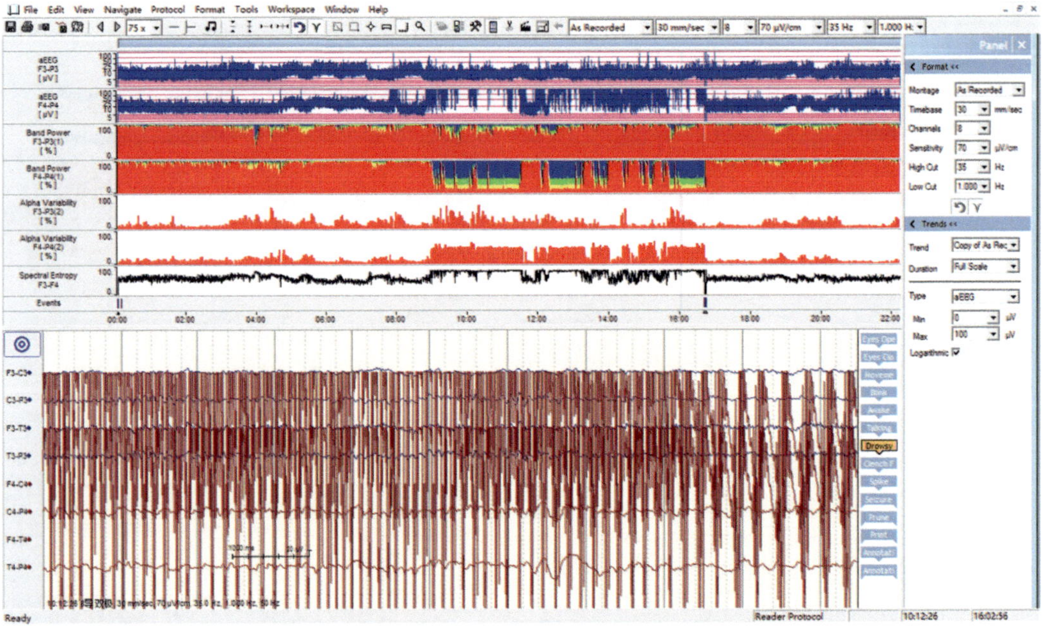

**Fig. 2.43** The above picture shows that when the electrode at point T4 falls off, the EEG shows a high-amplitude fast wave, and the trend graph shows that all the leads are affected by the poor electrode contact

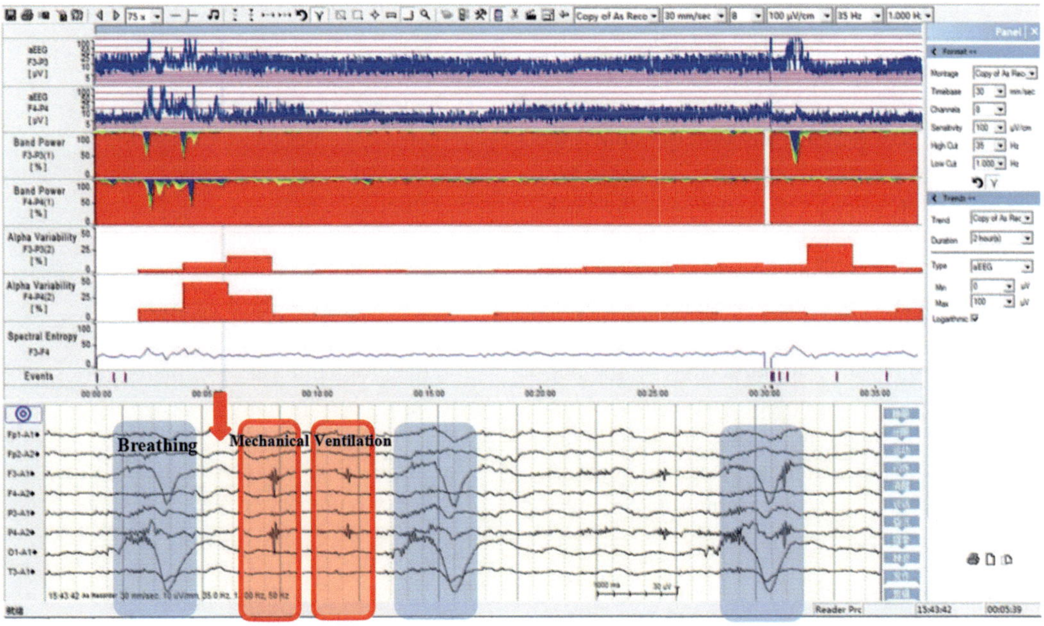


**Fig. 2.44** Vibrations and mechanical movements of the ventilator cause the increased amplitude of aEEG of the trend graph

## References


1. Scheuer ML, Wilson SB. Data analysis for continuous EEG monitoring in the ICU: seeing the forest and the trees. J Clin Neurophysiol. 2004;21(5):353–78.
2. Thakor NV, Tong S. Advances in quantitative electroencephalogram analysis methods. Annu Rev Biomed Eng. 2004;6:453–95.
3. Maynard DE. EEG analysis using an analogue frequency analyser and a digital computer. Electroencephalogr Clin Neurophysiol. 1967;23(5):487.
4. Jordan KG. Continuous EEG monitoring in the neuroscience intensive care unit and emergency department. J Clin Neurophysiol. 1999;16(1):14–39.
5. Thorngren-Jerneck K, Hellstrom-Westas L, Ryding E, et al. Cerebral glucose metabolism and early EEG/aEEG in term newborn infants with hypoxic-ischemic encephalopathy. Pediatr Res. 2003;54(6):854–60.
6. Al NN, Edwards AD, Cowan FM, et al. Assessment of neonatal encephalopathy by amplitude-integrated electroencephalography. Pediatrics. 1999;103(6 Pt 1):1263–71.
7. Hellstrom-Westas L, Rosen I. Continuous brain-function monitoring: state of the art in clinical practice. Semin Fetal Neonatal Med. 2006;11(6):503–11.
8. Sundt TJ, Sharbrough FW, Piepgras DG, et al. Correlation of cerebral blood flow and electroencephalographic changes during carotid endarterectomy: with results of surgery and hemodynamics of cerebral ischemia. Mayo Clin Proc. 1981;56(9):533–43.
9. Ingvar DH, Sjolund B, Ardo A. Correlation between dominant EEG frequency, cerebral oxygen uptake and blood flow. Electroencephalogr Clin Neurophysiol. 1976;41(3):268–76.
10. Ingvar DH. Cerebral metabolism, cerebral blood flow and EEG. Electroencephalogr Clin Neurophysiol. 1967:25–102.
11. Vespa PM, Nuwer MR, Juhasz C, et al. Early detection of vasospasm after acute subarachnoid hemorrhage using continuous EEG ICU monitoring. Electroencephalogr Clin Neurophysiol. 1997;103(6):607–15.
12. Shannon CE. A mathematical theory of communication. Bell Syst Tech J. 1948;27(3):379–423.
13. Johnson R, Shore J. Which is the better entropy expression for speech processing: -S log S or log S?. IEEE Trans Acoustics Speech Signal Process. 1984;32(1):129–37.
14. Viertio-Oja H, Maja V, Sarkela M, et al. Description of the entropy algorithm as applied in the Datex-Ohmeda S/5 entropy module. Acta Anaesthesiol Scand. 2004;48(2):154–61.
15. Kwon MY, Lee SY, Kim TY, et al. Spectral entropy for assessing the depth of propofol sedation. Korean J Anesthesiol. 2012;62(3):234–9.
16. Nuwer M. Assessment of digital EEG, quantitative EEG, and EEG brain mapping: report of the American Academy of Neurology and the American Clinical Neurophysiology Society. Neurology. 1997;49(1):277–92.
17. Claassen J, Hirsch LJ, Kreiter KT, et al. Quantitative continuous EEG for detecting delayed cerebral ischemia in patients with poor-grade subarachnoid hemorrhage. Clin Neurophysiol. 2004;115(12):2699–710.

# Part II

# Interpretation and Clinical Significance of Abnormal EEG in Severely Ill Patients

# Common Abnormal EEG in Neurocritical Ill Patients

# 3

Qun Wang, Feng Li, Xiaoyi Li, and Ying Zhang

## Contents



Q. Wang
Department of Neurology, Beijing Tiantan Hospital, Capital Medical University, Beijing, China
e-mail: wangq@ccmu.edu.cn

F. Li (✉)
Department of Neurology, The First Affiliated Hospital of Chongqing Medical University, Chongqing, China

X. Li
Department of Neurophysiology, Guizhou Provincial People's Hospital, Guiyang, Guizhou, China

Y. Zhang
Department of Neurology, Xi'an International Medical Center Hospital, Xian, Shaanxi, China



X. Wang et al. (eds.), *Multi-Modal EEG Monitoring of Severely Neurologically Ill Patients*,
https://doi.org/10.1007/978-981-16-4493-1_3

**Abstract**

Critically ill patients have a high risk of various types of nerve damage, and if not detected and treated in time, this may lead to permanent neurological dysfunction. EEG is extremely sensitive to the evaluation of cerebral cortical function in patients with brain injury and can promote the early recognition and management of abnormal conditions in critically ill patients. Therefore, correct identification of abnormal EEG waveforms in critically ill patients and understanding of its clinical guiding significance are the basis of critically ill EEG interpretation and the difficult issues with which clinicians deal their work. This chapter, combined with the EEG legend, introduces how to identify epileptiform discharge, periodic discharge (PD), ictal-interictal continuum (IIC), abnormal slow-wave activity, and special coma EEG, such as α and β coma, BS pattern, nonreactive low-voltage slow activity, and ECS. This chapter focuses on explaining the pathological mechanism of each abnormal waveform, the possible disease direction, and the guiding significance for clinical treatment and prognostic judgment, providing a reference for clinicians to read and interpret severely abnormal EEGs.

**Keywords**

Epileptiform discharge · PD · Slow-wave activity · BS · Unresponsive EEG · ECS

## 3.1 Common Abnormal Discharge Patterns in Severely Ill Patients

Frequent seizures in severely ill patients, or in those who evolve into SE, will seriously damage neurons, leading to secondary brain function injury, resulting in poor prognosis and high mortality and greatly increasing the medical and economic burden of society. cEEG monitoring can effectively reflect the activity of neurons in patients and plays an important role in monitoring epileptic seizures. According to the spatial distribution, the common epileptic discharges in critically ill patients can be divided into generalized or diffuse discharges, unilateral discharges, and multifocal discharges.

### 3.1.1 Generalized or Diffuse Discharges (Figs. 3.1, 3.2, 3.3, 3.4, and 3.5)

#### 3.1.1.1 Generalized Epileptiform Discharges (GEDs)

GEDs refer to bilateral, synchronous, and symmetrical abnormal discharge activities [1]. According to the relevant standards of the International League Against Epilepsy (ILAE) [2], GEDs are defined as “originating at a certain point in the brain and rapidly spreading into a bilaterally distributed network, including cortex and subcortical structure, but not necessarily the entire cortex,” which indicates that GEDs may originate from subcortical structures (such as the

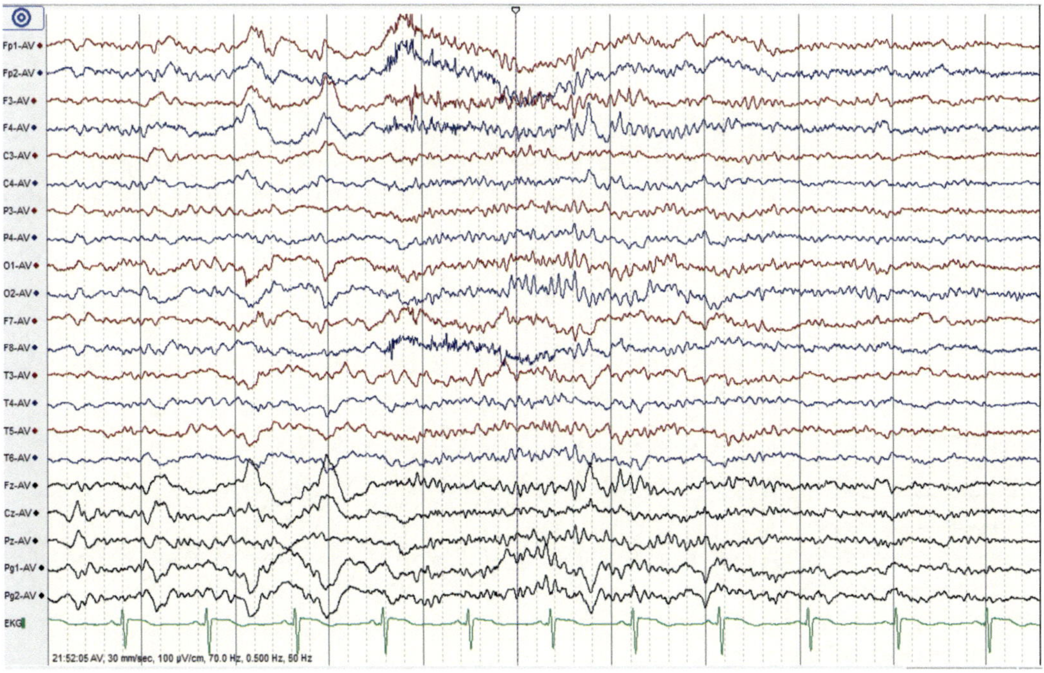


**Fig. 3.1** The EEG of a 35-year-old female, showing low-voltage patterns after a widespread burst of low amplitude and fast rhythm (calibration: 1 s, 70 μV)

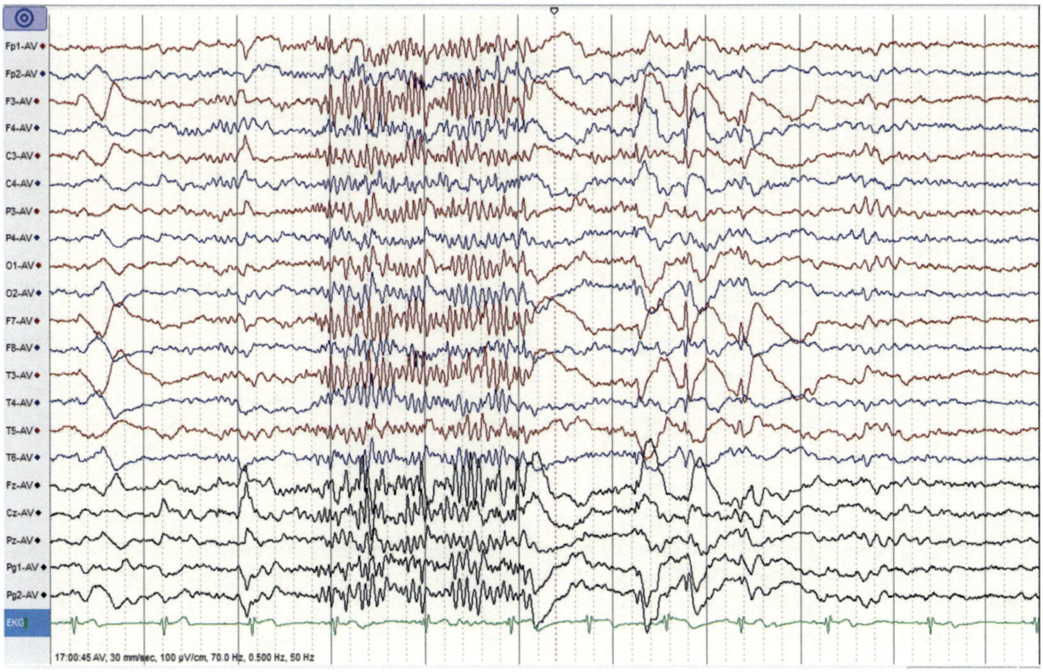


**Fig. 3.2** A 16-year-old boy's EEG showing a widespread spike wave followed by a spike slow wave (calibration: 1 s, 100 μV)

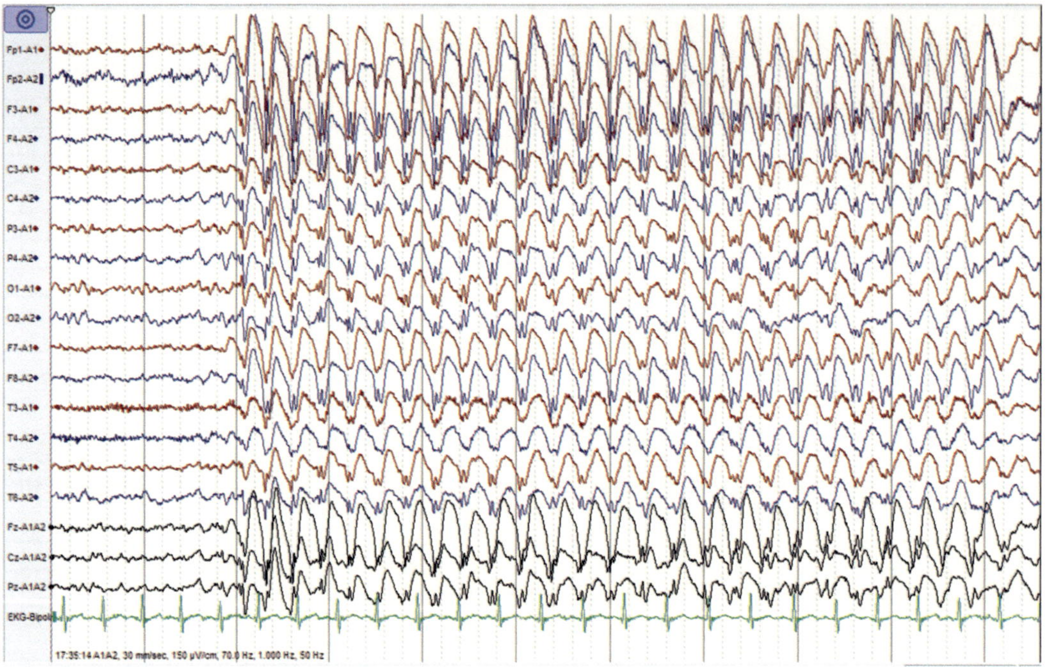

**Fig. 3.3** The EEG of a 15-year-old boy, showing a widespread intermittent spike wave of 3 Hz lasting 8 s (calibration: 1 s, 150 μV)

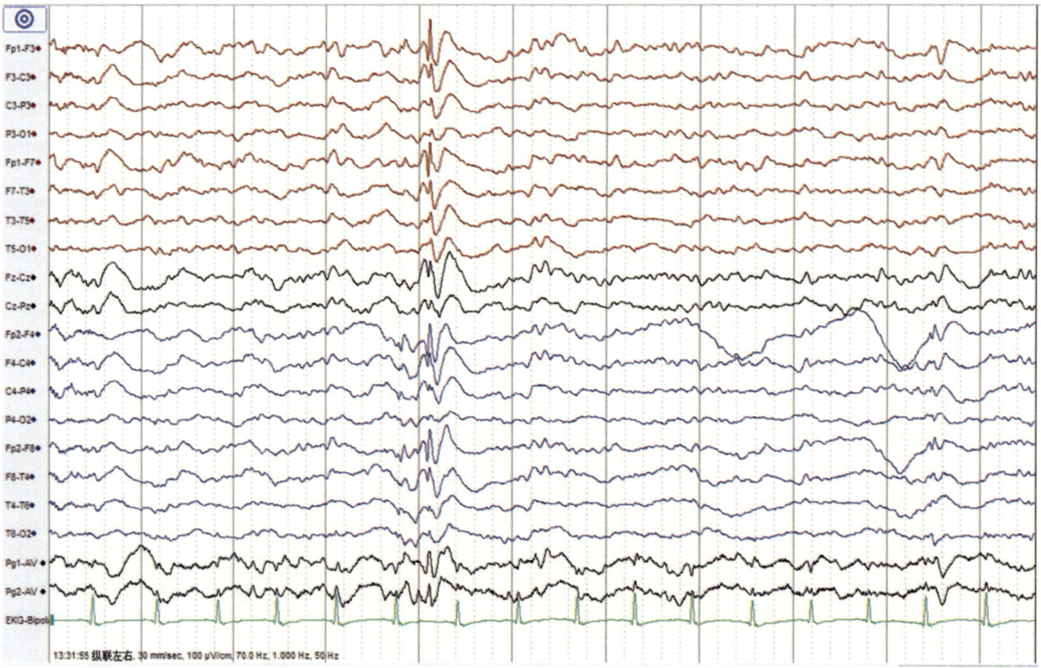

**Fig. 3.4** A 2-year-old boy's EEG showing widespread single-spike slow waves (calibration: 1 s, 100 μV)

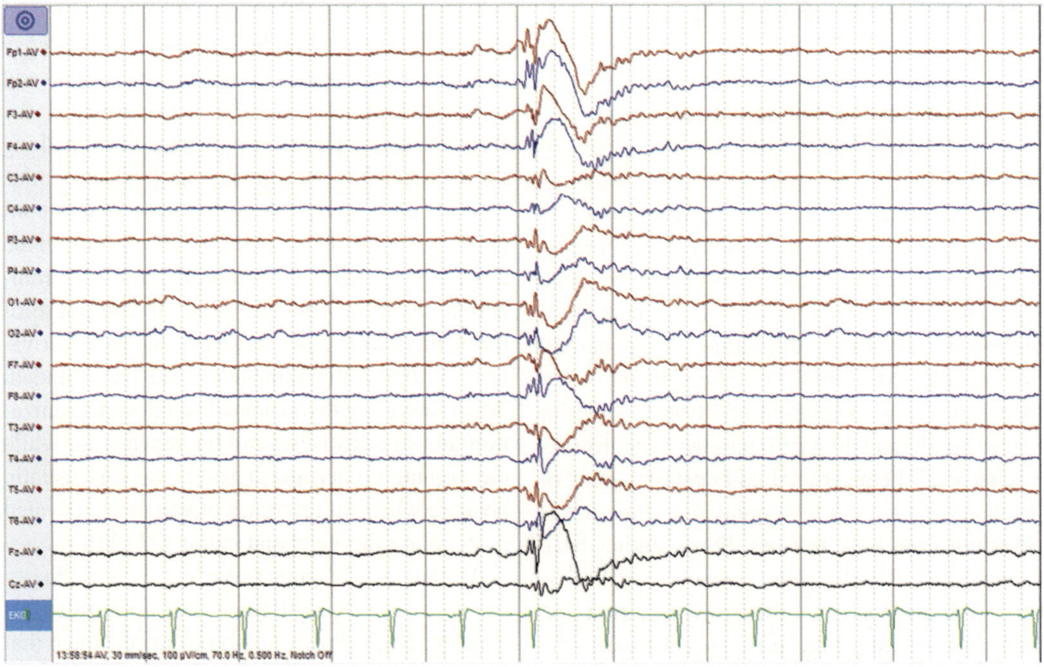


**Fig. 3.5** A 19-year-old male's EEG showing widespread single multiple spike slow waves (calibration: 1 s, 100 μV)

thalamus) or a certain local cortex. Therefore, they can be divided into primary and secondary GEDs according to their different origins. The common mechanism may be that brains with GEDs have diffusely increased excitability, and any local discharge may quickly activate the bilateral cortical-subcortical network (such as the thalamus-cortical loop), resulting in widespread discharges [3–5].

The electrophysiological characteristics of GEDs are usually dominated by generalized spike slow-wave complexes and multispike slow-wave complexes, with higher amplitudes on the frontal lobe, such as absence seizures and general myoclonic seizures [6–9]. There are differences in the incidence of GEDs in different diseases. Studies have shown that attention-deficit hyperactivity disorder (ADHD) is significantly related to epileptiform discharges. Among children with ADHD, approximately half (48.3%) of EEGs can be abnormal [10], and the incidence of GEDs can be 8.3%–28.1% [11, 12]. Among patients with malformation of cortical development (MCD), the incidence of GEDs is 22.7% [13]. Relevant investigation reports show that healthy children can also have widespread abnormal discharges, although the incidence is very low [14].

In addition, related studies have shown that GEDs are closely related to disease prognosis. Jayalakshmi S et al. [15] showed that in patients with MCDs, the occurrence of GEDs is related to developmental delay, cerebellar malformations, and ectopic disease. Borges MA [16] analyzed the emergency EEGs of 681 patients with different causes and found that the 3-month survival rate of patients with GEDs was 50%. Gomez-Ibanez A et al. [17] analyzed the factors affecting the adverse prognosis of patients with idiopathic generalized epilepsy and showed that GEDs (especially the appearance of multispike waves) are considered to be one of the factors affecting their poor prognosis. Ruijter B J et al. [18] conducted qEEG analysis on patients with HIE and showed that patients with GEDs, which are accompanied by higher background continuity and discharge frequency and lower relative discharge power and discharge period, have a good prognosis.

#### 3.1.1.2 Diffuse Discharge (Fig. 3.6)

### 3.1.2 Unilateral Discharges (Figs. 3.7 and 3.8)

Unilateral abnormal discharge mode refers to unilateral or bilateral synchronous and asymmetric abnormal discharge mode, which can be focal, regional, or hemispheric [1]. The mechanism of unilateral abnormal discharge is generally through the long bundle of fibers in the brain (occipito-frontal commissural fiber or superior longitudinal fasciculus) to achieve synchronous discharge of the prefrontal and occipital areas of one hemisphere, and the conduction direction is generally from back to front. Some studies have adopted a display that reduces the screen display time limit and increases the time resolution and then measures the time difference between the peaks of the two parts before and after and the distance between the two point electrodes. The conduction velocity of the spike wave is 6.7~19.2 m/s, and most of the spikes in the occipital area appear 11~32 ms earlier [9, 19]. In recent years, related studies have found that epilepsy initiated in the back of the head (such parietal and occipital regions) is easily transmitted to the frontal or temporal lobes from back to front along the superior and inferior longitudinal fasciculus and cingulate gyrus. However, there is less conduction from front to back [20]. Therefore, in the clinical judgment of occipital-frontal synchronization, attention should be paid to the phase of the spike wave, and reference electrode activation or dipole phenomena should be excluded. Spike waves with occipito-frontal synchronization are all negative in the reference lead, while the frontal synchronized spike wave is usually positive when the reference electrode is activated or there is a dipole phenomenon [21, 22].

Unilateral abnormal electrical activity due to various causes has different electrophysiological characteristics. Previous studies have shown that the secondary occipito-frontal synchronization spike wave is a developmental EEG phenomenon that is related to the maturation process of the brain and is common in focal epilepsy in children

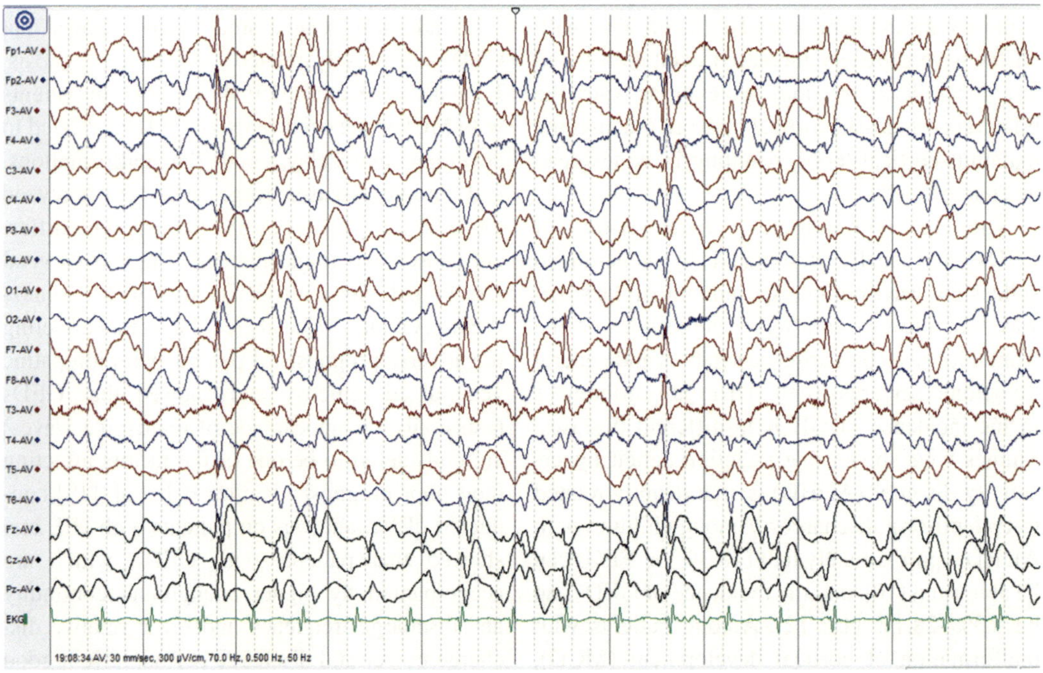


**Fig. 3.6** A 5-year-old girl's EEG showing high-amplitude spike slow waves of 2–2.5 Hz across the head (calibration: 1 s, 300 μV)

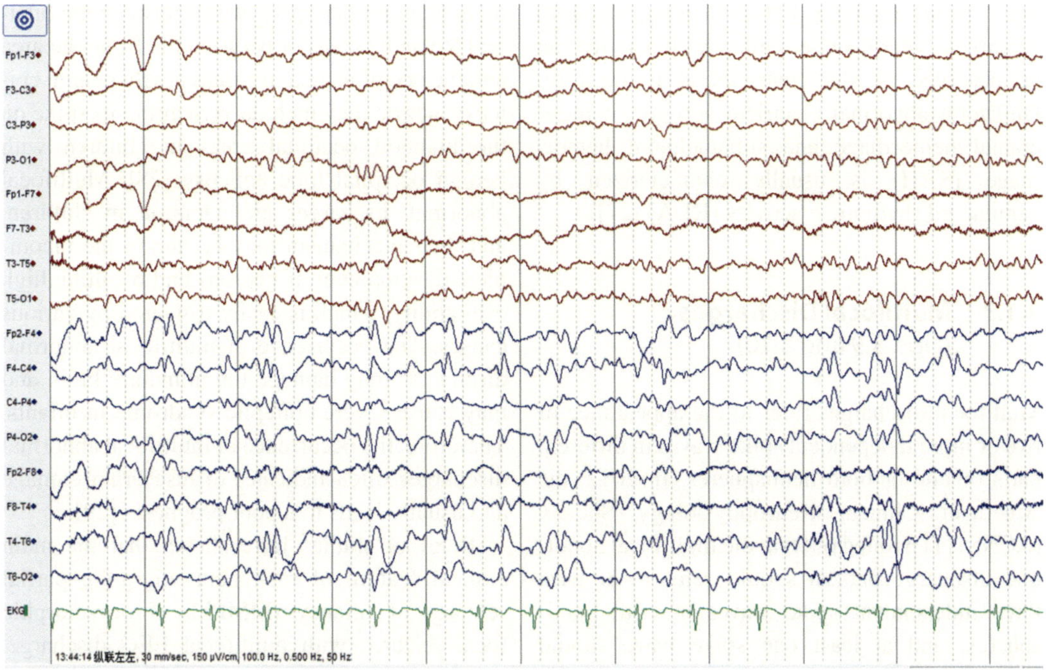


**Fig. 3.7** The EEG of an 8-year-old male, showing continuous spike and slow waves with varying amplitudes in the right hemisphere (calibration: 1 s, 150 μV)

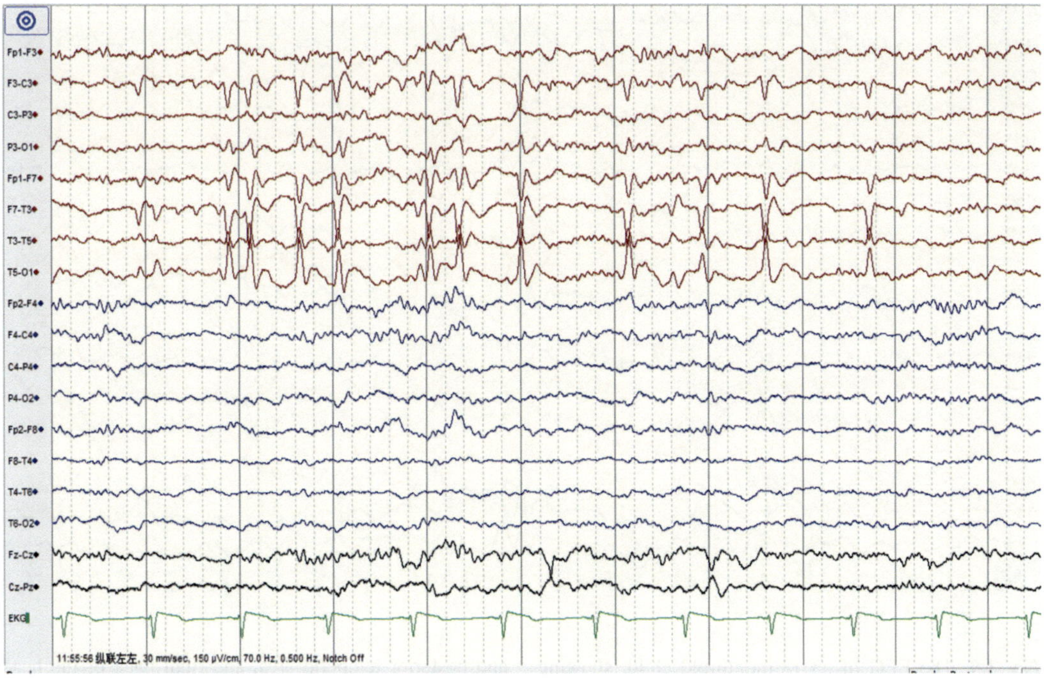


**Fig. 3.8** A 27-year-old male's EEG showing intermittent spike waves and spike slow waves in the left hemisphere (calibration: 1 s, 150 μV)

with various etiologies [23–25]. In patients with cerebrovascular disease, unilateral β activity can be observed on the contralateral lesion [26]. Unilateral abnormal electrical activity of intracranial hemorrhage and subarachnoid hemorrhage (SAH) is usually characterized by hemilateral rhythmic δ activity (RDA) [27].

### 3.1.3 Multifocal Discharges (Figs. 3.9 and 3.10)

Multifocal discharges refer to the appearance of two or more independent spike waves in different parts of one or both hemispheres. In 2012, the American Clinical Neurophysiology Society (ACNS) [1] pointed out that the multifocal abnormal discharge pattern should refer to at least three independent spike waves in both hemispheres, and at least one spike wave should appear in each hemisphere. However, the various definitions of multifocal spike waves do not include migratory spike waves between the bilateral Rolandic areas or between the Rolandic area and the occipital area in children with benign epilepsy, nor do they include asynchronous spike on the bilateral occipital areas in children with benign occipital lobe epilepsy [28]. Multifocal abnormal discharges are common in children, and their mechanism may be due to the incomplete development of neurons and resulting high excitability, which is easily triggered by various causes. The occurrence of multifocal abnormal discharges may damage the immature brain and may cause severe epileptic syndrome in infants. Therefore, the occurrence of multifocal abnormal discharges often indicates diffuse brain damage and usually leads to a poor prognosis [29].

Relevant studies have shown that the main clinical feature of malignant migrating partial seizures of infancy (MMPSI) is polymorphic focal seizures with multifocal EEG discharge. MMPSI has obvious drug resistance, which can eventually lead to severe axial hypotonia and

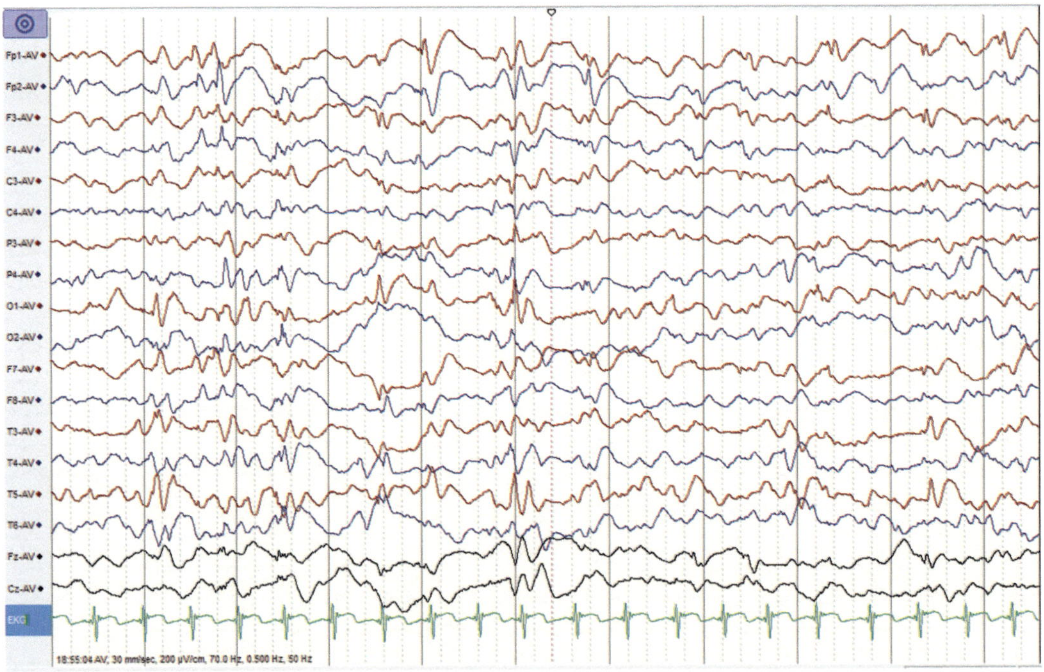


**Fig. 3.9** The EEG of an 18-month-old child, showing spike slow waves and sharp slow waves that appear asynchronously in the bilateral frontal area, left occipital and posterior temporal area, and right back of the head (calibration: 1 s, 200 μV)

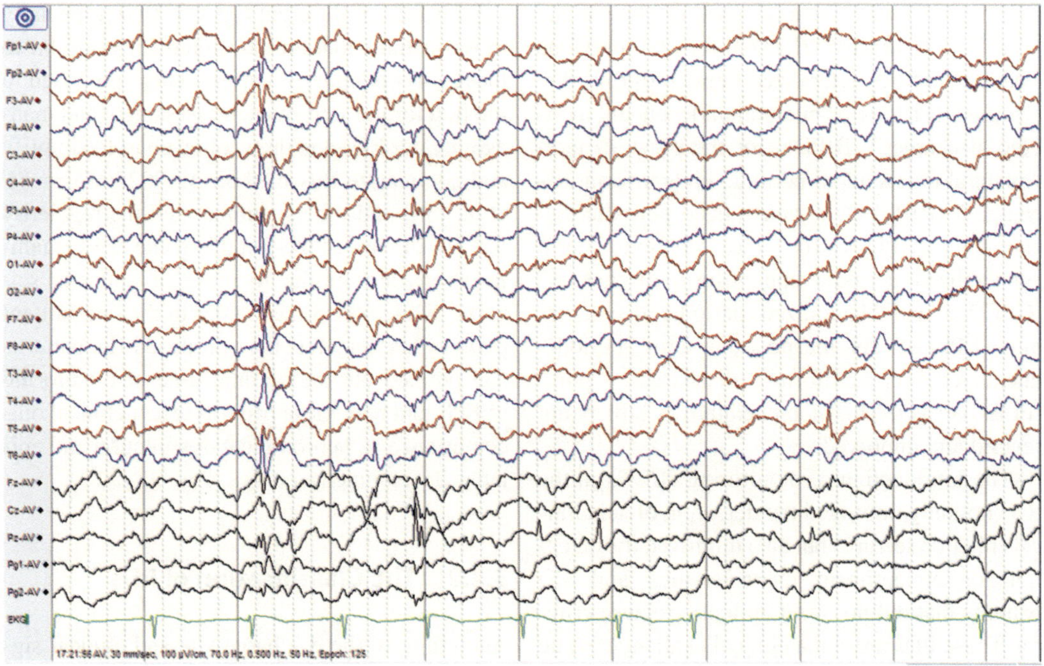

**Fig. 3.10** The EEG of a 6-year-old girl, showing the release of spike slow waves and spike slow waves that appear asynchronously in the left parietal and posterior temporal areas, right central and parietal regions, temporal region, and midline parietal areas (calibration: 1 s, 100 μV)

signs of pyramidal and extrapyramidal tracts, accompanied by poor prognosis, such as unconscious movements and strabismus [30]. Recent studies have also shown that children with new-onset refractory status epilepticus (RSE) and febrile infection-related epilepsy syndrome (FIRES) can also have multifocal abnormal discharge in the chronic stage of disease development and usually have a poor prognosis. A total of 66%–100% of survivors suffer from intellectual disability, and the mortality rate can reach 30% [31, 32]. Riikonen et al. [33] also pointed out that multifocal abnormal discharges can be seen in children with spasms and can be one of the important potential factors affecting the prognosis of children. Early recognition and intervention can improve prognosis.

However, it should be noted that the phenotype and EEG characteristics of children's clinical onset will change with the development of the brain. Therefore, early recognition of multifocal abnormal discharges and timely treatment can help improve prognosis.

## 3.2 PDs

PDs are an EEG pattern that reflects brain dysfunction and seizure predisposition. In 2005, the ACNS proposed a new definition of PDs, stating that a "waveform with relatively uniform shape and duration and quantifiable intervals, and at least in 6 cycles to appear at almost regular intervals," is called PDs [34]. The waveform of this discharge does not exceed three phases or any number of phases for duration of <0.5s. It can be sharp waves, spikes, slow waves, TWs, etc.; and the interval fluctuation during the cycle is not more than 50%. Because high-amplitude PDs are likely to cause epileptic seizures and convulsive status epilepticus (CSE) or nonconvulsive status epilepticus (NCSE), some scholars believe that these discharges are epileptic and advocate the use of antiepileptic drugs (AEDs) to control the occurrence of these discharges [35, 36]. However, sometimes the discharges are not epileptiform, and there is no definite epileptogenesis. Therefore, the Critical Care Monitoring Committee of the

ACNS put forward the new terms of "lateralized periodic discharges" (LPDs) for the previous term "periodic lateralized epileptiform discharges" (PLEDs), "bilateral independent periodic discharges" (BIPDs) for the previous term "bilateral independent periodic epileptiform discharges" (BIPLEDs), "generalized periodic discharges" (GPDs) for the previous term "generalized periodic epileptiform discharges" (GPEDs), and "lateralized periodic discharges plus (LPDs+)" for the previous term "periodic lateralized epileptiform discharges plus" (PLEDs+) [1]. This nomenclature is still being revised and improved.

The introduction of monitoring cEEGs in the ICU not only improved the detection of subclinical epileptic seizures but also improved the detection of epileptiform characteristics and PD patterns that did not meet epileptic seizure criteria. These PDs present a clinical challenge: some patterns may reflect brain damage that has already occurred, while others may cause new brain damage and therefore require treatment. However, in general, PDs are a common EEG pattern, and their exact significance and clinical value are still being explored [37].

### 3.2.1 The Discovery and Historical Evolution of PDs

In 1950, Cobb et al. [38] reported the "periodic" EEG of a patient with subacute progressive encephalitis and attributed the periodicity of its discharge to the separation of cortical and subcortical structures, believing that it was caused by large white matter lesions. In 1964, Chatrian et al. [39] first used LPDs to describe the electrical activity of the brain consisting of sharp waves and/or spikes, which may be followed by complex waves with slow waves or other waveforms at periodic intervals. In 1974, the IFSECN first came up with the official terminology of LPDs as periodic, in which the discharges occur in sequence at approximately regular frequencies or at roughly regular intervals, typically between one and a few seconds [40]. In 2018, Bauerschmidt et al. [41] retrospectively analyzed the clinical significance of different types of PDs, especially those features that are physiologically similar to those of epileptic seizures. They proposed a method for the step-by-step assessment and management of PDs and drew a flowchart to simplify and summarize this method. In 2020, Zahar SF et al. [36] and others summarized the regularity of PDs. In view of the fact that some cEEG manifestations are similar to those of epileptic seizures, while others are similar to the intermittent period after seizures, they proposed IIC patterns and pointed out the optimal time of monitoring cEEGs and how these patterns affect clinical outcomes such as neurological dysfunction and epilepsy development.

### 3.2.2 The Classification of PDs

According to the discharge site and clinical significance, the ACNS's Standardized Critical Care EEG Terminology [1] proposed that periodic EEGs can be divided into the following four types.

#### 3.2.2.1 LPDs

LPDs refer to lateralized patterns and bilateral synchronous and asymmetric patterns, including focal, regional, and hemispherical patterns [34]. Reiher et al. [42] put forward that there are two subclasses of LPDs: LPDs proper, which are characterized by a relatively stable discharge period, simple and uniform discharge structure, and nonphasic rhythmic discharge; and LPDs+, which are associated with low-amplitude rhythmic activity and have variable discharge periodicity. Chong et al. [43] summarized their findings of 24-h cEEG and found that LPDs rarely occur alone. The common EEG pattern is the conversion between LPD proper and LPDs+, and patients with these patterns have a high risk of seizures.

#### 3.2.2.2 BIPDs

BIPDs refer to two independent (nonsynchronous) lateral patterns, and one lateral pattern should appear on each hemisphere [1]. Compared with LPDs, BIPDs may manifest as bilateral unsynchronized composite waves, which are usually different in morphology, amplitude, repetition rate, and most affected site [44].

#### 3.2.2.3 GPDs

GPDs are a kind of discharge with a relatively uniform shape and duration. These discharges are usually bilateral, bisynchronous, and symmetrical periodic complex waves, accounting for at least 50% of the standard 30-min EEG. Although they may be more prominent in specific areas and have different shapes, they are usually characterized by high-amplitude spikes or sharp waves [1, 43–45]. GPDs represent a rare EEG pattern. In EEG, the total incidence rate is between 0.4 and 1% [46].

In 1971, Gaches et al. [47] divided GPDs into periodic short-interval discharges (PSIDDs) and periodic long-interval discharges (PLIDDs). Many scholars also agree with this division, and the period of PSIDDs is smaller than that of PLIDDs [48].

#### 3.2.2.4 Others

**TWs**

GPDs also include TWs. Foley et al. [49] first described this EEG pattern in 1950 and called it "blunted and spike waves"; then, according to morphological characteristics, Bickford et al. [50] proposed that, regardless of whether there are two or three phases, with each phase longer than the previous phase and the positive phase of highest amplitude, this pattern is called TWs. In the case of three phases, the polarity should be negative-positive-negative. TWs are usually displayed more clearly in bipolar montages and usually appear in diffuse low-amplitude slow-activity backgrounds. Some composite waves have a particularly sharp component. The first component is similar to spikes, while others are monophasic, biphasic, or polyphasic slow waves or sharp waves, but the positive phase part is prominent, and the time limit is wider [51].

The waveforms of TWs in corresponding parts of each cerebral hemisphere are basically the same, and they can be sporadic or distributed periodically. A study showed that widespread and bisynchronous discharges occurred in most patients, 60% of which were prominent in the frontal area, 40% were mainly distributed in the posterior head or diffusely; 9% were located on one side, and most of them were located in the same hemisphere of injury; local TWs were also found, especially in the frontal and central regions, but sometimes in the temporal region [52]. In widespread TWs, the main positive phase components can have a 25–140 ms phase difference in the frontal-occipital region, of which 73% of the longitudinal bipolar waves have anterior-posterior phase differences, and only 27% of the referential montages have phase differences [52, 53]. However, whether the difference actually exists or is caused by montages is still unclear.

**Stimulus-Induced Rhythmic, Periodic, or Ictal Discharges (SIRPIDs)**

SIRPIDs are a special brain electrical pattern that may appear as PDs [1]. In this EEG pattern, the rhythmic, periodic, or paroxysmal abnormal discharges are mainly induced by alertness stimulation, such as auditory stimulation, chest pressing, physical examination, sputum suction, turning over, and other nursing work; and they differ from those induced by light, sound, or pain stimulation seen in EEGs [51].

Since Hirsch et al. first reported SIRPIDs in 2004 [54], they have been mentioned in the literature, but there are few clinical studies. Therefore, whether SIRPIDs need active treatment and which medicines should be used are still questions to be solved.

**PDs Plus**

PDs plus are defined as the occurrence of superimposed RDA or superimposed fast activity on the basis of PDs. For example, BIPDs with superimposed RDA in one hemisphere only would be classified as BIPDs +R [1].

### 3.2.3 Prevalence

Lee JW et al. [55] conducted a multicenter study of 280 critically ill patients and found that 35.7% had PDs. Foreman B et al. [56] investigated 200 patients with an average age of 66 years. A study of 56% of comatose patients found that 46% had PDs in EEGs and epileptic seizures during hospitalization. Husari et al. [57] evaluated 5742 EEGs from 4772 patients and found that the EEGs of 41% of patients contained at least one kind of PD, the most common of which were LPDs, with an incidence rate of 14%. According to this, approximately 35–41% of the patients with severe illness had PDs and rhythmic discharges in EEGs; therefore, the incidence of PDs in the EEGs from patients with severe illness might be 35–46%.

### 3.2.4 Clinical Characteristics of PDs

#### 3.2.4.1 LPDs

**LPDs and Brain Injury**

LPDs are the most common and periodic EEG pattern reported in current studies [43]. Chatrian et al. [39] found through the study of pathological specimens that any brain lesion may cause LPDs. Studies have shown that within 2~3 weeks after acute brain injury, the amplitude of LPDs will decrease gradually, the repetition rate will gradually decrease, and then discharges will stop [43]. The reason may be that, in acute brain injury, neuron dysfunction causes a disturbance in neurotransmitter transmission, leading to PDs, but these neurons return to normal or die after a period of time, and then LPDs will appear on EEGs. Therefore, LPDs are considered to be the nonspecific results of acute partial and transient denervation in local cortical regions [58]. In brain injury, the periodic phenomenon of the discharges in this unstable state may be related to the injury process and the related LPDs caused by the synchronization of the pre-existing local field potentials to enhance excitatory neurotransmission and the inactivation of inhibitory neurotransmission.

Many scholars have suggested that acute or subacute destructive lesions in the brain and the resulting structural brain damage are important causes of LPDs [59]. Rapid growth of brain tumors (such as pleomorphic glioblastoma), brain abscesses, infections of the CNS (related to viral encephalitis, herpes simplex virus), Creutzfeldt–Jakob disease, hematomas, mitochondrial encephalomyopathy, demyelinating disease, HIE, toxic metabolic encephalopathy, migraine and fat embolism, lipidosis, congenital protein C deficiency, and so on may cause LPDs [43, 58–62].

The cause of LPDs is not clear. PDs have been shown to lead to an overexcitation state with high metabolism and high perfusion, which may lead to local metabolic failure [63]. Subramaniam, T et al. [64] also found that, during the uptake of F-deoxyglucose (FDG), patients with an increased frequency of LPDs in EEGs were associated with increased FDG metabolic activity.

**LPDs and Epilepsy**

Vineet Punia et al. [65] conducted a long-term follow-up of 38 patients with LPDs in cEEGs, age ≥18 years old, and no history of epilepsy to understand the relationship between LPDs and epilepsy. The results showed that 33 patients (85%) had epileptic seizures, among whom 7 patients (18%) had intermittent epileptic seizures on EEGs. The LPDs of these patients were usually continuous, and their amplitude was twice that of the background activity. The patients were followed up for 1–12 months after discharge. Among them, 11 patients (31%) developed epilepsy, but only 3 patients showed interictal epileptiform discharges on EEGs. The authors believe that LPDs can be used as a marker of epileptic seizures in approximately 18% of patients. Rodriguez et al. [66] also found similar results in 4772 patients. The risk of epileptic seizures in LPDs was higher than that in other EEG manifestations. When PDs plus (low-amplitude rhythm or sharp waves/spikes discharges) appeared, the correlation of seizures was further increased. Fedele Dono et al. [67] reported the case of a patient with sudden speech disorder accompanied by hypersecretion and sensory abnormalities, and the EEGs of this patient showed LPDs superimposed on fast activity. After intravenous antiepileptic treatment, EEG activity returned to normal, and all neurological symptoms disappeared completely. These authors believe that although the relationship between LPDs and seizures is still controversial, when they are associated with LPDs+ and high periodic frequency, they support the characteristics of epileptic seizures. In summary, Sully K E et al. [68] found that in coma patients, patients in whom LPDs lasted for more than 5 days had a higher frequency of SE and a poor prognosis. It is not clear whether LPDs are the manifestation of epileptic seizures or the interictal or postepileptic manifestations. Some scholars believe that PDs may be a seizure-related phenomenon, but the frequency of LPDs is lower than the expected frequency of NCSE [69], and LPDs are not always related to epileptic seizures and SE. Therefore, although in some patients LPDs are a pattern of epileptic seizure, they are generally considered to occur in the interval between epileptic seizures [36, 43, 70].

#### 3.2.4.2 GPDs

GPDs are generalized discharges with a relatively uniform shape and duration and a quantifiable interval [1]. In recent decades, our understanding of these waveforms has greatly improved.

**GPDs and Brain Injury**

In critically ill patients, especially those in the ICU, PDs are very common in routine EEGs, and most patients have obvious acute or subacute brain injury. In patients with HIE, acute cerebrovascular disease, SE, intracranial infection, craniocerebral trauma, and toxic metabolic encephalopathy, EEGs show PDs, and the ratio of lactate/pyruvate in the CSF of patients with PDs is increased, suggesting that brain tissue hypoxia may be caused by "metabolic crisis" [71]. In addition, Moseley et al. [72] believe that brain injury may trigger GPDs, which in turn will aggravate metabolic stress, which may lead to severe disability or even death. However, Carneiro F et al. [73] studied 41 epileptic patients with GPDs and compared them with 82 epileptic patients without GPDs. The results showed that GPDs were not a sign of drug resistance and could not explain the specific etiology of epilepsy.

**GPDs and Prognosis**

A study of comatose patients in the ICU showed that the detection rate of GPDs was 3.2–17%. Patients with GPDs had a poor prognosis, with mortality rate as high as 34–41%. The mortality rate of patients with GPDs was the highest (46%) [74]. Han-Tao Li et al. [75] also found that the frequent occurrence of GPDs was related to patients' deaths, which suggested that this EEG pattern could cause brain tissue hypoxia, aggravate metabolic stress, and cause additional brain damage. Neville et al. [76] studied a total of 113 patients with GPDs, whose average age was 70.4 years; 60 of these patients died (53.1%).

The interval time of GPDs has also been reported as one of the important factors affecting the prognosis of patients. A prolonged activity time or shortened intermittent period of attack leads to higher mortality. In patients with infectious diseases and cerebrovascular diseases, the mortality rate of patients with short-term GPDs (within 1 month) is 50%, while the mortality of patients with long-term GPDs is lower. Therefore, the appearance of short-term GPDs can be used as one of the parameters to determine poor prognosis in patients [77].

#### 3.2.4.3 BIPDs

The prevalence and incidence rate of BIPDs is not clear. The detection rate of BIPDs in ICUs is 4–22%, and the routine EEG detection rate is 0.1% [78]. BIPDs are usually associated with acute structural brain damage. When white matter abnormalities and cortical atrophy occur at the same time, there is a higher incidence of BIPDs [79, 80].

Osman G et al. [81] explored the clinical relevance of BIPDs and their relationship with seizures and prognosis. Eighty-five patients with BIPDs were retrospectively analyzed and compared with 85 controls. The most common causes were stroke, CNS infection, and hypoxic brain injury. Compared with nonperiodic discharges, patients with BIPDs were more likely to have seizures (45 vs. 8%). The mortality of patients with BIPDs (36%) was higher than that of controls (18%). In multivariate analysis, BIPDs were still associated with mortality and poor outcome. Therefore, it is believed that BIPDs are caused by bilateral acute brain injury and are associated with high-risk seizures and adverse outcomes. To understand the value of BIPDs, Brin Freund et al. [82] conducted a retrospective, multicenter study of 25 patients with a GCS of 6.5 and a modified Rankin Scale (mRS) of 3.9 who underwent EEG monitoring. The average monitoring time was 287 h (range: 0.75–3.216), and the results showed that the most common causes of BIPDs were cardiac arrest, CNS infection, and acute/chronic ischemic/hemorrhagic stroke. In neuroimaging, most of these patients had subcortical injuries and cortical injuries. The PD frequency of most patients was 0.5–2 Hz, located in the prefrontal region. Of the 25 patients, 18 had clinical or EEG seizures. Patients with BIPDs with a history of epilepsy ($P$ = 0.08) and acute metabolic dysfunction ($P$ = 0.08) had more epileptic seizure trends, especially those with acute structural lesions. Epileptic seizures were predicted by bilateral symmetrical frequency ($P$ = 0.02), and seizures were more likely when the PD frequency was less than 2 Hz ($P$ = 0.08). Two of the 25 patients survived and were discharged from the hospital. To understand the relationship between PDs and NCSE in posterior leukoencephalopathy, Bastide, L et al. [40] studied 37 eligible patients. The results showed that 23 patients (62%) had PDs or NCSE, and the authors believed that the two were closely related. The main manifestation of PDs is LPDs or BIPDs of the posterior head. BIPDs are often closely related to the seizures of acute patients [43]. The incidence of epilepsy in different studies was 28–78%, with 90% of clinical low-power seizures. The common types were generalized seizures and focal seizures with or without consciousness impairment and SE [83–85].

The common causes of BIPDs are mainly HIE and CNS infection. Other causes include stroke involving both hemispheres, cerebral atrophy, brain tumors, AE of different causes, metabolic encephalopathy, etc. [86]. The prognosis of patients with BIPDs may be worse than that of patients with LPDs when acute lesions and nervous system injury occur, but there are also reports of benign BIPDs [80, 87, 88].

#### 3.2.4.4 TWs

Extensive periodic TWs are usually anterior head dominant [43, 45]. The occurrence of TWs was initially reported to be related to hepatic encephalopathy [49]; later, TWs were found to occur in any toxic metabolic or structural encephalopathy (uremia, hyponatremia, hypercalcemia, nonketotic hyperosmolar coma, hypoglycemia, hyperthyroidism, etc.), Creutzfeldt-Jakob disease, carbon monoxide poisoning, HIE, toxic encephalopathy, stroke, craniopharyngioma, glioma at the level of thalamus, cortical and subcortical metastatic tumors, Binswanger subcortical encephalopathy, elderly psychiatric patients receiving lithium salt treatment, etc. [80, 89]. The three most common causes of TWs are hepatic encephalopathy, renal failure, and hypoxia damage. The mechanism is not clear. It is speculated that TWs may be related to biochemical metabolism disorder in vivo, and the specificity of their etiological diagnosis is controversial.

Some scholars divide TWs into two types: typical and atypical [53]. Typical TW features are bilateral symmetrical synchronization, anterior head protrusion, frontal-occipital location difference, and group or continuous occurrence, while atypical TWs lack one or more of the above characteristics. Typical TWs are more common in hepatic encephalopathy (hepatic coma), while atypical TWs can appear in liver disease or other metabolic encephalopathies, CNS degeneration diseases, cerebrovascular diseases, and supratentorial and infratentorial tumors, but these distinctions have not been widely confirmed. At present, most EEG workers believe that either typical or atypical TWs can occur in various toxic metabolic encephalopathies, including hepatic encephalopathy, uremia, hyperammonemia caused by valproic acid, severe water electrolyte imbalance, hypercalcemia, hypoxia, hypoglycemia, hyperthyroidism, myxedema, Hashimoto's encephalopathy, and accidental hypothermia. There is no specific species or combination of several characteristics to distinguish hepatic encephalopathy from other metabolic or nonmetabolic encephalopathies. Therefore, this term is used only to describe the special shape of TWs with sharp and slow complexes [44].

It is difficult to distinguish between NCSE and toxic metabolic encephalopathy when patients have confusion or decreased consciousness and slow response and show rhythmic spikes similar to TWs in EEGs. In these patients, benzodiazepines are recommended to verify EEG changes in NCSE, and even frequent TWs may be eliminated by benzodiazepines [90]. Boulanger et al. [91] compared 87 EEGs of 71 patients with TWs and 27 EEGs of 13 patients with NCSE. The frequency of epileptic discharges related to NCSE was faster, and the first component of discharges lasted for a shorter time, had spike wave components, and had less extensive background slowing. Noxious or auditory stimuli often increase TWs and have no effect on epileptiform patterns. These EEG characteristics and responses to stimuli help to distinguish TWs from generalized NCSE [84].

#### 3.2.4.5 SIRPIDs

SIRPIDs may be detected in patients owing to different causes, but the mechanism of this pattern has not been clarified. Some scholars have proposed that the possible mechanism is that the deep initial epileptogenic focus is stimulated to induce discharge, and the thalamic cortex projection function is dysfunctional or overexpressed [54, 92]. Braksick Sherri A et al. [93] studied 416 patients and found that the incidence of SIRPIDs was 10.3%, in which hypoxic brain injury, the use of AEDs, and epileptic discharge on EEGs were independently related to the occurrence of SIRPIDs. Alvarez V et al. [94] monitored the cEEGs of 114 patients who received therapeutic hypothermia after cardiac arrest. By evaluating the changes in neuron-specific enolase (NSE) concentration in serum, it was found that NSE was related to the occurrence of SIRPIDs, suggesting that SIRPIDs are more likely to be a manifestation of damage. The study also found that patients with SIRPIDs had a poor prognosis at 3 months and that SIRPIDs combined with intermittent or unresponsive EEG background activity also indicated poor prognosis. Therefore, SIRPIDs are considered to be a manifestation of brain function damage and an important risk factor for death. The clinical study of Rodriguez et al. [66] included a small number of cases of this pattern. The results showed that the incidence of epileptic seizures in the stimulation-induced pattern was not significantly different from that in the spontaneous discharge pattern and that both SIRPIDs and spontaneous discharge might respond to benzodiazepines. Although in long-term EEG monitoring, it is time-consuming to use video data to evaluate the correlation between each rhythmic, periodic, or subclinical seizure pattern and external stimuli; quantitative analysis brings some interesting hints to clinical practice. Johnson et al. [95] compared and analyzed the data of 25 patients with SIRPIDs and 25 patients with spontaneous discharge by using FFT and proposed that the termination pattern of SIRPID patients was "sputtering" or "periodic tapering termination," while the clinically confirmed epileptic seizures showed a "sudden" termination pattern. In addition, patients with SIRPIDs were more likely to have systemic infection, poisoning, or metabolic disorders. In this study, the SIRPID termination pattern had high sensitivity and specificity for the rapid differentiation of the two types of discharges.

#### 3.2.4.6 Case

(1) A male, 52 years old, day 3 after herpes simplex virus encephalitis, showing unilateral inactivity in the limbs, confusion. EEG and magnetic resonance imaging (MRI) showed characteristic features (Fig. 3.11a–b). The course of the disease was more than 1 month, and the epileptic seizure reoccurred once after stopping valproic acid. Re-examination of EEG shows that the amplitudes of PDs were lower than the previous one. Comparison of the same level of head MRI, the lesion was not enlarged (Fig. 3.11c–d). Re-examination after 6 months. The general condition was good. EEG background basically returned to normal (Fig. 3.11e–f).

(2) A patient with anti-neurexin-3α antibody encephalitis, on the 8th day of the onset, focal and generalized seizures were observed. EEG showed BS pattern (Fig. 3.12). On the 10th day of the onset, EEG and symptoms

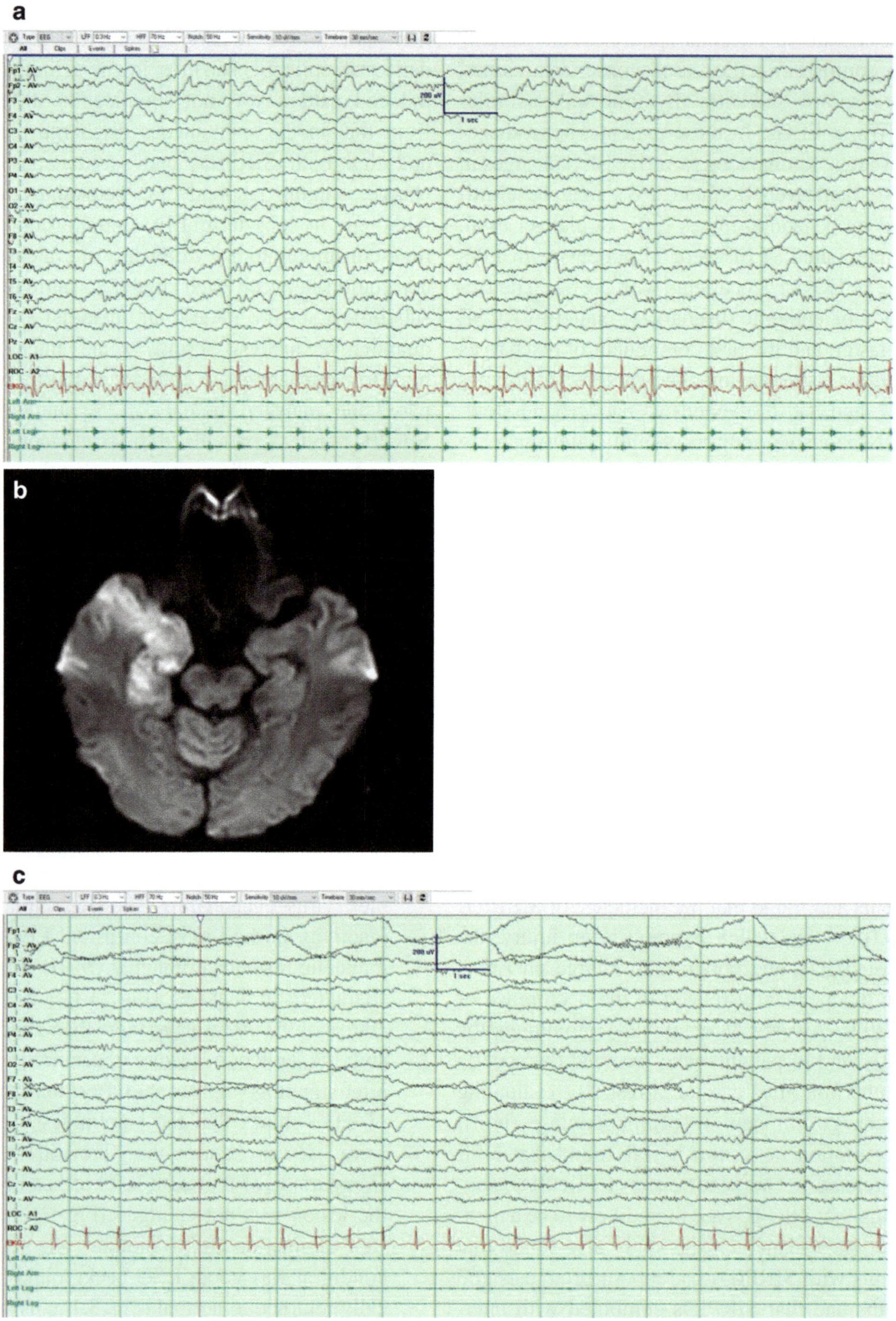

**Fig. 3.11** (**a**) Day 3 EEG from a patient with herpes simplex virus encephalitis, showing unilateral inactivity in the limbs, confusion, and PDs in the right temporal area. (**b**) MRI FLAIR image of the head long signal of the cortex and hippocampus in the right temporal area. (**c**) The course of the disease was more than 1 month, and the epileptic seizure reoccurred once after stopping valproic acid. The EEG shows that the amplitudes of PDs in the right temporal area of the EEG were lower than the previous one. (**d**) Comparison of the same level of MRI of the head; the lesion was not enlarged compared to the front. (**e**) Re-examination after 6 months. The general condition was good. The background is generally normal. No abnormal waves are seen. (**f**) No significant improvement in head MRI

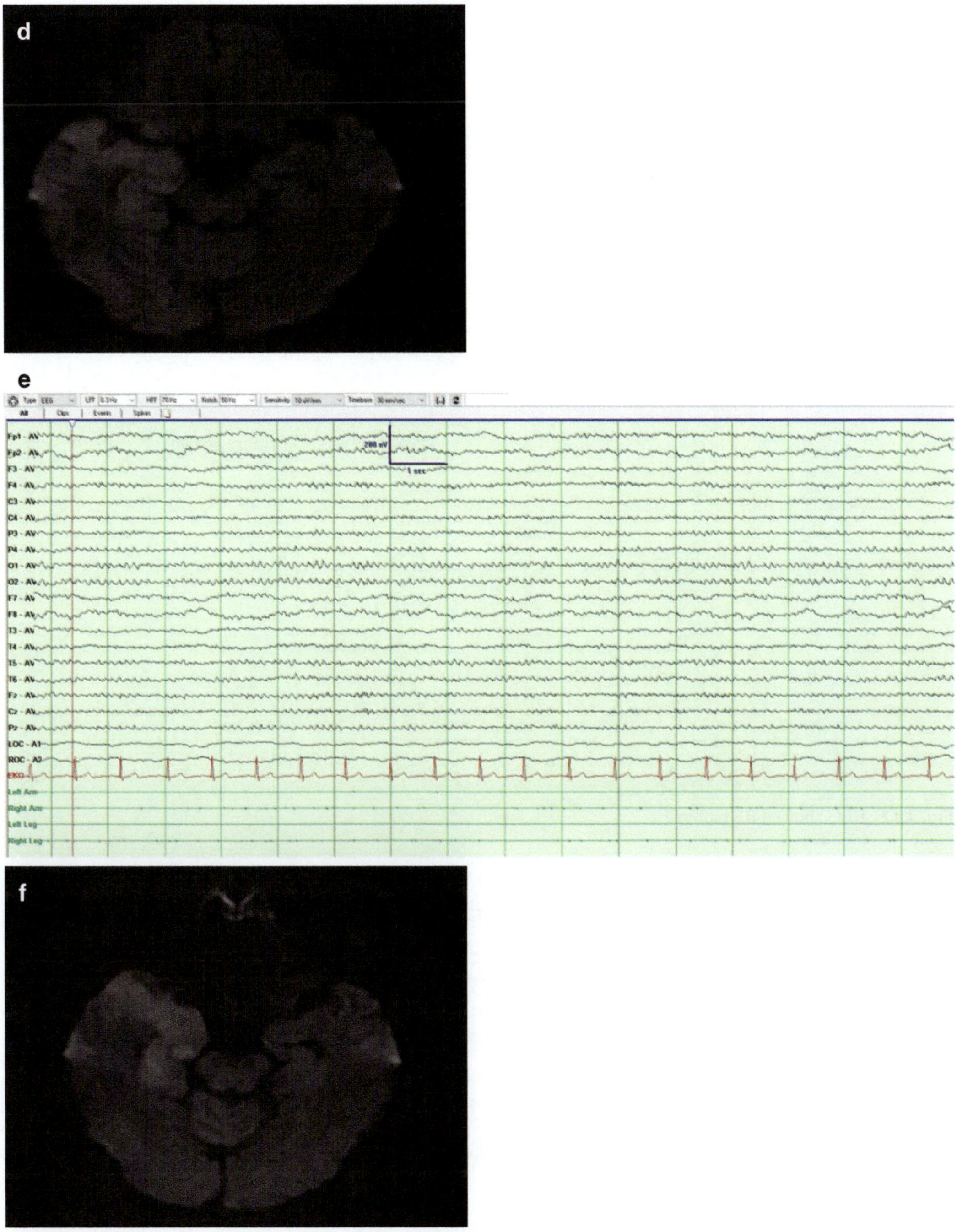

**Fig. 3.11** (continued)

did not improve. In the later stage, the EEG further evolved into periodic waveform (Fig. 3.13), and the prognosis was not good.

(3) An elderly male was after surgery for left temporal glioma. He could spontaneously open his eyes (Fig. 3.14a–b).

(4) EEG from a 50-year-old male who suffered from hydrogen sulfide poisoning and HIE (Fig. 3.15a–b).

## 3.3 IIC in cEEG Monitoring

cEEG monitoring has been used in neurological ICUs since the 1950s, specializing in reflecting functional defects of the brain in real time. In the neurological unit, cEEG has been used to detect seizures, assess the extent of brain damage, evaluate treatment planning, and estimate prognosis [96]. Compared with routine EEG, cEEG moni-

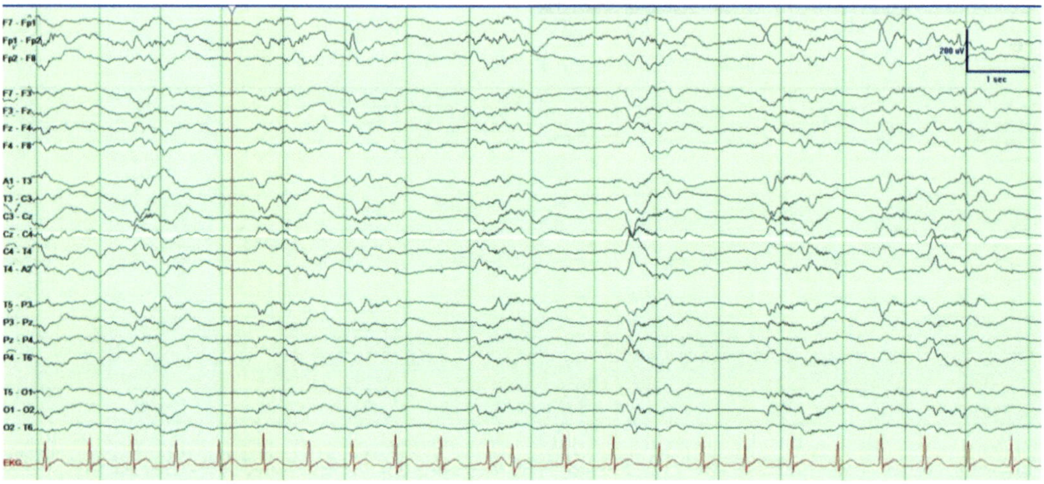

**Fig. 3.12** EEG showed BS pattern

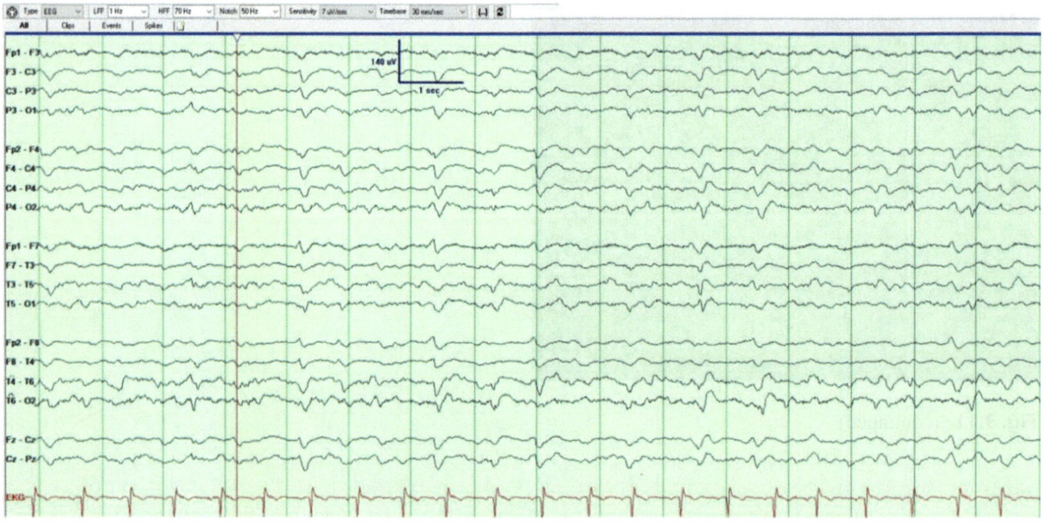

**Fig. 3.13** EEG showed a periodic waveform and bipolar longitudinal connection

a

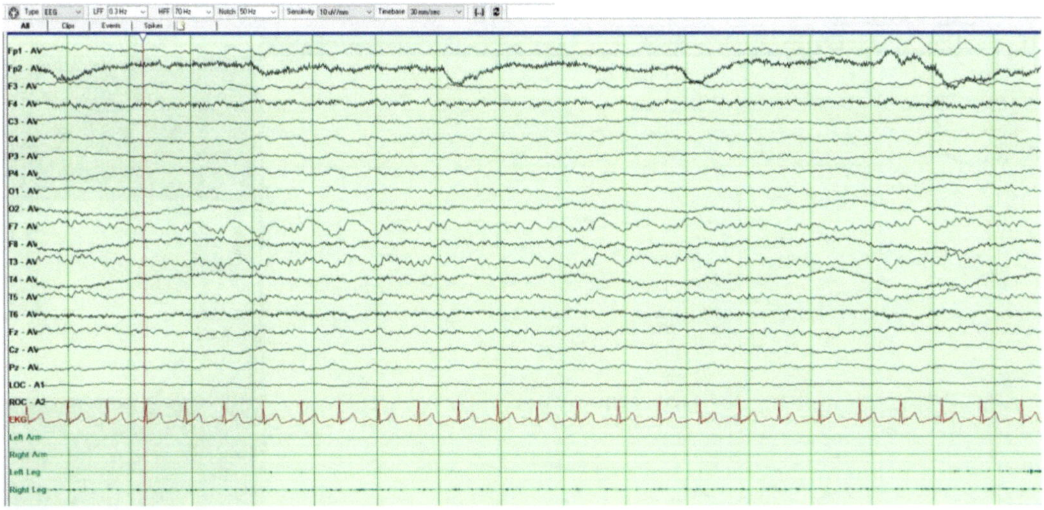


b

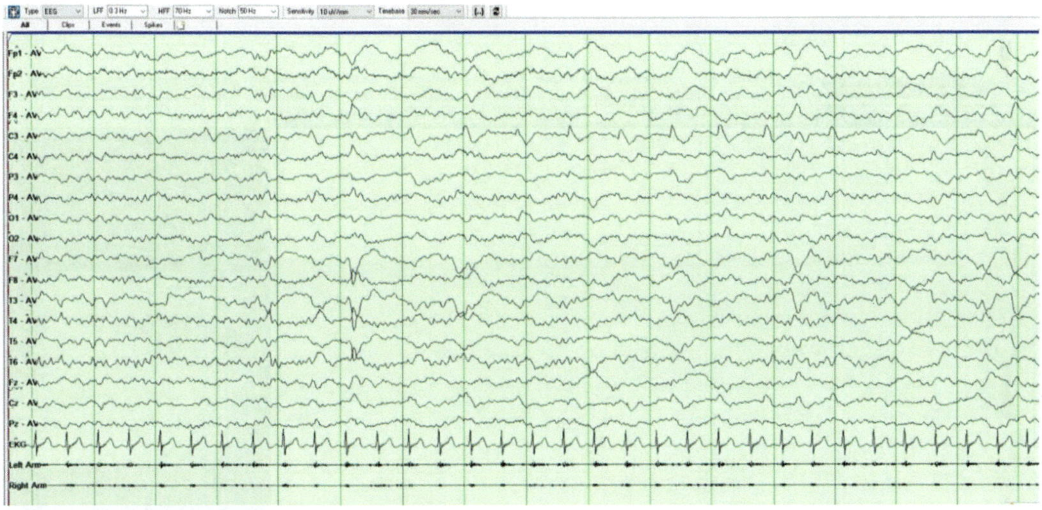


**Fig. 3.14** (**a**) EEG from 1 week after surgery showed a focal slow wave in the left temporal area. (**b**) EEG from 2 weeks after surgery showed epileptic seizures. A paroxysmal slow wave in the left temporal area with spike-wave LPDs in the left central area

toring lasts more than 24 h, which significantly improves the detection rate of subclinical epilepsy and directs more attention to abnormal situations that are not clearly defined.

Approximately one-third of PDs or rhythmic discharges in the NICU show an epileptic form [55], though diagnostic criteria for EEG seizures have not yet been established [69, 97]. The spectrum of these ambiguous patterns is called the IIC [43]. Although no guidelines have been put forward to diagnose an IIC pattern until now, a range of different patterns and their clinical characteristics have been studied to some extent, and some of the research detected an association with an increased risk of seizures or poor outcomes.

a

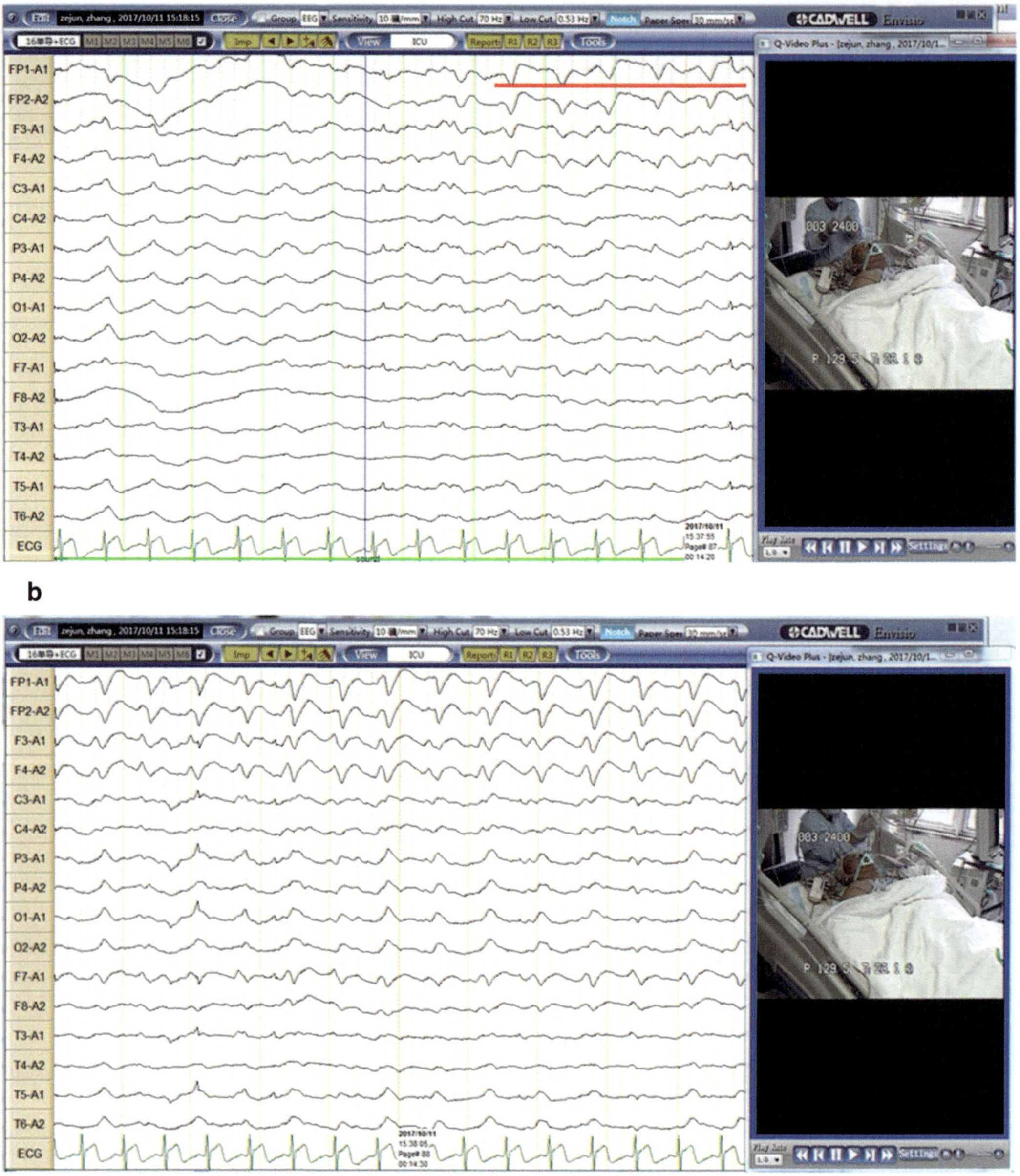


**Fig. 3.15** (**a**) The EEG before stimulation showed 1.5–2.0 Hz low-medium amplitude diffuse slow-wave activity. (**b**) After sound stimulation, the frontal area leads showed continuous emission of moderate-amplitude 1.5–2.0 Hz sharp slow waves. This discharge had a significant time-locking relationship with the stimulus, and background activity resumed within a short time after the stimulus

## 3.3.1 Background

### 3.3.1.1 IIC Definition

As its name implies, the IIC refers to abnormal patterns that conform neither to ictal nor to interictal discharges, which are currently difficult to classify. This concept was first proposed by Pohlmann Eden et al. in 1996 [98]. Common characteristics of an IIC pattern are PDs or rhythmic discharges, most of which are at frequencies between 1 and 2.5 Hz and sometimes with plus modifiers. Some specific patterns also have fluctuating or evolving features similar to the onset of epileptic discharges [1]. According to the Salzburg diagnostic criteria for NCSE, proposed by Beniczky et al., those patterns that meet criteria for an electrographic seizure or NCSE are not included in the scope of the IIC [97]. In addition, interictal patterns, for example, PDs or rhythmic discharges with a frequency less than 1 Hz, should also be excluded.

An IIC pattern is more "malignant" than other EEG patterns because it may be associated with increased neuronal pressure and secondary brain injury. At present, there are no clear guidelines for the management of these potentially harmful EEG patterns, which creates clinical difficulties for ICU doctors. One study reviewed various IIC models and their associated characteristics, seizure risk, and outcomes and proposed a clinical management approach based on available data and expert advice. The study pointed out that if the EEG pattern was found to be interictal, there was no need for drug treatment, and the monitoring time should be more than 24 h to exclude inconclusive seizures. Given the potential risk of epileptic seizures when using anesthesia infusion, these treatments are usually directed only to specific seizure patterns, such as NCSE. However, under certain circumstances, narcotic drugs are allowed for patients with refractory epilepsy [99].

In terms of pathophysiological processes, Pohlmann [98] took LPD as an example and regarded it as a kind of EEG phenomenon indicating a relatively dynamic neurobiological process, revealing the constant state between the ictal and the interictal stages. Within this range, whether seizures occur is affected by potential neuronal damage, metabolic disorders, and individual susceptibility to epilepsy.

In recent years, hemodynamic monitoring, positron emission tomography-computed tomography (PET-CT), and other imaging studies have also explained the pathophysiological process of an IIC pattern from another perspective. For example, a prospective small sample cohort study designed by Struck included 18 subjects who underwent F-deoxyglucose positron emission tomography (FDG-PET) and cEEG examination, and IIC patterns were captured in all of the subjects during the FDG uptake period. The study compared different patterns along the IIC and found that during the FDG uptake period, the discharge tended to be ictal [100]. Further research on LPDs found that the higher the frequency of discharge, the more FDG-PET suggests increasing metabolism [101].

#### 3.3.1.2 Patterns Along the IIC

PDs discharge at a relatively uniform morphology, duration, and interval. According to the definition of PDs, each discharge lasts ≤0.5 s or recurs up to 3 times/s [1]. The background of intervals between two discharges is usually low voltage. On the basis of location, PDs can be further classified as LPDs, BIPDs, and GPDs. PDs are described as proper PDs (without plus modifiers), PDs with superimposed fast rhythm ("PDs + F"), PDs with rhythm-like δ activity ("+ R"), and PDs in which the previous two exist simultaneously ("+ FR").

RDA is characterized as patterns with relatively uniform shape and duration without intervals and discharge at a frequency less than 4 Hz. RDA can also be further classified as lateralized rhythmic δ activity (LRDA) (Fig. 3.16) and generalized rhythmic δ activity (GRDA) (Fig. 3.17a, b) according to where the discharges occur. Similar to PD, RDAs are also associated with plus modifiers, such as fast rhythms ("+ F"), superimposed sharp waves or spikes ("+ S"), and both ("+ FS") [1].

Another special rhythmic discharge are brief (potentially) ictal rhythmic discharges (B(I) RDs). [This term was proposed by Yoo et al. and has not yet been included in the ACNS's Standardized Critical Care EEG Terminology (2012 version).] B(I)RDs were previously researched in newborns and are also called brief rhythmic discharges (BRDs) or brief electroencephalogram rhythmic discharges (BERDs). Yoo et al. first put forward this term, aiming at emphasizing its potential episodic characteristics. The frequency of these rhythmic discharges is always higher than 4 Hz, but they last less than 10 s

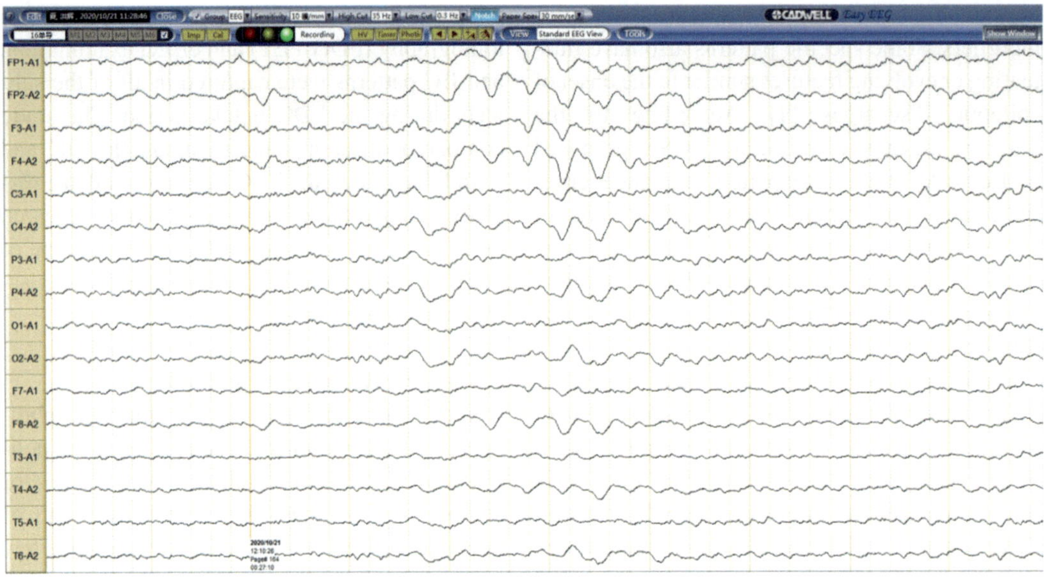


**Fig. 3.16** The EEG of a 33-year-old female with alcoholic encephalopathy, showing moderate-amplitude LRDA at 2–3 Hz in the right hemisphere

(mostly less than 4 s) [102] (Fig. 3.18a–c). B(I) RDs exist in unilateral or bilateral hemispheres and most often show θ waves without evolution.

SIRPIDs were first discovered during nursing procedures in the ICU [54] (Fig. 3.19a–c). Whether SIRPIDs have ictal features or are associated with seizures is still inconclusive. Research has found that SIRPIDs are more common in patients in a coma or with cardiac arrest and in those who receive mild hypothermia treatment. Other than stimulation induction, there is nothing special about the SIRPID pattern compared with the others above. Therefore, the new standard EEG terminology updated in 2012 treats stimulation as an additional feature of patterns. Such waveforms can be written as SI-LPDs, SI-GPDs, etc., to distinguish them from spontaneous patterns. SIRPIDs and focally evolving RDA are referred to together as stimulus-evolving RDA (SI-Evolving LRDA) [1].

For such waveforms, the following mainly discusses the correlation between the IIC pattern and the risk of seizures, the short-term and long-term prognosis implications for patients, and the treatment strategies based on this.

### 3.3.2 Risks of Seizure and Prognosis Related to Patterns Along the IIC

#### 3.3.2.1 LPDs

LPDs are one of the most common patterns in cEEG monitoring in critically ill patients, accounting for 6.2–8.6% of patterns [55] (Fig. 3.20). Common causes are unilateral structural injuries, such as strokes, infections, and tumors [103]. Among them, acute stroke is more common. Hartings et al. [104] found that in rat models, LPDs originate from the ischemic penumbra rather than the central region of the infarction. A retrospective study involving 102 patients with cerebral hemorrhage found that approximately 13% of patients developed LPDs [105].

LPDs are characterized by episodic waveforms. Many studies have found that certain seizure symptoms are time locked to LPDs, especially motor symptoms such as myoclonus [106]. However, the study also found that the time-lock relationship between LPDs and motor symptoms recorded in the central region cannot prove the ictal characteristics of LPDs. In addi-

a

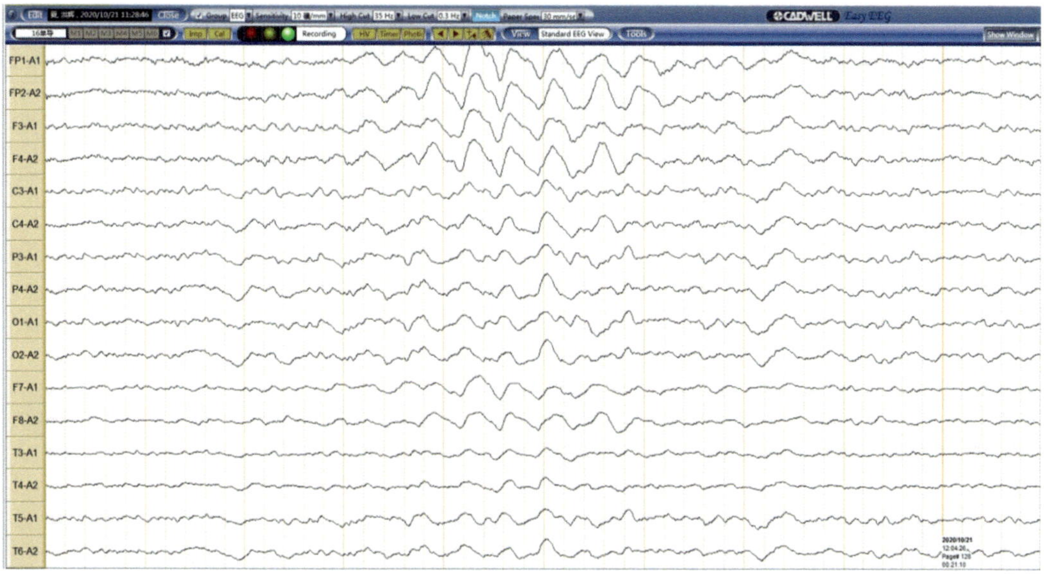


b

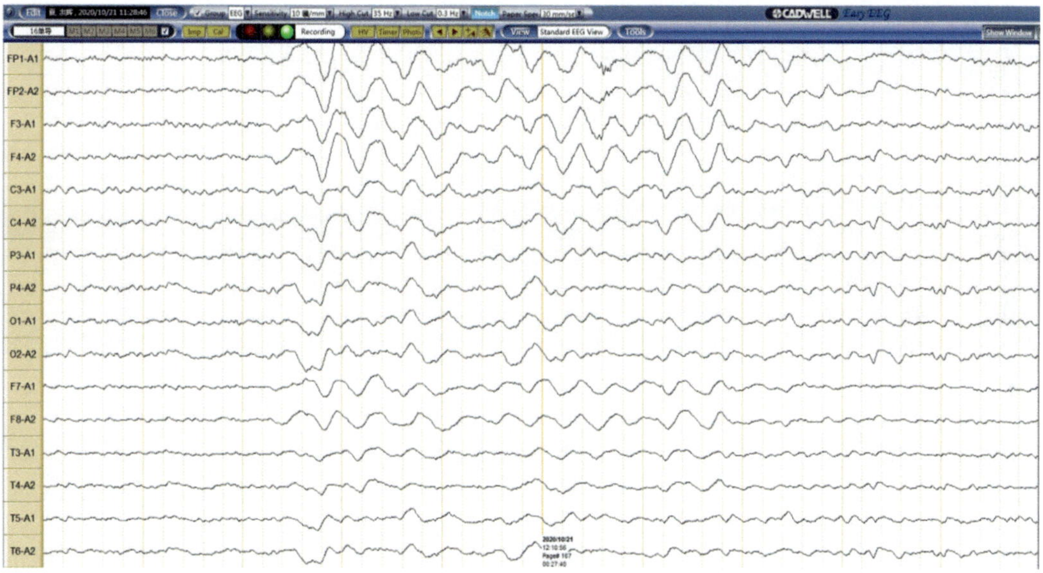


**Fig. 3.17** (**a**) The EEG of a 38-year-old female with carbon monoxide poisoning, showing RDA at approximately 3 Hz. (**b**) GRDA, showing the obvious frontal area

tion, imaging and serological tests also suggest that LPDs on EEG changes are synchronized in different stages of seizures. Struck A F et al. [100] enrolled 18 patients who underwent cEEG monitoring and FDG-PET. High metabolism on FDG-PET was found to effectively predict clinical or EEG seizures.

In the ICU, a multicenter study involving 4772 patients found that LPDs were clearly a risk factor for seizures (OR = 8.61, 95% CI [7.08–10.49], $P < 0.001$). The risk was greater (OR = 16.40, 95% CI [8.97–30.64], $P < 0.001$) when LPDs were observed at a frequency higher than 2 Hz, and LPDs (LPDs +) with superimposed modifiers

**a**

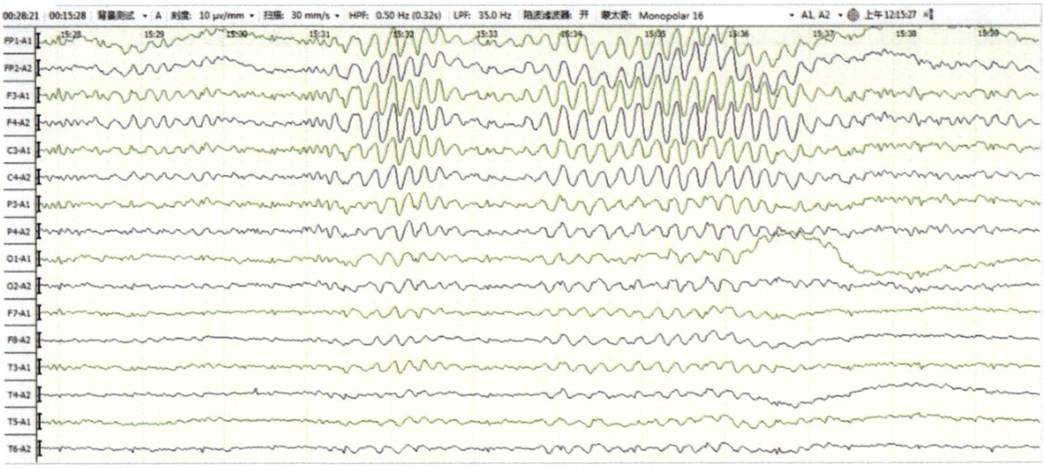

**b**

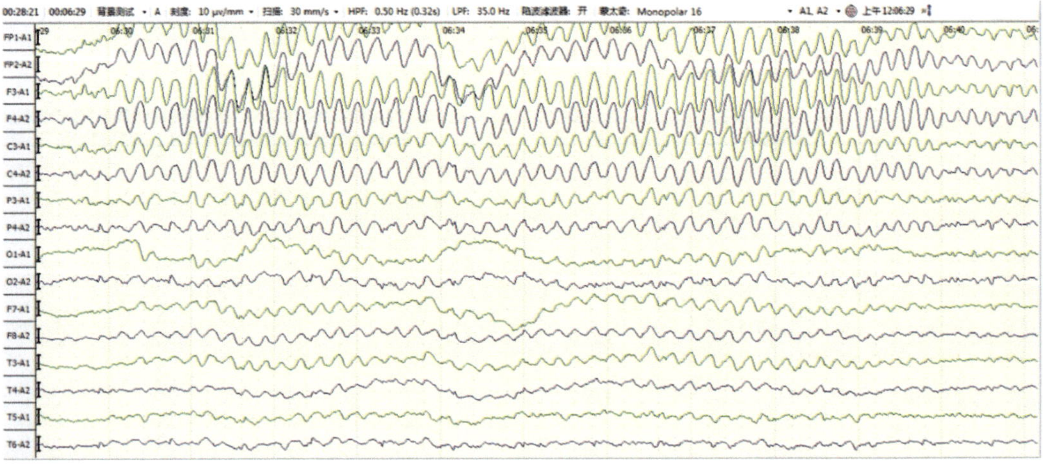

**c**

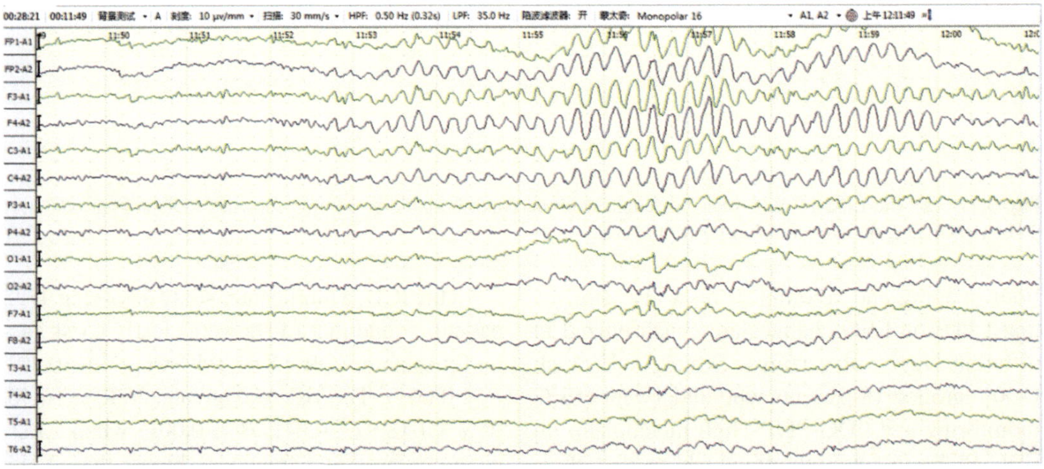

**Fig. 3.18** (**a**) The EEG of a 32-year-old male with acute alcoholism, showing rhythmic θ activity at approximately 4 Hz in all EEG leads but mostly in the frontal lead. (**b**) Rhythmic θ activity lasts for nearly 10 s. (**c**) Rhythmic θ activity with mid-wave amplitude of approximately 4 Hz is evident in bilateral frontal area leads

also significantly increased the risk of seizures (OR = 2.00, 95% CI [1.44–2.78], $P < 0.001$) [66]. Earlier studies also confirmed that seizures and SE were seen in 74% of patients with LPDs+, compared to only 6% in proper LPDs without plus modifiers [42]. Further comparing the different components of the LPD stack, LPDs +R had the highest risk of seizures and seizure status (OR = 13, 95% CI [5.3–36.52]; $P < 0.000$), followed by LPDs + F (OR = 5.16, 95% CI [2.08–13.07], $P = 0.0004$) [107].

The appearance of LPDs is related to a number of data indicating poor prognosis, such as hospital mortality, the length of hospital stay, and

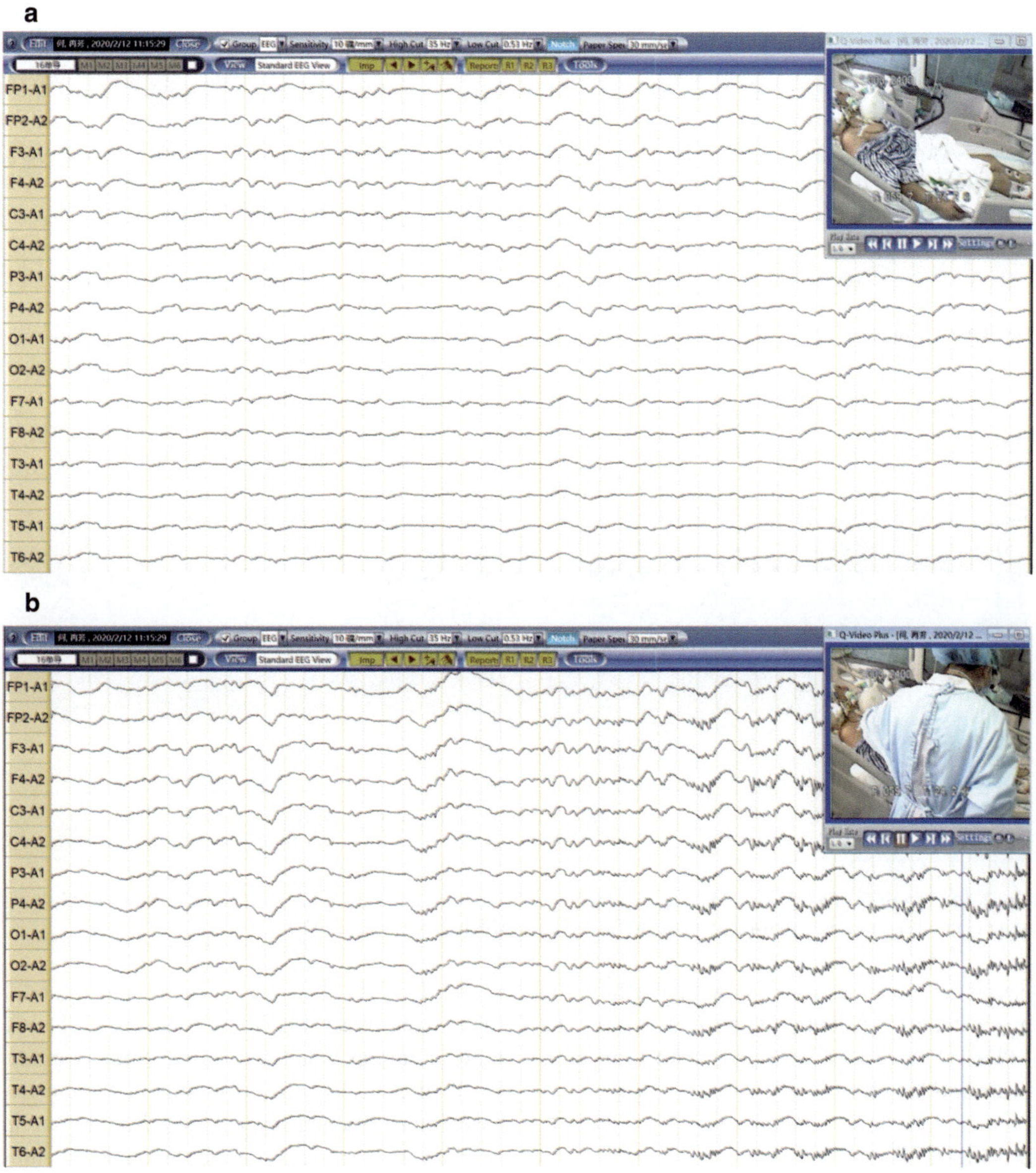


**Fig. 3.19** (**a**) A 55-year-old male with fulminant myocarditis underwent CPR. EEG background activity shows diffuse low- to medium-amplitude slow waves in all leads. (**b**) Rhythmic discharge induced by pain stimulation. (**c**) The patient presented with clinically generalized myoclonic seizures after stimulation, and EEG showed poly spike waves and multi spike-slow waves in all leads

c

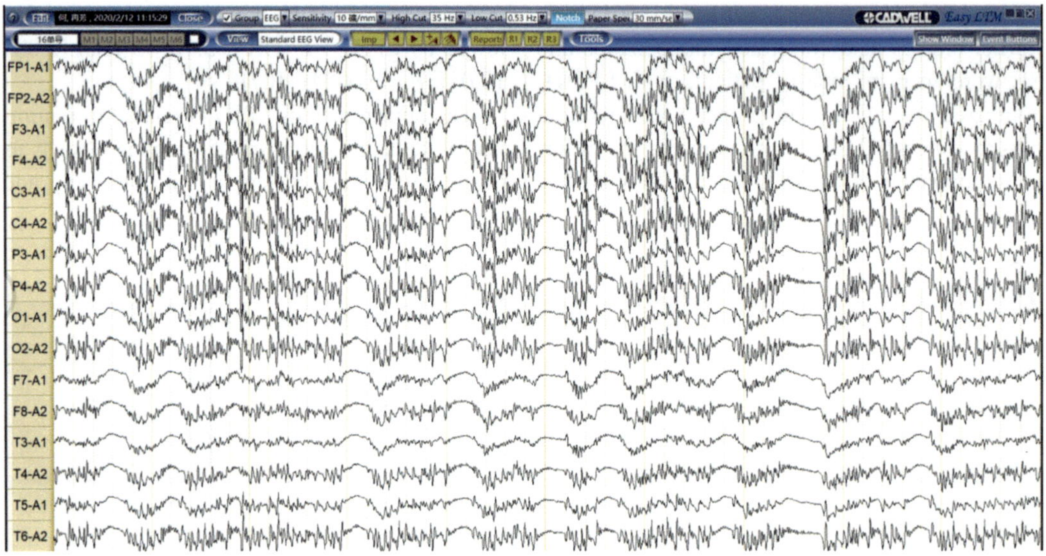

**Fig. 3.19** (continued)

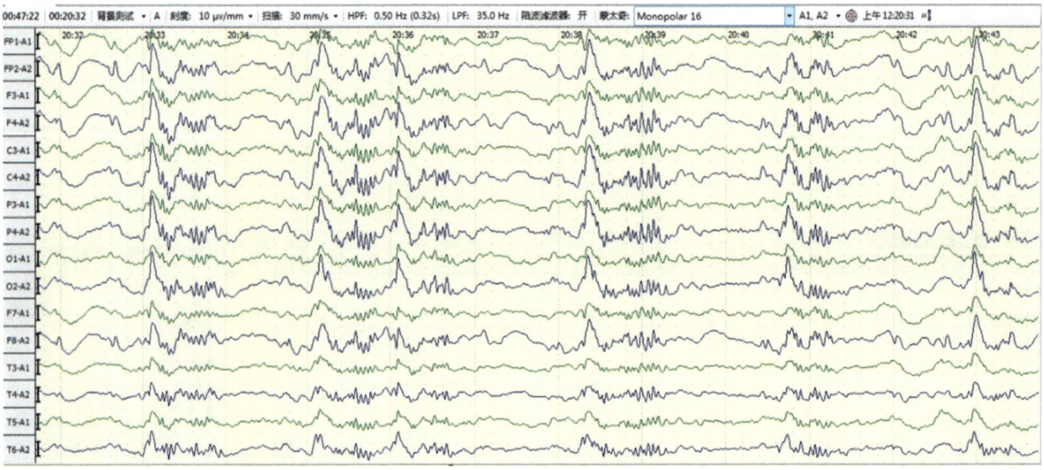

**Fig. 3.20** The EEG of a 67-year-old male with meningeal carcinoma and a disturbance of consciousness. EEG shows a right lateral sharp wave followed by periodic fast activity, which appeared as LPD + F

neural functional recovery in 1 year. Furthermore, many studies in recent years have also found that LPDs are associated with poor short-term prognosis of SAH [108].

### 3.3.2.2 GPDs

GPDs are a type of bilateral synchronous discharge. The amplitude is usually >100 μV, each episode lasts no more than 3 s, and the frequency is mostly 1 Hz (Fig. 3.21). There is also a relatively fixed interval between episodes. GPDs are more common when the whole brain is extensively affected by drug poisoning, metabolic diseases, acute brain injury, etc.; but they are rare in cerebral hemorrhage or brain trauma. Most studies suggest that the probability of GPDs appearing in severe brain injury EEG monitoring is approximately 0.8–1.8%. A case-control study

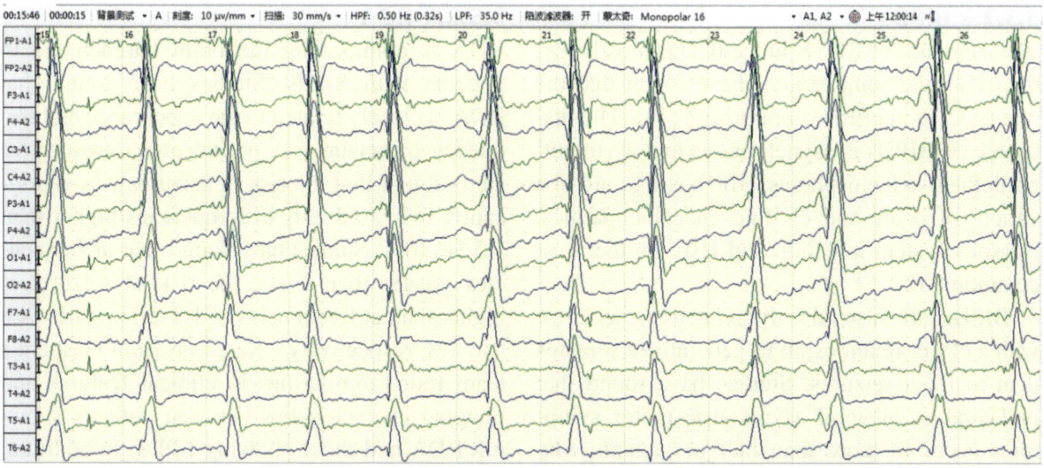


**Fig. 3.21** The EEG of a 74-year-old male who presented with HIE. The EEG shows a generalized periodically sharp wave, GPD

by Professor Foreman's team found that the incidence of GPDs in severe brain injury EEG monitoring was as high as 4.8%. The study also found that the incidence of seizures in the GPD group was 46%, which was higher than the 34% in the control group ($p = 0.014$). The occurrence rate of NCSE in the GPD group was 21.5%, which was also higher than the 6.5% in the control group ($p < 0.001$) [56]. GPDs may appear in the late stage or just after the onset of generalized SE, but they are unable to predict the occurrence of generalized SE [56, 109, 110].

Similar to LPDs, GPDs with other superimposed components or at a frequency greater than 1.5 Hz are more likely to be a risk factor for seizures. Rodriguez and his colleague found that GPDs at frequencies below 1.5 Hz had a lower correlation with seizures, while GPDs at frequencies above 2 Hz were highly associated with seizures (OR = 3.30, 95% CI, 1.79–5.87, $P = 0.04$) [66]. The study also found that GPDs had a certain correlation with seizures when combined with modifiers; in contrast, no correlation was found without superimposed rhythmic, fast, or sharp activity.

The prognosis of patients with GPDs also suggests higher morbidity and mortality, which are more obvious in patients with neonatal HIE and brain trauma. There are also opinions that GPDs are a byproduct of primary injury and do not affect the prognosis itself. For example, the above study [56] by Professor Foreman found that GPDs were not an independent risk factor for poor prognosis (GCS score of 4–5), although the GPD group had a longer hospital stay in the ICU after excluding factors such as age and etiology. The prognosis of patients with a severe past medical history is poor. In addition, studies have found that GPDs often co-occur with LPDs. This also makes the clinical characteristics of GPDs difficult to judge.

TWs are a special type of GPD. They were first discovered in patients with hepatic encephalopathy and later were found in many metabolic diseases, such as hyponatremia, hypothyroidism, lithium poisoning, and hypertensive encephalopathy [111]. TWs have a close relationship with seizures and are very sensitive to benzodiazepines. However, although benzodiazepines can reduce the appearance of TWs on EEGs, they are unable to improve clinical performance; therefore, benzodiazepines can be used to distinguish TWs from NCSE [90]. Studies have found that TWs are associated with an increase in in-hospital mortality (OR = 4.5, 95% CI, 1.57–12.7, $p = 0.005$) [112]. However, Professor Foreman's research suggests that, unlike other PDs, the presence of TWs does not predict an increased risk of subsequent seizures [113].

#### 3.3.2.3 BIPDs

The incidence of BIPDs in the ICU is mostly less than 1%, and some studies have found that the rate is 3.5% in cEEG monitoring [114]. The discharge of BIPDs is asynchronous and asymmetric in the two hemispheres. BIPDs are found in a variety of acute and chronic encephalopathies. Nervous system infection and HIE are the most common [103].

BIPDs are also closely related to seizures, with a closer relationship to generalized seizures than to focal seizures. Studies have found that unilateral or bilateral asymmetric motor symptoms occur in more than half of patients who have BIPDs detected by EEG [87]. Previous research that focused on patients with BIPDs found that the incidence of seizures was 43–78% [79, 87]. For example, De la Paz and Brenner found that the incidence of seizures was 78% in 18 patients with EEGs showing BIPDs [115]. Snodgrass and his team analyzed 147 patients with cardiac arrest, CNS infection, and delayed epilepsy, which accounted for 10% of seizures, and 4 of them subsequently developed a state of epilepsy [116].

Many studies have suggested that the emergence of BIPDs may herald a poor prognosis. Coma is also more common in patients who have not been monitored for BIPDs. Fitzpatrick and colleagues included 96 patients with LPD in cEEG monitoring. The study found that the overall hospital mortality was 27%, while the mortality of patients with BIPDs was 52% [87]. Orta found that the neurological recovery of such patients in 1 year was not satisfactory [79]. At the same time, there were a few cases reporting the occurrence of "benign" BIPDs. Professor Fushimi reported the case of a 64-year-old male patient who had a seizure after pneumonia. MRI of the head indicated bilateral hippocampal ischemic infarction. Since then, the EEG was monitored for 6 consecutive months, and multiple BIPDs were monitored without significant changes in symptoms or consciousness before or later [80].

#### 3.3.2.4 RDA

RDA is common in the brain parenchyma in patients with SAHs. Studies have found that RDA is closely related to the appearance and frequency of seizures. A multicenter retrospective study found that the risk of seizures was significantly increased only at frequencies higher than 1.5 Hz [66]. Studies have found that at frequencies greater than 2 Hz, the risk of seizures is higher than at frequencies of 1.5–2 Hz (OR = 4.0 and 1.8, respectively). Research from Gaspard's team found similarities in clinical features and imaging characteristics between patients showing RDA and those showing LPDs. In addition, they also found differences among patients showing RDA, patients showing LPDs, and patients showing arrhythmic abnormal discharges. The results showed that the latter lesions were more limited to subcortical white matter, which also suggested that the common pathophysiological mechanism of RDA and LPDs may be damaged cortical-subcortical circuits [27].

LRDA is common in a variety of CNS injuries, mostly in intracranial and SAHs. Many studies have found that the clinical features of LRDA are very similar to those of LPDs, but the presence of LDRA indicates a greater risk of seizures, especially nonconvulsive seizures (NCSs) [27]. In a study of 4772 patients, it was found that LRDA plus was related to an increased risk of seizures (OR = 3.57, 95% CI, 2.25–5.63; $p < 0.001$), and the presence of LRDA alone was not a clear risk factor [66].

GRDA is more common in patients with infections or metabolic diseases. Because GRDA mostly occurs in the bilateral frontal lobe, it is often called frontal intermittent rhythmic δ activity (FIRDA). This bilateral symmetric, simultaneous discharge of GRDA confined to the prefrontal lobe is highly associated with structural damage and diffuse encephalopathy but hardly indicates the concurrence of seizures [27, 117, 118]. The study from Ettore included 36 patients and found that the incidence of epileptiform discharges in the EEG in the FIRDA group

(5%) was significantly lower than that in the control group (40%) during the same period (Fisher's $p < 0.05$) [118]. A multicenter retrospective study involving 927 patients found that GRDA was not associated with seizures even with plus modifiers superimposed or at a frequency greater than 2 Hz [66].

Temporal intermittent rhythmic δ activity (TIRDA), a special form of GRDA, is usually confined to the medial temporal lobe, especially in patients with medial temporal lobe sclerosis. TIRDA is associated with late-onset epilepsy, and this form of epileptic attack is more suggestive of complex partial seizures [117].

#### 3.3.2.5 SIRPIDs

SIRPIDs are a kind of stimulation-induced abnormal EEG finding. The incidence of SIRPIDs being monitored in hospitals is approximately 10–34%, and they are more likely to occur in severe patients [119]. Hirsch et al. [54] found that the most common cause of SIRPIDs is SAH. Cerebral hemorrhage and SE are also independent predictors of SIRPIDs. Other studies have confirmed that cerebral hypoxia injury and traumatic brain injury (TBI) are strongly associated with SIRPIDs [93, 120]. In current clinical studies of SIRPIDs, standardized stimuli include auditory stimuli and tactile stimuli. Some studies have suggested that the sequence of stimuli does not affect EEG responsiveness. Bilateral nipple pinching is the most likely to induce SIRPIDs [121].

There is much debate about the relevance of SIRPIDs to seizures. The study designed by Hirsch and Braksick suggests that SIRPIDs are associated with a higher risk of seizures in EEGs in severe patients [54, 93]. However, a prospective study by Alsherbini and his team concluded that there was no significant correlation [120]. Another large multicenter study found that stimulation-induced abnormal EEG patterns will not significantly increase the risk of seizures compared to spontaneous IIC patterns [66].

Studies have found that SIRPIDs are more responsive to benzodiazepines and can achieve improvements in EEGs and clinical status, which supports their seizure characteristics. Professor Alvarez reported that the appearance of SIRPIDs after mild hypothermia treatment in coma patients due to cardiac arrest suggested a poor prognosis (Cerebral Performance Category (CPC) score of 3–5) [94], and another study found that SIRPIDs were not an independent risk of increased mortality and poor prognosis. Increases in morbidity and mortality were affected by the severity of the primary disease [93]. Professor Ong performed long-range EEG monitoring of comatose patients for more than 10 days and found that the appearance of SIRPIDs was independent of consciousness and prognosis [77].

#### 3.3.2.6 B(I)RDs

B(I)RDs have rarely been studied in adults in the past. In 2014, Yoo J et al. [102] found that B(I) RDs were present in approximately 2% of patients under cEEG monitoring in neurological wards. Regarding the etiology, acute brain injury occurred in all but one of the patients, and tumors and strokes were the most common cause. In this study, the incidence of seizures was significantly higher in the B(I)RD group (75%) than in the control group (25%) ($P < 0.01$). Of the 15 people who had seizures, 14 had B(I)RDs before the first seizure occurred. Although there was no significant difference, the prognosis of the B(I)RD group appeared to be worse than that of the control group [102].

In addition, Struck et al. proposed a risk factor scoring system for seizures, referred to as 2HELPS2B. In this scoring system, the presence of B(I)RDs is one of the highest scoring risk factors [122]. A study in a newborn treatment algorithm found that B(I)RDs clearly predicted an increase in mortality, with a similar risk to seizures [123].

### 3.3.3 Treatment Algorithm

Until now, there has been no consensus for the treatment of patterns within the IIC. Most studies on the IIC have resulted in intervention options.

Many factors were taken into consideration, including the severity of the primary disease, the clinical manifestations corresponding to patterns, the risk of seizures, and the degree of neural functional damage, to assess the dose of medication. In this process, the researchers used their experience in the treatment of NCSE and NCSs to draw some conclusions on the IIC pathophysiology mechanism.

First, clinicians need to judge whether suspicious abnormal patterns fall into the IIC. Research has found that approximately 1/4 of seizures occur 24 h after primary disease onset. Therefore, cEEG monitoring is usually required for 24–48 h [56, 124, 125]. For coma patients, monitoring for 48 h is necessary [126]. Professor Johnson [103] suggests monitoring for 24–48 h when some IIC patterns that are known to have a greater correlation with seizures are detected, such as LPDs, LRDA, BIPDs, and SIRPIDs, without relevant clinical symptoms or high-risk features, such as frequency >2 Hz or superimposed plus modifiers. Medications are not recommended unless the release of EEG epilepsy waves or clinical symptoms worsens. If the patterns are accompanied by the abovementioned high-risk characteristics, benzodiazepines or AEDs could be used experimentally [103]. For GRDA, considering that the risk of seizures is low, there is no need for additional treatment if no clinical symptoms are present. GPDs are mostly related to toxic or metabolic abnormalities, and further screening is needed for the existence of a clear primary infection, poisoning, or metabolic disease. If no such cause is identified, experimental trials are also recommended, using benzodiazepines or additional AEDs [103].

#### 3.3.3.1 Use of AEDs

For the choice of experimental drugs, the curative effect and side effects need to be evaluated and compared between sedatives and nonsedatives. A study found that benzodiazepines may cause deep sedation and even respiratory depression. In a study of patients with persistent epilepsy, it was found that some patients had a poor long-term prognosis. Other studies suggest that the improvement of clinical symptoms by benzodiazepines is limited, and EEGs seldom return to normal background rhythm. In addition, the difference in baseline level of consciousness between patients also has a large impact on the results; therefore, benzodiazepines are not recommended as a first-line medication [71]. However, for cases in which patterns are still considered ictal, it is recommended to quickly titrate traditional AEDs and continuously monitor the EEGs for 24 h to capture delayed seizures. Once drug treatment is started, the dose should be increased stepwise, with close attention to EEG changes, and then the dosage should be adjusted accordingly.

Commonly used nonsedative AEDs include phenytoin and valproic acid. The use of the former is restricted in the ICU due to interactions with many other drugs [127], while the latter should also be used with caution because of its impairment of liver function. Other options include levetiracetam, lacosamide, and other first-line AEDs. Osman's study considered that the high metabolic demand caused by primary acute injury may cause secondary neuronal damage. The use of nonsedative AEDs for IIC patterns should be avoided. The subsequent treatment plan is also based on the abovementioned high-risk characteristics and their relation with seizures. For more efficiency, nonsedative AEDs can be added to therapeutic doses or, additionally, benzodiazepines according to the circumstances [128].

In addition to the treatment effect and clinical manifestations, neuroimaging, serological tests, and multimodal monitoring are used to help assess whether there is neuronal damage. In imaging studies, indications of the IIC are observed with restricted diffusion in diffusion-weighted imaging (DWI); hypermetabolism in FDG-PET [100]; elevated regional CBF in single-photon emission computed tomography (SPECT), which indicates increased focal blood flow velocity [129, 130]; and increased perfusion on computed tomography perfusion (CTP). These findings return to normal as LPDs disappear. Previous studies have confirmed the restricted diffusion on DWI in the peri-ictal period, seizures, and SE [131, 132]. The pathophysiological mechanism consists of increased energy metabolism, increased blood flow perfusion, and neuronal edema due to episodic activity. However, the above evidence is based on a clear status convulsion, and some studies have suggested that changes in DWI are unable to prove that neuronal damage is related to LPDs. For example, Narayanan's study found that patients with LPDs who had seizures presented restricted diffusion on DWI, while patients without seizures did not show DWI changes [132]. Therefore, the article recommends intervention only for patients with LPDs who present seizures. Patients with acute brain injury should complete neuroimaging before and after treatment and carefully analyze whether the changes in blood flow are caused by electrical discharges rather than the primary disease.

#### 3.3.3.2 Multimodal Monitoring

In patients with seizures, serological tests show increased levels of NSE and glutamate and an increased lactate-pyruvate ratio. The increase in NSE, although not very specific, can reflect the degree of neuronal damage and has been confirmed to exist in many types of seizures. With the widespread development of multimodal monitoring in ICUs, invasive detection methods also play an important role. For example, microdialysis technology can simultaneously detect parameters such as the partial brain tissue oxygen tension ($PbtO_2$), local blood flow, and perfusion pressure and can evaluate blood flow perfusion and brain tissue oxygen supply in areas where abnormal patterns are present. Witsch J and his colleagues enrolled 90 patients with spontaneous SAH for EEG and multimodal testing. They found that when the frequency of PD was higher than 2 Hz, $PbtO_2$ decreased, local blood flow increased, and perfusion pressure decreased [63]. At this time, active use of AEDs can help prevent secondary damage due to increased metabolic demands.

In addition, although intracranial electrodes are not routinely used in monitoring, their sensitivity is significantly higher than that of scalp electrodes [71]. For patients with seizures detected only by intracranial electrodes, active medication is also recommended [133]. Therefore, some scholars believe that for patients with unexplained coma, scalp electrodes may not be sufficient to reflect the degree of injury and PDs or NCSEs.

### 3.3.4 Conclusion

In summary, the mechanism of how an IIC pattern is generated and its clinical characteristics are affected by many factors. Among them, the primary etiology and different EEG backgrounds among individuals cannot be ignored. In addition, because most epileptic seizures in the ICU are nonconvulsive, the recognition of clinical symptoms may be inaccurate, and most studies are limited by the sample size, some conclusions are still controversial. Therefore, as many scholars and clinicians have implied, the diagnosis and treatment of IIC patterns should be individualized, and the conclusions of some clinical trials need to be considered dialectically. We should take an objective view of the contradictions in different studies, but at the same time, the results of larger and multicenter studies are still worth looking forward. In addition, clinicians and EEG professionals should pay more attention to such waveforms and work together to explore more of their clinical features and commonalities.

## 3.4 Abnormal Slow-Wave Activity

Slow waves are not necessarily pathological waveforms. Slow waves adapted to age and/or status are normal. In critically ill patients, slow waves are the most common nonspecific abnormal brain waves. The waveform of the abnormally slow wave can be a sine-like wave, or it can be a polymorphic slow wave or a complex slow wave with overlapping fast wave components, and generally the amplitude is high [134]. According to the location and mode of slow waves, this section will introduce four aspects: persistent nonrhythmic δ activity (PNDA), intermittent rhythmic δ activity (IRDA), paroxysmal high-amplitude δ activity (PHDA), and unresponsive low-voltage slow activity.

### 3.4.1 PNDA

PNDA is the most common EEG manifestation of coma resulting from various causes, but it lacks cause specificity [135] (Figs. 3.22 and 3.23). In the early stage of coma in critically ill patients, amplitude attenuation may occur when there is external stimulation, and the α rhythm gradually disappears. As the coma deepens, intermittent θ-band activity appears, similar to a normal early drowsiness pattern. Diffuse nonrhythmic δ activities will appear in the future. Afterwards, diffuse nonrhythmic δ activities appear, which are continuously issued for irregular δ activities with high to very high amplitudes of 1–3 Hz. The discharge waveform can be a single rhythm or a polymorphic slow wave with irregular waveforms, or it can be combined with some irregular low-amplitude fast waves (complex slow waves) on the slow wave and sometimes mixed with different numbers of spikes or sharp waves [136]. The appearance of PNDA suggests diffuse brain injury. The injury site often involves both the cerebral cortex and the subcortical white matter. However, the involvement of the pure cortex or deep gray matter nuclei rarely manifests as obvious pleomorphic δ waves. Studies have shown

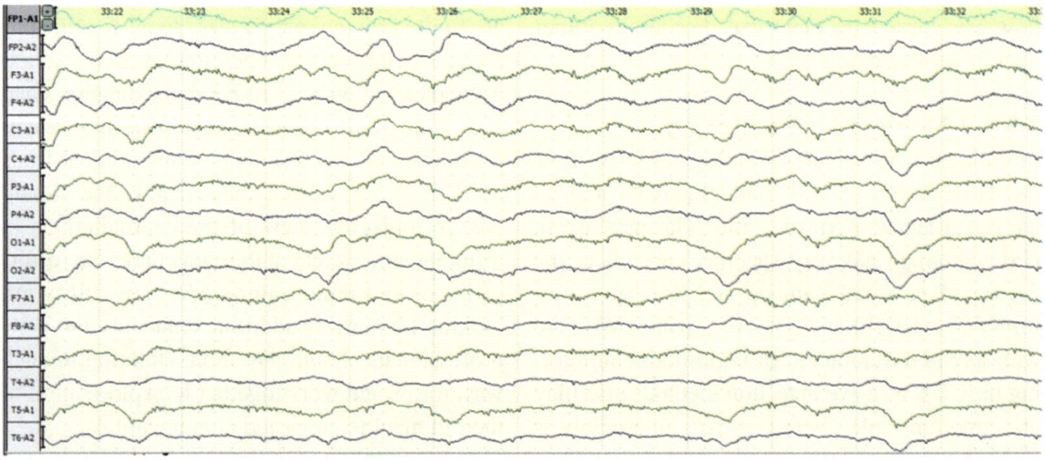


**Fig. 3.22** EEG from a 29-year-old female patient with anti-*N*-methyl-D-aspartate receptor (anti-NMDAR) encephalitis. She was admitted to the hospital due to repeated limb twitching for 3 days, and the patient had obvious hypoventilation. The EEG shows diffuse nonrhythmic δ activity

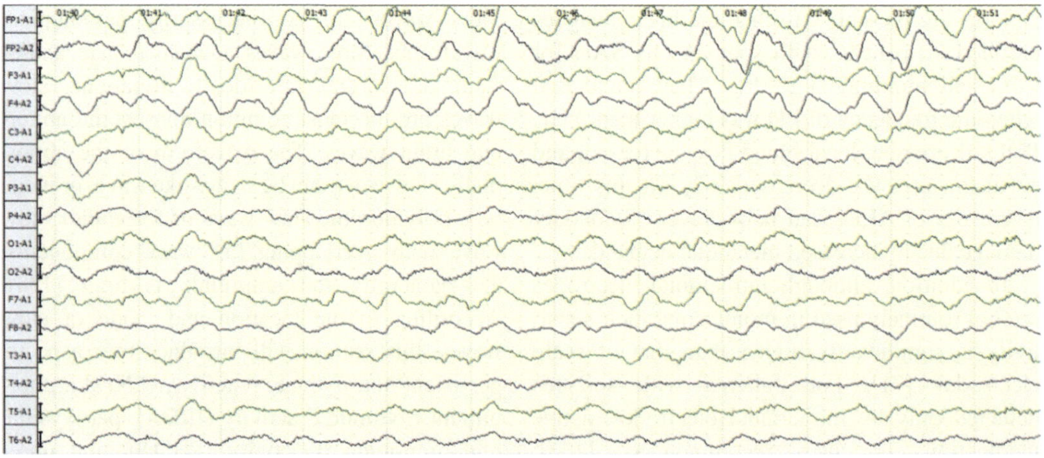


**Fig. 3.23** EEG from a 49-year-old male patient with HIE. The patient was in a superficial coma after undergoing CPR due to fulminant myocarditis. The EEG shows diffuse nonrhythmic δ activity of 1–2 Hz

that the loss of afferent impulses caused by subcortical lesions is an important reason for persistent diffuse slow waves [137].

PNDA is common in the active phase of acute disease and is rare in chronic stable lesions. The degree and number of slow waves often reflect the severity of diffuse encephalopathy [138]. Slow waves dominated by the δ band indicate more serious damage and are often accompanied by disturbances in consciousness, while slow waves with significantly reduced amplitude often reflect more serious damage [139]. In a prospective observational cohort study, 110 patients with sepsis were studied using early standard EEGs (20 min). The slow wave dominated by the δ band was associated with the later development of delirium in severe patients and the increased risk of death in patients, and early standard EEGs helped to predict mortality and identify patients who may develop delirium [140]. A recent study showed that, in children with Sturge–Weber syndrome, persistent severe diffuse nonrhythmic asymmetry slowing may be related to the occurrence of subclinical RSE [141].

### 3.4.2 IRDA

IRDA refers to an EEG pattern that erupts with intermittent, rhythmic monomorphic slow-wave activity. The frequency is usually 1–4 Hz, and the duration is at least 2 s. IRDA appears repeatedly and intermittently throughout the record, sometimes manifesting as migratory asymmetry (Fig. 3.24). The appearance of IRDA is mostly related to status. When patients are alert or with eyes opened, the number or amplitude decreases. However, when patients' eyes are closed, or when hyperventilation or drowsiness occurs, the number increases or the amplitude increases. IRDA disappears after the onset of stage I of NREM sleep but can reappear during REM stage of sleep. According to different parts of the cortex, IRDA can be divided into FIRDA, TIRDA, and occipital intermittent rhythmic δ activity (OIRDA). Among them, FIRDA and OIRDA have the most prominent volatility [142].

In 1945, Cobb et al. [143] first proposed that RDA is nonspecific pathological brain-wave activity that is seen in a variety of neurological diseases. As the understanding of IRDA has deepened, most current researchers believe that IRDA is mainly related to two factors, brain metabolism and brain structure. Metabolic factors include liver and kidney dysfunction, high blood ammonia, hyperlacticaemia, blood sugar or electrolyte disorders, anemia, infection, thyroid function, etc. Watemberg N et al. [144] found that 32% of FIRDA patients have diabetes and 18% of patients have renal failure. It has been reported that 90–98% of patients with Hashimoto encephalopathy may have a nonspecific slow-

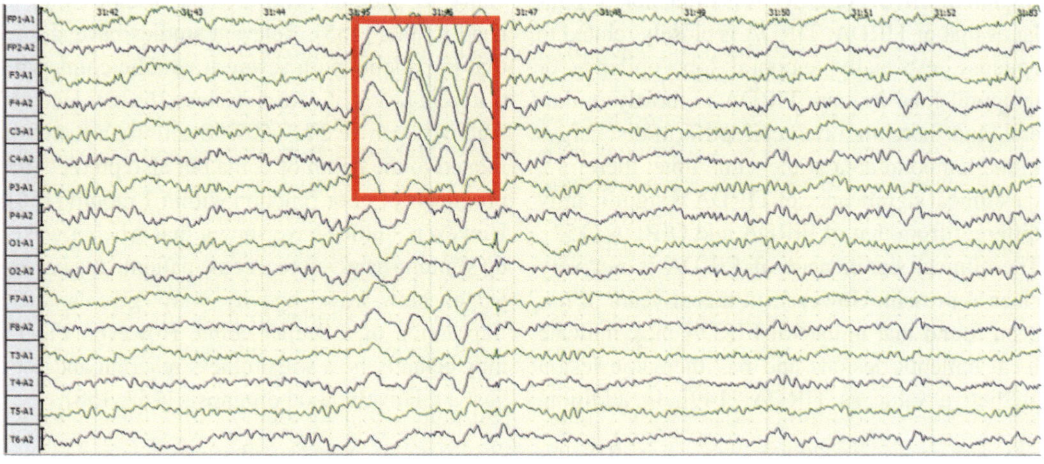


**Fig. 3.24** The EEG of a 45-year-old woman with intracranial infection. The background of EEG is α activity, and IRDA of approximately 2 Hz with medium to high amplitude can be seen in bursts, which last approximately 2 s

down of background activity, and FIRDA may even occur [145]. Structural factors include tumors in the posterior fossa or third ventricle, intracranial hypertension, hydrocephalus, subcortical lesions, generalized or focal epilepsy, basilar-type migraine, corticobasal ganglionic degeneration, progressive supranuclear palsy, Creutzfeldt–Jakob disease, dementia with Lewy bodies, stroke, juvenile Huntington disease, Salmonella infection of the CNS, subacute sclerosing panencephalitis, etc. [118, 146, 147]. There are many theories about the pathophysiological mechanism of IRDA, but they lack direct clinical evidence. The final common pathway may be an abnormality of the thalamus-cortex interaction.

The incidence of IRDA in EEG monitoring in the NICU is 0.4–17.3%, and there is no significant difference in incidence between men and women [148, 149]. IRDA is a nonspecific abnormality with a wide range of origins. The difference in location has nothing to do with the cause. In most cases, IRDA has no obvious relationship with the lesion location. OIRDA is more common in children and is related to brain maturity. IRDA can also be seen in some patients with epilepsy, such as those with typical absence seizures, generalized tonic-clonic seizures (GTCSs), myoclonia with absences, myoclonus, and atonic seizures [148–151]. TIRDA manifests as 2.5–4 Hz δ and slow θ activities and rhythmic or semirhythmic intermittent firing, and the waveform and rhythm of FIRDA or OIRDA is often not as regular as that of TIRDA. TIRDA is closely related to epilepsy, especially temporal lobe epilepsy or temporal lobe lesions. TIRDA is mostly unilateral, and there are often epileptiform discharges in the temporal area at the same time; therefore, the clinical significance of TIRDA is significantly different from that of FIRDA and OIRDA [152]. The clinical significance of FIRDA is not very clear at present. However, in recent years, it has been found that unilateral FIRDA may indicate focal epileptic lesions and has the same lesion predictive value as TIRDA [149]. In addition, IRDA is often accompanied by slower background activities in patients, and some have disturbances in consciousness, especially those with metabolic encephalopathy (Fig. 3.25a, b). IRDA can also occur when healthy people hyperventilate. In this case, IRDA is the normal response of the CNS to changes in the blood partial pressure of carbon dioxide and should not be interpreted as an abnormal phenomenon. Therefore, the EEG phenomenon of IRDA should be explained in combination with specific clinical conditions.

### 3.4.3 PHDA

PHDA mainly manifests as paroxysmal and extensive bilateral δ activity for a long period of time. The frequency of δ activity is 1–2 Hz, with high amplitude. Most PHDA is nonrhythmic and can spontaneously appear or be induced by external stimuli. PHDA is similar to the more continuous K-complex, which can last for several seconds to several minutes. Patients with PHDA often have clinical manifestations of trying to communicate, such as muscle movement and restlessness [153] (Figs. 3.26 and 3.27).

Previous studies have shown that PHDA can occur in very preterm infants with gestational age less than 30 weeks, and slow-wave activity can gradually decrease with increasing gestational age [154]. In severely ill adult patients, PHDA is common in various intracranial lesions, especially in patients who are unconscious due to head trauma [155]. Relevant studies have shown that in patients with severe traumatic coma with different levels of consciousness, the incidence of δ activity can be 27.8–50%. δ activity not only is related to the depth of coma but also predicts the prognosis of poor function within 1 month [156]. However, studies have shown that when a wake-up stimulus is given to a coma patient, this paroxysmal slow-wave activity may give a false impression of a deeper coma. However, PHDA may actually be a wakefulness reaction and suggest a relatively good prognosis [157, 158].

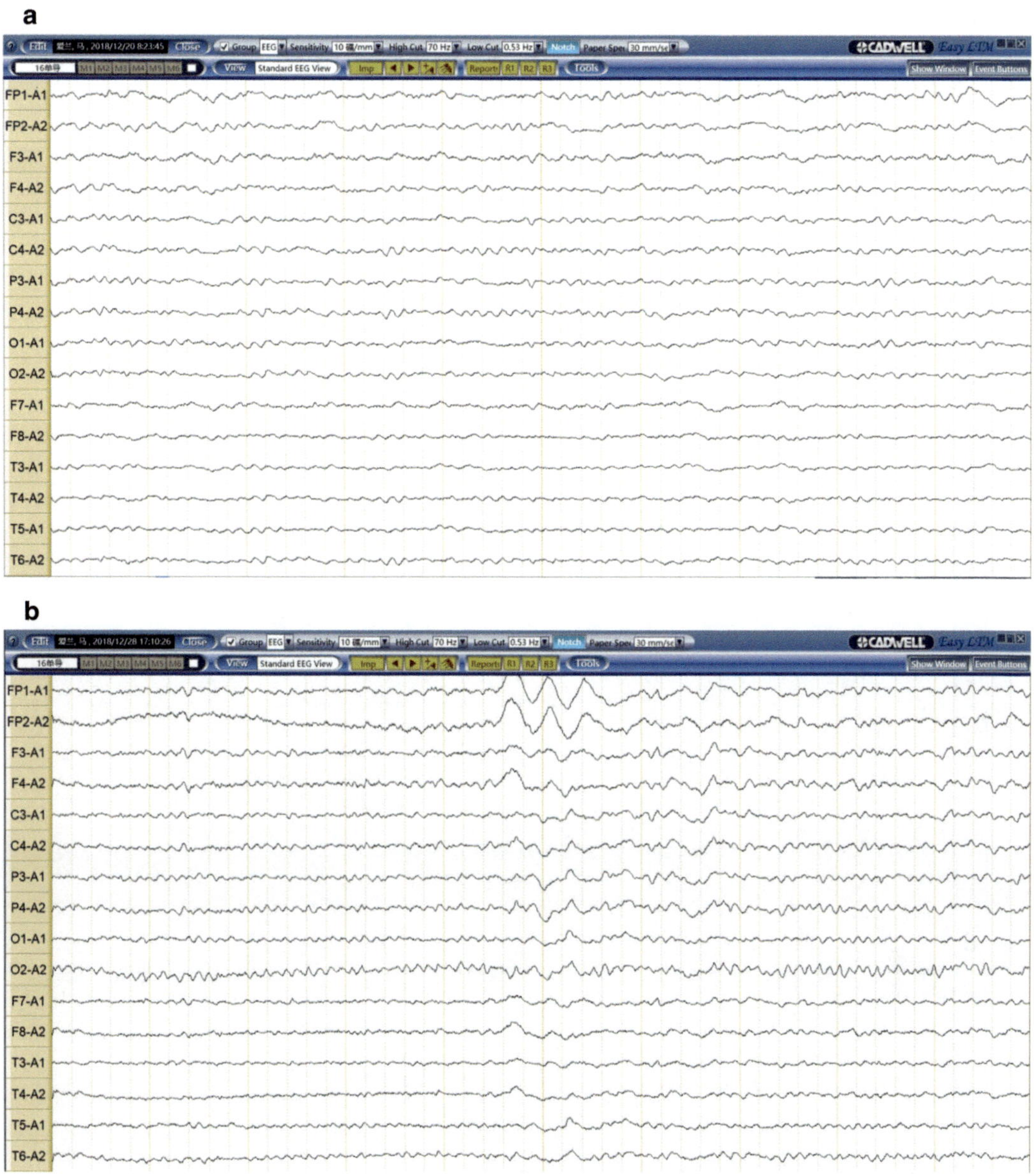


**Fig. 3.25** (**a**) The EEG of a 46-year-old unconscious man with carbon monoxide poisoning. The EEG background is accompanied by slightly more slow-wave activity. (**b**) EEG showing IRDA, which is prominent in the frontal area

## 3.5 α Coma and β Coma

### 3.5.1 Introduction

α or β coma is a rhythmic brain electrical activity in which the EEG background is dominated by a certain frequency band when the patient is in a coma. α or β coma is a pathological abnormal brain electrical activity. Most of this brain electrical activity lacks responsiveness to external stimuli. In addition, α or β coma related to the patient prognosis.

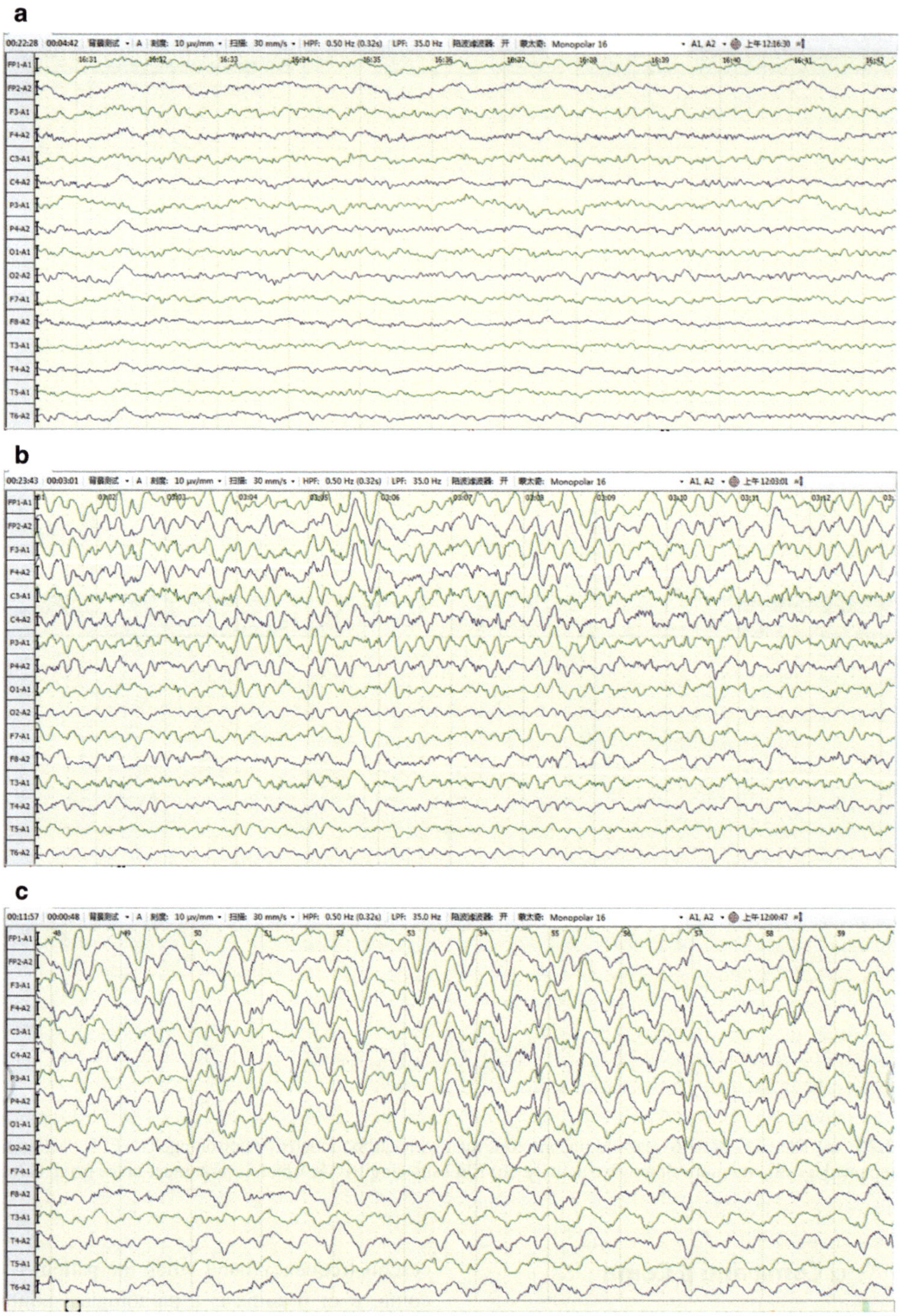


**Fig. 3.26** (**a**) EEG from a 46-year-old man with impaired consciousness after TBI. The background activity of EEG is diffuse slow-wave activity, which is obvious on the right. (**b**) The patient has paroxysmal irritability. The EEG shows high-amplitude δ activity in each lead, and the frontal leads are significant. (**c**) EEG showing that δ activity lasts from a few seconds to a few minutes. (**d**) During EEG monitoring, the patient exhibited irritability and was unable to cooperate with the physical examination. After 5 days, the patient's consciousness improved, and he partially complied with the instructions

d

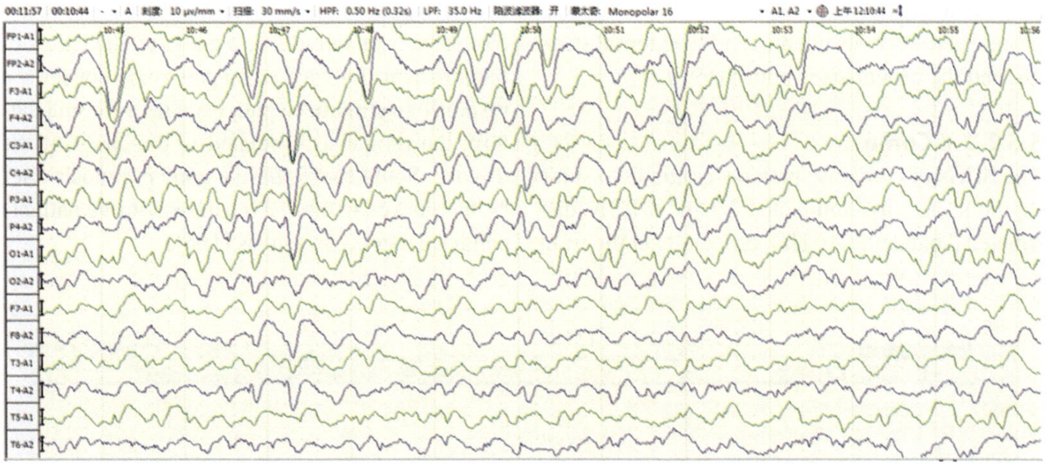

**Fig. 3.26** (continued)

### 3.5.2 Historical Evolution

α coma was first described by Loeb in 1953 [159]. Since then, many scholars have observed this pattern on the EEGs of patients with coma due to multiple causes. The etiology of α coma is different, as are the distribution of α activity, the response to external stimuli, and the prognosis [160–163].

β coma was initially seen only in the brain electrical activity of patients with sedative-drug overdose. Later, it was found that there are similar patterns of β coma in a variety of etiologies, such as HIE and brainstem diseases. The prognosis of patients with a β coma EEG pattern depends on the etiology of their coma and their EEG response to external stimuli [164–167].

### 3.5.3 Concepts

#### 3.5.3.1 α Coma

The EEGs of patients with coma continue to show rhythmic activity dominated by the widely distributed α band (8–13 Hz), and its amplitude is 10–50 μV, especially in the front of the head; this α rhythm can be mixed with θ waves and δ waves, and the α rhythm can be superimposed on the slow wave [166]. The EEGs of most patients with an α coma pattern do not show a response to external stimuli, such as eye opening or closing, light, sound, and pain. Most α coma patterns are related to a poor prognosis (Fig. 3.28).

The α activity of α coma is different from the α rhythm in normal awake and quiet states in terms of spatial distribution, modulation amplitude, and responsiveness to stimuli; and it is not a generalization or advancement of a normal α rhythm.

The α coma pattern is a short-lived pattern that can be transformed into a θ coma, pleomorphic δ coma, BS pattern coma, or β coma pattern after a few days, and it can also coexist with other patterns. During the course of disease, the EEG background activity of some patients with α coma can also switch between different rhythms [166].

The distribution of α activity in α coma pattern depends largely on the cause. Reactive α patterns are usually seen in patients with overdose, and some patients with these patterns can completely recover [168]. α coma can also be seen in patients with toxic encephalopathy. α coma due to poisoning is usually caused by barbiturates, benzodiazepines, anesthetics, and anxiolytics. The responsiveness of the EEG background is usually retained, and the prognosis is good [169, 170]. In contrast, coma patients have obvious α coma patterns at the back of the head, which are more common in brainstem lesions, and the prognosis is poor. α coma is widely observed in patients with HIE after CPR; usually, EEG background activity does not respond to external stimuli, and the prognosis is poor [169, 171].

#### 3.5.3.2 β Coma

The EEGs of comatose patients continue to show rhythmic activity dominated by the widely distributed β band (12–16 Hz), especially at the front of the head, and this rhythmic activity can be β activity alone or β activity mixed with spindle-like activity, α activity, or δ activity. The EEGs of most patients with a β coma pattern do not show a response to stimuli. In patients with a β coma pattern, the prognosis is related to the cause of the disease. Some causes have a good prognosis after being relieved in time. Even unresponsive patients can have a good prognosis [166].

a

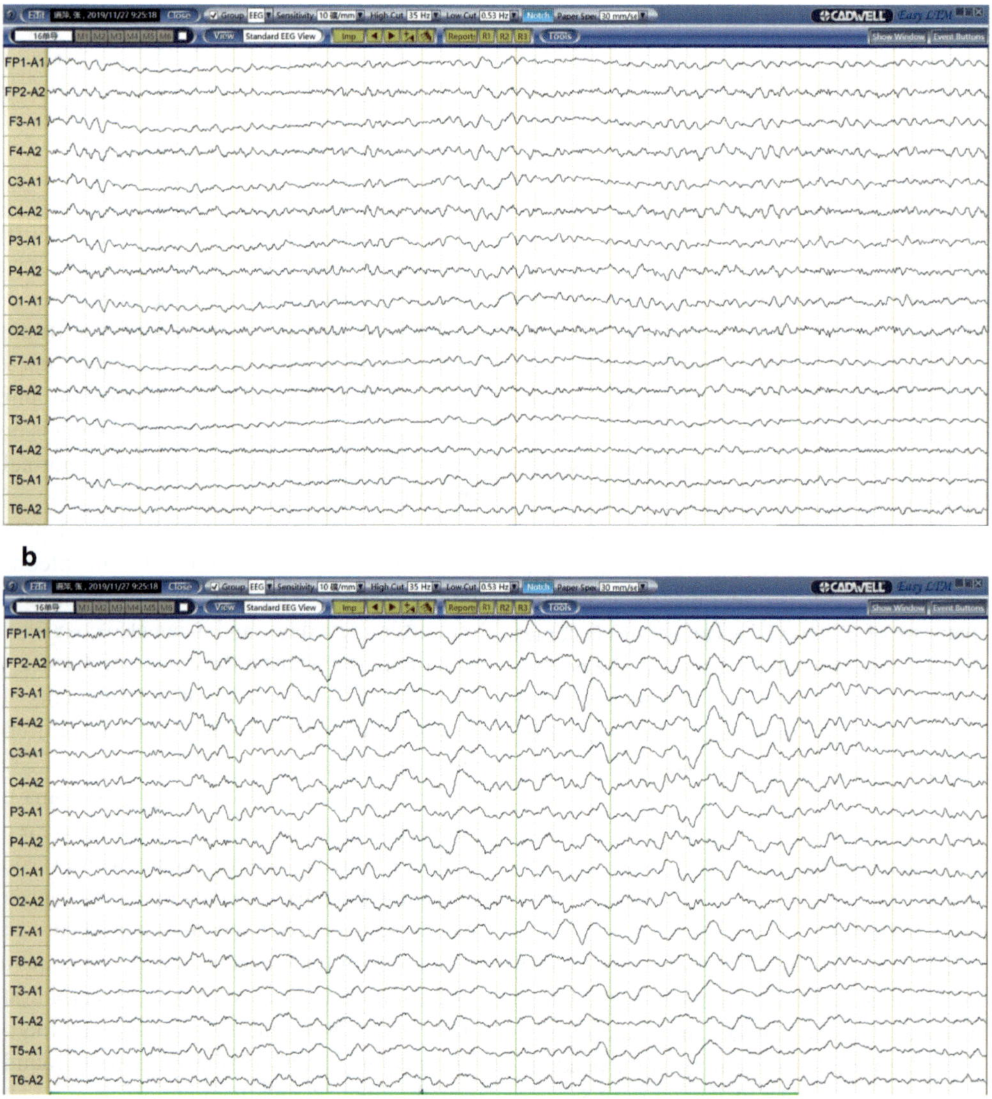


**Fig. 3.27** (**a**) The EEG of a 38-year-old woman with alcoholic encephalopathy. The EEG shows increased background slow-wave activity when she was irritable. (**b**) Intermittent long-range δ activity of 2.0–3.0 Hz with medium amplitude. (**c**) The EEG background activity on the second day was normal, the intermittent slow-wave activity disappeared, and the patient was conscious

c

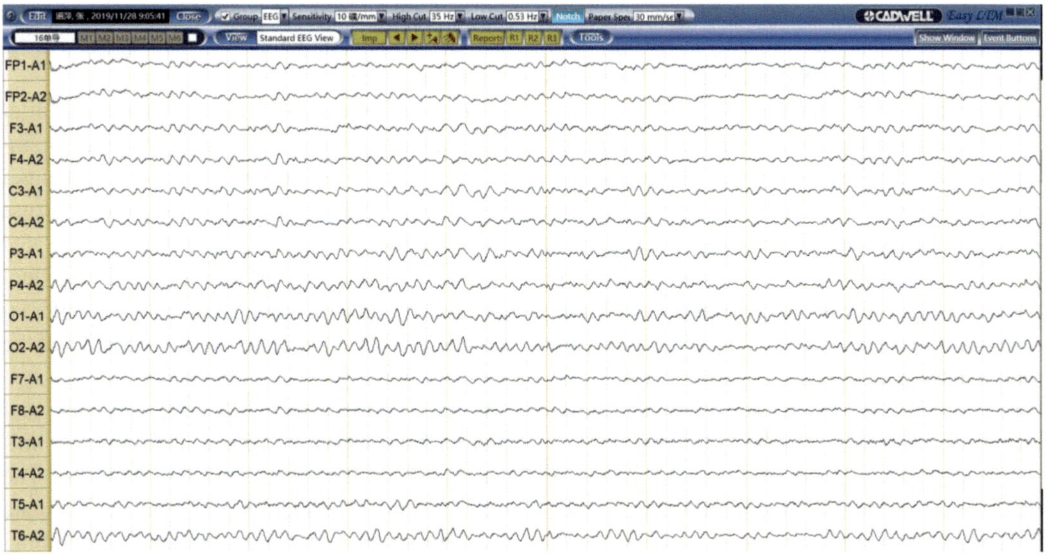

**Fig. 3.27** (continued)

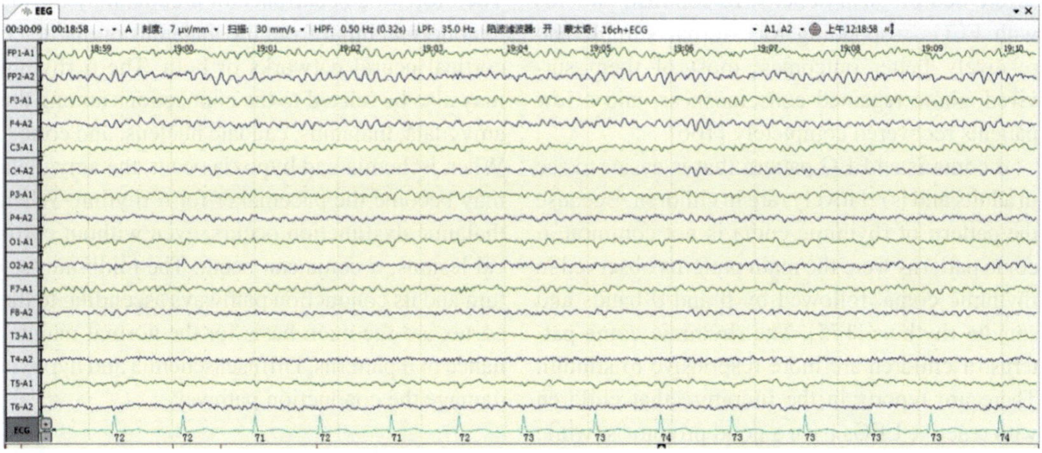

**Fig. 3.28** EEG from a 45-year-old male after CPR, showing diffuse α activity at approximately 8 Hz in each lead and no response to sound, light, or pain stimulation

### 3.5.4 The Clinical Significance and Related Pathological Mechanisms of α Coma and β Coma

#### 3.5.4.1 α Coma

It was originally thought that coma accompanied by α coma patterns appeared only in patients with cerebrovascular disease in the pons and midbrain. Later, it was reported in the literature that this pattern could also be seen after successful CPR from cardiac arrest, brain hypoxia, brain trauma, metabolic encephalopathy, drug or chemical toxic encephalopathy, atresia syndrome, encephalitis, and thalamic tumors, even in 2-year-old children with acute brain injury or hypoglycemia, generally indicating a poor prognosis [163, 172, 173]. The prognosis is related to the etiology and the degree of brain injury.

**Hypoxic Encephalopathy**

There are many reports of α coma in patients with hypoxic encephalopathy, mainly focusing on the prognosis of patients. Most survivors have residual neurological dysfunction [163, 174].

EEG activity in patients with hypoxic encephalopathy is based on α activity, which is diffuse and widespread, especially in the frontal area. There are also some patients whose EEG background activity shows a coexistence of α and θ activities. α activity is mostly transient and rarely responds to external stimuli. However, compared with α activity caused by brainstem vascular disease in α coma, α pattern after hypoxia has more changes and reactivity and lasts longer.

The responsiveness of EEG background activity to external stimuli is the main factor in judging prognosis. A study reported that the prognosis of patients with anergy was poor, most of them died, and most of the survivors were left with severe neurological deficits. In contrast, patients with EEGs responding to external stimuli had relatively better outcomes, most of them survived, some regained consciousness, and a few patients recovered completely [166].

α coma is an EEG pattern that is easier to see in adults and is relatively rare in children. Because the pattern of rhythmic coma is not common, α coma patterns were the main patterns observed in rhythmic coma, followed by β and θ bands and spindle rhythms [175]. The rhythmic coma patterns of children are more responsive to stimuli. There are reports in the literature that children with reactive EEGs have a good prognosis, while those with nonresponsive EEGs have a poor prognosis [176]. It has been reported that the prognosis of children with α coma is similar to that of children with other types of rhythmic coma patterns, such as α, θ, β, or spindle rhythm patterns. Studies have shown that an unresponsive α coma pattern has higher predictive value in adults [170].

It is recommended to perform EEG monitoring immediately after coma onset because, in addition to α activity during coma, EEG activity before α activity has predictive value. All reports showed that the initial brain electrical activity of patients with α coma after hypoxia was equipotential or BS, and most of these patients died. The initial brain electrical activity was θ and/or δ activity, and the patients with subsequent α coma were all awake [177].

The observation of patients with α coma after hypoxia who died did not reveal obvious brainstem abnormalities but diffuse abnormal changes that are typical after cerebral hypoxia. Diffuse abnormalities can damage the structures related to α activity and rhythm formation. The production of a normal α rhythm is related to the interaction between the thalamus–cortex system and the cortex–cortex system, and the cortex–cortex system has a greater effect [178, 179]. Animal model studies have shown that the transmission of similar rhythms to the cortex can cause α rhythm. The cortex receives periodic input signals to simulate the activity of the thalamus. When the incoming signal disappears, the system is disrupted, causing contact disorder or a loss of contact [180]. Therefore, the occurrence of α coma may be due to abnormal input from the thalamus or disrupted cortical neural networks or both. The α rhythm may also be related to the connections among the amygdala, thalamus, caudate nucleus, and cortex. When ischemia and hypoxia occur, the amygdala may become the pacemaker for α rhythm. When thalamic dysfunction occurs, even without cortical lesions, α coma can occur. The midbrain tectum and its conduction pathways ascending to the cortex are the main basis for the normal maintenance of α patterns. Diffuse ischemia and hypoxia damage the conduction pathway.

**HIE After CPR**

The incidence of α coma pattern after CPR is approximately 12%, and α coma pattern can be seen in adults, children, and infants [163, 171]. α activity is widely distributed, prominently in the forehead area; the waveform is mostly sinusoidal; and the amplitude of the wave is rarely changed. α waves can be mixed with varying amounts of θ or δ waves. The EEGs of these patients rarely respond to sound, light, or other harmful stimuli.

Most patients with α coma after CPR have a poor prognosis, and the prognosis is related to the duration of CPR. A short duration of CPR allows survival, but there will be severe neurological deficits. The mortality rate is high, and only a few of these patients survive or recover completely [171]. However, there are reports in the literature that there is no significant difference in the prognosis of patients with or without α coma. The prognosis mainly depends on the cause and the response of α coma pattern to stimulation.

The α coma pattern often appears within a few hours to 4 days after the coma, and even up to 6–9 days. The pattern will change with the change in the condition. When the condition is aggravated, the pattern can convert to periodic activity or BS and finally ECS [177]. Some patients continue to have varying degrees of extensive or focal abnormalities, and these patients can progress into a vegetative state (VS) [181]. When the condition improves, the α coma pattern first changes to a pattern with extensive theta activity and then gradually to a normal physiological rhythm; when awake, the α rhythm is limited to the occipital and posterior temporal regions, and the α rhythm has regulation and amplitude modulation phenomena, with eye-opening and eye-closing reactions and light-driven responses, and a normal sleep pattern and wake-up cycle.

**Overdose**

Drug overdose can also cause α coma. α coma due to drug overdose is related to the following drugs: amitriptyline, imipramine, barbiturates, benzodiazepines (diazepam, lorazepam, medazepam, nitrazepam), chloromethylthiazole, clomethiazole, glutamine, trimethoprim, and anesthetics [176]. It has been reported that an overdose of bupropion can also cause α coma, which can completely recover after a short period of time [173, 182]. The α rhythm of α coma caused by drug overdose is short-lived, usually predominantly or diffusely distributed in the frontal area, and nonresponsive, but the prognosis is good. The α rhythm of α coma can fully recover to normal rhythm within a few days.

Benzodiazepines are taken as an example to analyze α coma caused by overdose. Benzodiazepines mainly act on the limbic system and brainstem, reduce the spontaneous and induced neuronal electrical activity of the hippocampus and dorsal locus coeruleus of the pons, and inhibit the arousal system. Benzodiazepines may also cause a link disorder between the reticular structure and the nonspecific nucleus of the thalamus. These midline nuclei directly or indirectly affect the occurrence of cortical EPSPs, resulting in α electrical activity recorded on scalp EEGs [165]. The mechanism of the widespread α activity, particularly in the front of the head, that causes α coma may be as follows: dysfunction in the ventral and precentral thalamic nuclei and nonspecific nuclei of the hypothalamus that mainly connect with the frontal cortex selectively causes the ascending reticulothalamic activity to decrease or disappear.

**Cerebrovascular Disease and Brain Trauma**

The α activity of patients with α coma caused by brainstem stroke is especially observed at the back of the head, with variability and reactivity. The analysis of α-coma-related studies of brainstem lesions showed that the mortality rate was high, which was related to lesion etiology and the coexistence of multiple etiologies [183]. The prognosis of patients with α coma from brainstem vascular disease is very poor. Most patients die soon after awakening, and a few patients may have neurological dysfunction of varying degrees. Individual patients with α coma with vertebrobasilar artery ischemia can fully recover [159, 184].

α coma caused by brainstem vascular disease or TBI is found mainly in the transitional parts of the midbrain and pons in the brainstem, and these diseases or injuries mostly cause structural destructive lesions. The possible causes of the destructive brainstem lesions leading to α coma are as follows: (**a**) Damage to the bilateral pontine cover, base of the pontine and midbrain, as well as damage to the reticular structure, can block the reticulothalamic pathway, producing α activity. (**b**) Lesions located at or below the pons-midbrain transition can damage the pons or midbrain tegmental part and the midbrain tegmental part of the ascending conduction beam, which is the site where normal α rhythm is maintained. (**c**) Damage to the pontine reticular structure, especially bilateral damage, will reduce the level of consciousness. Vascular α activity is usually a transient phenomenon with poor reactivity. When the brainstem is damaged, the α rhythm of the α coma is not reactive. This can be used to identify atresia syndrome, because the α rhythm of atresia syndrome is reactive [183].

#### 3.5.4.2 β Coma

**Overdose**

β coma can be seen in patients with sedative drug overdose or sedative drug withdrawal, and it is most common in sedative-hypnotic overdose. For example, high-dose benzodiazepine and barbiturate poisoning can cause widespread fast-wave activity in the β band. β activity is often issued in a spindle-like rhythm, with the highest amplitude in front of the head [185]. The EEG background activity's response to stimuli depends on the depth of the coma. Reactivity can be retained, but there is no response in deep coma. If acute poisoning is treated promptly, the prognosis is good. Patients with unresponsive β coma may also have a good prognosis.

In severely ill patients, intravenous midazolam has the same effect as other benzodiazepines; namely, it activates β activity at therapeutic doses. At high doses, intravenous midazolam causes diffuse slow waves and increases in 10–16 Hz activity and 10–30 Hz fast activity. High doses of intravenous midazolam rarely causes α coma [165].

**Brain Injury**

β coma can also be seen in patients with brain trauma, often with poor prognosis. Brain injury may be related to β coma through the following mechanism: Oscillating waves passing through the skull during brain trauma can cause diffuse brain tissue damage; cerebrovascular traction, squeezing, and tearing; and secondary brain damage, such as blood-brain barrier damage and inflammation. These effects lead to increased release of sex factors, excess free radicals, and increases in glutamate neurotransmitters and $Ca2+$ and $Na+$, all of which can enter neurons, and, among other effects, damage mitochondria, leading to neuronal necrosis, cerebral edema, and increased ICP. The above factors lead to extensive brain damage, affecting nonspecific nuclei of the thalamus, pons, midbrain tegmentum, and other areas [178].

**Brainstem Disease**

Early EEGs from patients with brainstem focal damage caused by acute and severe vertebrobasilar artery blood supply disorder can manifest low-amplitude β activity. These patients all die in a short time after the appearance of β coma. Animal experiments have found that, when the transitional part of the pons and midbrain is cut off or the brainstem is strongly stimulated, low-amplitude fast activity can be seen. The effect of acute brainstem damage is similar to that of a cut brainstem or strong stimulation of the brainstem [186]. The formation of the β coma pattern may also be located in the lower brainstem, which is related to damage to the synchronization function of the lower brainstem. The ascending activation system of the brainstem network structure is blocked, but the cortex is not damaged or the damage is light [187, 188].

#### 3.5.4.3 Cases

(1) α coma (Figs. 3.29, 3.30, 3.31, and 3.32)
(2) β coma (Fig. 3.33)

## 3.6 BS Pattern in EEG

BS is a phenomenon that occurs in EEGs, and it is characterized by alternating high-amplitude fulminant activity and electrical attenuation (low voltage $\geq 10\ \mu V$ but less than 50% of background voltage) or electrical suppression (low voltage $<10\ \mu V$). Electrical attenuation or electrical suppression usually exceeds 50% of the recording time. The outbreak parts are mostly irregular slow waves, with a voltage of 150–350 μV, mixed with multifocal spikes. The duration of the outbreak must exceed 0.5 s on average, and the longest can reach 30 s. The suppression parts are almost flat, and the interval between two bursts is mostly 5–10 s (Fig. 3.34). In recent years, BS has often been used to predict the prognosis of diseases, and the methodology to identify BS has also been greatly improved [189–195].

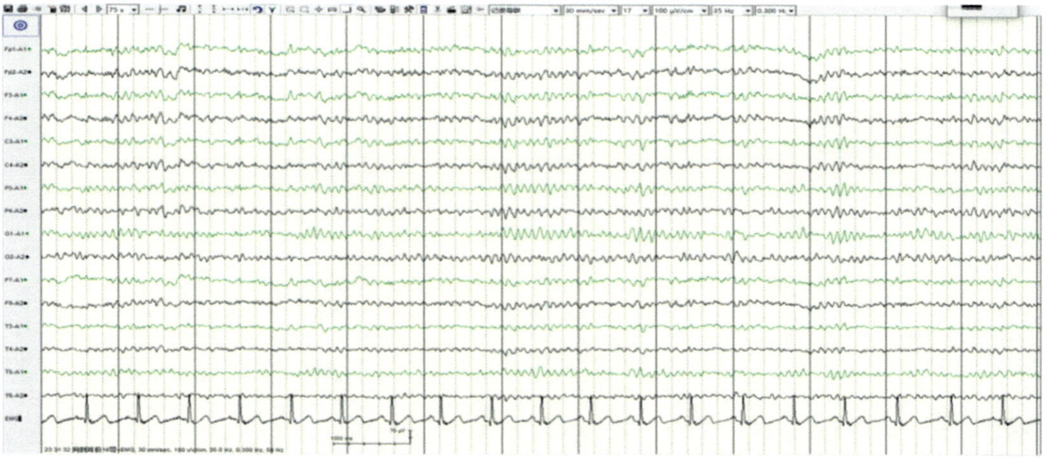

**Fig. 3.29** EEG from a healthy adult in the awake period: the waveform is regular; the amplitude is medium; the α rhythm of the occipital lobe is sinusoidal; and bilateral symmetry, regulation, and amplitude modulation are good

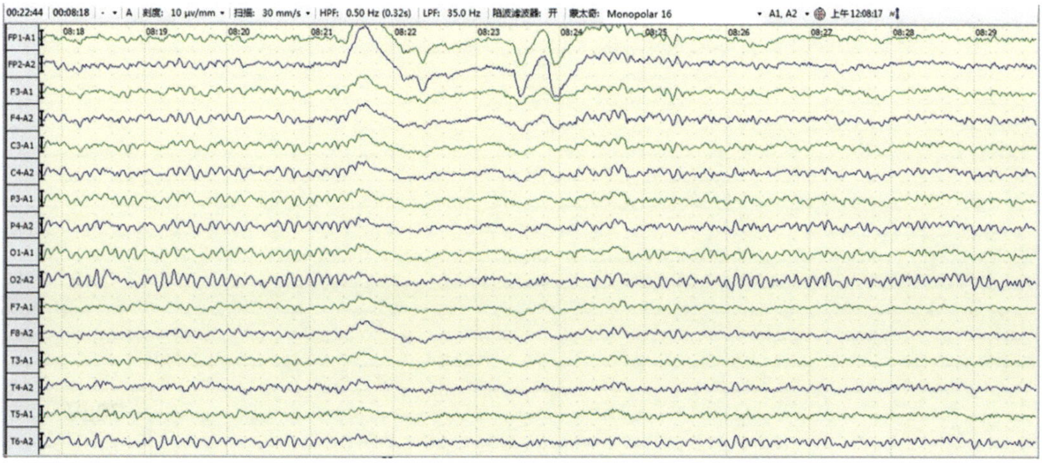

**Fig. 3.30** In a healthy state, the α rhythm of the occipital lobe disappears after the eyes open and appears after the eyes close

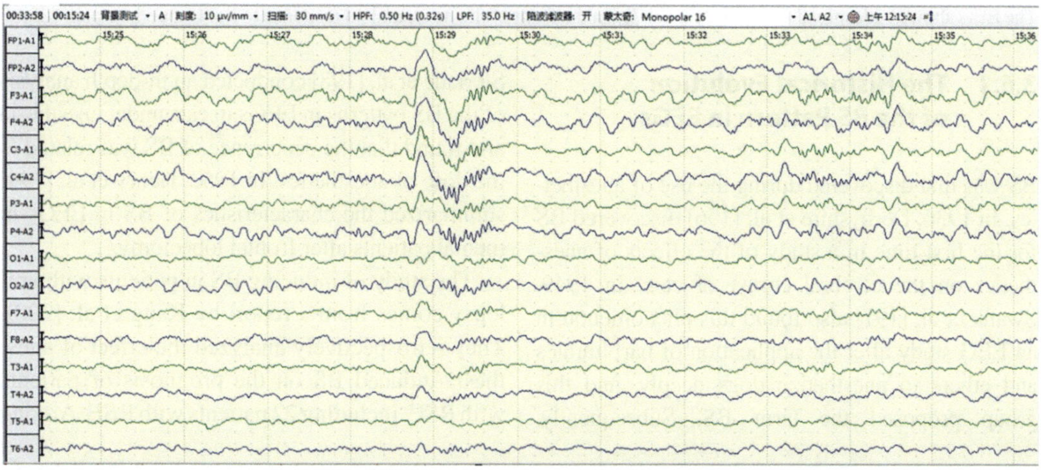

**Fig. 3.31** A normal sleep-wake cycle and apical, spindle, and K-C waves are visible in stage II sleep

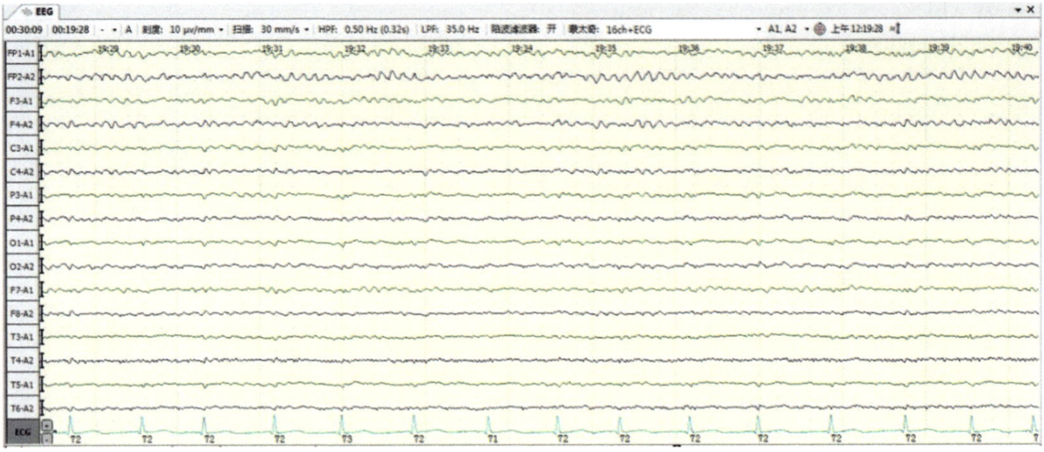


**Fig. 3.32** EEG from a 41-year-old male comatose patient at 12 h after CPR after cardiac arrest, showing a wide distribution of α activity, especially in the anterior part of the head. There was no response to light, sound, or pain

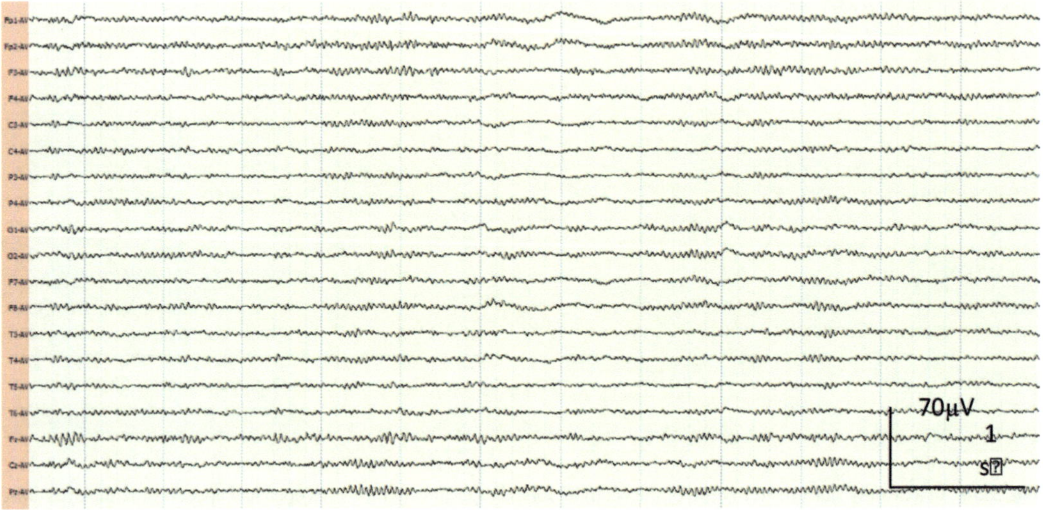


**Fig. 3.33** EEG from a 34-year-old female patient found to be in a coma 6 h after taking a large amount of estazolam. The EEG shows widespread β activity, especially in the front of the head, and no response to light, sound, or pain stimuli

### 3.6.1 The Historical Evolution of the BS Pattern in EEGs

BS was first discovered during the use of anesthetics. In 1936, Derbyshire et al. [196] discovered BS for the first time in a study of the effects of anesthetics on the cerebral cortex of cats. In 1949, Swank et al. [197] also found this phenomenon in an EEG study after the application of barbiturates and ethers to anesthetize dogs deeply, and this group proposed the term BS. Subsequently, Steriade et al. [198] conducted an in-depth analysis of the BS patterns in EEGs in cats under anesthesia and found that the occurrence of BS was related to the dose of anesthetics. In 1952, Henry et al. [199] summarized the characteristics of BS in EEGs in mental patients after frontal lobectomy.

The study of inducing BS in patients with epilepsy comes from a report by Kang et al. [200]. They retrospectively analyzed the effect of anesthesia-induced BS on the prognosis of patients with RSE, including 22 patients with RSE. Among

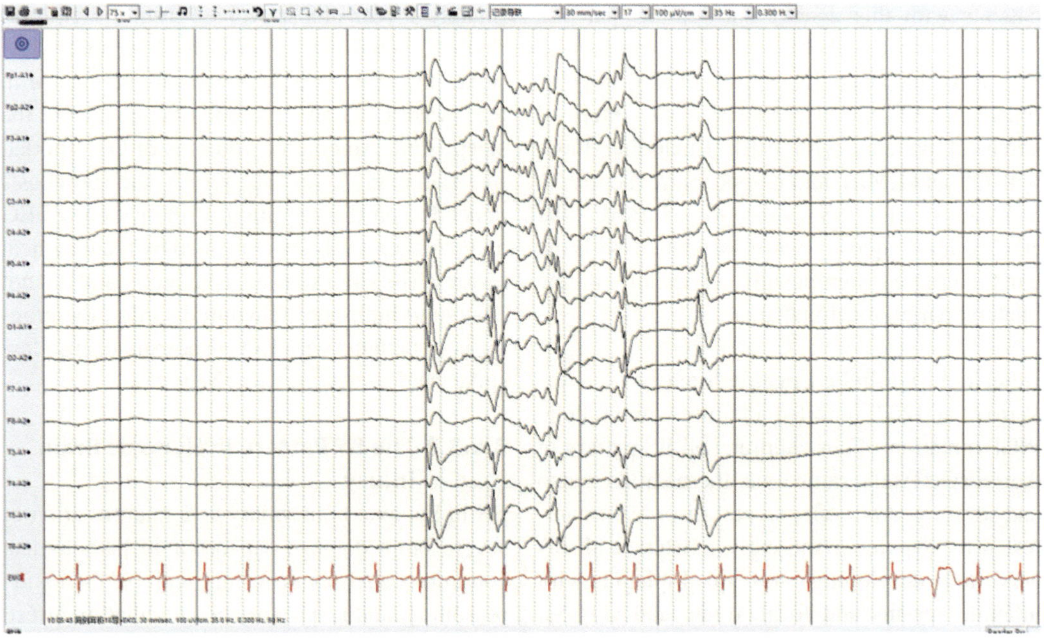

**Fig. 3.34** EEG from a 51-year-old male who was injured in a car accident and in a deep coma, showing a generalized SE pattern, with a burst time of approximately 4 s followed by a long-term full suppression waveform

them, 6 patients (27.5%) were found to have BS, but it had nothing to do with the prognosis, which promoted research on the clinical significance of BS in EEGs.

### 3.6.2 The Possible Mechanism of BS Patterns

The pathophysiological mechanism of BS in EEGs is unclear. Existing studies suggest that BS is related to the disorder of cortex-subcortical regulation, the interruption of contact, and excessive discharge of subcortical neurons caused by cortical damage [201]. It is also speculated that there are remnants of neurons in the white matter of the brain that are necessary for the development of neonatal cortical tissue and that undergo apoptosis gradually after birth. Such remnant neurons can lead to the interruption of cortical-subcortical contact and BS [202]. Chakravarty et al. [191] believe that the burst pattern and suppression pattern are related to the consumption and regeneration of adenosine triphosphate (ATP) resources, respectively, in the cortical network.

### 3.6.3 The BS Pattern in Different Diseases

#### 3.6.3.1 The BS Pattern in Epileptic Encephalopathy

**Early Myoclonic Encephalopathy (EME)**

EME is a rare and severe epileptic encephalopathy. In 1978, Aicardi et al. [203] found for the first time that BS may appear in the EEGs of patients with EME, manifesting as pseudoperiodic burst activity under a low-voltage background rhythm. Subsequently, Liu et al. [204] studied the clinical and EEG characteristics of EME and found that the manifestations in the EEGs of these patients were repetitive, paroxysmal, short-term bursts and long-term suppression. One out of three patients showed bilateral brain BS asynchrony. It is suggested that BS is an important manifestation of EME in childhood.

**Ohtahara Syndrome (OS)**

OS is also known as early infantile epileptic encephalopathy (EIEE). In 1976, it was first described by Ohtahara et al, so it is called OS [201, 205]. This group found that the EEGs in patients with this disease showed BS patterns similar to those of EME, which can be seen in both wake and sleep. Later, Toda et al. [206] also found that BS can also appear in the interictal EEGs of patients with EIEE (including those with OS and EME), and it appears frequently. In 6 patients with BS with OS or EME, the 80–150 Hz frequency wave associated with the burst increased significantly, especially in the bilateral parieto-occipital area.

**Inherited Metabolic Encephalopathy**

Vetro et al. [207] reported a family with biallelic PIGP mutations. Four children had BS pattern in their EEGs. At the same time, these children also had severe neurodevelopmental disorders, manifested by hypotonia and early movement disorders and developing into quadriplegia with infantile spasms and focal, tonic, and GTCSs. Two of the children died between the ages of 2 and 12 years old; the other two children were 2 years and 7 months and 7 years and 4 months old. Gene sequencing revealed that they had PIGP homozygous c.384del mutations, and functional studies revealed that the expression of GPI-AP CD16 in the granular cell membrane of individuals was reduced. The authors believe that PIGP mutations have the characteristics of EIEE, and CD16 is a valuable marker for the diagnosis of hereditary glycosylphosphatidylinositol (GPI) defects.

**The Laws of BS Patterns in Epileptic Encephalopathy**

The prognosis of EME and OS is extremely poor, and the mortality rate is high. Approximately 1/3 of the children will die within 1 year. Many cases of OS transform into Lennox–Gastaut syndrome or West syndrome at 3–6 months [201, 202, 208]. When OS changes to West syndrome, gradual changes in EEGs from BS to high-grade rhythm disorder can be observed. At the beginning of the transition, the amplitude of the suppressing phase increases gradually; the disappearance of BS during wakefulness precedes that during sleep, which means that when the awake EEG shows a high rhythm disorder, the EEG during sleep continues to show BS [206]. Furthermore, at approximately 1 year old, it evolved from a high-level rhythm disorder to a diffuse slow spike-slow wave. In the process of evolution, the change in the awake EEG also preceded the change in the sleep EEG. Among the 16 cases of OS reported by Yamatogi Y et al. [208], the prognosis depended on the evolution of the patient's EEG and whether it was accompanied by focal cortical lesions. The EEG showed asymmetry and did not change to high-grade rhythm disorder; the prognosis of patients with EEGs showing diffuse low spikes and slow waves was better.

#### 3.6.3.2 The BS Pattern in Hypoxic Brain Injury

BS in hypoxic brain injury as a manifestation of severe brain damage can occur in pathological conditions such as drowning, carbon monoxide poisoning, and respiratory and circulatory arrest. Neonatal patients with severe HIE can also further develop ECS and brain death on this basis. Survivors mostly have neurological sequelae of varying degrees [209].

BS, as a manifestation of severe brain damage, is helpful in determining the prognosis of the disease. Barbella et al. [193] analyzed the characteristics of 522 patients with successful cardiac arrest and CPR. A total of 147 (28%) patients showed BS in their EEGs, and 10 of them (7%) had a good prognosis. Of these patients, 129 (88%) died, and the authors suggested that BS has value in the prediction of the prognosis of this type of disease. Amorim et al. [210] retrospectively analyzed the clinical characteristics and the EEGs of 373 patients who resumed spontaneous circulation after cardiac arrest. They found that the positive predictive value for the poor prognosis of patients with both nonresponse and outbreak suppression EEG performance was 100% (95% CI [0.96–1.00]), and the false-positive rate was 0% (95% CI [0.00–0.11]). At the same time, they also found that simple BS in patients without SE or seizures after taking anesthetics could not independently predict poor prognosis. Westhall et al. [211] used conventional EEG to predict the prognosis of patients after CPR, and they found that BS during resuscitation is a highly malignant pattern in EEGs, and the prognosis of these patients is poor. In a study on whether the background type in EEGs can predict the prognosis of patients with coma after cardiac arrest, Hofmeijer et al. [194] found that in the first 24 h of onset, most patients with constant BS and persistent anergy and low voltage in EEGs had a poor prognosis. The ability to quickly restore cEEG patterns within 12 h may indicate a good prognosis. The relationship between BS and HIE is also supported by evidence-based medical research. Awal et al. [212] conducted a meta-analysis on the relationship between background activity in EEGs and neurodevelopment in a neonate with HIE. Thirty-one studies were included, and it was found that patients with HIE who had BS had a poor prognosis (sensitivity 0.87 (95% CI [0.78–0.92]); specificity 0.82 (95% CI [0.72–0.88])).

Chalia et al. [213] also studied the relationship between BS and changes in cerebral hemodynamics and found that significant changes in oxygen and deoxy-protein concentrations corresponding to transient bursts in EEGs were seen in six infants.

#### 3.6.3.3 The Effect of Anesthetics on BS Patterns

BS is a manifestation of severe suppression of neuronal electrical activity under deep anesthesia. Existing studies have shown that ether, barbiturates, and various anesthetics may induce BS in the EEGs of deeply anesthetized humans and animals [1] (Fig. 3.35). Recovery can be achieved with the withdrawal of anesthetics. If the degree of anesthesia is deepened, the electrical activity of neurons on the EEG may disappear. In addition, drug-resistant refractory CSE requires the use of anesthetics to induce BS to control seizures. Therefore, the effect of anesthetics on BS needs to be excluded when evaluating the prognosis of patients [214].

Hogan et al. [215] analyzed the relationship among disease, anesthetics, BS, and prognosis in 471 neurocritical patients. They found that the severity of disease and BS were related to patient prognosis. Although propofol could cause BS, it had no obvious effect on the mortality of the disease. Its prognostic impact is achieved by affecting BS. Therefore, they believe that BS seems to cause death, but it is mainly the impact of serious diseases rather than iatrogenic using propofol. Martinez-Bermejo et al. [216] analyzed the relationship between neonatal BS and the etiology and prognosis of disease. They found that 30 patients who experienced BS with no administration of piperidines (including 14 patients with HIE, 4 patients with meningitis, 4 patients with OS, 2 patients with EME, 3 patients with multiple organ failure, 1 patient with nonketotic hyperglycinemia, 1 patient with leucine hyperplasia, and 1 patient with narcotic drug use) all had a poor prognosis, and those with a BS pattern due

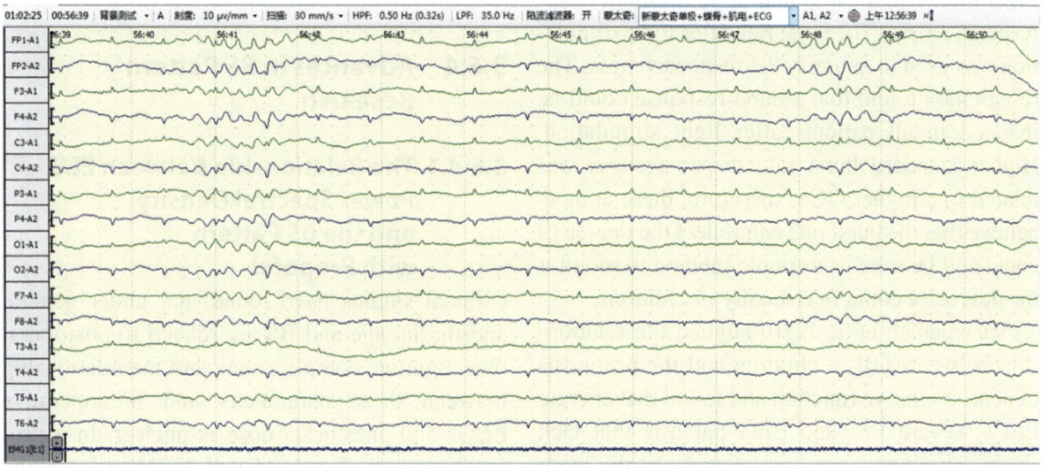


**Fig. 3.35** The EEG of a patient with SE, showing the BS pattern after the administration of 100 mg propofol

to the use of piperidines (3 patients) had a relatively good prognosis, indicating that the effect of anesthetics needs to be excluded when BS occurs in the disease.

#### 3.6.3.4 The BS Pattern and Postanesthesia Delirium

Among patients recovering from general anesthesia, delirium is the most common brain dysfunction. Not only is the pathophysiological cause unclear, but the relationship between BS and delirium in intraoperative EEGs is also unclear. To understand the relationship between them, many scholars have carried out relevant analyses [217, 218]. In a cohort study on whether BS is an effective predictor of delirium under sedation, Andresen et al. [217] found that the duration of BS during coma is an independent predictor of delirium after coma or deep sedation, but this view is not widely accepted. Koch et al. [218] conducted a prospective, observational cohort study. Ninety-seven children were included in the study, 40 of whom developed delirium, and 57 children did not have delirium. The results showed that there was no significant difference in the incidence of BS in the EEG and the duration of delirium between the two groups.

#### 3.6.3.5 The BS Pattern in Brain Injury

Nita et al. [219] monitored the EEGs of children in the ICU in a coma with brain injury due to different causes. Five patients with BS were given intermittent light stimulation to evaluate their responsiveness. The burst rate after light stimulation was used to quantify the responsiveness. The researchers found that a burst response could be induced in all patients after light stimulation. Higher standard burst rate responsiveness was related to a higher GCS; therefore, these authors believe that the burst rate can reflect the degree of coma and be used as a simple method to monitor the degree of coma in critically ill children.

Vaewpanich et al. [220] studied the relationship between TBI in children and the prognosis of neurocognitive function and found that anergic EEGs, severe BS, and EEG patterns that lack sleep structure are associated with poor prognosis.

#### 3.6.3.6 The BS Pattern in the Dying State

At the end of life, patients often have respiratory and circulatory failure, which, in turn, affects the CNS, and BS may appear on EEGs. As the disease progresses, the suppression period becomes increasingly longer, the burst wave decreases, the amplitude of the wave is gradually reduced, and the wave becomes simpler and finally develops into an ECS state. Zhou et al. [221] used a clustering method to analyze the changes in the EEG spectrum during BS and found that BS is a manifestation of the plurality of states of brain function. Kang et al. [222] monitored the EEGs of patients in the ICU with consciousness disorders and found that those with BS and persistent $\theta$ rhythm on background activities had a higher mortality rate.

#### 3.6.3.7 The BS Pattern in Metabolic Encephalopathy

Hyperammonemia is a common cause of metabolic encephalopathy and is related to many factors. Patients with hyperammonemic encephalopathy may also manifest BS on EEG. Leidi et al. [223] reported a case of an 81-year-old white male who initially showed drowsiness and then went into a coma. The EEG showed intermittent BS. He was diagnosed with hyperammonemic encephalopathy. He recovered well after supportive treatment. An examination of his EEG showed that his brain activity was normal.

### 3.6.4 Advances in BS Pattern Research

#### 3.6.4.1 The Relationship Between EEG Power Spectral Density and the BS Pattern with Propofol

Clinical studies have found that under general anesthesia, age and BS are related to postoperative cognitive complications, but the relationship between these parameters and intraoperative EEGs and anesthesia dose is unclear. In a prospective study, Touchard et al. [224] analyzed the relationship between propofol dose and $\alpha$-band power spectral density in the EEGs of 59 patients. They found that BS could be induced in the first few minutes of general anesthesia. At this time, the power spectral density in the EEG was reduced significantly ($p = 0.001$), which is considered to be a marker of brain damage and is negatively correlated with age.

#### 3.6.4.2 The Use of FDG-PET Combined with the BS Pattern to Predict the Effect of Drug Treatment

Akbik et al. [225] conducted a study on the use of FDG-PET combined with BS to predict the efficacy of AEDs in six patients with seizures and severe neurological damage. The inclusion of each patient was based on the absence of BS in the FDG-PET results. When BS appeared on an EEG, FDG-PET examination was performed. The results showed that the drugs could effectively inhibit the FDG-PET high-metabolism area, and the effect was good. If the drug had no effect on the high-metabolic area, the effect was poor.

In conclusion, BS, as a severely abnormal EEG pattern, can well reflect the functional activity of brain neurons and can evaluate the depth of anesthesia induction and the severity of life-threatening pathological conditions. In the treatment of RSE, BS can be used as an important marker for drug use.

## 3.7 Nonreactive Low-Voltage Slow Activity and ECS

Patients with severe neurological diseases often suffer from brain injury. Different degrees of consciousness disturbance may occur because of differences in damage location and degree. EEG changes often occur earlier than clinical symptoms, and early judgments on brain function can be made on the basis of these changes. In clinical practice, EEGs mostly present nonspecific changes due to the degree of consciousness disorder resulting from various causes and the different parts of the brain injured; among these changes, diffuse slow-wave activity is one of the most common. The length of the slow-wave activity cycle is closely related to the degree of coma, which has been proven by increasing evidence. In patients with extreme coma, the amplitude of slow waves decreases and waves become flat, showing low-voltage slow-wave activity [226, 227].

Nonreactive low-voltage slow activity is mainly characterized by θ and δ activity continuously lower than 20 μV (Figs. 3.36, 3.37, 3.38,

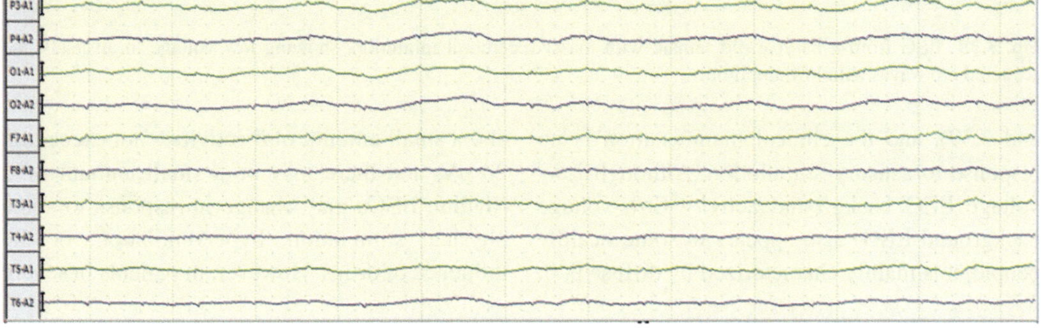


**Fig. 3.36** EEG from a 68-year-old male with HIE, showing diffuse δ activity below 20 μV

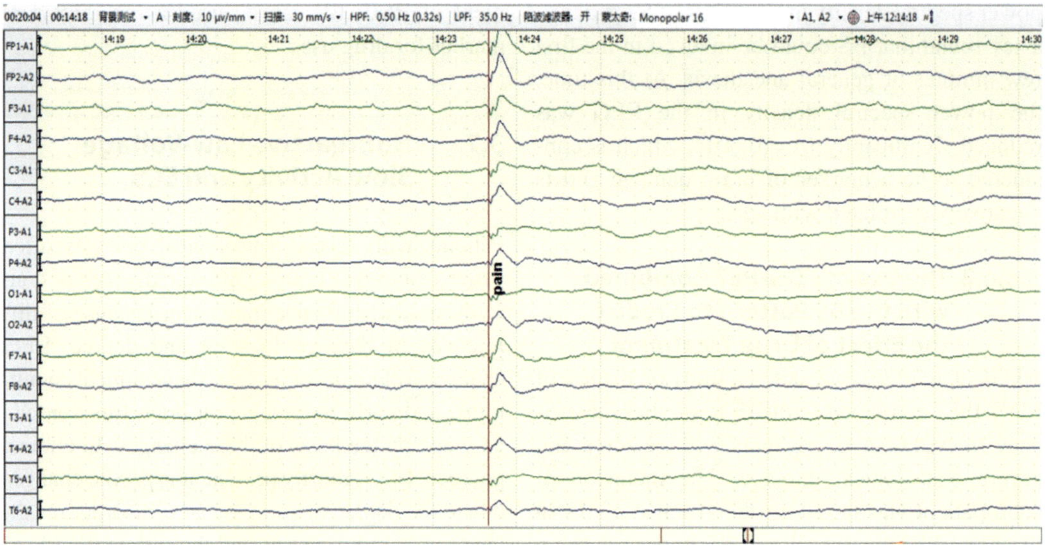


**Fig. 3.37** Sound, light, and pain stimulation was repeated, but the EEG showed no obvious change, and reactivity disappeared, indicating nonreactive low-voltage slow activity

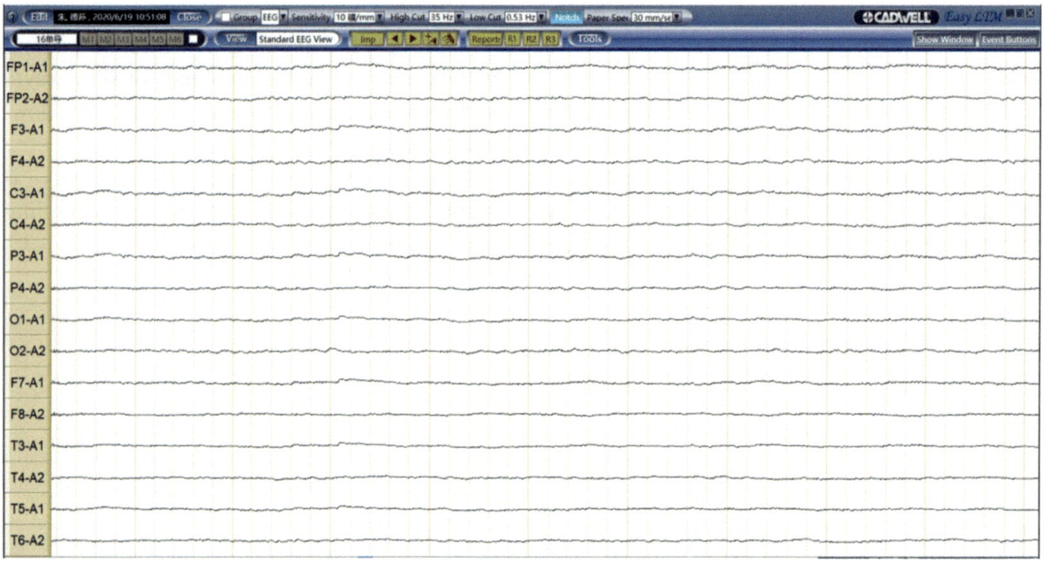


**Fig. 3.38** EEG from a 68-year-old female with massive cerebral infarction, showing low voltage in all leads and scattered δ/β waves with low amplitude

and 3.39), and the clinical manifestation is no response to sensory stimulation. Although low-voltage EEG background activity (low-voltage background EEG) also appears in some healthy people, it is mainly characterized by diffuse β, θ, and a small amount of δ activities not exceeding 20 μV, and there may be a small amount of α rhythm. EEGs may change in response to some physical stimulation, hyperventilation, or the influence of drugs. However, in patients in severe

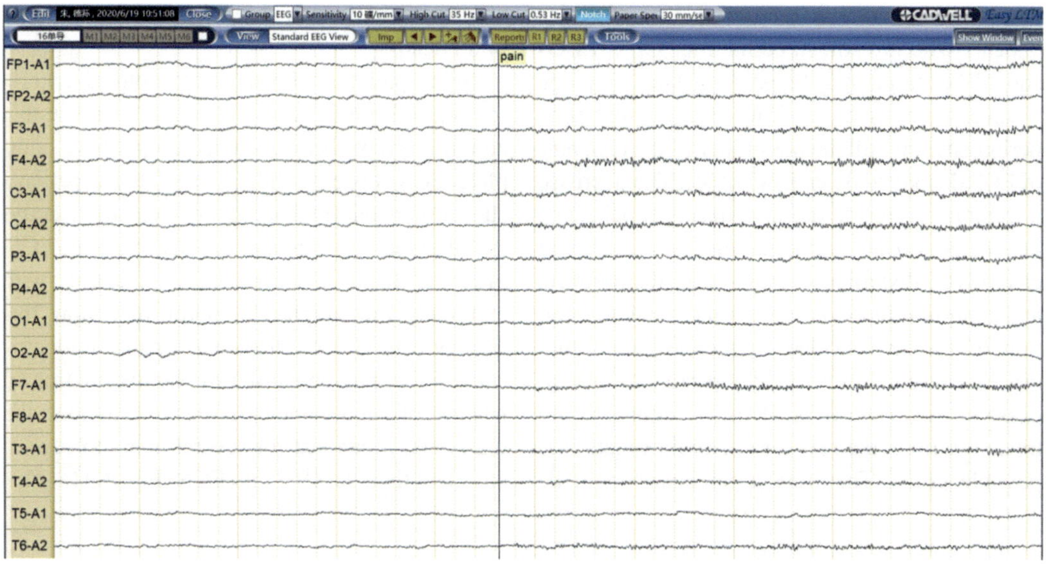


**Fig. 3.39** EMG artifacts were found in each lead after pain stimulation, and the reactivity disappeared

condition, the appearance of nonreactive low-voltage slow activity often indicates extensive and serious injury to the cerebral cortex, which is considered the prelude of ECS or clinical chronic VS and is often used as a predictor of the prognosis of the nervous system in patients with hypoxic coma. Studies have pointed out that in patients with cardiac arrest, EEGs with especially nonreactive low-voltage slow activity, with voltage <10 μV, are highly malignant, and their specificity for predicting adverse results can reach 100% [211, 228, 229]. Another prospective cohort study showed that nonreactive low-voltage activity in EEGs from the first day to the third day after admission was an independent predictor of death [142]. In addition, for children with HIE, the occurrence of low-voltage slow activity can also predict their neurodevelopmental disorder and death [230, 231]. Therefore, EEGs with nonreactive low-voltage slow activity are of great value for guiding medical staff to judge the prognosis of severe patients in clinical work.

ECS, also known as electrocerebral inactivity (ECI), refers to the complete disappearance of all EEG activity caused by spontaneous or physiological stimulation. In China's "Criteria and Technical Specifications for Determining Brain Death" (Adult Quality Control Edition), published in 2019, an EEG indicating brain death is defined as follows: EEG shows ECS when the parameter setting requirements (such as impedance <5 kΩ and sensitivity 2 μV/mm) are met, the EEG activity of at least 8 leads has an amplitude ≤2 μV for at least 30 min, and there is no response after stimulation [212].

The EEGs of patients with brain death mostly show sustained ECS, indicating the loss of cerebral cortex function; however, this does not mean that brain injury is irreversible. ECS can still be restored in a certain period of time. Sedative intoxication often causes BS or ECS. Although the inhibition interval can last for several minutes or even longer in severe cases, there is still the possibility of recovery [232]. ECS may appear at 17.8 ± 4 °C, and there is still the possibility of reversal within a certain time after rewarming without other complications [233]. EEG quickly shows ECS after cardiovascular diseases cause sudden cardiac arrest. The EEG activity gradually recovers within 12 or 72 h after CPR, and then consciousness is recovered. Therefore, in patients who are still in coma after CPR, EEGs should be monitored 12 or 72 h later to judge whether there is brain death. Before that time period, there is still the possibility of the recovery of ECS displayed on an EEG [234]. The decrease in cerebral perfusion pressure during shock; serious metabolic and endocrine diseases, including electrolyte disturbance, acid-base disturbance, and abnormal blood gas; and functional attenuation of the liver, kidney, pancreas, and other organs caused by severe hypoperfusion can all cause or aggravate ECS. If these conditions are treated in time, the recovery of brain function is possible [142]. Therefore, clinicians should be alert to various reversible factors when judging brain death.

Some patients who meet the clinical criteria for brain death in whom all kinds of reversible conditions have been excluded do not have complete ECS. Instead, the EEGs of these patients show other abnormal background electrical activity of wide low-voltage activity or near ECS, often a focal or multifocal potential with extremely low amplitude and/or very slow frequency (Fig. 3.40). This weak abnormal electrical activity may be caused by the distribution of islands of pathological tissues throughout the brain, and it can last for several hours to several days and then develop into ECS (Fig. 3.41a–e).

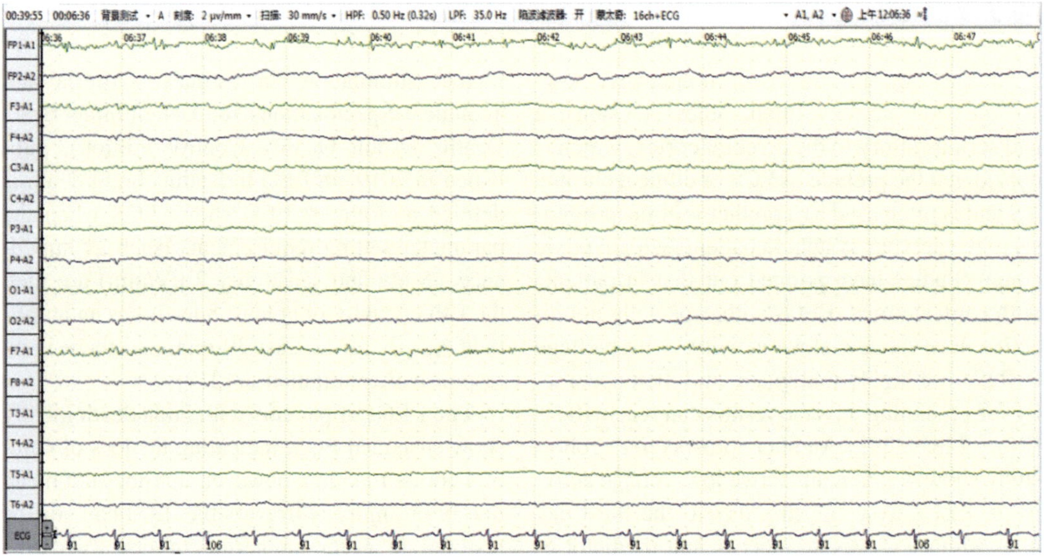


**Fig. 3.40** Sensitivity of 2 μV/mm. In each lead, a small amount of EEG activity was observed

a

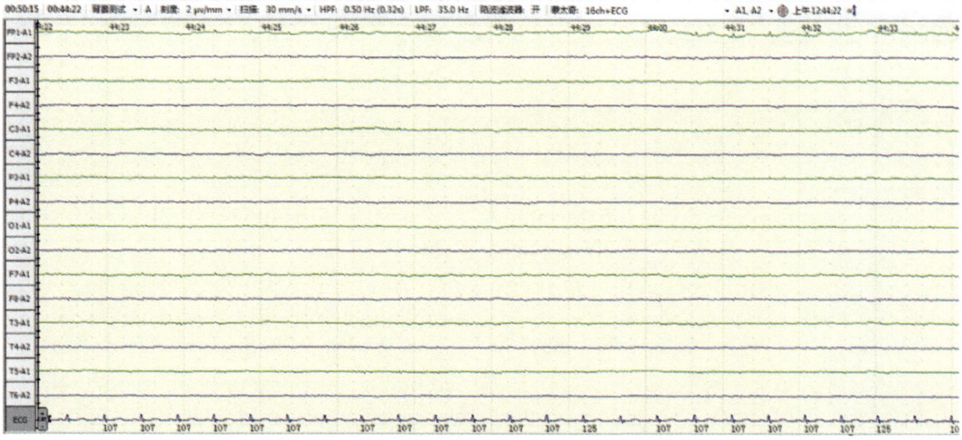

b

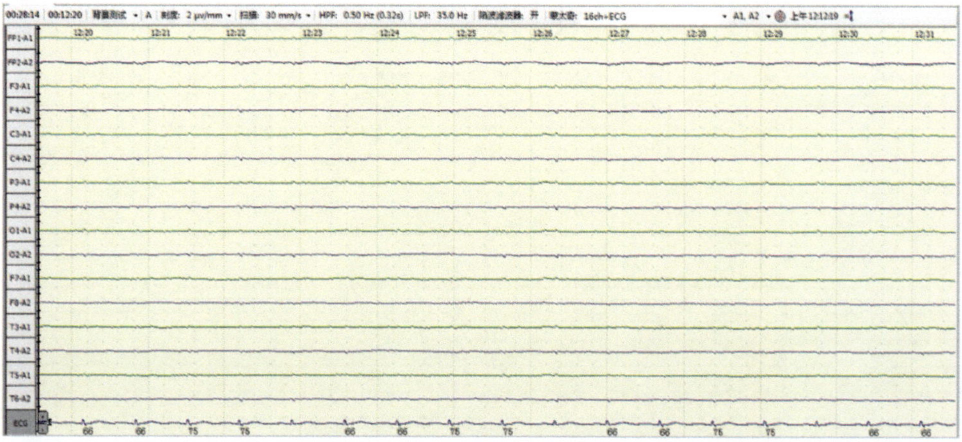

c

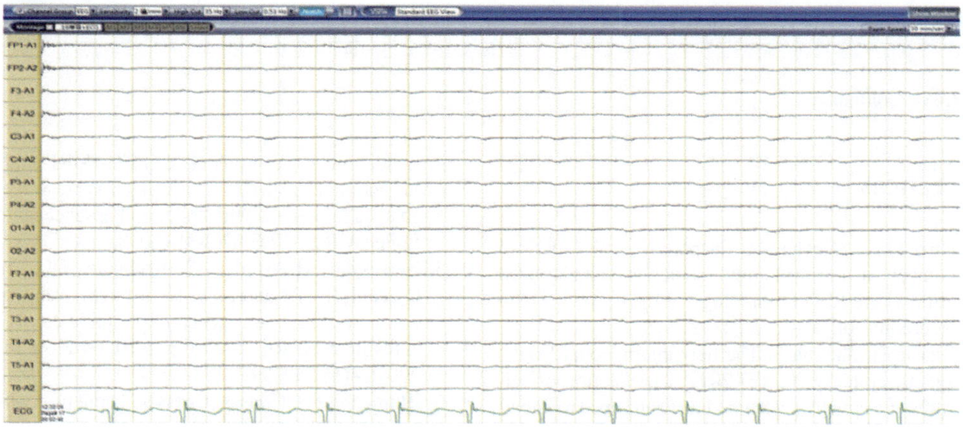

**Fig. 3.41** (**a**) Male, 40 years old, after CPR, brain death status, continuous ECS in each EEG lead. (**b**) Sensitivity of 2 μV/mm. In each lead, ECS was observed. (**c**) Male, 61 years old, injured in a car accident. EEG was seen in ECS. (**d**) EEG showing ECS lasted for 3 days, and the patient died. (**e**) Female, 45 years old. EEG of the car accident injury was seen in the continuous ECS, and there was no obvious EEG activity

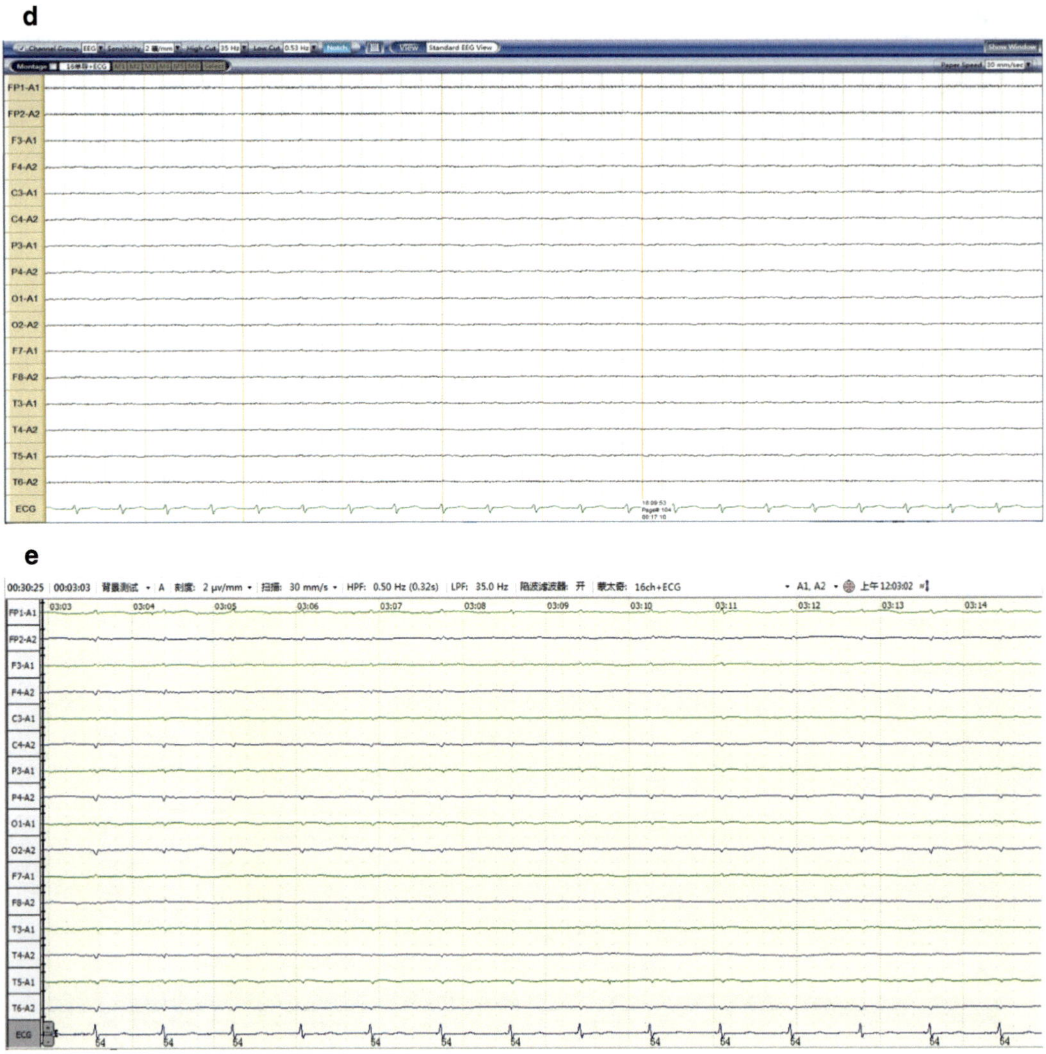


**Fig. 3.41** (continued)

## References


1. Hirsch LJ, LaRoche SM, Gaspard N, et al. American clinical neurophysiology society's standardized critical care EEG terminology: 2012 version. J Clin Neurophysiol. 2013;30(1):1–27.
2. Bhasin H, Sharma S. The new international league against epilepsy (ILAE) 2017 classification of seizures and epilepsy: what pediatricians need to know! Indian J Pediatr. 2019;86(7):569–71.
3. Moeller F, Muthuraman M, Stephani U, et al. Representation and propagation of epileptic activity in absences and generalized photoparoxysmal responses. Hum Brain Mapp. 2013;34(8):1896–909.
4. Li Q, Luo C, Yang T, et al. EEG-fMRI study on the interictal and ictal generalized spike-wave discharges in patients with childhood absence epilepsy. Epilepsy Res. 2009;87(2-3):160–8.
5. Nersesyan H, Hyder F, Rothman DL, et al. Dynamic fMRI and EEG recordings during spike-wave seizures and generalized tonic-clonic seizures in WAG/Rij rats. J Cereb Blood Flow Metab. 2004;24(6):589–99.
6. Blumenfeld H. Consciousness and epilepsy: why are patients with absence seizures absent? Prog Brain Res. 2005;150:271–86.
7. Blumenfeld H. Cellular and network mechanisms of spike-wave seizures. Epilepsia. 2005;46(Suppl 9):21–33.

8. Carney PW, Masterton RA, Harvey AS, et al. The core network in absence epilepsy. Differences in cortical and thalamic BOLD response. Neurology. 2010;75(10):904–11.
9. Westmoreland BF. Epileptiform electroencephalographic patterns. Mayo Clin Proc. 1996;71(5):501–11.
10. Kanazawa O. Reappraisal of abnormal EEG findings in children with ADHD: on the relationship between ADHD and epileptiform discharges. Epilepsy Behav. 2014;41:251–6.
11. Kartal A, Aksoy E, Deda G. The effects of risk factors on EEG and seizure in children with ADHD. Acta Neurol Belg. 2017;117(1):169–73.
12. Lee EH, Choi YS, Yoon HS, et al. Clinical impact of epileptiform discharge in children with attention-deficit/hyperactivity disorder (ADHD). J Child Neurol. 2016;31(5):584–8.
13. Mathew T, Srikanth SG, Satishchandra P. Malformations of cortical development (MCDs) and epilepsy: experience from a tertiary care center in south India. Seizure. 2010;19(3):147–52.
14. Grant AC, Chau L, Arya K, et al. Prevalence of epileptiform discharges in healthy 11- and 12-year-old children. Epilepsy Behav. 2016;62:53–6.
15. Jayalakshmi S, Dhondji M, Vooturi S, et al. Interictal EEG patterns in malformations of cortical development and epilepsy. Clin Neurol Neurosurg. 2020;196:106022.
16. Borges MA, Botos HJ, Bastos RF, et al. Emergency EEG: study of survival. Arq Neuropsiquiatr. 2010;68(2):174–8.
17. Gomez-Ibanez A, McLachlan RS, Mirsattari SM, et al. Prognostic factors in patients with refractory idiopathic generalized epilepsy. Epilepsy Res. 2017;130:69–73.
18. Ruijter BJ, van Putten MJ, Hofmeijer J. Generalized epileptiform discharges in postanoxic encephalopathy: quantitative characterization in relation to outcome. Epilepsia. 2015;56(11):1845–54.
19. Plummer C, Wagner M, Fuchs M, et al. Clinical utility of distributed source modelling of interictal scalp EEG in focal epilepsy. Clin Neurophysiol. 2010;121(10):1726–39.
20. Lengler U, Kafadar I, Neubauer BA, et al. fMRI correlates of interictal epileptic activity in patients with idiopathic benign focal epilepsy of childhood. A simultaneous EEG-functional MRI study. Epilepsy Res. 2007;75(1):29–38.
21. Plummer C, Wagner M, Fuchs M, et al. Dipole versus distributed EEG source localization for single versus averaged spikes in focal epilepsy. J Clin Neurophysiol. 2010;27(3):141–62.
22. Motomura E, Inui K, Ohoyama K, et al. Electroencephalographic dipole source modeling of frontal intermittent rhythmic delta activity. Neuropsychobiology. 2012;65(2):103–8.
23. Fogarasi A, Boesebeck F, Tuxhorn I. A detailed analysis of symptomatic posterior cortex seizure semiology in children younger than seven years. Epilepsia. 2003;44(1):89–96.
24. Xiao YH, Liao JX, Huang J, et al. Interictal epileptiform discharges in children with epilepsy. Zhongguo Dang Dai Er Ke Za Zhi. 2008;10(3):322–4.
25. Nariai H, Beal J, Galanopoulou AS, et al. Scalp EEG Ictal gamma and beta activity during infantile spasms: evidence of focality. Epilepsia. 2017;58(5):882–92.
26. Hooshmand H, Morganroth R, Corredor C. Significance of focal and lateralized beta activity in the EEG. Clin Electroencephalogr. 1980;11(3):140–4.
27. Gaspard N, Manganas L, Rampal N, et al. Similarity of lateralized rhythmic delta activity to periodic lateralized epileptiform discharges in critically ill patients. JAMA Neurol. 2013;70(10):1288–95.
28. Morikawa T. Rolandic discharges in benign childhood epilepsy with centrotemporal spikes, and in other forms of partial epilepsies. Epileptic Disord. 2000;2(Suppl 1):S23–8.
29. Al-Sulaiman A. Electroencephalographic findings in children with cerebral palsy: a study of 151 patients. Funct Neurol. 2001;16(4):325–8.
30. Coppola G. Malignant migrating partial seizures in infancy. Handb Clin Neurol. 2013;111:605–9.
31. Specchio N, Pietrafusa N. New-onset refractory status epilepticus and febrile infection-related epilepsy syndrome. Dev Med Child Neurol. 2020;62(8):897–905.
32. Fox K, Wells ME, Tennison M, et al. Febrile infection-related epilepsy syndrome (FIRES): a literature review and case study. Neurodiagn J. 2017;57(3):224–33.
33. Riikonen R. Infantile spasms: outcome in clinical studies. Pediatr Neurol. 2020;108:54–64.
34. Hirsch LJ, Brenner RP, Drislane FW, et al. The ACNS subcommittee on research terminology for continuous EEG monitoring: proposed standardized terminology for rhythmic and periodic EEG patterns encountered in critically ill patients. J Clin Neurophysiol. 2005;22(2):128–35.
35. Garzon E, Fernandes RM, Sakamoto AC. Serial EEG during human status epilepticus: evidence for PLED as an ictal pattern. Neurology. 2001;57(7):1175–83.
36. Zafar SF, Subramaniam T, Osman G, et al. Electrographic seizures and ictal-interictal continuum (IIC) patterns in critically ill patients. Epilepsy Behav. 2020;106:107037.
37. Lin L, Drislane FW. Lateralized periodic discharges: a literature review. J Clin Neurophysiol. 2018;35(3):189–98.
38. COBB W, HILL D. Electroencephalogram in subacute progressive encephalitis. Brain. 1950;73(3):392–404.

39. Chatrian GE, Shaw CM, Leffman H. The significance of periodic lateralized epileptiform discharges in EEG: an electrogranphic, clinical and pathological study. Electroencephalogr Clin Neurophysiol. 1964;17:177–93.
40. Bastide L, Legros B, Rampal N, et al. Clinical correlates of periodic discharges and nonconvulsive seizures in posterior reversible encephalopathy syndrome (PRES). Neurocrit Care. 2018;29(3):481–90.
41. Bauerschmidt A, Rubinos C, Claassen J. Approach to managing periodic discharges. J Clin Neurophysiol. 2018;35(4):309–13.
42. Reiher J, Rivest J, Grand'Maison F, et al. Periodic lateralized epileptiform discharges with transitional rhythmic discharges: association with seizures. Electroencephalogr Clin Neurophysiol. 1991;78(1):12–7.
43. Chong DJ, Hirsch LJ. Which EEG patterns warrant treatment in the critically ill? Reviewing the evidence for treatment of periodic epileptiform discharges and related patterns. J Clin Neurophysiol. 2005;22(2):79–91.
44. Brenner RP. EEG in convulsive and nonconvulsive status epilepticus. J Clin Neurophysiol. 2004;21(5):319–31.
45. Brenner RP, Schaul N. Periodic EEG patterns: classification, clinical correlation, and pathophysiology. J Clin Neurophysiol. 1990;7(2):249–67.
46. Hirsch LJBR. Periodic discharges and other controversial EEG patterns. In: Hirsch LJ, Brenner RP, editors. Atlas of EEG in critical care. Chichester: Wiley-Blackwell; 2010. p. 129–60.
47. Gaches J. Periodic activity in the EEG. Rev Electroencephalogr Neurophysiol Clin. 1971;1(1):9–33.
48. Praveen-kumar S, Sinha S, Taly AB, et al. Electroencephalographic and imaging profile in a subacute sclerosing panencephalitis (SSPE) cohort: a correlative study. Clin Neurophysiol. 2007;118(9):1947–54.
49. Foley JM, Watson CW, Adams RD. Significance of the electroencephalographic changes in hepatic coma. 1950.
50. Bickford RG, Butt HR. Hepatic coma: the electroencephalographic pattern. J Clin Invest. 1955;34(6):790–9.
51. Kaplan PW, Sutter R. Affair with triphasic waves-their striking presence, mysterious significance, and cryptic origins: what are they? J Clin Neurophysiol. 2015;32(5):401–5.
52. Emmady P D, Murr N. EEG triphasic waves. 2020.
53. Kaplan P, Schlattman DK. Typical versus atypical triphasic waves. J Clin Neurophysiol. 2013;30(2):211.
54. Hirsch LJ, Claassen J, Mayer SA, et al. Stimulus-induced rhythmic, periodic, or ictal discharges (SIRPIDs): a common EEG phenomenon in the critically ill. Epilepsia. 2004;45(2):109–23.
55. Lee JW, LaRoche S, Choi H, et al. Development and feasibility testing of a critical care EEG monitoring database for standardized clinical reporting and multicenter collaborative research. J Clin Neurophysiol. 2016;33(2):133–40.
56. Foreman B, Claassen J, Abou KK, et al. Generalized periodic discharges in the critically ill: a case-control study of 200 patients. Neurology. 2012;79(19):1951–60.
57. Husari KS, Johnson EL. Periodic discharges: how to approach, when to treat. J Clin Neurophysiol. 2020;37(5):411–21.
58. Garcia-Morales I, Garcia MT, Galan-Davila L, et al. Periodic lateralized epileptiform discharges: etiology, clinical aspects, seizures, and evolution in 130 patients. J Clin Neurophysiol. 2002;19(2):172–7.
59. Neufeld MY, Vishnevskaya S, Treves TA, et al. Periodic lateralized epileptiform discharges (PLEDs) following stroke are associated with metabolic abnormalities. Electroencephalogr Clin Neurophysiol. 1997;102(4):295–8.
60. Sekiguchi K, Akiyoshi K, Okazaki N, et al. PLEDs in an infant with congenital protein C deficiency: a case report. Clin Neurophysiol. 2010;121(5):800–1.
61. de Los RE, McJunkin JE, Glauser TA, et al. Periodic lateralized epileptiform discharges in La Crosse encephalitis, a worrisome subgroup: clinical presentation, electroencephalogram (EEG) patterns, and long-term neurologic outcome. J Child Neurol. 2008;23(2):167–72.
62. Gandelman-Marton R, Rabey JM, Flechter S. Periodic lateralized epileptiform discharges in multiple sclerosis: a case report. J Clin Neurophysiol. 2003;20(2):117–21.
63. Witsch J, Frey HP, Schmidt JM, et al. Electroencephalographic periodic discharges and frequency-dependent brain tissue hypoxia in acute brain injury. JAMA Neurol. 2017;74(3):301–9.
64. Subramaniam T, Jain A, Hall LT, et al. Lateralized periodic discharges frequency correlates with glucose metabolism. Neurology. 2019;92(7):e670–4.
65. Punia V, Vakani R, Burgess R, et al. Electrographic and clinical natural history of lateralized periodic discharges. J Clin Neurophysiol. 2018;35(1):71–6.
66. Rodriguez RA, Vlachy J, Lee JW, et al. Association of periodic and rhythmic electroencephalographic patterns with seizures in critically ill patients. JAMA Neurol. 2017;74(2):181–8.
67. Dono F, Russo M, Carrarini C, et al. Lateralized periodic discharges in insular status epilepticus: a case report of a periodic EEG pattern associated with ictal manifestation. Clin Neurophysiol Pract. 2019;4:27–9.
68. Sully KE, Husain AM. Generalized periodic discharges: a topical review. J Clin Neurophysiol. 2018;35(3):199–207.
69. Leitinger M, Beniczky S, Rohracher A, et al. Salzburg consensus criteria for non-convulsive status epilepticus—approach to clinical application. Epilepsy Behav. 2015;49:158–63.
70. Rodriguez V, Rodden MF, LaRoche SM. Ictal-interictal continuum: a proposed treatment algorithm. Clin Neurophysiol. 2016;127(4):2056–64.

71. Vespa P, Tubi M, Claassen J, et al. Metabolic crisis occurs with seizures and periodic discharges after brain trauma. Ann Neurol. 2016;79(4):579–90.
72. Moseley BD. Association of periodic discharges with reduced brain tissue oxygenation: no longer straddling the fence? JAMA Neurol. 2017;74(3):266–7.
73. Carneiro F, Bentes C, Peralta AR. Etiology and clinical impact of interictal periodic discharges on the routine outpatient scalp EEG. J Clin Neurophysiol. 2020;38:202–7.
74. Milani P, Malissin I, Tran-Dinh YR, et al. Prognostic EEG patterns in patients resuscitated from cardiac arrest with particular focus on generalized periodic epileptiform discharges (GPEDs). Neurophysiol Clin. 2014;44(2):153–64.
75. Li HT, Wu T, Lin WR, et al. Clinical correlation and prognostic implication of periodic EEG patterns: a cohort study. Epilepsy Res. 2017;131:44–50.
76. Jadeja N, Zarnegar R, Legatt AD. Clinical outcomes in patients with generalized periodic discharges. Seizure. 2017;45:114–8.
77. Ong C, Gilmore E, Claassen J, et al. Impact of prolonged periodic epileptiform discharges on coma prognosis. Neurocrit Care. 2012;17(1):39–44.
78. Gross DW, Wiebe S, Blume WT. The periodicity of lateralized epileptiform discharges. Clin Neurophysiol. 1999;110(9):1516–20.
79. Orta DS, Chiappa KH, Quiroz AZ, et al. Prognostic implications of periodic epileptiform discharges. Arch Neurol. 2009;66(8):985–91.
80. Fushimi M, Matsubuchi N, Sekine A, et al. Benign bilateral independent periodic lateralized epileptiform discharges. Acta Neurol Scand. 2003;108(1):55–9.
81. Osman G, Rahangdale R, Britton JW, et al. Bilateral independent periodic discharges are associated with electrographic seizures and poor outcome: a case-control study. Clin Neurophysiol. 2018;129(11):2284–9.
82. Freund B, Gugger JJ, Reynolds A, et al. Clinical and electrographic correlates of bilateral independent periodic discharges. J Clin Neurophysiol. 2018;35(3):234–41.
83. Shaikh AG, Gulati D, Wu S, et al. Independent and symmetric seizures from parasagittal cortex: is this a feature of profound hypoglycemia? Epilepsy Behav. 2012;25(2):263–5.
84. Andraus ME, Andraus CF, Alves-Leon SV. Periodic EEG patterns: importance of their recognition and clinical significance. Arq Neuropsiquiatr. 2012;70(2):145–51.
85. Roos KL, Tuite PJ, Below ME, et al. Reversible cortical blindness (Anton's syndrome) associated with bilateral occipital EEG abnormalities. Clin Electroencephalogr. 1990;21(2):104–9.
86. Aye SM, Lim KS, Ramli NM, et al. Periodic lateralized epileptiform discharges (PLEDs) in cerebral lupus correlated with white-matter lesions in brain MRI and reduced cerebral blood flow in SPECT. Lupus. 2013;22(5):510–4.
87. Fitzpatrick W, Lowry N. PLEDs: clinical correlates. Can J Neurol Sci. 2007;34(4):443–50.
88. Iyer R S, Ramalingam R, Akhtar S, et al. Bilateral independent periodic lateralised epileptiform discharges at presentation followed by rapid recovery: novel observations from a case of Epstein-Barr virus encephalitis. BMJ Case Rep. 2019;12(7).
89. Nicolai J, van Putten MJ, Tavy DL. BIPLEDs in akinetic mutism caused by bilateral anterior cerebral artery infarction. Clin Neurophysiol. 2001;112(9):1726–8.
90. Fountain NB, Waldman WA. Effects of benzodiazepines on triphasic waves: implications for nonconvulsive status epilepticus. J Clin Neurophysiol. 2001;18(4):345–52.
91. Boulanger JM, Deacon C, Lecuyer D, et al. Triphasic waves versus nonconvulsive status epilepticus: EEG distinction. Can J Neurol Sci. 2006;33(2):175–80.
92. Kaplan PW, Duckworth J. Confusion and SIRPIDs regress with parenteral lorazepam. Epileptic Disord. 2011;13(3):291–4.
93. Braksick SA, Burkholder DB, Tsetsou S, et al. Associated factors and prognostic implications of stimulus-induced rhythmic, periodic, or ictal discharges. JAMA Neurol. 2016;73(5):585–90.
94. Alvarez V, Oddo M, Rossetti AO. Stimulus-induced rhythmic, periodic or ictal discharges (SIRPIDs) in comatose survivors of cardiac arrest: characteristics and prognostic value. Clin Neurophysiol. 2013;124(1):204–8.
95. Johnson EL, Kaplan PW, Ritzl EK. Termination patterns of stimulus-induced rhythmic, periodic, or ictal patterns and spontaneous electrographic seizures. Clin Neurophysiol. 2017;128(11):2279–85.
96. Recommendations for electroencephalography monitoring in neurocritical care units. Chin Med J (Engl). 2017;130(15):1851–55.
97. Beniczky S, Hirsch LJ, Kaplan PW, et al. Unified EEG terminology and criteria for nonconvulsive status epilepticus. Epilepsia. 2013;54(Suppl 6):28–9.
98. Pohlmann-Eden B, Hoch DB, Cochius JI, et al. Periodic lateralized epileptiform discharges—a critical review. J Clin Neurophysiol. 1996;13(6):519–30.
99. Cormier J, Maciel CB, Gilmore EJ. Ictal-interictal continuum: when to worry about the continuous electroencephalography pattern. Semin Respir Crit Care Med. 2017;38(6):793–806.
100. Struck AF, Westover MB, Hall LT, et al. Metabolic correlates of the ictal-interictal continuum: FDG-PET during continuous EEG. Neurocrit Care. 2016;24(3):324–31.
101. Lee JW. The EEG ictal-interictal continuum-a metabolic roar but a whimper of a functional outcome. Epilepsy Curr. 2019;19(4):234–6.
102. Yoo JY, Rampal N, Petroff OA, et al. Brief potentially ictal rhythmic discharges in critically ill adults. JAMA Neurol. 2014;71(4):454–62.
103. Johnson EL, Kaplan PW. Population of the ictal-interictal zone: the significance of periodic and

rhythmic activity. Clin Neurophysiol Pract. 2017;2:107–18.
104. Hartings JA, Williams AJ, Tortella FC. Occurrence of nonconvulsive seizures, periodic epileptiform discharges, and intermittent rhythmic delta activity in rat focal ischemia. Exp Neurol. 2003;179(2):139–49.
105. Claassen J, Jette N, Chum F, et al. Electrographic seizures and periodic discharges after intracerebral hemorrhage. Neurology. 2007;69(13):1356–65.
106. Sen-Gupta I, Schuele SU, Macken MP, et al. "Ictal" lateralized periodic discharges. Epilepsy Behav. 2014;36:165–70.
107. Newey CR, Sahota P, Hantus S. Electrographic features of lateralized periodic discharges stratify risk in the interictal-ictal continuum. J Clin Neurophysiol. 2017;34(4):365–9.
108. Claassen J, Hirsch LJ, Frontera JA, et al. Prognostic significance of continuous EEG monitoring in patients with poor-grade subarachnoid hemorrhage. Neurocrit Care. 2006;4(2):103–12.
109. Akman CI, Riviello JJ. Generalized periodic epileptiform discharges in critically ill children: a continuum of status epilepticus or an epiphenomenon? J Clin Neurophysiol. 2011;28(4):366–72.
110. Tanaka H, Khoo HM, Dubeau F, et al. Association between scalp and intracerebral electroencephalographic seizure-onset patterns: a study in different lesional pathological substrates. Epilepsia. 2018;59(2):420–30.
111. Faigle R, Sutter R, Kaplan PW. Electroencephalography of encephalopathy in patients with endocrine and metabolic disorders. J Clin Neurophysiol. 2013;30(5):505–16.
112. Sutter R, Stevens RD, Kaplan PW. Clinical and imaging correlates of EEG patterns in hospitalized patients with encephalopathy. J Neurol. 2013;260(4):1087–98.
113. Foreman B, Mahulikar A, Tadi P, et al. Generalized periodic discharges and 'triphasic waves': a blinded evaluation of inter-rater agreement and clinical significance. Clin Neurophysiol. 2016;127(2):1073–80.
114. Claassen J, Mayer SA, Kowalski RG, et al. Detection of electrographic seizures with continuous EEG monitoring in critically ill patients. Neurology. 2004;62(10):1743–8.
115. de la Paz D, Brenner RP. Bilateral independent periodic lateralized epileptiform discharges. Clinical significance. Arch Neurol. 1981;38(11):713–5.
116. Snodgrass SM, Tsuburaya K, Ajmone-Marsan C. Clinical significance of periodic lateralized epileptiform discharges: relationship with status epilepticus. J Clin Neurophysiol. 1989;6(2):159–72.
117. Normand MM, Wszolek ZK, Klass DW. Temporal intermittent rhythmic delta activity in electroencephalograms. J Clin Neurophysiol. 1995;12(3):280–4.
118. Accolla EA, Kaplan PW, Maeder-Ingvar M, et al. Clinical correlates of frontal intermittent rhythmic delta activity (FIRDA). Clin Neurophysiol. 2011;122(1):27–31.
119. Johnson EL, Kaplan PW, Ritzl EK. Stimulus-induced rhythmic, periodic, or ictal discharges (SIRPIDs). J Clin Neurophysiol. 2018;35(3):229–33.
120. Alsherbini KA, Plancher JM, Ficker DM, et al. Stimulus-induced rhythmic, periodic, or ictal discharges in coma-incidence and interrater reliability of continuous EEG after a standard stimulation protocol: a prospective study. J Clin Neurophysiol. 2017;34(4):375–80.
121. Tsetsou S, Novy J, Oddo M, et al. EEG reactivity to pain in comatose patients: importance of the stimulus type. Resuscitation. 2015;97:34–7.
122. Struck AF, Ustun B, Ruiz AR, et al. Association of an electroencephalography-based risk score with seizure probability in hospitalized patients. JAMA Neurol. 2017;74(12):1419–24.
123. Nagarajan L, Palumbo L, Ghosh S. Brief electroencephalography rhythmic discharges (BERDs) in the neonate with seizures: their significance and prognostic implications. J Child Neurol. 2011;26(12):1529–33.
124. Punia V, Garcia CG, Hantus S. Incidence of recurrent seizures following hospital discharge in patients with LPDs (PLEDs) and nonconvulsive seizures recorded on continuous EEG in the critical care setting. Epilepsy Behav. 2015;49:250–4.
125. Swisher CB, Shah D, Sinha SR, et al. Baseline EEG pattern on continuous ICU EEG monitoring and incidence of seizures. J Clin Neurophysiol. 2015;32(2):147–51.
126. Struck AF, Osman G, Rampal N, et al. Time-dependent risk of seizures in critically ill patients on continuous electroencephalogram. Ann Neurol. 2017;82(2):177–85.
127. Morselli PL, Franco-Morselli R. Clinical pharmacokinetics of antiepileptic drugs in adults. Pharmacol Ther. 1980;10(1):65–101.
128. Osman GM, Araujo DF, Maciel CB. Ictal interictal continuum patterns. Curr Treat Options Neurol. 2018;20(5):15.
129. Assal F, Papazyan JP, Slosman DO, et al. SPECT in periodic lateralized epileptiform discharges (PLEDs): a form of partial status epilepticus? Seizure. 2001;10(4):260–5.
130. Smith CC, Tatum WO, Gupta V, et al. SPECT-negative SIRPIDs: less aggressive neurointensive care? J Clin Neurophysiol. 2014;31(3):e6–e10.
131. Cianfoni A, Caulo M, Cerase A, et al. Seizure-induced brain lesions: a wide spectrum of variably reversible MRI abnormalities. Eur J Radiol. 2013;82(11):1964–72.
132. Narayanan J. Can diffusion-weighted imaging be used as a tool to predict seizures in patients with PLEDS? Epileptic Disord. 2016;18(4):440–6.
133. Waziri A, Claassen J, Stuart RM, et al. Intracortical electroencephalography in acute brain injury. Ann Neurol. 2009;66(3):366–77.
134. Munro KE, Sakata S, Toyoizumi T. Theta oscillations alternate with high amplitude neocortical pop-

ulation within synchronized states. Front Neurosci. 2019;13:316.
135. Lowenstein DH, Aminoff MJ. Clinical and EEG features of status epilepticus in comatose patients. Neurology. 1992;42(1):100–4.
136. Chen J, Xie L, Hu Y, et al. Nonconvulsive status epilepticus after cessation of convulsive status epilepticus in pediatric intensive care unit patients. Epilepsy Behav. 2018;82:68–73.
137. Trinka E, Leitinger M. Which EEG patterns in coma are nonconvulsive status epilepticus? Epilepsy Behav. 2015;49:203–22.
138. Yildirim M, Konuskan B, Yalnizoglu D, et al. Electroencephalographic findings in anti-N-methyl-d-aspartate receptor encephalitis in children: a series of 12 patients. Epilepsy Behav. 2018;78:118–23.
139. Lee H, Mizrahi MA, Hartings JA, et al. Continuous electroencephalography after moderate to severe traumatic brain injury. Crit Care Med. 2019;47(4):574–82.
140. Azabou E, Magalhaes E, Braconnier A, et al. Early standard electroencephalogram abnormalities predict mortality in septic intensive care unit patients. PLoS One. 2015;10(10):e139969.
141. Bello-Espinosa LE. Infraslow status epilepticus: a new form of subclinical status epilepticus recorded in a child with Sturge-Weber syndrome. Epilepsy Behav. 2015;49:193–7.
142. Desai JD, Toczek MT, Mitchell WG. Frontal intermittent rhythmic delta activity (FIRDA): is there a clinical significance in children and adolescents? Eur J Paediatr Neurol. 2012;16(2):138–41.
143. Cobb WA. Rhythmic slow discharges in the electroencephalogram. J Neurol Neurosurg Psychiatry. 1945;8:65–78.
144. Watemberg N, Alehan F, Dabby R, et al. Clinical and radiologic correlates of frontal intermittent rhythmic delta activity. J Clin Neurophysiol. 2002;19(6):535–9.
145. Gayatri NA, Whitehouse WP. Pilot survey of Hashimoto's encephalopathy in children. Dev Med Child Neurol. 2005;47(8):556–8.
146. Brigo F. Intermittent rhythmic delta activity patterns. Epilepsy Behav. 2011;20(2):254–6.
147. Muellbacher W, Mamoli B. Prolonged impaired consciousness in basilar artery migraine. Headache. 1994;34(5):282–5.
148. Cerrahoglu ST, Bekdik SP, Arkali BN, et al. Electroencephalographic features associated with intermittent rhythmic delta activity. Neurophysiol Clin. 2019;49(3):227–34.
149. Dericioglu N, Khasiyev F, Arsava EM, et al. Frontal intermittent rhythmic delta activity (FIRDA) in the neurological intensive care: prevalence, determinants, and clinical significance. Clin EEG Neurosci. 2018;49(4):272–7.
150. Desai J, Mitchell WG, Rosser T, et al. Clinical associations of occipital intermittent rhythmic delta activity. J Child Neurol. 2012;27(4):503–6.
151. Gullapalli D, Fountain NB. Clinical correlation of occipital intermittent rhythmic delta activity. J Clin Neurophysiol. 2003;20(1):35–41.
152. Serafini A, Issa NP, Rose S, et al. TIRDA originating from lateral temporal cortex in a patient with mTLE is not related to hippocampal activity. J Clin Neurophysiol. 2016;33(6):e34–8.
153. Ondo WG, Verma A. Physiological assessment of paroxysmal dystonia secondary to subacute sclerosing panencephalitis. Mov Disord. 2002;17(1):154–7.
154. Vecchierini MF, Andre M, D'Allest AM. Normal EEG of premature infants born between 24 and 30 weeks gestational age: terminology, definitions and maturation aspects. Neurophysiol Clin. 2007;37(5):311–23.
155. Claassen J, Vespa P. Electrophysiologic monitoring in acute brain injury. Neurocrit Care. 2014;21(Suppl 2):S129–47.
156. Beridze M, Khaburzania M, Shakarishvili R, et al. Dominated EEG patterns and their prognostic value in coma caused by traumatic brain injury. Georgian Med News. 2010;186:28–33.
157. Rosen I, Hagerdal M. Electroencephalographic study of children during ketamine anesthesia. Acta Anaesthesiol Scand. 1976;20(1):32–9.
158. Morimoto Y, Matsumoto A, Koizumi Y, et al. Changes in the bispectral index during intraabdominal irrigation in patients anesthetized with nitrous oxide and sevoflurane. Anesth Analg. 2005;100(5):1370–4.
159. Loeb C, Poggio G. Electroencephalograms in a case with ponto-mesencephalic haemorrhage. Electroencephalogr Clin Neurophysiol. 1953;5(2):295–6.
160. Kaplan PW, Genoud D, Ho TW, et al. Etiology, neurologic correlations, and prognosis in alpha coma. Clin Neurophysiol. 1999;110(2):205–13.
161. Berkhoff M, Donati F, Bassetti C. Postanoxic alpha (theta) coma: a reappraisal of its prognostic significance. Clin Neurophysiol. 2000;111(2):297–304.
162. Homan RW, Jones MG. Alpha-pattern coma in a 2-month-old child. Ann Neurol. 1981;9(6):611–3.
163. Fernandez-Torre JL, Lopez-Delgado A, Hernandez-Hernandez MA, et al. Postanoxic alpha, theta or alpha-theta coma: clinical setting and neurological outcome. Resuscitation. 2018;124:118–25.
164. Sarma GR, Kumar A, Roy AK, et al. Post-cardiorespiratory arrest beta-alpha coma: an unusual electroencephalographic phenomenon. Neurol India. 2003;51(2):266–8.
165. Carroll WM, Mastaglia FL. Alpha and beta coma in drug intoxication uncomplicated by cerebral hypoxia. Electroencephalogr Clin Neurophysiol. 1979;46(1):95–105.
166. Husain AM. Electroencephalographic assessment of coma. J Clin Neurophysiol. 2006;23(3):208–20.
167. RamachandranNair R, Sharma R, Weiss SK, et al. A reappraisal of rhythmic coma patterns in children. Can J Neurol Sci. 2005;32(4):518–23.

168. Jones BN, Binnie CD, Fung D, et al. Reversible coma with an EEG pattern normally associated with wakefulness. Electroencephalogr Clin Neurophysiol. 1972;33(1):107–9.
169. Tomassen W, Kamphuisen HA. Alpha coma. J Neurol Sci. 1986;76(1):1–11.
170. Synek VM. Prognostically important EEG coma patterns in diffuse anoxic and traumatic encephalopathies in adults. J Clin Neurophysiol. 1988;5(2):161–74.
171. Sorensen K, Thomassen A, Wernberg M. Prognostic significance of alpha frequency EEG rhythm in coma after cardiac arrest. J Neurol Neurosurg Psychiatry. 1978;41(9):840–2.
172. Mundi JP, Betancourt J, Ezziddin O, et al. Dilated and unreactive pupils and burst-suppression on electroencephalography due to buproprion overdose. J Intensive Care Med. 2012;27(6):384–8.
173. Pourmand R, Markand ON. Drug-induced alpha coma. J Neurol Neurosurg Psychiatry. 1985;48(3):283–4.
174. Fossi S, Amantini A, Grippo A, et al. Anoxic-ischemic alpha coma: prognostic significance of the incomplete variant. Neurol Sci. 2004;24(6):397–400.
175. Martinez BA, Lopez-Martin V, Arcas J, et al. Alpha coma: clinical, electroencephalographic and aetiological correlation in childhood. Rev Neurol. 2001;33(12):1101–5.
176. Ostojic S, Vukovic R, Milenkovic T, et al. Alpha coma in an adolescent with diabetic ketoacidosis. Turk J Pediatr. 2017;59(3):318–21.
177. Janati A, Erba G. Electroencephalographic correlates of near-drowning encephalopathy in children. Electroencephalogr Clin Neurophysiol. 1982;53(2):182–91.
178. Steriade M, Gloor P, Llinas RR, et al. Report of IFCN committee on basic mechanisms. Basic mechanisms of cerebral rhythmic activities. Electroencephalogr Clin Neurophysiol. 1990;76(6):481–508.
179. Da SF, van Lierop TH, Schrijer CF, et al. Organization of thalamic and cortical alpha rhythms: spectra and coherences. Electroencephalogr Clin Neurophysiol. 1973;35(6):627–39.
180. Gurvitch AM, Zarzhetsky Y, Trush VD, et al. Experimental data on the nature of postresuscitation alpha frequency activity. Electroencephalogr Clin Neurophysiol. 1984;58(5):426–37.
181. Alving J, Moller M, Sindrup E, et al. 'alpha pattern coma' following cerebral anoxia. Electroencephalogr Clin Neurophysiol. 1979;47(1):95–101.
182. Bolen RD, Campbell Z, Bonilha L, et al. Alpha coma related to intentional bupropion overdose. J Neurol Sci. 2016;365:48–9.
183. Patterson JR, Grabois M. Locked-in syndrome: a review of 139 cases. Stroke. 1986;17(4):758–64.
184. Chase TN, Moretti L, Prensky AL. Clinical and electroencephalographic manifestations of vascular lesions of the pons. Neurology. 1968;18(4):357–68.
185. Herkes GK, Wszolek ZK, Westmoreland BF, et al. Effects of midazolam on electroencephalograms of seriously ill patients. Mayo Clin Proc. 1992;67(4):334–8.
186. Pais-Roldan P, Edlow BL, Jiang Y, et al. Multimodal assessment of recovery from coma in a rat model of diffuse brainstem tegmentum injury. Neuroimage. 2019;189:615–30.
187. Sumskii LI. Alpha and beta coma in a brain lesion at the pontomesencephalic level. Fiziol Cheloveka. 1984;10(3):473–6.
188. Moruzzi G, Magoun HW. Brain stem reticular formation and activation of the EEG. Electroencephalogr Clin Neurophysiol. 1949;1(4):455–73.
189. Westover MB, Gururangan K, Markert MS, et al. Diagnostic value of electroencephalography with ten electrodes in critically ill patients. Neurocrit Care. 2020;33:479–90.
190. Jafarian A, Freestone DR, Nesic D, et al. Identification of a neural mass model of burst suppression. Conf Proc IEEE Eng Med Biol Soc. 2019;2019:2905–8.
191. Chakravarty S, Baum TE, An J, et al. A hidden semi-Markov model for estimating burst suppression EEG. Conf Proc IEEE Eng Med Biol Soc. 2019;2019:7076–9.
192. Rubin DB, Angelini B, Shoukat M, et al. Electrographic predictors of successful weaning from anaesthetics in refractory status epilepticus. Brain. 2020;143(4):1143–57.
193. Barbella G, Novy J, Marques-Vidal P, et al. Prognostic role of EEG identical bursts in patients after cardiac arrest: multimodal correlation. Resuscitation. 2020;148:140–4.
194. Hofmeijer J, van Putten MJ. EEG in postanoxic coma: prognostic and diagnostic value. Clin Neurophysiol. 2016;127(4):2047–55.
195. Liang Z, Wang Y, Ren Y, et al. Detection of burst suppression patterns in EEG using recurrence rate. Sci World J. 2014;2014:295070.
196. Derbyshire A, Rempel B, Forbes A. Effect of anesthetics on action potentials in cerebral cortex of the cat. Amer J Physiol. 1936;116:577–96.
197. Swank RL, Watson CW. Effects of barbiturates and ether on spontaneous electrical activity of dog brain. J Neurophysiol. 1949;12(2):137–60.
198. Steriade M, Amzica F, Contreras D. Cortical and thalamic cellular correlates of electroencephalographic burst-suppression. Electroencephalogr Clin Neurophysiol. 1994;90(1):1–16.
199. Henry CE, Scoville WB. Suppression-burst activity from isolated cerebral cortex in man. Electroencephalogr Clin Neurophysiol. 1952;4(1):1–22.
200. Kang BS, Jung KH, Shin JW, et al. Induction of burst suppression or coma using intravenous anesthetics in refractory status epilepticus. J Clin Neurosci. 2015;22(5):854–8.
201. Ohtahara S, Ohtsuka Y, Oka E. Epileptic encephalopathies in early infancy. Indian J Pediatr. 1997;64(5):603–12.

202. Donat JF. The age-dependent epileptic encephalopathies. J Child Neurol. 1992;7(1):7–21.
203. Aicardi J, Goutieres F. Neonatal myoclonic encephalopathy (author's transl). Rev Electroencephalogr Neurophysiol Clin. 1978;8(1):99–101.
204. Liu CT, Yin F, Huang R, et al. The clinical and electroencephalographic characteristics of early myoclonic encephalopathy. Zhonghua Er Ke Za Zhi. 2012;50(12):899–902.
205. Ohtahara S, Ohtsuka Y, Yamatogi Y, et al. The early-infantile epileptic encephalopathy with suppression-burst: developmental aspects. Brain Dev. 1987;9(4):371–6.
206. Toda Y, Kobayashi K, Hayashi Y, et al. High-frequency EEG activity in epileptic encephalopathy with suppression-burst. Brain Dev. 2015;37(2):230–6.
207. Vetro A, Pisano T, Chiaro S, et al. Early infantile epileptic-dyskinetic encephalopathy due to biallelic PIGP mutations. Neurol Genet. 2020;6(1):e387.
208. Yamatogi Y, Ohtahara S. Early-infantile epileptic encephalopathy with suppression-bursts, Ohtahara syndrome; its overview referring to our 16 cases. Brain Dev. 2002;24(1):13–23.
209. Hong SY, Hsin YL, Lee IC. An infant with congenital central hypoventilation syndrome: transient burst suppression electroencephalogram. Pediatr Neonatol. 2016;57(4):357–8.
210. Amorim E, Rittenberger JC, Zheng JJ, et al. Continuous EEG monitoring enhances multimodal outcome prediction in hypoxic-ischemic brain injury. Resuscitation. 2016;109:121–6.
211. Westhall E, Rossetti AO, van Rootselaar AF, et al. Standardized EEG interpretation accurately predicts prognosis after cardiac arrest. Neurology. 2016;86(16):1482–90.
212. Awal MA, Lai MM, Azemi G, et al. EEG background features that predict outcome in term neonates with hypoxic ischaemic encephalopathy: a structured review. Clin Neurophysiol. 2016;127(1):285–96.
213. Chalia M, Lee CW, Dempsey LA, et al. Hemodynamic response to burst-suppressed and discontinuous electroencephalography activity in infants with hypoxic ischemic encephalopathy. Neurophotonics. 2016;3(3):31408.
214. Bloom J, Wyler D, Torjman MC, et al. High incidence of burst suppression during propofol sedation for outpatient colonoscopy: lessons learned from neuromonitoring. Anesthesiol Res Pract. 2020;2020:7246570.
215. Hogan J, Sun H, Aboul NH, et al. Burst suppression: causes and effects on mortality in critical illness. Neurocrit Care. 2020.
216. Martinez-Bermejo A, Roche C, Lopez-Martin V, et al. Neonatal EEG trace of burst suppression. Etiological and evolutionary factors. Rev Neurol. 2001;33(6):514–8.
217. Andresen JM, Girard TD, Pandharipande PP, et al. Burst suppression on processed electroencephalography as a predictor of postcoma delirium in mechanically ventilated ICU patients. Crit Care Med. 2014;42(10):2244–51.
218. Koch S, Rupp L, Prager C, et al. Emergence delirium in children is related to epileptiform discharges during anaesthesia induction: an observational study. Eur J Anaesthesiol. 2018;35(12):929–36.
219. Nita DA, Moldovan M, Sharma R, et al. Burst-suppression is reactive to photic stimulation in comatose children with acquired brain injury. Clin Neurophysiol. 2016;127(8):2921–30.
220. Vaewpanich J, Reuter-Rice K. Continuous electroencephalography in pediatric traumatic brain injury: Seizure characteristics and outcomes. Epilepsy Behav. 2016;62:225–30.
221. Zhou DW, Westover MB, McClain LM, et al. Clustering analysis to identify distinct spectral components of encephalogram burst suppression in critically ill patients. Conf Proc IEEE Eng Med Biol Soc. 2015;2015:7258–61.
222. Kang X, Jiang H, Wu C, et al. Application of continuous video-electroencephalographic monitoring in patients with consciousness disorders in intensive care unit. Zhonghua Yi Xue Za Zhi. 2015;95(21):1663–6.
223. Leidi A, Pisaturo M, Fumeaux T. Malnutrition-related hyperammonemic encephalopathy presenting with burst suppression: a case report. J Med Case Rep. 2019;13(1):248.
224. Touchard C, Cartailler J, Leve C, et al. EEG power spectral density under Propofol and its association with burst suppression, a marker of cerebral fragility. Clin Neurophysiol. 2019;130(8):1311–9.
225. Akbik F, Robertson M, Das AS, et al. The PET sandwich: using serial FDG-PET scans with interval burst suppression to assess ictal components of disease. Neurocrit Care. 2020;33:330–1.
226. Jiang M, Su Y, Liu G, et al. EEG pattern predicts awakening of comatose patients after cardiopulmonary resuscitation. Resuscitation. 2020;151:33–8.
227. Rossi SD, Visani E, Panzica F, et al. Sleep patterns associated with the severity of impairment in a large cohort of patients with chronic disorders of consciousness. Clin Neurophysiol. 2018;129(3):687–93.
228. Sandroni C, D'Arrigo S, Cacciola S, et al. Prediction of poor neurological outcome in comatose survivors of cardiac arrest: a systematic review. Intensive Care Med. 2020;46:1803–51.
229. Azabou E, Fischer C, Mauguiere F, et al. Prospective cohort study evaluating the prognostic value of simple EEG parameters in postanoxic coma. Clin EEG Neurosci. 2016;47(1):75–82.
230. Han Y, Fu N, Chen W, et al. Prognostic value of electroencephalography in hypothermia-treated neonates with hypoxic-ischemic encephalopathy: a meta-analysis. Pediatr Neurol. 2019;93:3–10.
231. Qian SY, Wang Q, Su YY. Interpretation of criteria and practical guidance for determination of brain death in children. Zhonghua Er Ke Za Zhi. 2019;57(11):826–9.

232. Caronna E, Vilaseca A, Maria GGR, et al. Long-term prognosis related to deep sedation in refractory status epilepticus. Acta Neurol Scand. 2020.
233. Stecker MM, Cheung AT, Pochettino A, et al. Deep hypothermic circulatory arrest: I. Effects of cooling on electroencephalogram and evoked potentials. Ann Thorac Surg. 2001;71(1):14–21.
234. Scarpino M, Carrai R, Lolli F, et al. Neurophysiology for predicting good and poor neurological outcome at 12 and 72 h after cardiac arrest: the ProNeCA multicentre prospective study. Resuscitation. 2020;147:95–103.

# Abnormal EEG Background Activity

4

Xuefeng Wang and Yin Yan

## Contents



**Abstract**

Background activity refers to the brain's electrical activity that is recorded when the subject is in a normal or pathological basic state. Abnormal background activities include reduction or disappearance of normal brain wave activity, changes in the frequency of brain electrical activity (increased slow waves or increased fast waves), changes in rhythm (absence of normal rhythm or abnormal rhythmic activity), changes in amplitude (significant increase or decrease), obvious waveform distortion (e.g., polymorphic slow waves),

X. Wang
Department of Neurology, The First Affiliated Hospital of Chongqing Medical University, Chongqing, China

Y. Yan (✉)
Department of Neurology, Chongqing University Central Hospital, Chongqing Emergency Medical Center, Chongqing, China



X. Wang et al. (eds.), *Multi-Modal EEG Monitoring of Severely Neurologically Ill Patients*,
https://doi.org/10.1007/978-981-16-4493-1_4

etc., as well as abnormal spatial and temporal distribution of brain electrical activity. Abnormal background activity is a nonspecific abnormality that is related to the severity of diffuse or local brain dysfunction but lacks the specificity of etiology or pathology. Background activity analysis in ICU patients is different from that of non-ICU patients. It has particularity and complexity, especially in patients with impaired consciousness and ICU patients who cannot record awake patterns. The judgment of their background activities also needs to consider the symmetry, continuity, and reactivity of background activities. This chapter describes in detail the related concepts and interpretation methods of EEG symmetry, continuity, and reactivity in combination with illustrations. At the same time, it introduces its clinical guidance value for the evaluation of brain function and prognosis of critically ill patients, which lays the foundation for EEG analysis of critically ill patients.

**Keywords**

ICU · EEG · Background activity · Symmetry · Continuity · Reactivity

## 4.1 EEG Symmetry

### 4.1.1 The Clinical Significance of Mild/Significant Amplitude Asymmetry

According to the amplitude and frequency difference of the two sides, the EEG background activity can be divided into (**a**) symmetrical activity; (**b**) slight asymmetrical activity (in the reference lead record, the amplitude is asymmetric, with the difference between the two sides being less than 50%, or the frequency is asymmetric, with the difference between the two sides being 0.5~1 Hz); and (**c**) obviously asymmetrical activity (the wave amplitude difference between the two sides is ≥50%, or the frequency difference is >1 Hz) [1]. Asymmetrical amplitudes in the EEGs of both sides are common when there are unilateral pathological changes in brain structures, such as cerebral ischemia, intraparenchymal hemorrhage, prenatal or postpartum ischemic injury, congenital brain malformations, and tumors, among which cerebral ischemia is especially common in patients [2]. In hemispheric infarction, metabolism may slow down in both hemispheres, but there are obvious differences between hemispheres in the recovery time and rate of brain function. EEG changes in the infarcted hemisphere may be related to the reperfusion of the infarcted brain area, the dynamic changes in cerebral edema, and the functional recovery of surviving neuronal cells, while the changes in the contralateral hemisphere are more related to intracellular acidosis caused by brain edema and the improvement in hypoxia in tissue cells [3–5].

The asymmetry of amplitude/frequency in the EEGs of both sides has early diagnostic value for acute cerebral infarction. Petty et al. [6] found that within 48 h of the onset of the first lacunar infarction, a unilateral severe abnormality in the EEG can help rule out lacunar infarction or infarction limited to the brainstem. In the study of Macdonell et al. [7], the EEG characteristics of 91 patients with acute cerebral infarction were observed, and it was found that the EEGs showed that unilateral abnormal changes were related to cortical infarction. In the early state of disease, the fast-wave activity may be slightly weakened in the infarcted hemisphere; as the disease progresses, polymorphic δ activity appears in the temporal and frontotemporal areas of the affected hemisphere, and the α and β activities on the side of the lesion are diminished or missing [8]. A study on acute large-area cerebral infarction by Schneider et al. [9] found that more than 56% of patients' EEGs revealed unilateral severe abnormalities, and they found a unique EEG pattern of acute large-area cerebral infarction (regional attenuation without δ, RAWOD); in this pattern, all frequency waves in a wide area are weakened, and no δ waves appear.

In addition, asymmetry in the activity of the cerebral hemispheres has suggestive significance for the prognosis of severe patients. Amrein et al.

[10] showed that an increase in the α band ratio after hemispheric infarction is significantly correlated with an improvement in clinical symptoms after stroke, and an increase in the δ activity ratio or a gradual increase in bilateral asymmetry is associated with continuous deterioration of brain function in the infarcted brain area and an important manifestation of poor prognosis [11]. Asymmetrical activity in EEGs is an indicator of the long-term prognosis of severely ill patients. Nazish et al. [12] found that asymmetrical background activity is associated with disease-related sequelae after discharge from the hospital in critically ill patients with different etiologies of illness. Bentes et al. [13] showed for the first time that asymmetrical background activity in EEGs is an independent predictor of epilepsy 1 year after stroke.

### 4.1.2 Gap Effect

In 1979, Cobb et al. [14] first recorded epileptiform scalp brain waves on skull defects, which are called the notch rhythm. The characteristics of the notch rhythm in EEGs are usually focal, asymmetrical, high-amplitude activity; arched waveforms, sometimes similar to sharp or spike waves; irregular rhythm waves, or waves that are similar to sharp waves or spikes, which can appear individually; and prominence in the central and temporal areas [15, 16] or other parts of the brain with skull defects. During sleep, the notch rhythm waveform appears as a higher-amplitude and faster-frequency wave, corresponding to brain waves at different stages of sleep. For example, the notch rhythm can be expressed as an increase in the amplitude of the brain waves that occur in the second stage of sleep [17, 18]. There is a difference between the gap rhythm and the "third rhythm." The "third rhythm" refers to the α and fast θ (6~11 Hz) rhythms recorded in the temporal lobe of some patients with intact skulls that are distinguishable from those of the occipital area and the physiological rhythms of the α rhythm and the μ rhythm in the central area [19, 20].

The occurrence of the notch rhythm is related to changes in local skull resistance caused by various reasons. Changes in skull electrical resistance can lead to the appearance of the notch rhythm. The reasons may include skull defects, skull disease (such as Langerhans histiocytosis, multiple myeloma, skull metastasis, skull bone tuberculosis), or surgical repair and other factors [21, 22]. For changes in skull resistance caused by different reasons, the amplitude and frequency of the notch rhythm recorded on the corresponding scalp on the opposite side will have different characteristics. When the skull is missing or the resistance of the repair material is significantly lower than that of the skull (such as titanium mesh), stronger brain electrical activity can be recorded on the scalp than on the corresponding scalp on the opposite side, with higher brainwave amplitude and faster frequency. When the resistance of the repair material is similar to that of the skull (such as autologous bone), scalp EEG cannot record the gap rhythm; if the resistance of the repair material is greater than that of the skull (polymethyl methacrylate or polyether ether ketone), the gap rhythm will have a decreased amplitude and slowed frequency [23, 24]. It should be noted that the notch rhythm is not caused by the abnormality of the brain, but because of the abnormality of the skull, the resistance is reduced, thereby reducing the filtering effect of the corresponding part. Therefore, the notch rhythm is usually regarded as a benign EEG variation. Identification is particularly critical for the diagnosis and treatment of clinical diseases.

To date, there is little literature about the gap rhythm, the epidemiology of the gap rhythm is not clear, and whether the gap rhythm can be recorded after skull repair is still controversial. Clinically, it is not uncommon for skull defects to be associated with abnormal brain tissues in the corresponding parts. The scalp EEG recorded on the skull defect area may include the notch rhythm, epileptic discharge, and other pathological slow-wave abnormal activities [15, 16, 25, 26]. Therefore, based on the overall situation of the patient, correctly interpreting the benign variations of EEGs, avoiding confusion with interictal epileptiform discharges, paroxysmal fast-wave activity, β activity, low-amplitude slow-wave activity, and myoelectric artifacts, is essential to avoid missed and overdiagnosed epilepsy.

### 4.1.3 The Clinical Significance of the Front-Back Gradient and Front-Back Inverse Gradient

The anterior-posterior gradient refers to a clear and continuous (lasting at least 1 min) voltage difference and frequency difference appearing from front to back at any point in the record, which indicates that the amplitude is lower and the frequency is faster in the front lead, while the rear lead has a higher amplitude and slower frequency. The posterior-anterior gradient refers to the voltage difference and frequency difference from the back to the front [1].

The clinical significance of the anterior-posterior gradient in different diseases is different. Hunter et al. [27] monitored the qEEGs of patients with Huntington disease and showed that Huntington disease patients showed a loss of relative α and δ power before and after normal anterior-posterior gradients compared with healthy subjects. The relative loss of the α- anterior-posterior gradient was related to a decrease in the patient's total functional capacity and cognitive dysfunction. Relative δ anterior-posterior gradient loss was related to low total functional capacity, more severe motor symptoms, and more trinucleotide CAG repetitions. Previous studies have shown that the slowing of the predominant α rhythm in the posterior part of EEGs is a biomarker for patients with Lewy body dementia [28]. However, a recent multicenter European cohort study [29] showed that in patients with dementia with Lewy bodies, the anterior EEG and dominant rhythms in the posterior part are all front α (5.5–7.5 Hz), but the lead of the dominant rhythm is slower than the posterior rhythm. The study's authors believe that the formation of this anterior-posterior inverse gradient may be caused by thalamic cortical rhythm disturbance, which is closely related to the patient's cognitive impairment. In addition, the anterior-posterior gradient of EEGs is also correlated with different sleep stages. In NREM sleep, the forward guide frequency of the 2 Hz band is higher than the backward guide frequency, while the forward guide frequency of the 4~10 Hz band is lower than the backward guide frequency. In REM sleep, most mid-to-high frequency bands have a backward advantage. This suggests that the front and back of the cerebral cortex may be involved in different sleep processes [30, 31].

## 4.2 EEG Continuity

### 4.2.1 Definition of EEG Continuity

EEG continuity is the maintenance of certain amplitude without obvious fluctuations during the recording process (Fig. 4.1a, b). According to the guidelines of the ACNS in 2012 [1], EEG continuity is defined as brain activity that has no obvious electrical attenuation (low voltage $\geq$10 μV but less than 50% of the background voltage) or inhibition (low voltage <10 μV). Research on the background EEG activity in coma patients after brain injury pointed out that EEG continuity is one of the most indicative features of brain function, and the continuous pattern is related to the recovery of consciousness [32]. Relevant evidence shows that for patients with brain injury, there is a correlation between the prognosis of neurological function and the time limit for the EEG to return to normal continuity [33]. Sugiyama et al. [34] explored the relationship between the neurological prognosis of coma survivors after cardiac arrest and the recovery time of CNV and determined the recovery time limit for predicting a good neurological prognosis. EEG recovery to CNV within 23 h after sudden arrest can predict a good neurological prognosis of the patient. The sensitivity was 89%, the specificity was 100%, the positive-predictive value was 100%, and the negative-predictive value was 86%. Oh et al. [35] reported that the time for cEEG recovery in patients with cardiac arrest is 24 h, which is the best value for predicting a good neurological prognosis. Although

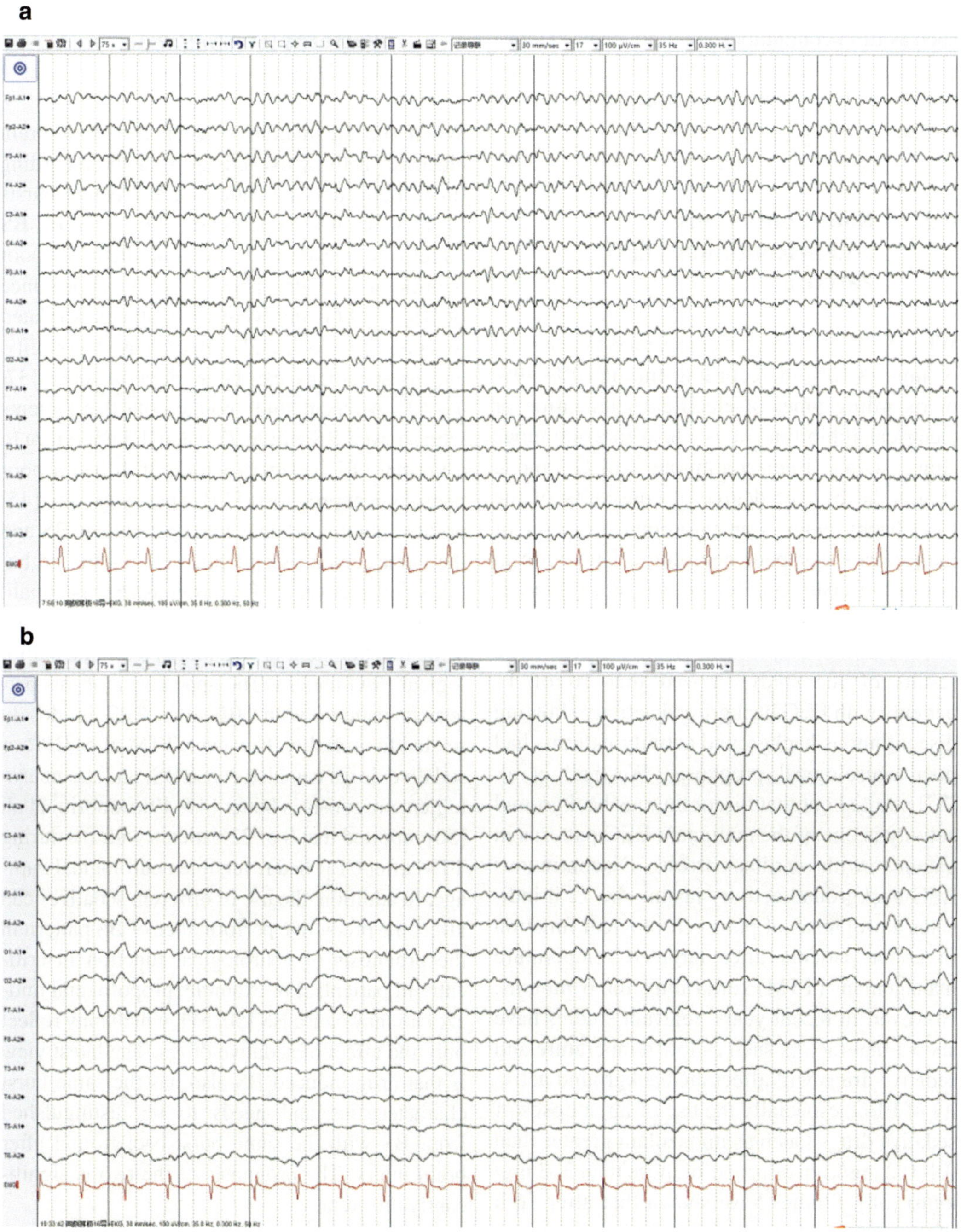

**Fig. 4.1** (**a**) An EEG with a continuous background pattern, showing certain amplitude without obvious fluctuation during the recording process. (**b**) Continuous background EEG

the CNV recovery time of approximately 24 h has good sensitivity and specificity to predict a good neurological prognosis, some patients within this time period still have a poor neurological prognosis in the two studies. In some patients with severe brain injury, although the background activity of EEG is continuous, it may still have a poor prognosis, such as α coma or θ coma. Therefore, in clinical practice, an indicator such as EEG continuity should not be used alone to predict the outcome, and multimodal evaluation should be combined to avoid evaluation errors.

### 4.2.2 Near-Continuous and Discontinuous EEG Patterns

When EEG activity is accompanied by a period of time (≤10% of recording time)/(10%~49% of recording time) of electrical attenuation or electrical inhibition, it is close to continuous (Fig. 4.2a, b)/discontinuous EEG mode (Fig. 4.3a, b). The degree of continuity of the EEG background is an important predictor of the prognosis of poor neurological function in critically ill patients. Benarous et al. [36] monitored the cEEGs of patients with hypoxic coma after cardiac arrest and resuscitation. The results of the study showed that 10 of 11 patients with EEG background activity showing discontinuous background activity patterns had poor neurological prognosis. Westhall et al. [37] pointed out that discontinuous background activity is one of the malignant EEG patterns in patients with cardiac arrest. Discontinuous EEG background activity lasting 48–72 h indicates a prognosis of poor neurological function in coma patients after targeted temperature management (TTM) rewarming for 6 months. However, in recent years, relevant studies have shown that factors such as low temperature and sedative drugs will affect the background activity of EEG, especially the use of large doses of sedative drugs (such as midazolam greater than 0.1–0.2 mg/kg/h or propofol more than 2–3 mg/kg/h) [38]. Studies have shown that after 16 h of therapeutic hypothermia, 50% of patients can have discontinuous background patterns, but the prognosis of patients is relatively good [39, 40]. Therefore, when using EEG to assess the prognosis of patients, it is necessary to exclude the influence of related reversible factors (such as sedative drugs or therapeutic hypothermia).

### 4.2.3 Discontinuous EEG of BS Patterns (See the Sect. 3.6 for Details)

When the attenuation or suppression of brain electrical activity exceeds 50% of the recording time, it appears as a pattern of alternating bursts of attenuation or suppression (Fig. 4.4a, b). BS pattern is considered to be a predictor of poor neurological prognosis [37, 41]. The appearance of BS on EEGs in severely ill patients is related to a poor prognosis and even increased mortality, and its specificity can be as high as 100% [37, 41–43]. A recent study pointed out that patients who showed BS within 72 h and did not return to a normal cEEG pattern within 36 h had a poor neurological prognosis [44]. Thenayan et al. [45] pointed out that when a coma patient has BS and the burst content is epileptic activity, the probability of recovery of consciousness is small. Hofmeijer et al. [46] proposed that BS with the same burst content is considered a unique pathological EEG pattern. The appearance of this pattern in patients with HIE after CPR is closely related to mortality. However, TTM after CPR or sedative drugs can also cause BS, and the neurological prognosis is better [47–49]. Amorim et al. [50] reported that 8 of 22 patients with BS during TTM after CPR had reversible neurological damage. In addition, the use of different sedatives can affect the predictive performance of BS pattern in the prognosis of neurological function in critically ill patients. For example, propofol and midazolam may cause BS [50, 51], which may reflect only the effect of sedative drugs. The latest view is that drug-induced BS also has the same burst characteristics and needs to be distinguished from BS with the same burst background after brain injury. The prognosis of the two is significantly different.

### 4.2.4 Suppression-State Background Mode

If the entire recorded EEG is composed of suppression (<10 μV), it is in an inhibited state (Fig. 4.5). Continuous suppression, or a resting

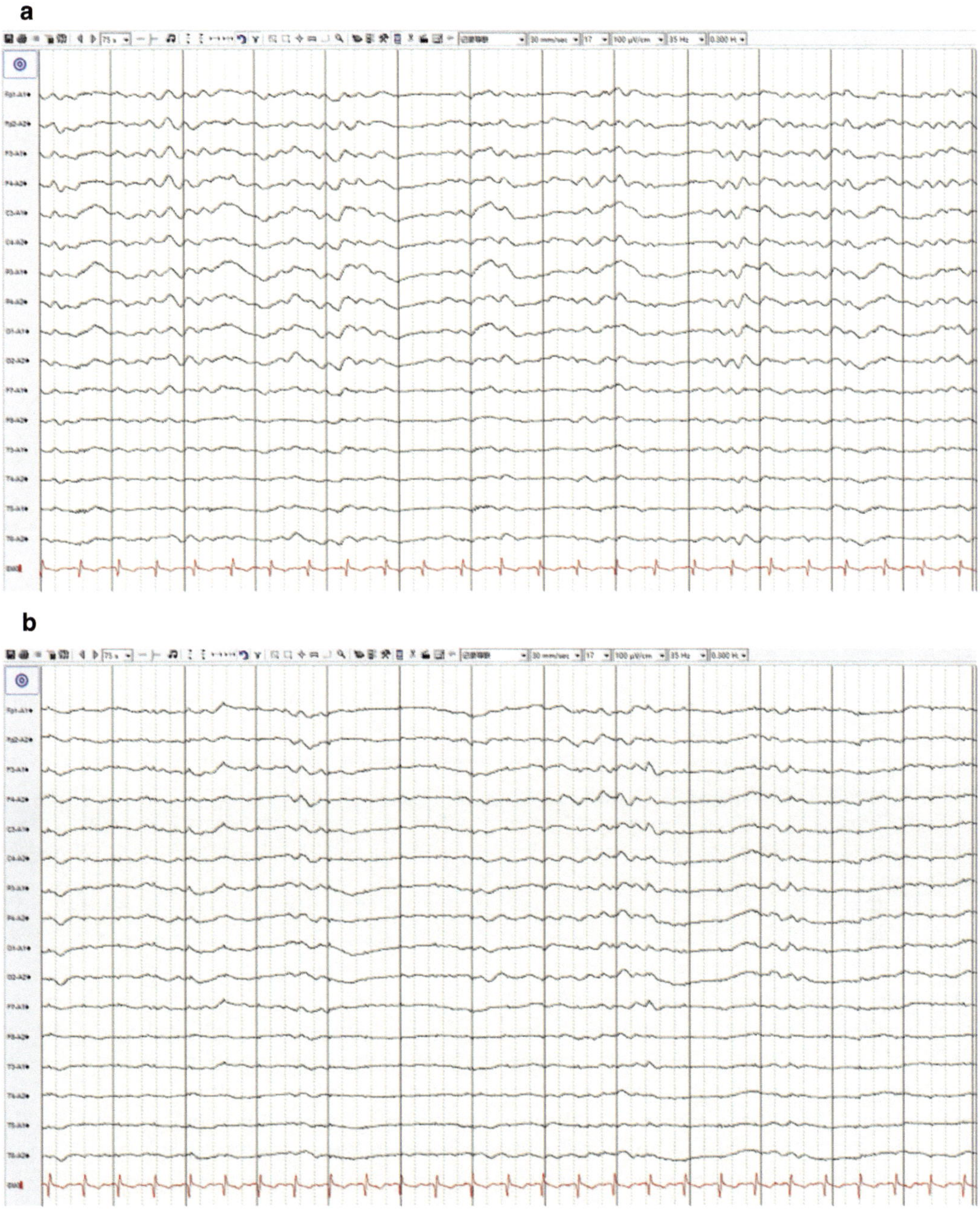

**Fig. 4.2** (**a**) An EEG showing a period of electrical attenuation or electrical suppression (≤10% of the recording time), which is close to a continuous background pattern. (**b**) Near-continuous EEG background pattern

EEG pattern, is closely related to adverse neurological outcomes. The study of Cloostermans et al. [48] showed that the continuous suppression of EEG patterns and isoelectric patterns 24 h after resuscitation can predict poor neurological prognosis with a specificity of 100%. The results of Guedes et al. [39] also showed that completely suppressed EEG background activity, as one of the highly malignant EEG patterns, is closely related to adverse neurological outcomes; its

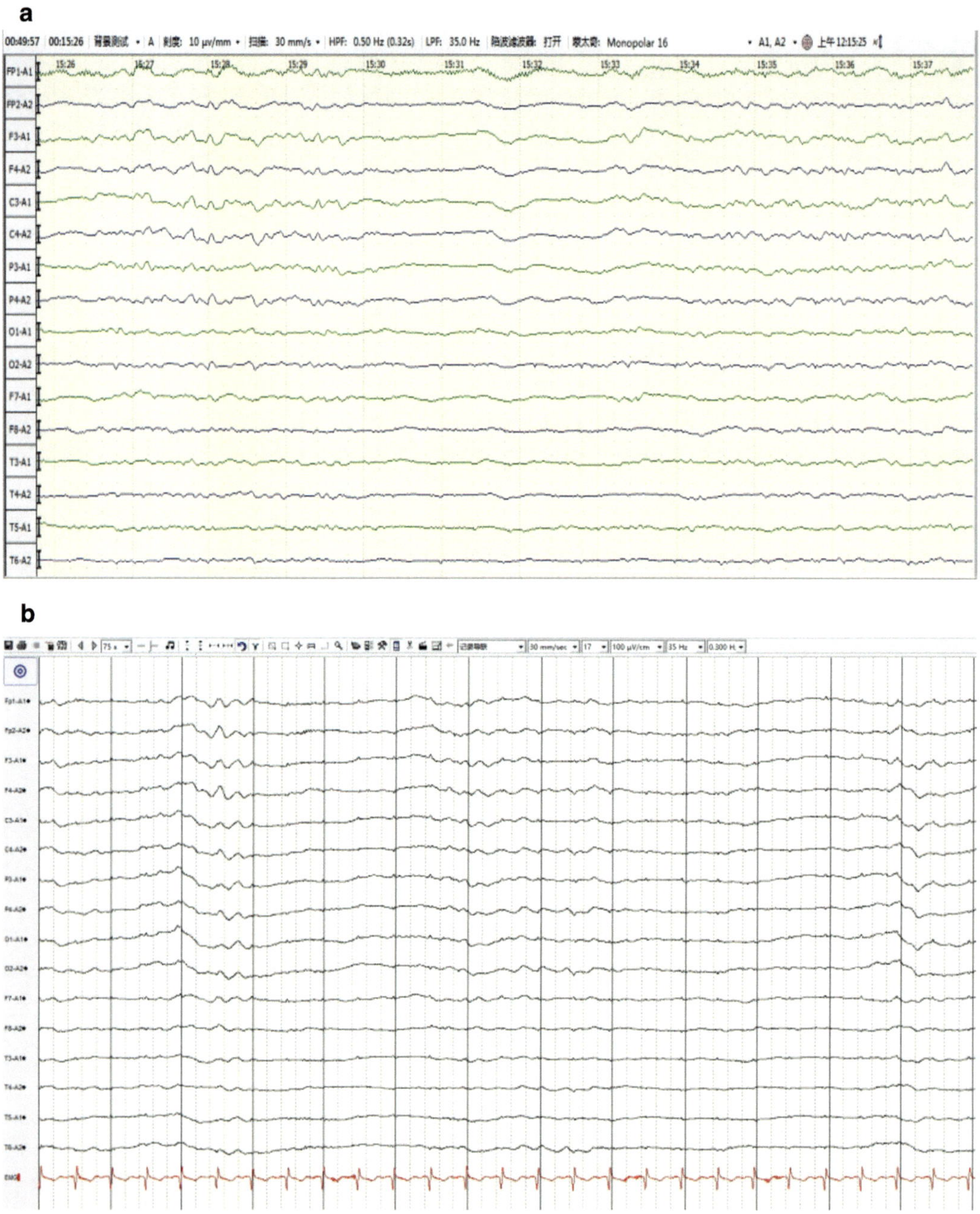


**Fig. 4.3** (**a**) An EEG showing a period of electrical attenuation or electrical suppression (10% to 49% of the recording time), which is a discontinuous background pattern. (**b**) Discontinuous EEG background pattern

specificity is as high as 100%, and the specificity for predicting death can reach 82.4%. However, in another study, Rundgren et al. [52] analyzed the EEG characteristics recorded within 8 h after cardiac arrest or immediately after rewarming. The results showed that patients with continuous

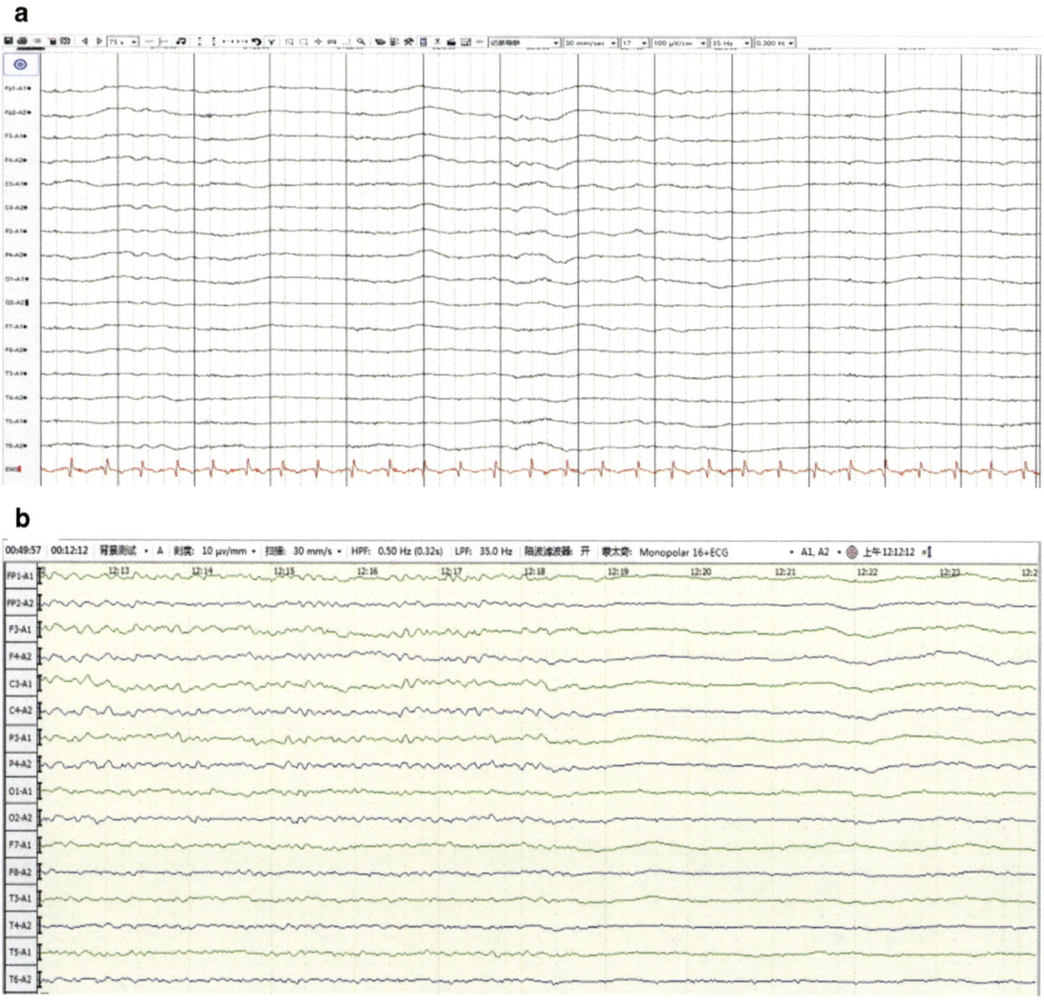

**Fig. 4.4** (**a**) An EEG showing the attenuation or suppression of activity for more than 50% of the recording time, which is an alternating pattern of bursts of attenuation or suppression. (**b**) Burst attenuation or BS pattern

suppression of EEG patterns (<10 μV) often regained consciousness. In the study of Bouwes et al. [53], three patients without EEG reactivity (EEG-R) after rewarming had a good outcome. This difference may be related to the interpretation of EEG-R and the time point of EEG recording. Therefore, the evaluation of the patient's prognosis requires dynamic follow-up. If suppressed or resting EEG patterns gradually evolve into continuous patterns, with the improvement of the slow-wave mode, the prognosis of the patient is more likely to be good.

## 4.3 EEG-R

### 4.3.1 The Definition of EEG-R

The responsiveness of an EEG refers to the changes in the frequency or amplitude of the EEG background waves after external stimuli (such as sound, light, pain), and it has a strict time-dependent relationship with the stimulus (Figs. 4.6 and 4.7). The anatomical basis of EEG-R depends on the completeness of all structures and functions from the brainstem network

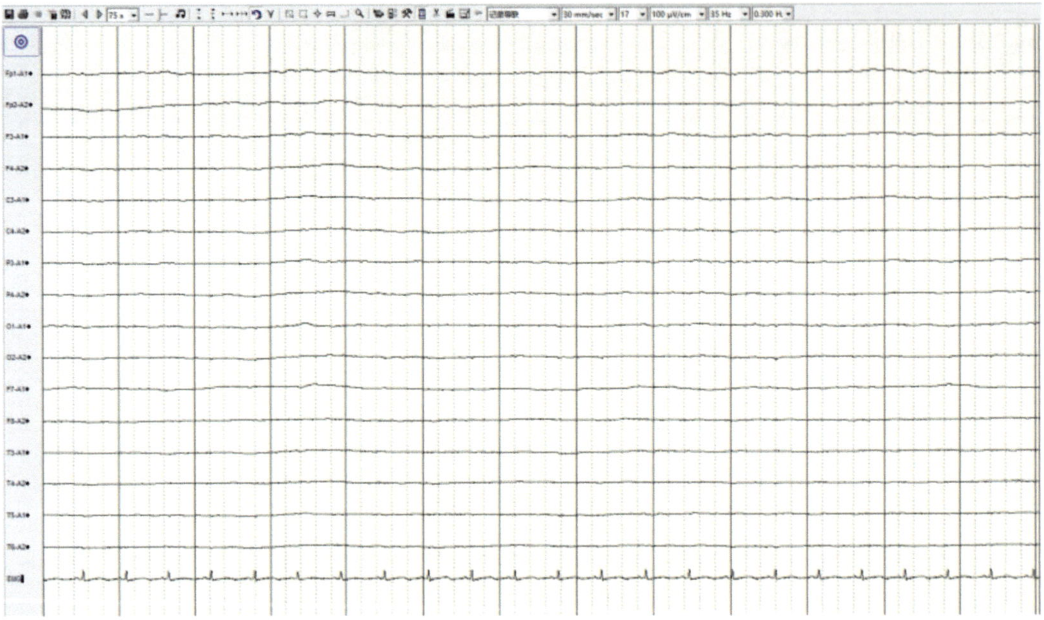

**Fig. 4.5** An EEG showing a suppression (<10 μV) for the whole recording time, which is a suppressed state

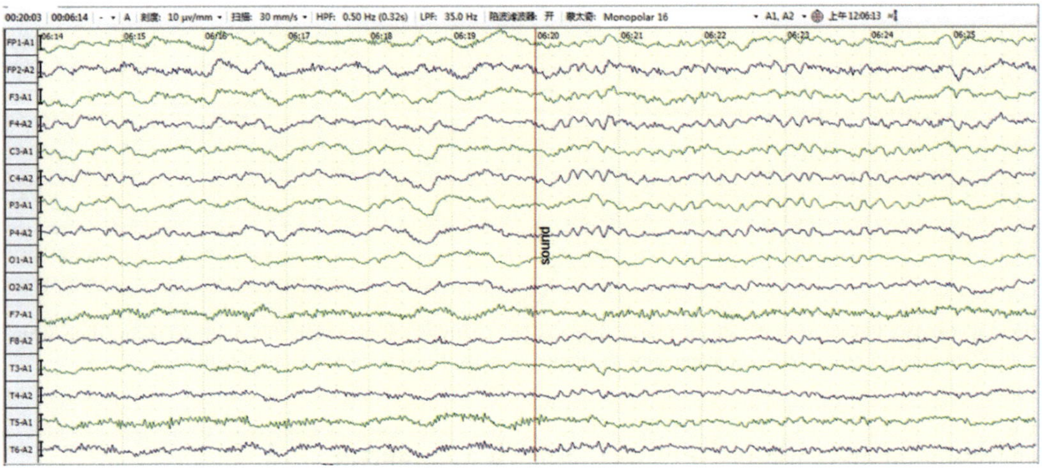


**Fig. 4.6** Brain-wave amplitude and frequency increase after sound stimulation. There is an obvious time-dependent relationship between stimulation and EEG-R

to the subthalamus, hypothalamus, and thalamus cortical system, reflecting the integrity of the overall network function of the cerebral cortex [54, 55]. Common exogenous stimuli include sound (calling or clapping the palms), visual stimulation (passively opening the eyes), or somatosensory stimuli (pressing the nail bed or pressing the supraorbital nerve until painful). Studies have pointed out that nipple pinching is more effective in causing EEG changes than acupuncture at the back of the nose or pressing nails [56].

### 4.3.2 The Prognostic Value of EEG-R for Adult Patients

Azabou E et al. [57] prospectively studied the early bedside EEG characteristics of 61 patients with coma after acute hypoxia. The EEG features

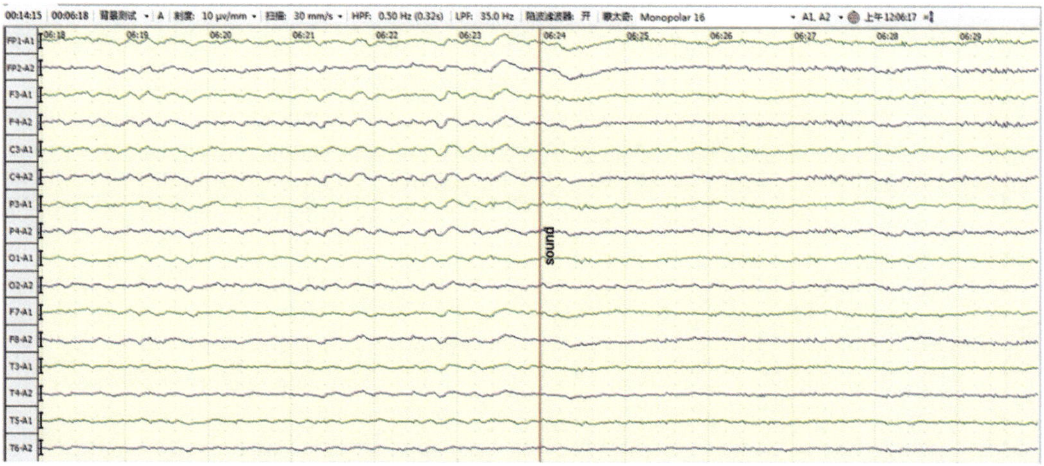


**Fig. 4.7** The amplitude of the whole lead decreases after sound stimulation, and there is an obvious time-dependent relationship between stimulation and EEG-R

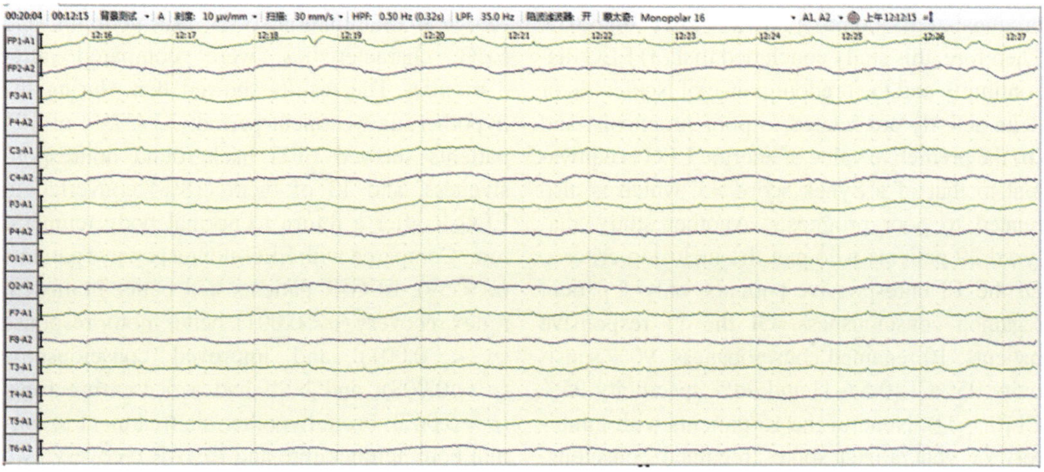

**Fig. 4.8** An EEG showing comprehensive low-voltage slow-wave activity as background activity

were divided into five types, namely, equal "waves," discontinuity, no response to strong sound or painful stimulation (Figs. 4.8 and 4.9), dominant δ frequency, and paroxysmal abnormalities. Variables such as sensitivity, specificity, positive-predictive value, negative-predictive value, and the AUC are used to predict poor prognosis. Poor prognosis is divided into death, persistent VS, minimally conscious state (MCS), and severe neurological disability. After the patients were in a coma for 1 year, the above variables were calculated, and the Synek score was also calculated. Fifty-six patients (91.8%) had a poor prognosis. The sensitivity, specificity, positive-predictive value, negative-predictive value, and nonresponsive EEG AUC predicted poor prognosis, with values of 84%, 80%, 98%, 31%, and 0.82, respectively; all these values were close to those of a Synek score >3, which were 82%, 80%, 98%, 29% and 0.81, respectively. Isoelectric activity, discontinuities, and δ activities were predominant; the specificity of predicting adverse consequences was 100%; and they all indicated poor prognosis. The lack of EEG-R was obviously related to the poor prognosis of coma after hypoxia, and its accuracy was comparable to that of a Synek score >3. Analyzing these EEG characteristics can help clinicians understand the

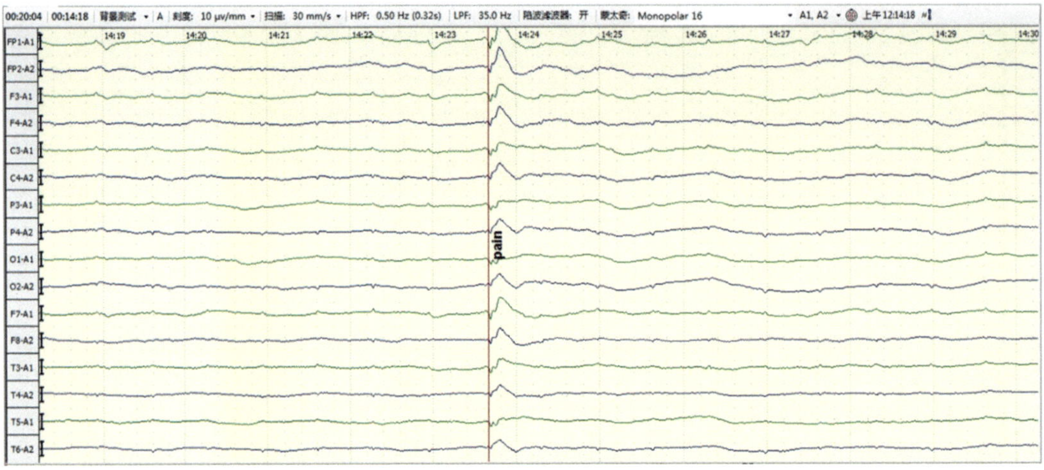

**Fig. 4.9** An EEG showing no changes in amplitude/frequency following sound and pain stimulation, which is an unresponsive EEG

prognosis of coma patients after hypoxia. Therefore, this study concluded that (**a**) EEG discontinuity and the predominance of isoelectric or delta activity are related to poor prognosis; and (**b**) the predictive value of anergic EEG is equivalent to that of a Synek score >3, which is also related to poor prognosis. Another study analyzed 29 patients who met the inclusion criteria. Of the 18 unresponsive patients, only 1 patient regained consciousness. Of the 11 responsive patients, 10 regained consciousness (90% sensitivity 95%CI [0.57–1] and 94% specificity 95% CI [0.7–1]). None of the 15 patients with inhibitory or generalized spikes regained consciousness, and none of their EEGs showed reactivity. The research results showed that EEG-R after cardiac arrest is a relatively good EEG feature. Extensive inhibition or extensive epileptiform activity and nonresponsiveness are associated with difficulty in recovering consciousness [45].

Elsa Juan et al. [58] observed EEG nonresponsiveness during hypothermia treatment, while EEG-R was restored after a return to normal body temperature; therefore, whether some patients are different from those who have never shown EEG-R remains unclear. The subjects of the study were patients with no EEG-R during hypothermia treatment and were unconscious adults whose EEGs were recorded after successful CPR from March 2009 to June 2014. The neurological examination, NSE, procalcitonin, and EEG characteristics were compared after 3 months. The results showed that, during the hypothermia treatment period, 72 (37%) of 197 patients showed EEG background nonresponsiveness, and 13 of them (18%) converted to EEG-R after a return to normal body temperature. Compared with EEG-nonresponsive patients ($n = 59$), EEG-R patients had better brainstem reflex recovery ($p < 0.001$), better motor response ($p < 0.001$), and improved consciousness ($p = 0.008$); and NSE had a decreasing trend ($p = 0.067$). From hypothermia treatment to normal body temperature and EEG-R recovery, two groups of patients could be distinguished, namely, the EEG-R group and the EEG nonresponse group. Patients with EEG-R and EEG nonresponse were dynamically changing, which makes us confident that patients who do not show EEG-R should continue to receive intensive treatment, even if these patients show no EEG-R during hypothermia treatment. Because there are still a small number of patients who later recover EEG-R, the prognosis is improved. Rossetti AO et al. [47] prospectively selected 61 patients who received hypothermia treatment after cardiac arrest. When studying EEG-R and serum NSE for the prognosis of patients with coma after hypoxia, it was found that serum NSE and EEG-R were significantly correlated (spearman rho = 0.45; $p < 0.001$). The average peak value of NSE was the highest in patients with an unresponsive EEG background ($p < 0.001$) and discontinuous pattern ($p = 0.001$). All patients with an unresponsive EEG background died. Among the survivors, 5 had NSE levels >33 μg/L. Therefore, the researchers believed that early EEG changes can reflect permanent neurological damage. After cardiac arrest, a lack of EEG-R in the background and the appearance of transient epileptiform discharges indicate a poor prognosis.

To explore the reliability of EEG-R in predicting the recovery of consciousness after acute brain injury. Logi F et al. [59] analyzed the EEGs of 50 patients with impaired consciousness, and all patients had a GCS ≤8. They suffered from TBI, cerebrovascular disease or hypoxia. According to the Synek classification method, their EEGs were divided into benign, malignant, and ambiguous categories. The EEG-R to painful stimuli was observed. The results found that 20% of EEG-R were benign, 38% were malignant, and 42% were classified as unclear. The prognosis of patients with an unclear EEG-R is difficult to judge. Forty-eight percent of the patients with unclear EEG-R underwent EEG-R testing, and after 5 months, 92% of them regained consciousness. For patients with EEG-R, the possibility of the recovery of consciousness was as high as 97%. Therefore, the researchers concluded that EEG-R is a good predictor of whether patients in a coma after acute brain injury can regain consciousness, with a specificity of up to 88.9%. A lack of EEG-R is without exception related to poor prognosis.

To study the role of temperature-stimulated EEG-R in patients with chronic consciousness disorder in judging the prognosis of patients with VS or MCS, Li et al. [60] studied the changes in functional magnetic resonance imaging (fMRI) and EEG-R after giving temperature stimulation to 22 patients. fMRI was performed after the stimulation of the foot. The hand was stimulated to check EEG-R. Each patient was followed up for 1 year. Among 22 patients, 1 was lost to follow-up, 10 had clinical improvement, and the remaining 11 had no clinical improvement. Eleven patients showed EEG-R, and 9 of them had improved prognosis. However, in 10 patients without EEG-R, 9 had no clinical improvement. Therefore, after temperature stimulation, fMRI and EEG-R could accurately predict the clinical outcome of the patients.

Kaplan PW et al. [61] discussed the prognostic value of spindle coma based on EEG-R and found that in 15 patients with spindle coma due to various causes, EEG-R to external stimuli indicated a good prognosis. All patients, regardless of the cause of the coma, survived if they demonstrated EEG-R. Neurological examination had no predictive value. The prognosis of patients with spindle coma caused by encephalopathy, seizures, and head injury is relatively good. However, patients with hypoxia, cardiac arrest, and structural brain disease have a poor prognosis. In the acute stage of coma caused by TBI, EEG spindle activity and reactivity are associated with a good prognosis [62]. Compared with the clinical and neuroimaging findings, an anergic EEG pattern can predict the risk of death in patients with triphasic encephalopathy, whereas the specific etiology and potential pathological changes cannot predict the clinical outcome [63].

### 4.3.3 The Prognostic Value of EEG-R in Children

To understand the EEG pattern of rhythmic coma in comatose children, we explored the prognostic value of the pattern of reactive rhythmic coma. According to the improved Young classification, Ramachandrannair R et al. [64] prospectively analyzed and classified the EEGs of children with coma between 2 months and 18 years of age from 1996 to 2003. After 1 year of follow-up, the children's clinical prognosis was scored according to the Paediatric Cerebral and Overall Performance Category Scale score. Fisher's exact test and Mann-Whitney test were used to compare clinical prognosis. The results showed that, of 63 EEGs from 38 children, 19 EEGs showed rhythmic patterns (30.2%, 9 α, 4 spindle, 4θ, and 2β coma patterns; the total number of children was 14). Sixty percent of the records with no reactivity pattern were related to a poor prognosis. Therefore, Ramachandrannair R et al. [64] believed that the EEG pattern of rhythmic coma in children with coma is common, and the clinical prognosis patients with reactive rhythmic coma pattern is better.

Rajesh Ramachandrannair et al. [65] retrospectively analyzed the EEGs of children with coma aged 2 months to 18 years between 1996 and 2003. Thirty-three children underwent EEG examination within 72 h after unconsciousness. The EEGs of 14 children were reactive, and 4 (28.6%) of these children had a poor prognosis. Nineteen children had no EEG-R; 13 (65%) of these children had a poor clinical prognosis, and 10 died. In the remaining surviving children, there was nerve damage. Therefore, children with responsive EEGs had a better clinical prognosis. EEG-R is a marker for predicting clinical prognosis that is independent of the etiology, coma score, or EEG pattern. An EEG study of comatose newborns showed that those with reactive outbreak inhibition had a better prognosis [66].

EEGs with an incomplete α coma pattern showed responsiveness to painful stimuli. Adult patients with this EEG pattern have a better prognosis than those with a complete α coma pattern with EEG-R. A 5-year-old child suffered from hypoxic brain injury after surgery. His EEG showed an incomplete α coma pattern, and the prognosis was improved. In addition, the prognosis of children with a hypoxic α coma pattern is better than that of adults [67].

### 4.3.4 It Is Feasible to Study EEG-R Using Quantitative Methods?

Most of the existing studies use visual methods to assess prognosis. This method is time-consuming, and clinicians are not always consistent in their judgments; therefore, these judgments are subjective. Thus, is it possible to use automatic analysis to make quantitative judgments on brain injury? Liu G et al. [68] retrospectively analyzed the EEG-R recordings in coma patients 1–3 days after CPR or after hypothermia treatment after their body temperature returned to normal. We analyzed the EEG-R recordings by visual and quantitative methods. The clinical results were tracked at 3 months, and the patients were divided into two groups: those with a recovery of consciousness and those with unrecovered consciousness. Ninety-six patients met the inclusion criteria. Of the 27 patients who had EEG-R on the basis of visual analysis of EEGs, 22 regained consciousness. Of the 69 patients who did not exhibit EEG-R on the basis of visual analysis of EEGs, 16 regained consciousness. The sensitivity and specificity of EEG-R determined by visual analysis were 58% and 91%, respectively. Using quantitative analysis, the AUC was 0.92 (95% CI [0.87–0.97]), which had the best margin of 0.10. Therefore, quantitative analysis of EEG-R is a better method to predict the recovery of consciousness in patients with hypoxic coma after CPR. Another study included 46 coma patients who were treated with hypothermia treatment after cardiac arrest. EEG background activity was quantitatively analyzed with the BS ratio and approximate entropy. The reactivity of the patient was identified through the change in the energy spectrum before and after stimulation. Automatic and visual analysis of the EEG background activity and reactivity showed that the agreement between the two was very high. In some specific populations, compared with approximate entropy, the BS ratio was more suitable for distinguishing BS and cEEG background activity. The automatically analyzed EEG background activity and reactivity were obviously related to prognosis. Our conclusion was that qEEG analysis can assess a patient's current state and clinical prognosis [69].

### 4.3.5 The Shortcomings of the Use of EEG-R to Judge Prognosis

The obvious shortcomings of using EEG-R to judge prognosis are the lack of clear diagnostic criteria and the unknown effects of sedative drugs [70]. There are deviations in the judgment of EEG-R among observers [71]. Previous studies have not fully defined and standardized the quality and quantity of stimuli. The measurement of responsiveness is often performed visually and under nonblinded conditions; therefore, there is a great risk of bias. Moreover, all studies on the use of EEG-R for prognostic judgment regard this EEG feature as an isolated feature. No research analyzes the background EEG activity. The EEG background activity pattern may already contain sufficient and reliable information for prognostic prediction [44, 72]. Therefore, the predictive value of reactivity is unknown. In fact, EEG-R may be related to continuous background patterns with circadian rhythms. At the same time, a nonreactive EEG may represent a low-voltage background activity pattern [57].

Furthermore, the predictive value of EEG-R for prognosis is not 100%. We studied adults in a coma who were hospitalized from February 2008 to November 2012 after successful CPR patients with EEG-R during hypothermia treatment were selected. The clinical prognosis was evaluated after 3 months and divided into survival and nonsurvival (no patient was in a VS). Univariate and multivariate analyses were used to compare demographic characteristics, clinical changes, EEG characteristics, serum NSE, and procalcitonin. A total of 290 patients were treated with hypothermia treatment after cardiac arrest, and 146 patients underwent EEG examination, 90 of whom had EEG-R, 77 (86%) survived, and 13 (14%) died (without recovering from coma). The nonsurviving population had a higher incidence of discontinuous EEGs ($P = 0.006$; $P = 0.026$ in multivariate analysis) and higher serum NSE peaks ($P = 0.021$; $P = 0.014$ in multivariate analysis). In contrast, the demographic characteristics and other clinical variables, including serum procalcitonin, of the nonsurviving population were not different from those of survivors. Therefore, discontinuous EEGs and high serum NSE were related to mortality after cardiac arrest, and the prognosis was poor, even though EEGs were reactive during hypothermia treatment [73].

In conclusion, EEG-R is correlated with prognosis. Coma patients with EEG-R are more likely to recover consciousness. Coma patients with no EEG-R are less likely to recover consciousness. However, there are limitations when using EEG-R to judge the prognosis of comatose patients. EEG-R, EEG background activity, and other indicators should be considered comprehensively to make a better judgment of the prognosis of coma patients.

## References


1. Hirsch LJ, LaRoche SM, Gaspard N, et al. American clinical neurophysiology society's standardized critical care EEG terminology: 2012 version. J Clin Neurophysiol. 2013;30(1):1–27.
2. Kharoshankaya L, Filan PM, Bogue CO, et al. Global suppression of electrocortical activity in unilateral perinatal thalamic stroke. Dev Med Child Neurol. 2014;56(7):695–8.
3. Tecchio F, Zappasodi F, Pasqualetti P, et al. Rhythmic brain activity at rest from rolandic areas in acute mono-hemispheric stroke: a magnetoencephalographic study. NeuroImage. 2005;28(1):72–83.
4. Lavy S, Melamed E, Portnoy Z. The effect of cerebral infarction on the regional cerebral blood flow of the contralateral hemisphere. Stroke. 1975;6(2):160–3.
5. Diedler J, Sykora M, Bast T, et al. Quantitative EEG correlates of low cerebral perfusion in severe stroke. Neurocrit Care. 2009;11(2):210–6.
6. Petty GW, Labar DR, Fisch BJ, et al. Electroencephalography in lacunar infarction. J Neurol Sci. 1995;134(1–2):47–50.
7. Macdonell RA, Donnan GA, Bladin PF, et al. The electroencephalogram and acute ischemic stroke. Distinguishing cortical from lacunar infarction. Arch Neurol. 1988;45(5):520–4.
8. COHN R, RAINES GN, Et A. Cerebral vascular lesions; electroencephalographic and neuropathologic correlations. Arch Neurol Psychiatr. 1948;60(2):165–81.
9. Schneider AL, Jordan KG. Regional attenuation without delta (RAWOD): a distinctive EEG pattern that can aid in the diagnosis and management of severe acute ischemic stroke. Am J Electroneurodiagnostic Technol. 2005;45(2):102–17.
10. Amrein I, Palvolgyi L, Debreczeni R, et al. Effect of mental arithmetic and verbal fluency on blood flow velocity in the middle cerebral arteries. Ideggyogy Sz. 2004;57(1–2):23–9.
11. Sinkin MV, Kaimovsky IL, Komoltsev IG, et al. Electroencephalography in acute stroke. Zh Nevrol Psikhiatr Im S S Korsakova. 2020;120(8. Vyp. 2):10–6.
12. Nazish S, Zafar A, Shariff E, et al. Clinical correlates of electroencephalographic patterns in critically ill patients. Clin EEG Neurosci. 2020:1428873148.
13. Bentes C, Martins H, Peralta AR, et al. Early EEG predicts poststroke epilepsy. Epilepsia Open. 2018;3(2):203–12.

14. Cobb WA, Guiloff RJ, Cast J. Breach rhythm: the EEG related to skull defects. Electroencephalogr Clin Neurophysiol. 1979;47(3):251–71.
15. Lee JW, Tanaka N, Shiraishi H, et al. Evaluation of postoperative sharp waveforms through EEG and magnetoencephalography. J Clin Neurophysiol. 2010;27(1):7–11.
16. Brigo F, Cicero R, Fiaschi A, et al. The breach rhythm. Clin Neurophysiol. 2011;122(11):2116–20.
17. Kadian R, Vemireddy LP, Kumar A. Breach rhythm. 2020.
18. Mari-Acevedo J, Yelvington K, Tatum WO. Normal EEG variants. Handb Clin Neurol. 2019;160:143–60.
19. Niedermeyer E. The "third rhythm": further observations. Clin Electroencephalogr. 1991;22(2):83–96.
20. Shinomiya S, Fukunaga T, Nagata K. Clinical aspects of the "third rhythm" of the temporal lobe. Clin Electroencephalogr. 1999;30(4):136–42.
21. van Doorn J, Cherian PJ. Neurological picture. Breach rhythm related to a solitary skull lesion caused by multiple myeloma. J Neurol Neurosurg Psychiatry. 2008;79(7):819.
22. Krause-Titz UR, Warneke N, Freitag-Wolf S, et al. Factors influencing the outcome (GOS) in reconstructive cranioplasty. Neurosurg Rev. 2016;39(1):133–9.
23. Khader BA, Towler MR. Materials and techniques used in cranioplasty fixation: a review. Mater Sci Eng C Mater Biol Appl. 2016;66:315–22.
24. Huang J, Peng Y, Yang J, et al. A study on correlation of pedestrian head injuries with physical parameters using in-depth traffic accident data and mathematical models. Accid Anal Prev. 2018;119:91–103.
25. Mader EJ, Miller D, Toler JM, et al. Focal epileptiform discharges can mimic electrode artifacts when recorded on the scalp near a skull defect. J Investig Med High Impact Case Rep. 2018;6:1559706839.
26. Lau S, Flemming L, Haueisen J. Corrigendum to "Magnetoencephalography signals are influenced by skull defects" [Clin. Neurophysiol. 125 (2014) 1653–1662]. Clin Neurophysiol. 2017;128(6):1116.
27. Hunter A, Bordelon Y, Cook I, et al. QEEG measures in Huntington's disease: a pilot study. PLoS Curr. 2010;2:N1192.
28. Bonanni L, Franciotti R, Nobili F, et al. EEG markers of dementia with Lewy bodies: a multicenter cohort study. J Alzheimers Dis. 2016;54(4):1649–57.
29. Franciotti R, Pilotto A, Moretti DV, et al. Anterior EEG slowing in dementia with Lewy bodies: a multicenter European cohort study. Neurobiol Aging. 2020;93:55–60.
30. Werth E, Achermann P, Borbely AA. Brain topography of the human sleep EEG: antero-posterior shifts of spectral power. Neuroreport. 1996;8(1):123–7.
31. De Gennaro L, Ferrara M, Curcio G, et al. Cortical EEG topography of REM onset: the posterior dominance of middle and high frequencies. Clin Neurophysiol. 2002;113(4):561–70.
32. Rundgren M, Rosen I, Friberg H. Amplitude-integrated EEG (aEEG) predicts outcome after cardiac arrest and induced hypothermia. Intensive Care Med. 2006;32(6):836–42.
33. Oh SH, Park KN, Kim YM, et al. The prognostic value of continuous amplitude-integrated electroencephalogram applied immediately after return of spontaneous circulation in therapeutic hypothermia-treated cardiac arrest patients. Resuscitation. 2013;84(2):200–5.
34. Sugiyama K, Kashiura M, Akashi A, et al. Prognostic value of the recovery time of continuous normal voltage in amplitude-integrated electroencephalography in out-of-hospital cardiac arrest patients treated with therapeutic hypothermia: a retrospective study. J Intensive Care. 2016;4:25.
35. Oh SH, Park KN, Shon YM, et al. Continuous amplitude-integrated electroencephalographic monitoring is a useful prognostic tool for hypothermia-treated cardiac arrest patients. Circulation. 2015;132(12):1094–103.
36. Benarous L, Gavaret M, Soda DM, et al. Sources of interrater variability and prognostic value of standardized EEG features in post-anoxic coma after resuscitated cardiac arrest. Clin Neurophysiol Pract. 2019;4:20–6.
37. Westhall E, Rossetti AO, van Rootselaar AF, et al. Standardized EEG interpretation accurately predicts prognosis after cardiac arrest. Neurology. 2016;86(16):1482–90.
38. Hawkes MA, Rabinstein AA. Neurological prognostication after cardiac arrest in the era of target temperature management. Curr Neurol Neurosci Rep. 2019;19(2):10.
39. Guedes B, Manita M, Rita PA, et al. Prognostic significance of specific EEG patterns after cardiac arrest in a Lisbon cohort. Clin Neurophysiol Pract. 2020;5:147–51.
40. Pati S, McClain L, Moura L, et al. Accuracy of limited-montage electroencephalography in monitoring postanoxic comatose patients. Clin EEG Neurosci. 2017;48(6):422–7.
41. Lamartine MM, Taccone FS, Depondt C, et al. The prognostic value of 48-h continuous EEG during therapeutic hypothermia after cardiac arrest. Neurocrit Care. 2016;24(2):153–62.
42. Sadaka F, Doerr D, Hindia J, et al. Continuous electroencephalogram in comatose postcardiac arrest syndrome patients treated with therapeutic hypothermia: outcome prediction study. J Intensive Care Med. 2015;30(5):292–6.
43. Sivaraju A, Gilmore EJ, Wira CR, et al. Prognostication of post-cardiac arrest coma: early clinical and electroencephalographic predictors of outcome. Intensive Care Med. 2015;41(7):1264–72.
44. Sugiyama K, Miyazaki K, Ishida T, et al. Categorization of post-cardiac arrest patients according to the pattern of amplitude-integrated electroencephalography after return of spontaneous circulation. Crit Care. 2018;22(1):226.
45. Thenayan EA, Savard M, Sharpe MD, et al. Electroencephalogram for prognosis after cardiac arrest. J Crit Care. 2010;25(2):300–4.

46. Hofmeijer J, Tjepkema-Cloostermans MC, van Putten MJ. Burst-suppression with identical bursts: a distinct EEG pattern with poor outcome in postanoxic coma. Clin Neurophysiol. 2014;125(5):947–54.
47. Rossetti AO, Carrera E, Oddo M. Early EEG correlates of neuronal injury after brain anoxia. Neurology. 2012;78(11):796–802.
48. Cloostermans MC, van Meulen FB, Eertman CJ, et al. Continuous electroencephalography monitoring for early prediction of neurological outcome in postanoxic patients after cardiac arrest: a prospective cohort study. Crit Care Med. 2012;40(10):2867–75.
49. Nolan JP, Soar J, Cariou A, et al. European resuscitation council and european society of intensive care medicine guidelines for post-resuscitation care 2015: Section 5 of the European resuscitation council guidelines for resuscitation 2015. Resuscitation. 2015(95):202–22.
50. Amorim E, Rittenberger JC, Baldwin ME, et al. Malignant EEG patterns in cardiac arrest patients treated with targeted temperature management who survive to hospital discharge. Resuscitation. 2015;90:127–32.
51. ter Horst HJ, Brouwer OF, Bos AF. Burst suppression on amplitude-integrated electroencephalogram may be induced by midazolam: a report on three cases. Acta Paediatr. 2004;93(4):559–63.
52. Rundgren M, Westhall E, Cronberg T, et al. Continuous amplitude-integrated electroencephalogram predicts outcome in hypothermia-treated cardiac arrest patients. Crit Care Med. 2010;38(9):1838–44.
53. Bouwes A, van Poppelen D, Koelman JH, et al. Acute posthypoxic myoclonus after cardiopulmonary resuscitation. BMC Neurol. 2012;12:63.
54. Young GB. The EEG in coma. J Clin Neurophysiol. 2000;17(5):473–85.
55. Rossetti AO, Oddo M, Logroscino G, et al. Prognostication after cardiac arrest and hypothermia: a prospective study. Ann Neurol. 2010;67(3):301–7.
56. Tsetsou S, Novy J, Oddo M, et al. EEG reactivity to pain in comatose patients: importance of the stimulus type. Resuscitation. 2015;97:34–7.
57. Azabou E, Fischer C, Mauguiere F, et al. Prospective cohort study evaluating the prognostic value of simple EEG parameters in postanoxic coma. Clin EEG Neurosci. 2016;47(1):75–82.
58. Juan E, Novy J, Suys T, et al. Clinical evolution after a non-reactive hypothermic EEG following cardiac arrest. Neurocrit Care. 2015;22(3):403–8.
59. Logi F, Pasqualetti P, Tomaiuolo F. Predict recovery of consciousness in post-acute severe brain injury: the role of EEG reactivity. Brain Inj. 2011;25(10):972–9.
60. Li L, Kang XG, Qi S, et al. Brain response to thermal stimulation predicts outcome of patients with chronic disorders of consciousness. Clin Neurophysiol. 2015;126(8):1539–47.
61. Kaplan PW, Genoud D, Ho TW, et al. Clinical correlates and prognosis in early spindle coma. Clin Neurophysiol. 2000;111(4):584–90.
62. Urakami Y. Relationship between, sleep spindles and clinical recovery in patients with traumatic brain injury: a simultaneous EEG and MEG study. Clin EEG Neurosci. 2012;43(1):39–47.
63. Sutter R, Stevens RD, Kaplan PW. Significance of triphasic waves in patients with acute encephalopathy: a nine-year cohort study. Clin Neurophysiol. 2013;124(10):1952–8.
64. RamachandranNair R, Sharma R, Weiss SK, et al. A reappraisal of rhythmic coma patterns in children. Can J Neurol Sci. 2005;32(4):518–23.
65. Ramachandrannair R, Sharma R, Weiss SK, et al. Reactive EEG patterns in pediatric coma. Pediatr Neurol. 2005;33(5):345–9.
66. Douglass LM, Wu JY, Rosman NP, et al. Burst suppression electroencephalogram pattern in the newborn: predicting the outcome. J Child Neurol. 2002;17(6):403–8.
67. RamachandranNair R, Weiss SK. Incomplete alpha coma pattern in a child. Pediatr Neurol. 2005;33(2):127–30.
68. Liu G, Su Y, Jiang M, et al. Electroencephalography reactivity for prognostication of post-anoxic coma after cardiopulmonary resuscitation: a comparison of quantitative analysis and visual analysis. Neurosci Lett. 2016;626:74–8.
69. Noirhomme Q, Lehembre R, Lugo ZR, et al. Automated analysis of background EEG and reactivity during therapeutic hypothermia in comatose patients after cardiac arrest. Clin EEG Neurosci. 2014;45(1):6–13.
70. Gilmore EJ, Gaspard N, Choi HA, et al. Acute brain failure in severe sepsis: a prospective study in the medical intensive care unit utilizing continuous EEG monitoring. Intensive Care Med. 2015;41(4):686–94.
71. Westhall E, Rosen I, Rossetti AO, et al. Interrater variability of EEG interpretation in comatose cardiac arrest patients. Clin Neurophysiol. 2015;126(12):2397–404.
72. Hofmeijer J, Beernink TM, Bosch FH, et al. Early EEG contributes to multimodal outcome prediction of postanoxic coma. Neurology. 2015;85(2):137–43.
73. Tsetsou S, Oddo M, Rossetti AO. Clinical outcome after a reactive hypothermic EEG following cardiac arrest. Neurocrit Care. 2013;19(3):283–6.

# Patterns and Clinical Significance of Abnormal Sleep EEG

# 5

Yuping Wang and Yicong Lin

## Contents



**Abstract**

ICU patients often exhibit severe sleep abnormalities, including reduced sleep periods, sleep fragmentation, poor sleep continuity, and circadian rhythm disturbances, which are closely related to the prognosis of patients' awakening. Sleep is an important part of brain function assessment in ICU patients. Sleep research in patients with severe brain injury can provide information for assessing the integrity of residual brain function in patients with impaired consciousness and has important clinical diagnostic and prognostic value. However, it is more difficult to measure and assess sleep in ICU patients. The assessment should include quantity, quality, and 24-h sleep distribution. However, the traditional sleep assessment method is not suitable for ICU patients, and there are great difficulties, especially in sleep analysis and quantification of sleep. This chapter focuses on specific manifestations of the common sleep waveforms, sleep structure and sleep cycle, and atypical sleep types of ICU patients in combination with legends from the clinical needs. It also introduces the relationship between sleep abnormalities and clinical prognosis, providing a reference for the evaluation of brain function and prognosis in patients with severe brain injury.

**Keywords**

ICU patients · Sleep EEG · Sleep structure · Sleep cycle · Atypical sleep · Pathological arousal · Brain function damage · Prognosis

Y. Wang (✉) · Y. Lin
Department of Neurology, Xuanwu Hospital, Capital Medical University, Beijing, China
e-mail: liny@xwhosp.org


X. Wang et al. (eds.), *Multi-Modal EEG Monitoring of Severely Neurologically Ill Patients*,
https://doi.org/10.1007/978-981-16-4493-1_5

ICU patients often have severe sleep disorders, which mainly manifest as reduced sleep periods, sleep fragmentation, poor sleep continuity, and circadian rhythm disturbance. The causes of abnormal sleep in critically ill patients can be roughly divided into two aspects: external causes and internal causes. External factors include the external environment (such as noise and light) and treatment measures (such as mechanical ventilation, drugs, and care). Internal factors include natural sleep before illness, emotional state, pain, and physiological state of severe illness. Sleep changes are mainly related to the destruction of the neurobiology of sleep and sleep dynamics, which will affect the restoration of sleep function.

Sleep measurement and the assessment of sleep in critically ill patients are more difficult. Sleep assessment should include an evaluation of the quantity (total length of sleep and the length of each sleep period) and quality (the degree of sleep fragmentation, the type of sleep EEG pattern) of sleep and the 24-h sleep distribution. Polysomnography (PSG) is a reliable method of sleep measurement, especially for patients with significant sleep abnormalities. In recent years, a certain degree of progress has been made in the clinical evaluation of sleep EEGs in critically ill patients, especially in terms of those with brain damage and the prognosis of critically ill patients, which has attracted increasing clinician attention.

## 5.1 Sleep Structure and Sleep Cycle

Sleep is the most basic physiological need of humans. When people sleep, swollen neurons begin to recover after a period of activity, their volume decreases, and the gap between cells becomes larger. CSF enters the intercellular space to wash and take away various metabolites produced when individuals are awake so that neurons can continue to work. When diseases damage the structure or function of sleep, sleep disorders will appear. EEG can be used to record brain activity related to damage to sleep function, and sleep EEGs are an electrophysiological marker of brain dysfunction. EEG is the best tool to detect sleep dysfunction. Human sleep EEGs can be divided into the NREM1-3 phase and the REM phase, and the EEG characteristics are shown in Figs. 5.1, 5.2, 5.3, 5.4, and 5.5.

In ICU patients, PSG lasting 16–24 h can provide better sleep quality analysis than EEG. Critically ill patients usually have severe sleep structure disturbances, including increased stage N1 and N2 of NREM sleep, decreased stage N3 NREM sleep and REM sleep, and increased sleep fragmentation [1–4]. The clinical research data of each care unit is slightly different, but the difference is not significant. For example, stage N1 and N2 NREM sleep accounted for 96% and 99%, respectively, of the total sleep time in surgical ICU patients [5–7]; 76% and 83%, respectively, in internal ICU patients; and 80% and 100%, respectively, in trauma ICU patients [8–10]. In critically ill patients [5], slow-wave sleep is reduced by 1%, or the total sleep time is reduced by 9% ± 18% [11]. However, some studies have shown that slow-wave sleep is extended by 25% [12] or close to the upper limit of normal (19% of the total sleep time) [13]. Severely ill patients show a moderate reduction (to 0–15% of the total sleep time) in REM-stage sleep [8, 14, 15]. Long-term PSG monitoring in surgical ICU patients showed that there was a significant reduction in slow-wave sleep and REM sleep during the first 2 days after surgery and a significant increase on the 3rd and 4th days [16]. This reduction in slow-wave and REM sleep may be mainly related to the use of benzodiazepines and opioids, because these drugs can inhibit REM sleep [17], and to the intermittent sleep of patients in the ICU. In addition, severely ill patients also have abnormal transitions between each sleep period [5, 9, 18].

The total sleep time of critically ill patients is usually within the normal range of 6–8 h. For patients who are administered sedative drugs, the total sleep time will be extended to 10.9–18.9 h

a

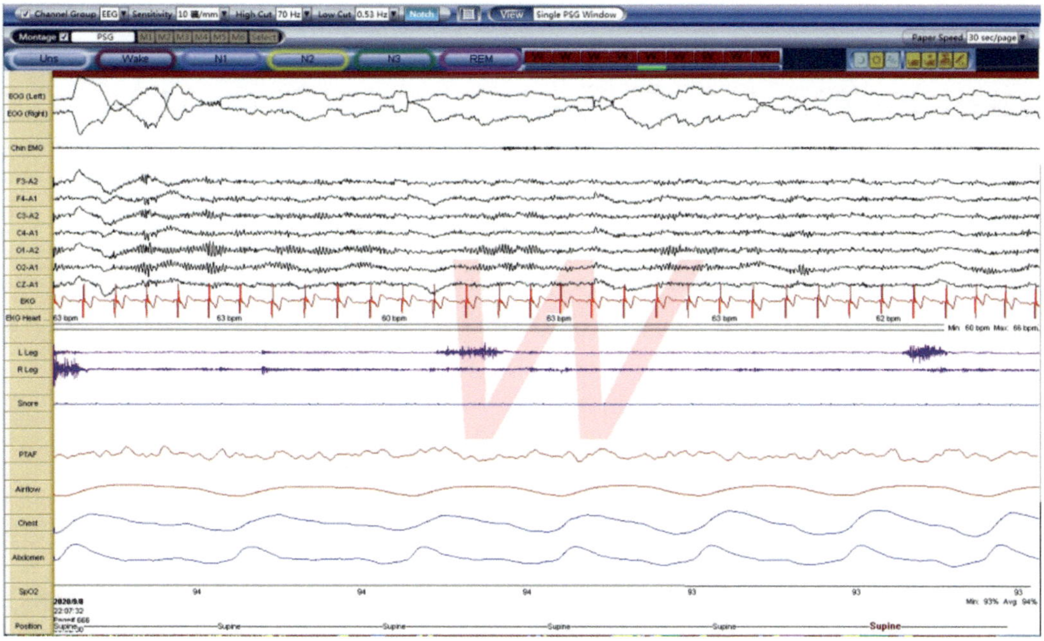

b

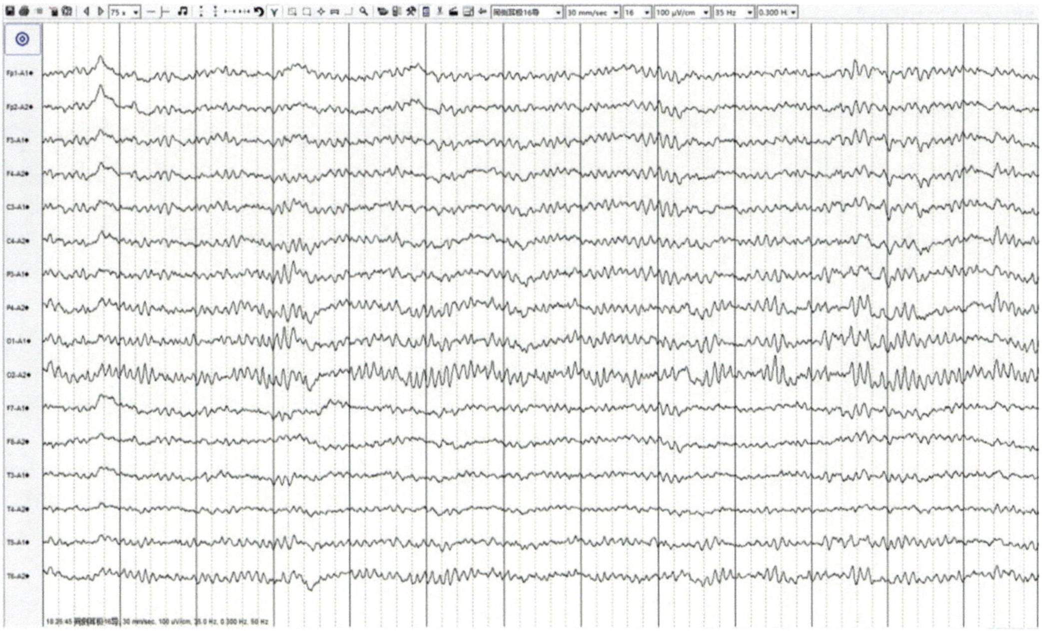

**Fig. 5.1** (**a**) The EEG of healthy adults during the awake period. (**b**) EEGs from healthy adults during the awake period, showing a regular waveform, moderate amplitude, sinusoidal α rhythm in the occipital region, bilateral symmetry, good amplitude modulation, and few fast waves and slow waves. No focal or generalized spike/sharp or slow-wave activity is observed

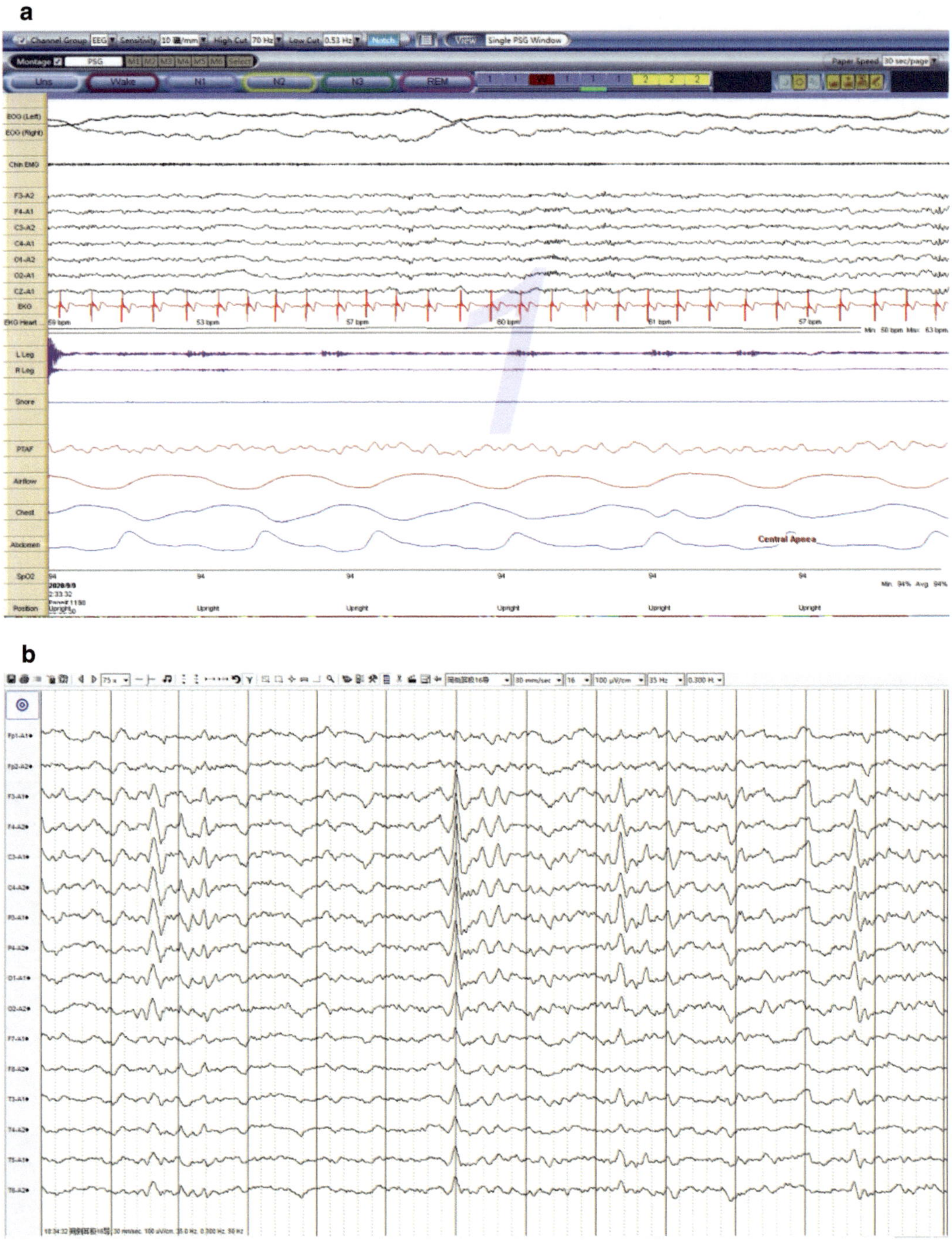


**Fig. 5.2** (**a**) The EEG performance of healthy adults during sleep (NREM 1 stage). (**b**) Sleep EEGs (NREM stage 1) from a healthy adult, showing apical sharp waves, mostly in the central and parietal lobes

[19], but the sleep of critically ill patients is often intermittently dispersed over 24 h. It has been reported that critically ill patients have approximately 30–60 awakenings within 1 h [7, 13], and the average sleep time before one awakening is approximately 3–15 min [11, 20]. Therefore, there is obvious sleep fragmentation in critically ill patients. According to Bonnet's sleep continu-

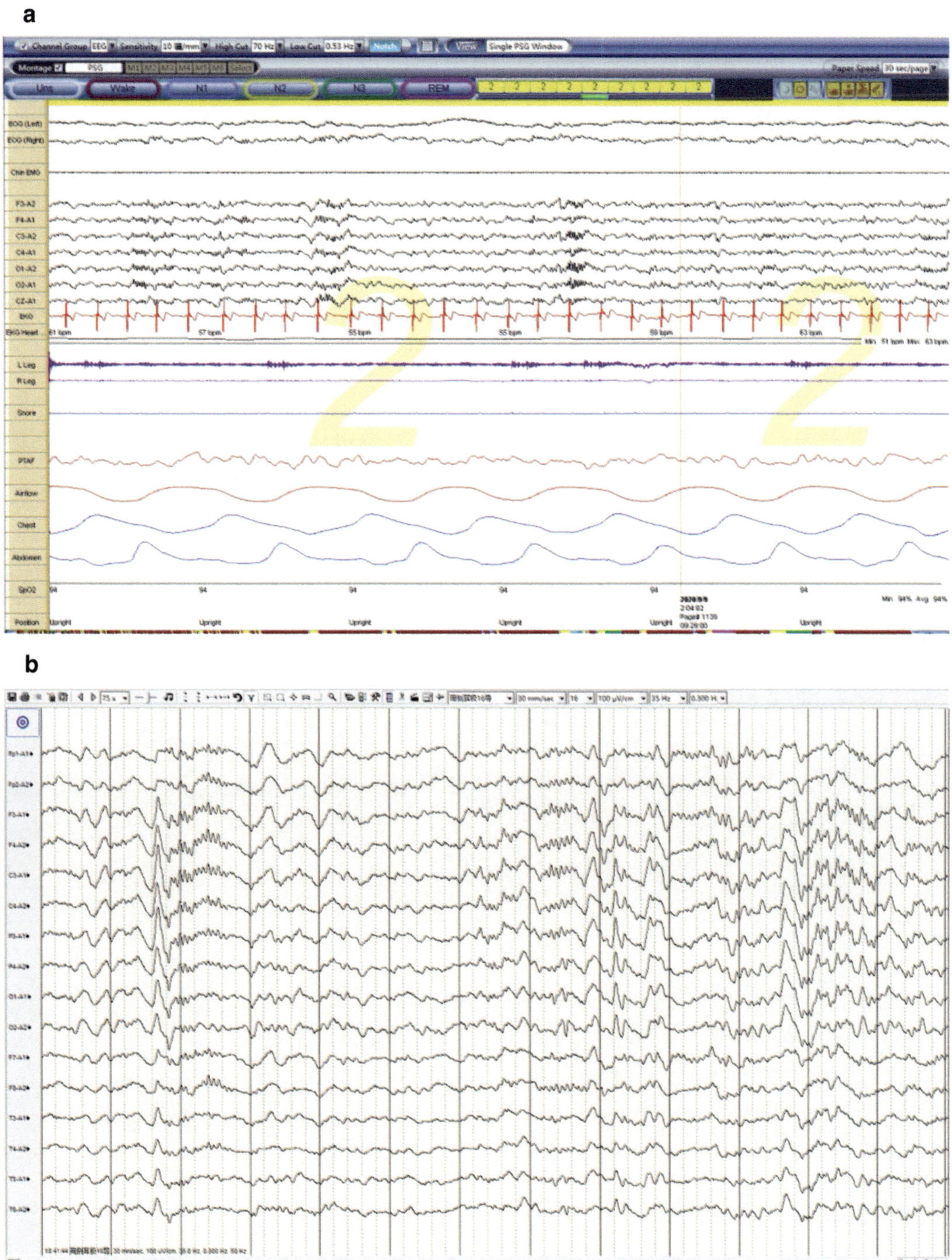

**Fig. 5.3** (**a**) The EEG performance of healthy adults during sleep (NREM stage 2). (**b**) Sleep EEGs (NREM stage 2) from a healthy adult, showing bilateral synchronous symmetry apical sharp waves, K-complex waves, and 14–16 Hz sleep spindles, mostly in the central and parietal lobes

ity theory [21], at least 10 min of uninterrupted sleep can produce restorative function. Therefore, significant sleep fragmentation in critically ill patients can have an adverse effect on restorative sleep. A study by Drouot et al. [22] showed that among patients with hypercapnic respiratory fail-

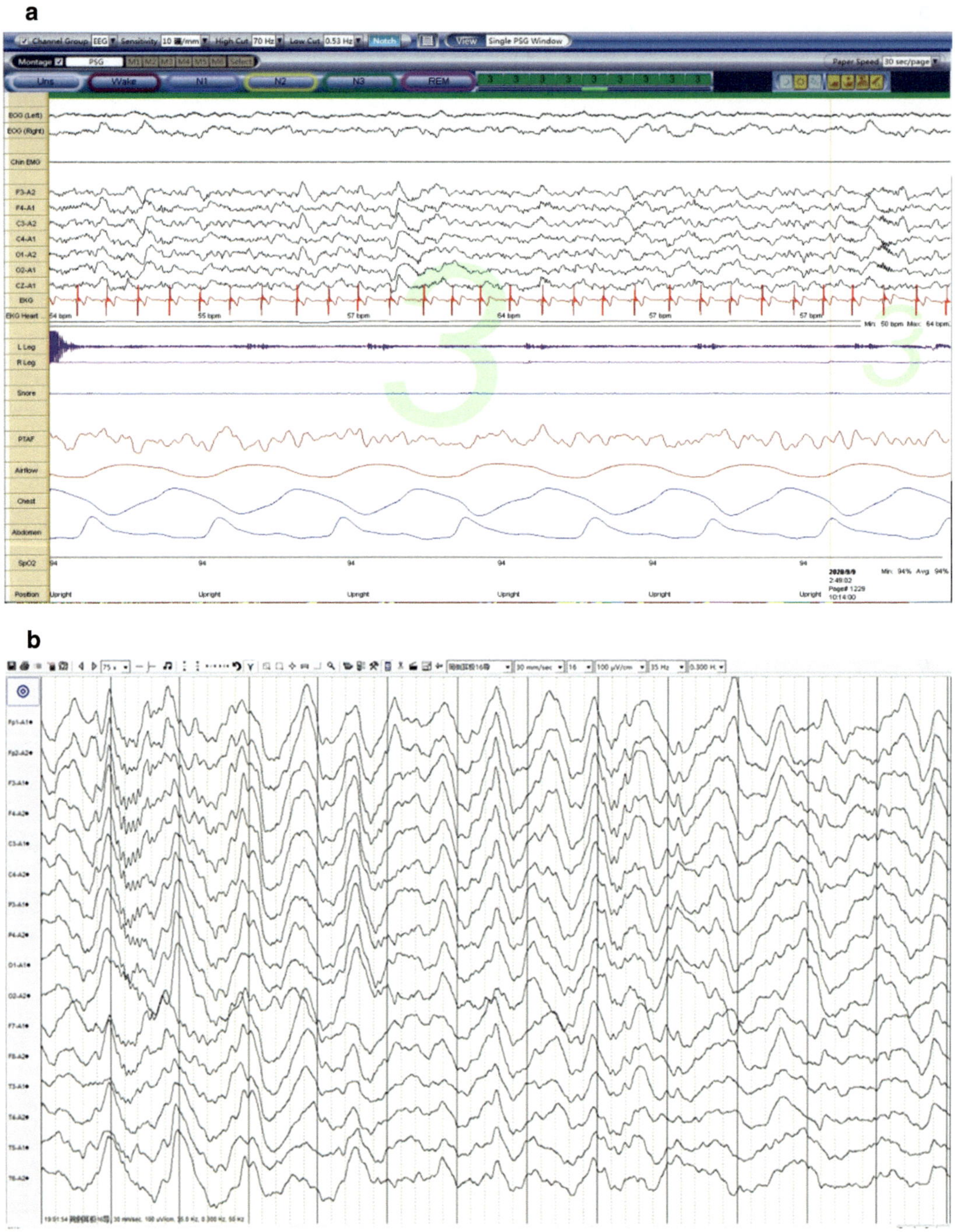


**Fig. 5.4** (**a**) The EEG performance of healthy adults during sleep (NREM stage 3). (**b**) Sleep EEGs (NREM stage 3) from healthy adults, characterized by δ rhythm, accounting for more than 50%, and the disappearance of sleep spindles

ure treated by noninvasive ventilation (NIV), patients in whom NIV treatment was successful had a higher percentage of short naps (that is, sleep lasting 10–30 min) than those in whom NIV treatment failed, and less sleep time was spent in sleep for less than 10 min. However,

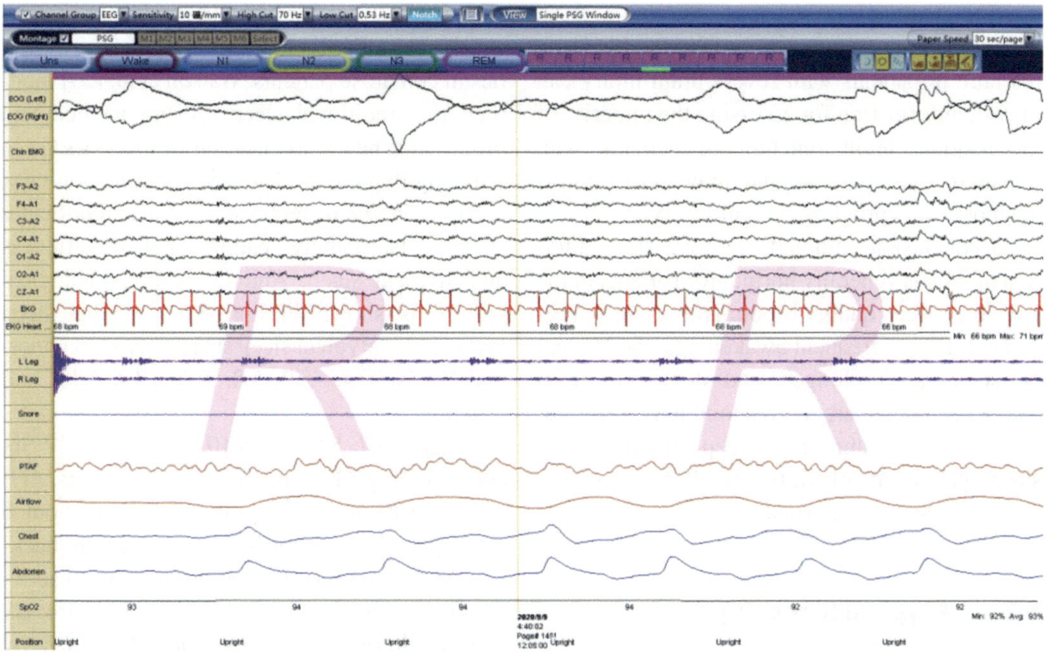


**Fig. 5.5** The EEG background activity is similar to that of N1 sleep EEGs, with low-voltage mixed frequency and intermittent α waves. The frequency is usually 1–2 Hz slower than that in the awake period. The EMG showed transient and irregular activity and REM

there was no difference in the amount of regular sleep (such as the total sleep time, sleep stage composition, and sleep fragmentation) between patients in whom NIV treatment was successful and patients in whom NIV treatment failed. It is worth noting that sleep abnormalities in critically ill patients often continue after leaving the ICU. A study has shown that the proportion of critically ill patients with insomnia is 18% before entering the ICU, 73% after entering the ICU, and 57% 6 months after leaving the ICU [23].

Severely ill patients have severe circadian rhythm abnormalities, and sleep cycle disturbance is one of the important factors affecting survival rate [14]. Valente et al. [24] proposed five types of sleep and arousal patterns based on the study of comatose patients: (**a**) monophasic pattern: continuous low-voltage θ-δ activity; (**b**) cycling alternating pattern: repeated alternation of low-voltage activity and burst high-amplitude monophasic δ waves but no sleep elements; (**c**) rudimentary sleep: basic NREM elements, namely, K complexes and/or sleep spindles; (**d**) NREM stage: structural elements of NREM; and (**e**) REM stage: structural elements of REM. The higher the classification level, the better the prognosis of consciousness-impaired patients [25].

In a PSG study of 20 patients with impaired consciousness [26], patients in a MCS, VS, or unresponsive wakefulness syndrome (UWS) had a sleep-wake pattern, which was circadian, ultradian, or nonrhythmic. Patients in a persistent VS may have or do not have a sleep cycle, and there was no significant difference in their clinical conditions. The absence of a sleep-wake cycle reflected brainstem damage in patients with impaired consciousness. The number of sleep spindles in patients with brain injury reflected the degree of damage to the thalamic cortex and was related to the clinical prognosis. Patients with clinical improvement within 6 months had a higher proportion of sleep spindles. Slow-wave sleep was present in eight patients in an MCS and three patients in a VS/UWS, but it was never due to by ischemic causes. All patients in an MCS or VS/UWS developed REM sleep. In short, the existence of an alternating cycle of open/closed eyes does not necessarily mean that the electrophysiological sleep structure is retained in patients with UWS or in those in an MCS. Sleep research in patients with severe brain injury can provide information for assessing the integrity of the residual brain function of patients with impaired consciousness and may have clinical diagnostic and prognostic significance.

In conclusion, although the total sleep duration of 24 h is generally normal for patients in the ICU, their sleep quality is poor and severely fragmented. Due to frequent awakenings, the N1 and N2 stages are prolonged, and slow-wave sleep and REM sleep are correspondingly reduced, resulting in an abnormal sleep structure. The sleep cycle is disturbed; that is, there is a severe circadian rhythm abnormality.

## 5.2 Atypical Sleep Types

Critically ill patients usually do not have normal sleep EEGs or the usual staging markers [11, 27, 28]; instead, they have θ and δ band EEG activity in the awake state, rapid transition between awake EEG features and NREM EEG features, REM in stage 2 sleep, low-amplitude fast rhythm similar to that induced by sedative drugs, and awakening mode in δ brush [9, 29].

The traditional sleep score currently in use was formulated by the American Academy of Sleep Medicine [30], and it is mainly based on normal EEGs and is not suitable for all critically ill patients. It is especially difficult to analyze and quantify sleep. A large number of critically ill patients lack standard sleep EEG types. In 2012, Drouot et al. [28] conducted a sleep EEG study on patients with respiratory failure who received NIV in the ICU and proposed the concepts of atypical sleep and pathological arousal. Atypical sleep refers to NREM sleep without sleep spindles or K complexes. Pathological wakefulness refers to the slowing of whole-brain activity (peak frequency is less than or equal to 7 Hz) accompanied by decreased EEG-R [28]. In 2013, Watson et al. [29] found that EEGs were separated from clinical behavior in 37 patients in the ICU. The EEGs were characterized by abnormal slow waves (θ or δ waves) in awakened patients and low-amplitude and high-frequency β activities in comatose patients. Watson et al. [29] modified the traditional sleep scoring method and proposed a new classification of sleep EEGs in critically ill patients. The new classification view is based on two different sleep states in critically ill patients, namely, pathological wakefulness and atypical sleep. Among them, pathological arousal is shown in Fig. 5.6. Atypical sleep includes six atypical sleep stages based on abnormal EEGs (Figs. 5.7, 5.8, 5.9, 5.10, 5.11, and 5.12).

Figures 5.7, 5.8, 5.9, 5.10, 5.11, and 5.12 Six atypical sleep EEGs in critically ill patients. *At1*: at least 10% α or θ activity with or without δ activity. *At2*: multiform δ activity with background β, α, or θ activity. *At3*: multiform δ activity without background β, α, or θ activity. *At4*: BS and the alternation of intermittent EEG activity and ECS. *At5*: low voltage with amplitude <20 μV. *At6*: no EEG activity.

Atypical sleep is found in 28–85% of critically ill patients [31, 32]. The pathological mechanism of each stage of atypical sleep needs to be confirmed by more clinical studies. There are many reasons for atypical sleep, and the first factor is hypercapnia. In the study of Drouot et al. [28] several patients developed hypercapnic respiratory failure, which may induce various brain dysfunctions. Similar EEG changes are also seen in healthy and conscious patients with hypercapnia. However, there was no difference in the arterial partial pressure of carbon dioxide ($PaCO_2$) between the atypical sleep or pathological arousal group and the normal sleep group, indicating that atypical sleep may also involve other factors. Sleep deprivation studies have shown that the α activity of awake EEGs decreases linearly, while theta and δ increase linearly [33]. The changes in the background EEG activity of patients with atypical sleep/pathological wakefulness are similar to those of healthy individuals with 24-h sleep deprivation [34, 35]. The characteristics of restorative sleep after sleep deprivation are a significant reduction in sleep

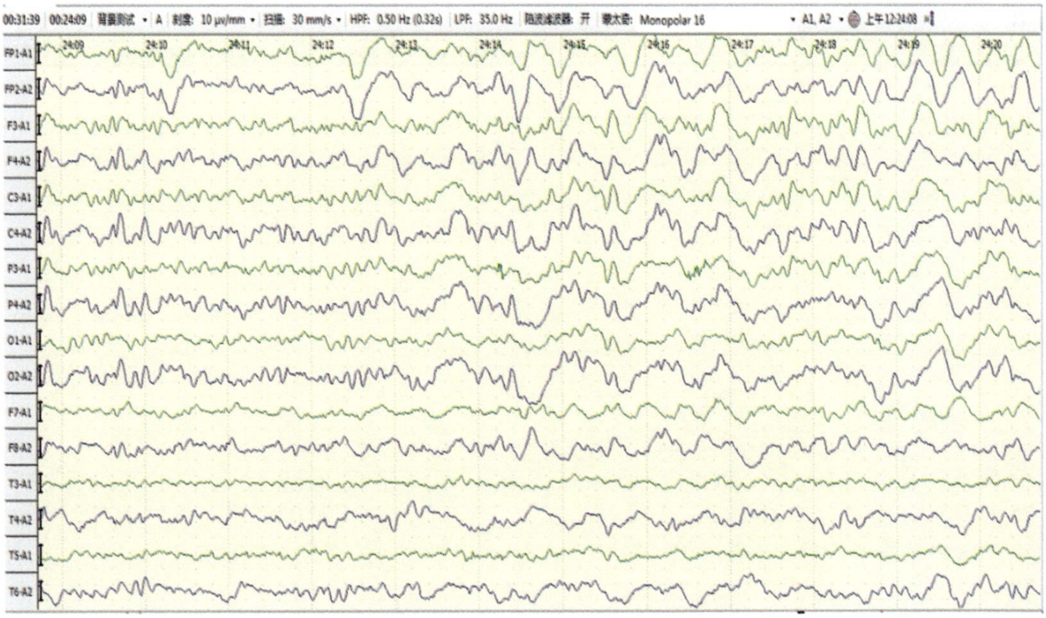


**Fig. 5.6** EEG showing δ waves. The patient is in an awake state and can execute simple instructions, which is the pathological arousal state

spindles and K complexes [36, 37]. Because patients in the ICU have sleep deprivation for several days or weeks [38, 39], atypical sleep may be a compensation mechanism, and deep sleep can restore sleep to the greatest extent. Since the number of sleep spindles decreases in atypical sleep, with increasing slow-wave activity and levels of arterial carbon dioxide, hypercapnia and sleep deprivation may be related to the generation of atypical sleep. However, the clear mechanism of atypical sleep production remains to be studied in the future.

## 5.3 Sleep Apnea

Obstructive sleep apnea syndrome (OSAS) is characterized by the partial or complete collapse of the upper airway during sleep, resulting in repeated cessation (apnea) or reduction (hypopnea) of airflow. Abnormal breathing causes sleep fragmentation and recurring nocturnal hypoxia. As a result, patients experience fatigue, daytime sleepiness, and cognitive dysfunction.

EEG can demonstrate the characteristics of EEG signal oscillation and is an indispensable tool in the clinical diagnosis and treatment of OSAS. The EEGs of OSAS patients showed more significant slow-wave activity throughout the cerebral cortex [40, 41]. Studies have found that the oxygen desaturation index of OSAS patients is positively correlated with the θ-band energy of the frontal, central, parietal, and temporo-occipital lobes [42], which may be related to sleep fragmentation. EEG source imaging analysis found a reduction in α activity in the right posterior cingulate gyrus and anterior cuneiform lobe, which reflects that intermittent chronic hypoxia may be related to emotion regulation, brain areas related to long-term memory, and default mode networks [43].

qEEG analysis technology can demonstrate more accurate changes in the brain electrical activity of patients with OSAS. In NREM, δ band activity gradually increases and generalizes, with the highest amplitudes in the postfrontal, central, and parietal regions. In REM, there is also an increase in the energy of the δ band, but it is not as significant as that in the NREM [44]. In the

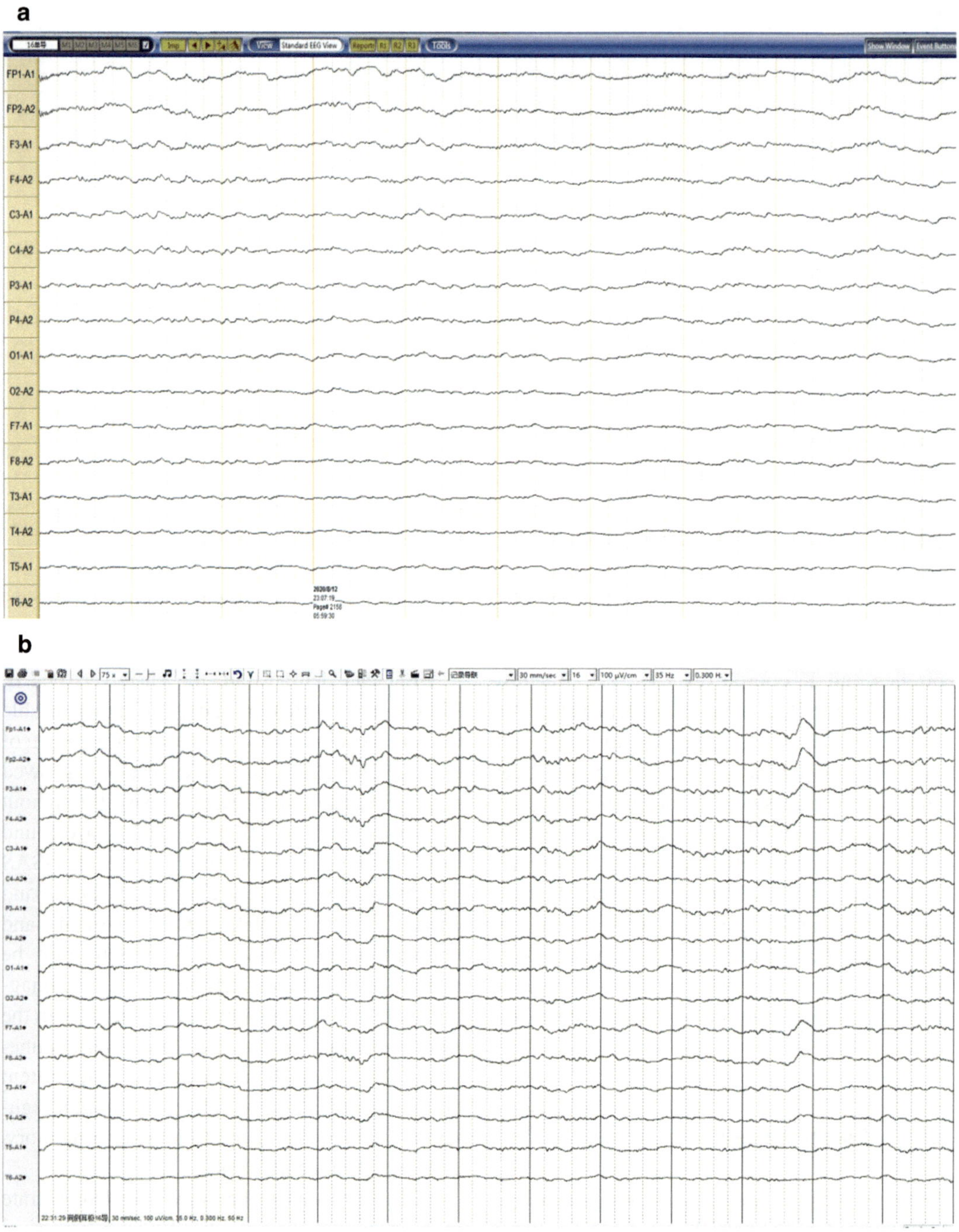


**Fig. 5.7** (**a**) At1. (**b**) At1

medium term of apnea, EEG activity in the frontal, central, and parietal regions slows down, and overall brain electrical activity decreases [45, 46]. However, multiple studies have found that there is no correlation between the increase in δ activity during apnea in REM sleep and oxygen desaturation, suggesting that slower EEG activity may not be caused by hypoxia [44, 45].

Continuous positive airway pressure (CPAP) is an effective measure for the treat-

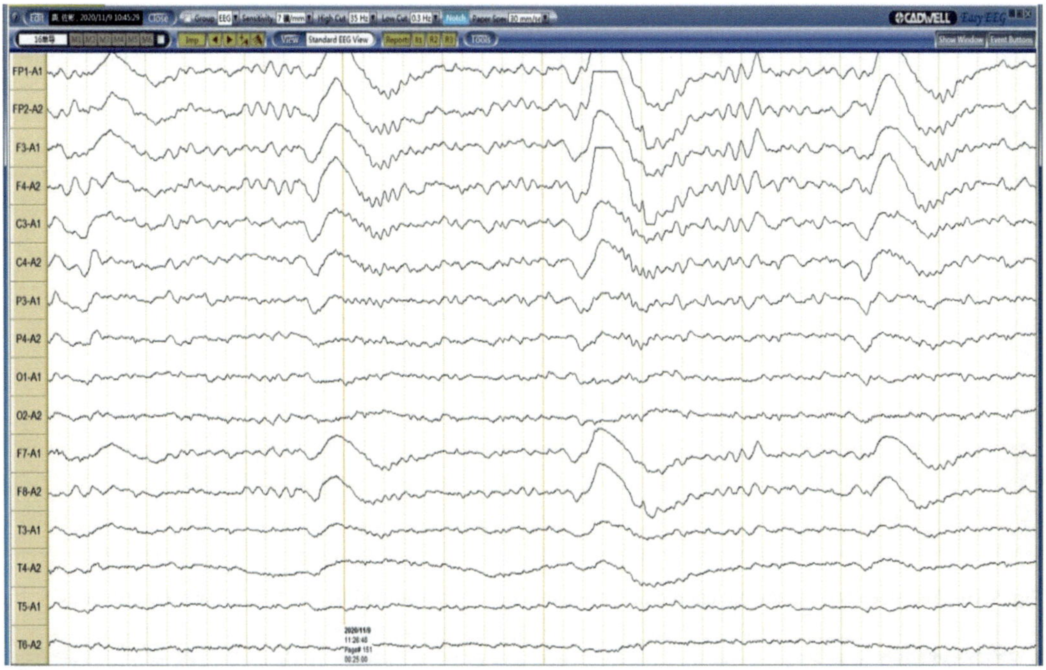


**Fig. 5.8** At2

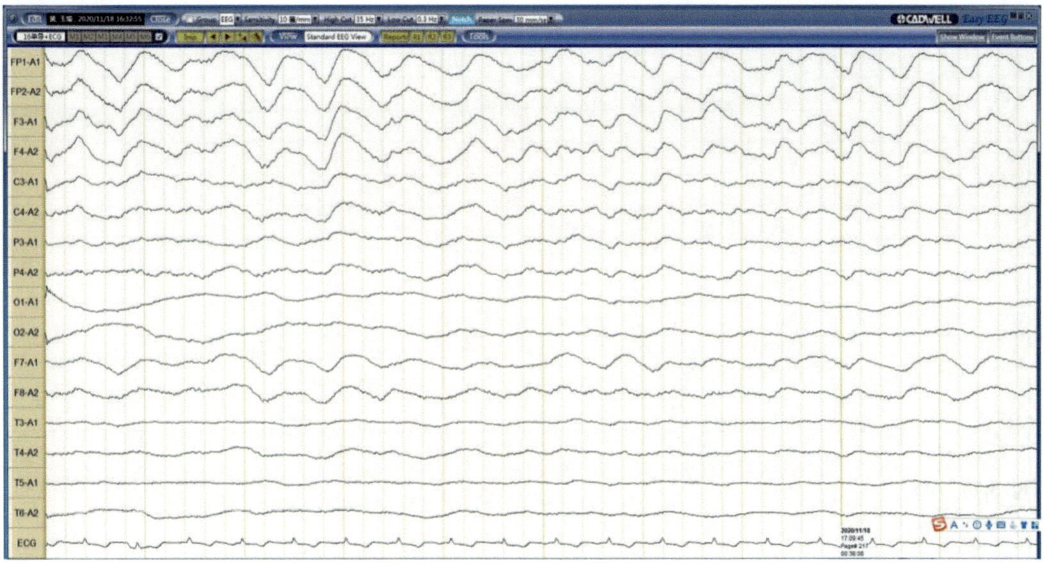


**Fig. 5.9** At3

ment of OSAS. After 3–6 months of CPAP treatment, in EEGs, the δ-band activity in the arousal and REM stages returned to normal [40, 47]. However, some studies have found that EEG activity is slower after CPAP treatment [42].

In conclusion, for OSAS patients, the most significant EEG feature is the slowing of extensive brain electrical activity during the arousal stage, which may be related to sleep fragmentation. CPAP treatment may correct EEG abnormalities and improve clinical symptoms.

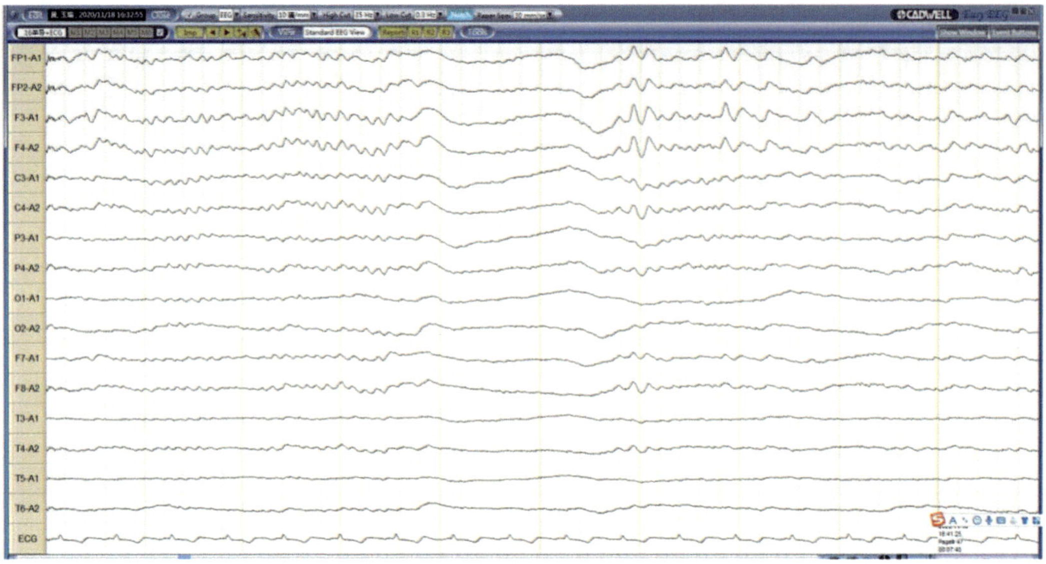


**Fig. 5.10** At4, sleep N1, but the patient did not respond to the external stimulus. The EEG shows a transient ECS

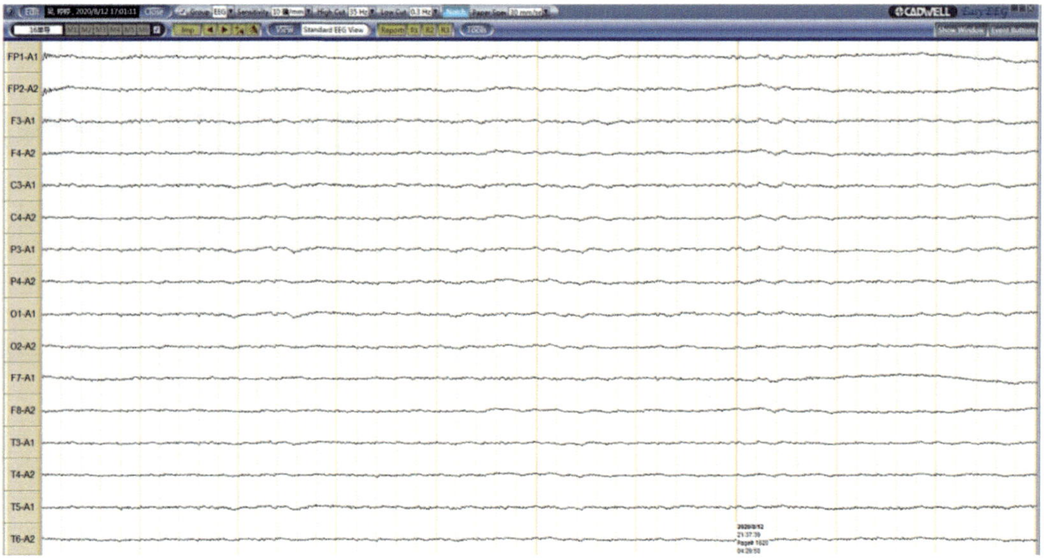


**Fig. 5.11** At5

## 5.4 Application of Abnormal Sleep in Brain Function Damage and Prognosis Judgment of Severely Ill Patients

At present, sleep research in critically ill patients is still in its infancy, and the evidence on the relationship between sleep and prognosis is insufficient. Some existing research results show that low-quality sleep in patients in the ICU has a negative impact on the prognosis of severe diseases. Patients in the ICU have poor mental status, reduced neurocognitive function and quality of life, and even fragmented sleep after discharge. The existence of multiple confounding factors has brought challenges to the study of sleep and disease prognosis in critically ill patients.

First, sleep deprivation can lead to abnormal immune function, affecting processes such as

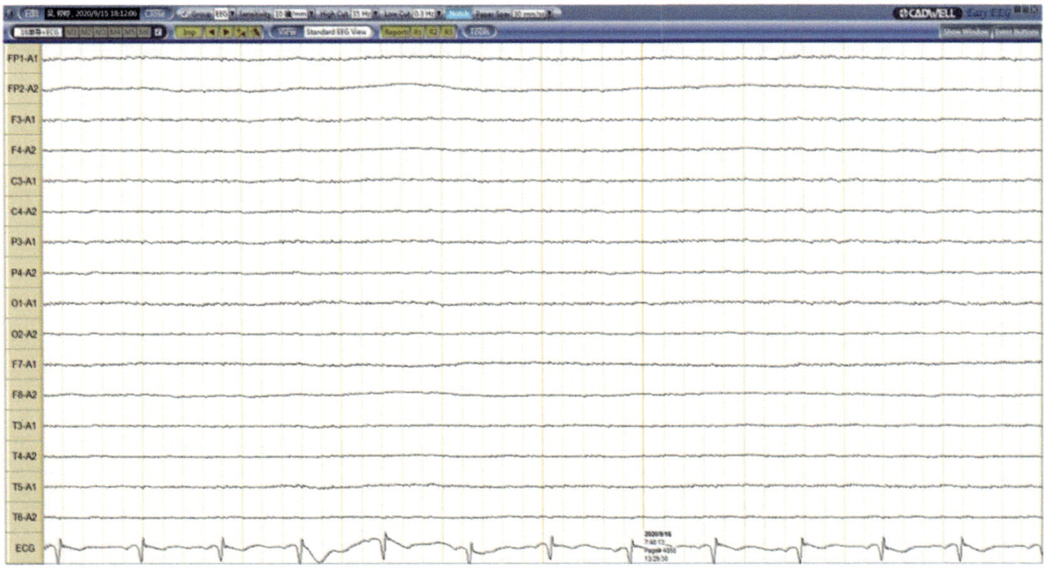


**Fig. 5.12** At6

oxygen consumption and carbon dioxide production, nitrogen balance, and cell metabolism. However, it is unclear whether this negative effect on the immune system is related to chronic or acute sleep disorders. Abnormal sleep can also cause sleep-related breathing abnormalities and neurocognitive dysfunction. Delirium and abnormal sleep are mutually causal factors. Delirium is present in 73.3% of patients in the ICU, and it is likely to be independently associated with sleep abnormalities [48] and is significantly related to high mortality [49]. In addition, abnormal sleep is also associated with more anxiety and depression, as well as reduced quality of life and prolonged mechanical ventilation [50–53].

EEG sleep structure is a potential clinical prognostic marker for critically ill patients. In the EEG sleep structure study of patients with post-traumatic coma in the subacute phase, the type of sleep-arousal structure could predict the probability of survival and functional recovery [24]. The EEGs of posttraumatic comatose patients show that the preservation of sleep structure is associated with a good prognosis [54]. A lack of normal sleep structure in patients with SAH is related to poor prognosis. A number of studies of critically ill patients have analyzed the relationship between the characteristics of sleep abnormalities and mortality and found that atypical sleep, a lack of K complexes, and a lack of sleep spindles are all significantly associated with high mortality [55, 56]. Abnormal sleep in critically ill patients may also be related to the recovery of spontaneous breathing. A prospective study [57] found that atypical sleep was an independent risk factor for prolonged ventilator weaning time. The weaning time of severely ill patients with atypical sleep and difficulty in weaning was significantly longer than that of other severely ill patients.

## Cases

1. A case of HIE. A 34-year-old woman with sudden cardiac arrest was transferred to the ICU after 5 min of CPR. Physical examination: tracheal intubation, coma, GCS score of 7 points, bilateral incomplete pupil dilation, bilateral weak light reflex, and pain stimulation. The woman had good sleep at usual (6–7 h/night with no benzodiazepines). The EEG activity was as follows: There was generalized θ activity, more spindle waves and some K-complex waves. The patient had an arousal response under sound and pain stimulation, and a background α rhythm appeared on the EEG. The EEG activity recovered to that of stage 2 sleep a few seconds after stimulation (Figs. 5.13, 5.14 and 5.15).

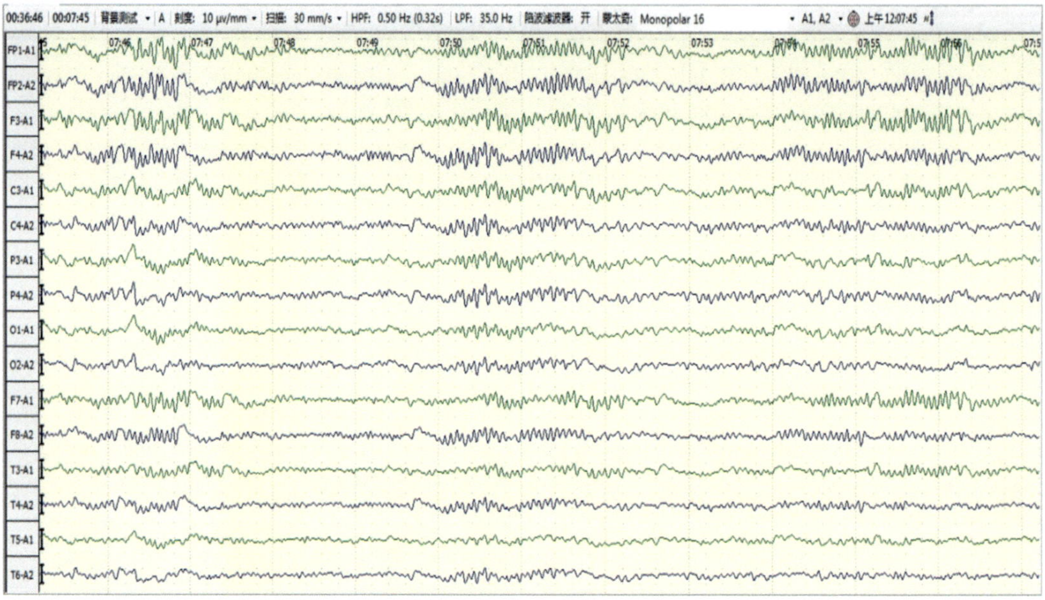


**Fig. 5.13** EEG from the patient with a disturbance of consciousness, continuously showing more spindles and some K-complex waves

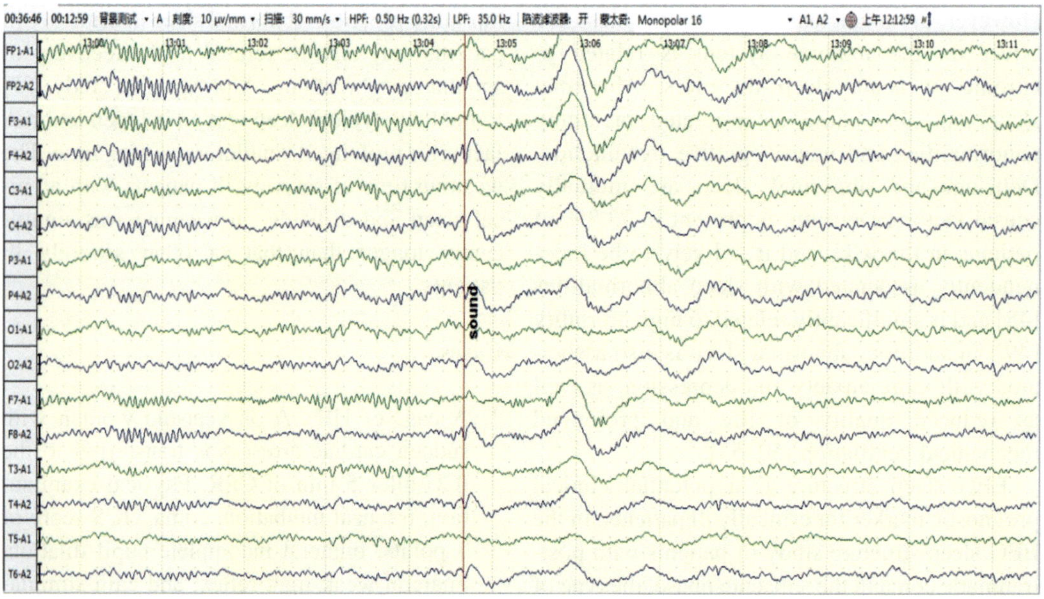


**Fig. 5.14** EEG showing a wake response after sound and pain stimulation

2. A case of herpes simplex virus type I meningoencephalitis. An 80-year-old male was admitted to the ICU with fever, dyspnea, and a disturbance of consciousness for 15 days. Physical examination: endotracheal intubation, ventilator-assisted ventilation of synchronized intermittent mandatory ventilation, MCS, ability to open eyes independently and blink and open mouth occasionally as required, limb intermittent myoclonus, clon-

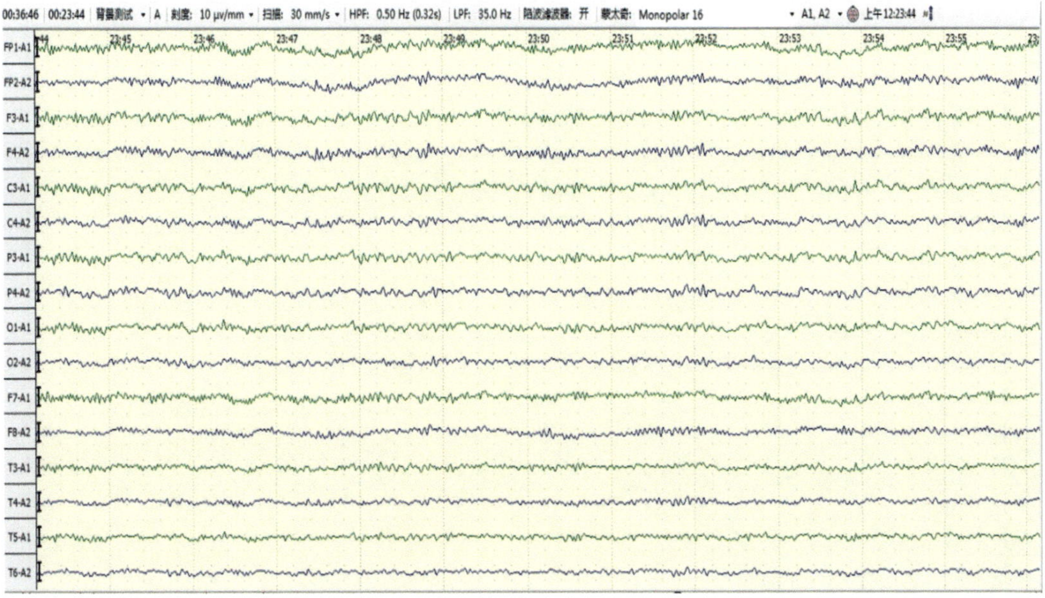

**Fig. 5.15** EEG showing the appearance of background α rhythm after stimulation; EEG activity recovered to that of stage 2 sleep several seconds after stimulation

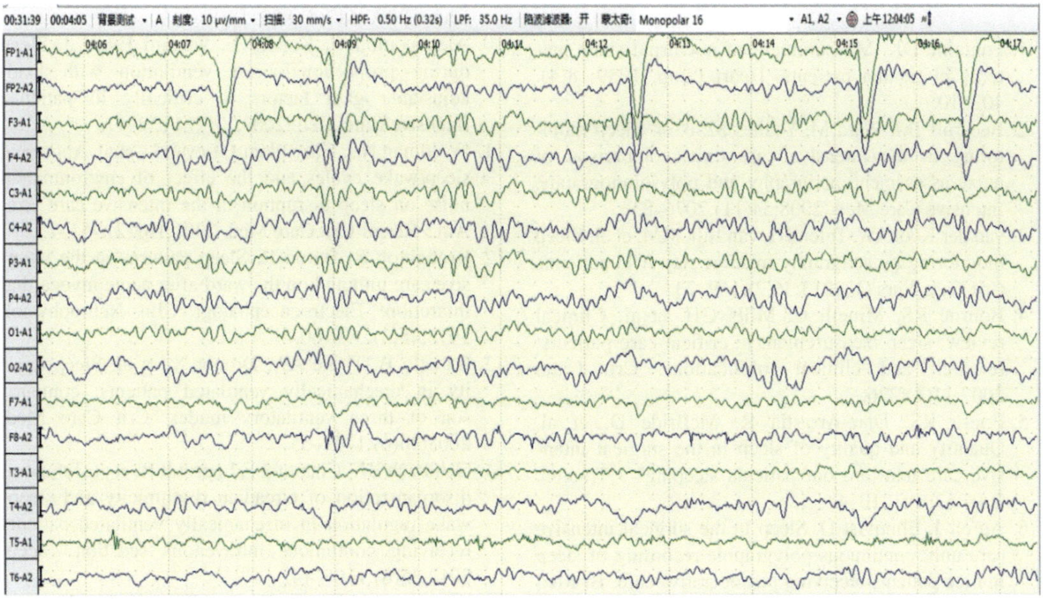

**Fig. 5.16** EEG during an awake phase

azepam 1 mg bid. The EEG activity was as follows: Figure 5.16 shows the EEG from an awake phase. The EEG shows a background α rhythm and generalized θ-δ waves, mostly in the right hemisphere. Figure 5.17 shows the EEG from a sleep phase. The EEG shows sleep spindles and some K-complex waves (Figs. 5.16 and 5.17).

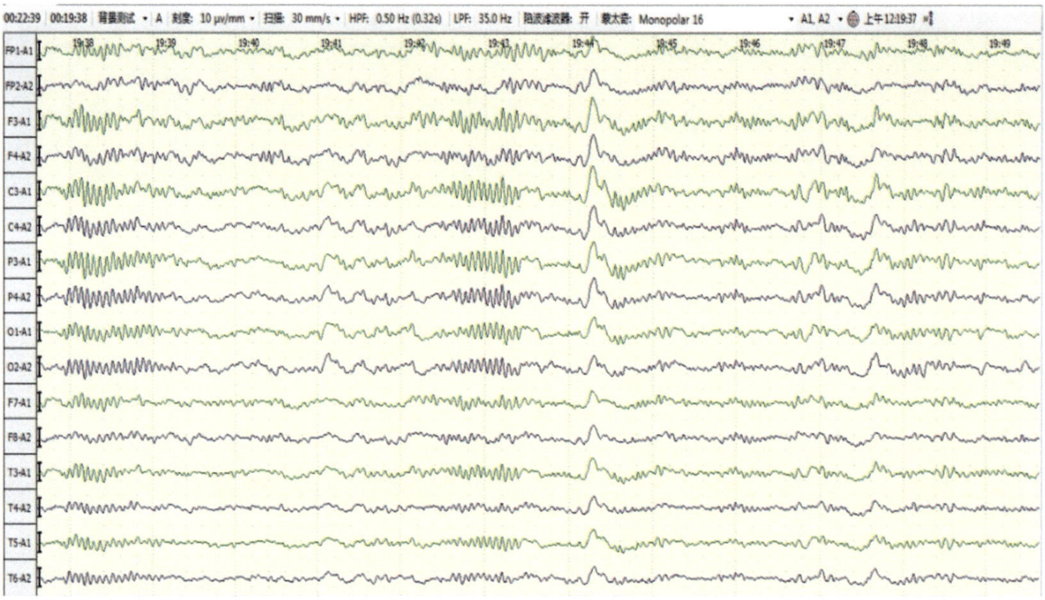


**Fig. 5.17** EEG during a sleep phase

## References


1. Fontaine DK. Measurement of nocturnal sleep patterns in trauma patients. Heart Lung. 1989;18(4):402–10.
2. Beecroft JM, Ward M, Younes M, et al. Sleep monitoring in the intensive care unit: comparison of nurse assessment, actigraphy and polysomnography. Intensive Care Med. 2008;34(11):2076–83.
3. van der Kooi AW, Tulen JH, van Eijk MM, et al. Sleep monitoring by actigraphy in short-stay ICU patients. Crit Care Nurs Q. 2013;36(2):169–73.
4. Bourne RS, Minelli C, Mills GH, et al. Clinical review: sleep measurement in critical care patients: research and clinical implications. Crit Care. 2007;11(4):226.
5. Friese RS, Diaz-Arrastia R, McBride D, et al. Quantity and quality of sleep in the surgical intensive care unit: are our patients sleeping? J Trauma. 2007;63(6):1210–4.
6. Aurell J, Elmqvist D. Sleep in the surgical intensive care unit: continuous polygraphic recording of sleep in nine patients receiving postoperative care. Br Med J (Clin Res Ed). 1985;290(6474):1029–32.
7. Edell-Gustafsson UM, Hetta JE, Aren CB. Sleep and quality of life assessment in patients undergoing coronary artery bypass grafting. J Adv Nurs. 1999;29(5):1213–20.
8. Gabor JY, Cooper AB, Crombach SA, et al. Contribution of the intensive care unit environment to sleep disruption in mechanically ventilated patients and healthy subjects. Am J Respir Crit Care Med. 2003;167(5):708–15.
9. Cooper AB, Thornley KS, Young GB, et al. Sleep in critically ill patients requiring mechanical ventilation. Chest. 2000;117(3):809–18.
10. Alexopoulou C, Kondili E, Vakouti E, et al. Sleep during proportional-assist ventilation with load-adjustable gain factors in critically ill patients. Intensive Care Med. 2007;33(7):1139–47.
11. Freedman NS, Gazendam J, Levan L, et al. Abnormal sleep/wake cycles and the effect of environmental noise on sleep disruption in the intensive care unit. Am J Respir Crit Care Med. 2001;163(2):451–7.
12. Broughton R, Baron R. Sleep patterns in the intensive care unit and on the ward after acute myocardial infarction. Electroencephalogr Clin Neurophysiol. 1978;45(3):348–60.
13. Cabello B, Thille AW, Drouot X, et al. Sleep quality in mechanically ventilated patients: comparison of three ventilatory modes. Crit Care Med. 2008;36(6):1749–55.
14. Gehlbach BK, Chapotot F, Leproult R, et al. Temporal disorganization of circadian rhythmicity and sleep-wake regulation in mechanically ventilated patients receiving continuous intravenous sedation. Sleep. 2012;35(8):1105–14.
15. Whooley MA, Stone B, Soghikian K. Randomized trial of case-finding for depression in elderly primary care patients. J Gen Intern Med. 2000;15(5):293–300.
16. Johns MW, Large AA, Masterton JP, et al. Sleep and delirium after open heart surgery. Br J Surg. 1974;61(5):377–81.
17. Harding SM. Sleep-related gastroesophageal reflux: evidence is mounting. Clin Gastroenterol Hepatol. 2009;7(9):919–20.

18. Richards KC. Effect of a back massage and relaxation intervention on sleep in critically ill patients. Am J Crit Care. 1998;7(4):288–99.
19. Hardin KA, Seyal M, Stewart T, et al. Sleep in critically ill chemically paralyzed patients requiring mechanical ventilation. Chest. 2006;129(6):1468–77.
20. Elliott R, McKinley S, Cistulli P, et al. Characterisation of sleep in intensive care using 24-hour polysomnography: an observational study. Crit Care. 2013;17(2):R46.
21. Bonnet MH. Performance and sleepiness as a function of frequency and placement of sleep disruption. Psychophysiology. 1986;23(3):263–71.
22. Drouot X, Bridoux A, Thille AW, et al. Sleep continuity: a new metric to quantify disrupted hypnograms in non-sedated intensive care unit patients. Crit Care. 2014;18(6):628.
23. McKinley S, Fien M, Elliott R, et al. Sleep and psychological health during early recovery from critical illness: an observational study. J Psychosom Res. 2013;75(6):539–45.
24. Valente M, Placidi F, Oliveira AJ, et al. Sleep organization pattern as a prognostic marker at the subacute stage of post-traumatic coma. Clin Neurophysiol. 2002;113(11):1798–805.
25. Yang XA, Song CG, Yuan F, et al. Prognostic roles of sleep electroencephalography pattern and circadian rhythm biomarkers in the recovery of consciousness in patients with coma: a prospective cohort study. Sleep Med. 2020;69:204–12.
26. Cologan V, Drouot X, Parapatics S, et al. Sleep in the unresponsive wakefulness syndrome and minimally conscious state. J Neurotrauma. 2013;30(5):339–46.
27. Watson PL. Measuring sleep in critically ill patients: beware the pitfalls. Crit Care. 2007;11(4):159.
28. Drouot X, Roche-Campo F, Thille AW, et al. A new classification for sleep analysis in critically ill patients. Sleep Med. 2012;13(1):7–14.
29. Watson PL, Pandharipande P, Gehlbach BK, et al. Atypical sleep in ventilated patients: empirical electroencephalography findings and the path toward revised ICU sleep scoring criteria. Crit Care Med. 2013;41(8):1958–67.
30. Silber MH, Ancoli-Israel S, Bonnet MH, et al. The visual scoring of sleep in adults. J Clin Sleep Med. 2007;3(2):121–31.
31. Urakami Y. Relationship between, sleep spindles and clinical recovery in patients with traumatic brain injury: a simultaneous EEG and MEG study. Clin EEG Neurosci. 2012;43(1):39–47.
32. Sutter R, Barnes B, Leyva A, et al. Electroencephalographic sleep elements and outcome in acute encephalopathic patients: a 4-year cohort study. Eur J Neurol. 2014;21(10):1268–75.
33. MH RT, WC D. Acute sleep deprivation. In: Kryger MH, Roth T, Dement WC, editors. Principles and practice of sleep medicine. Philadelphia: Elsevier Saunder; 2005. p. 51–66.
34. Naitoh P, Kales A, Kollar EJ, et al. Electroencephalographic activity after prolonged sleep loss. Electroencephalogr Clin Neurophysiol. 1969;27(1):2–11.
35. Rodin EA, Luby ED, Gottlieb JS. The electroencephalogram during prolonged experimental sleep deprivation. Electroencephalogr Clin Neurophysiol. 1962;14:544–51.
36. De Gennaro L, Ferrara M, Bertini M. Effect of slow-wave sleep deprivation on topographical distribution of spindles. Behav Brain Res. 2000;116(1):55–9.
37. Sforza E, Chapotot F, Pigeau R, et al. Effects of sleep deprivation on spontaneous arousals in humans. Sleep. 2004;27(6):1068–75.
38. Gabor JY, Cooper AB, Hanly PJ. Sleep disruption in the intensive care unit. Curr Opin Crit Care. 2001;7(1):21–7.
39. Weinhouse GL, Schwab RJ. Sleep in the critically ill patient. Sleep. 2006;29(5):707–16.
40. Morisson F, Decary A, Petit D, et al. Daytime sleepiness and EEG spectral analysis in apneic patients before and after treatment with continuous positive airway pressure. Chest. 2001;119(1):45–52.
41. Mathieu A, Mazza S, Petit D, et al. Does age worsen EEG slowing and attention deficits in obstructive sleep apnea syndrome? Clin Neurophysiol. 2007;118(7):1538–44.
42. Xiromeritis AG, Hatziefthimiou AA, Hadjigeorgiou GM, et al. Quantitative spectral analysis of vigilance EEG in patients with obstructive sleep apnoea syndrome: EEG mapping in OSAS patients. Sleep Breath. 2011;15(1):121–8.
43. Toth M, Faludi B, Wackermann J, et al. Characteristic changes in brain electrical activity due to chronic hypoxia in patients with obstructive sleep apnea syndrome (OSAS): a combined EEG study using LORETA and omega complexity. Brain Topogr. 2009;22(3):185–90.
44. Svanborg E, Guilleminault C. EEG frequency changes during sleep apneas. Sleep. 1996;19(3):248–54.
45. Morisson F, Lavigne G, Petit D, et al. Spectral analysis of wakefulness and REM sleep EEG in patients with sleep apnoea syndrome. Eur Respir J. 1998;11(5):1135–40.
46. Walsleben JA, O'Malley EB, Bonnet K, et al. The utility of topographic EEG mapping in obstructive sleep apnea syndrome. Sleep. 1993;16(8 Suppl):S76–8.
47. Lee SD, Ju G, Kim JW, et al. Improvement of EEG slowing in OSAS after CPAP treatment. J Psychosom Res. 2012;73(2):126–31.
48. Trompeo AC, Vidi Y, Locane MD, et al. Sleep disturbances in the critically ill patients: role of delirium and sedative agents. Minerva Anestesiol. 2011;77(6):604–12.
49. Scott BK. Disruption of circadian rhythms and sleep in critical illness and its impact on the development of delirium. Curr Pharm Des. 2015;21(24):3443–52.
50. White DP, Douglas NJ, Pickett CK, et al. Sleep deprivation and the control of ventilation. Am Rev Respir Dis. 1983;128(6):984–6.
51. Griffiths J, Fortune G, Barber V, et al. The prevalence of post traumatic stress disorder in survivors of ICU

treatment: a systematic review. Intensive Care Med. 2007;33(9):1506–18.
52. Schelling G, Stoll C, Haller M, et al. Health-related quality of life and posttraumatic stress disorder in survivors of the acute respiratory distress syndrome. Crit Care Med. 1998;26(4):651–9.
53. Scragg P, Jones A, Fauvel N. Psychological problems following ICU treatment. Anaesthesia. 2001;56(1):9–14.
54. Bergamasco B, Bergamini L, Doriguzzi T, et al. EEG sleep patterns as a prognostic criterion in post-traumatic coma. Electroencephalogr Clin Neurophysiol. 1968;24(4):374–7.
55. Boyko Y, Toft P, Ording H, et al. Atypical sleep in critically ill patients on mechanical ventilation is associated with increased mortality. Sleep Breath. 2019;23(1):379–88.
56. Knauert MP, Gilmore EJ, Murphy TE, et al. Association between death and loss of stage N2 sleep features among critically ill patients with delirium. J Crit Care. 2018;48:124–9.
57. Thille AW, Reynaud F, Marie D, et al. Impact of sleep alterations on weaning duration in mechanically ventilated patients: a prospective study. Eur Respir J. 2018;51(4).

# Part III

# Application of Multimodal EEG in Severely Ill Patients

# Application of Multimodal EEG in Coma Patients

6

Xin Tian and Feng Li

## Contents



**Abstract**

Patients with severe brain injury are mostly in a coma during the acute stage. Most comatose patients will recover their consciousness in a short period of time. However, some patients do not recover consciousness for a long time due to severe neurological deficits, eventually developing a persistent hyporesponsive state, VS, or even death. The medical expenses of patients who continue to be in a coma are enormous, conveying a heavy economic burden and huge psychological pressure to society and family members. Therefore, understanding the severity of brain damage in

X. Tian (✉) · F. Li
Department of Neurology, The First Affiliated Hospital of Chongqing Medical University, Chongqing, China
e-mail: xintian@cqmu.edu.cn



X. Wang et al. (eds.), *Multi-Modal EEG Monitoring of Severely Neurologically Ill Patients*,
https://doi.org/10.1007/978-981-16-4493-1_6

coma patients, early judgment of the prognosis of consciousness disturbance, and effective wake-up treatment are the focus of treatment in the NICU. This chapter briefly describes the methods of brain function assessment in patients with impaired consciousness, focusing on the application of multimodal EEG in patients with impaired consciousness, and helps critically ill doctors use multimodal EEG to accurately assess the brain functions of patients, providing effective information on patients with impaired consciousness to detect changes in their condition over time, observe treatment responses, and determine the severity of brain injury and early prognosis.

**Keywords**

Coma · Multimodal EEG · Abnormal EEG background activity · EEG-R · Sleep · Evoked potential (EP) · aEEG · Bispectral index (BIS)

Neurologically severely ill patients often experience severe brain damage due to cerebrovascular disease, brain injury, cardiac arrest, anesthesia accidents, etc. Relevant epidemiological surveys show that the incidence of moderate to severe brain injury is approximately 15/100,000 per year [1]. Most of these patients have consciousness disorder, which is related to their prognosis. Studies have found that the 6-month mortality rate of patients with severe brain injury and consciousness disorder is approximately 46%, and 15% are in a persistent VS. Among the survivors of severe brain injury, 52% regain consciousness but with disability, and only 7% fully recover [2].

Consciousness is the response of the human brain to internal and external environmental stimuli. When the response of the human brain changes, there would be a disturbance of consciousness. This disturbance of consciousness may be an abnormality of the brain's ascending network activation system, or it may be defects in the content of cortical consciousness. Mild disturbances of consciousness can recover without nervous system sequelae, whereas severe cases can lead to death. Understanding the degree of brain damage and judging the prognosis of consciousness disorder often become important clinical tasks. Multimodal EEG has unique advantages in this respect.

## 6.1 Methods to Evaluate Brain Function in Patients with Impaired Consciousness and the Significance of Multimodal EEG Evaluation

The fatality rate and disability rate of patients with brain injury are high, and some patients with chronic consciousness disorder have huge medical expenses, resulting in large economic burdens for patients' families and society. For such patients, medical staff and family members need to know whether the patient's consciousness disorder can be restored and how it can recover. Therefore, accurate and objective prognosis judgments can provide a basis for making reasonable and effective medical decisions.

The significance of evaluating brain function in patients with acute coma lies in judging the condition; improving objective, accurate, and reliable indicators for predicting the outcome; reducing blindness; improving the success rate of treatment; and reducing the mortality and disability rates. There are currently more than 20 methods to assess brain injury, including clinical observation; imaging; monitoring neuroelectrophysiology, ICP, CBF, and $PbtO_2$; and neuroendocrine therapy. These methods play an important role in the judgment of brain function and prognosis, but there are certain limitations to each method.

At present, clinical observation mainly relies on the inference and interpretation of patients' behavioral responses, and behavioral judgments based on clinical scales are currently the most commonly used evaluation methods. However, clinical observation is affected by the drugs administered, its objectivity and accuracy are poor, and its results are easily affected by the experience of the evaluator and the level of training received. Serum biochemical indicators are relatively objective, but they are mainly applicable to the acute stage of partial brain injury. Over the course of a disease, neuroimaging has played an increasingly important role in the judgment of brain function in disorders of consciousness in recent years and has received great attention, but its examination costs are expensive. Neuroimaging instruments are not available everywhere and they cannot be brought into the ICU, it is difficult to complete neuroimaging tests at the bedside, and the use of neuroimaging is greatly restricted. Neuroelectrophysiological monitoring is still the most important evaluation tool in the NICU. It provides a continuous, real-time, noninvasive brain function monitoring technology and has certain advantages in disease judgment, treatment monitoring, and short-term prognosis. Fast, convenient, systematic, and accurate tools to judge the severity of brain injury and predict prognosis will provide an important basis for subsequent reasonable and effective medical decisions.

## 6.2 The Application of Multimodal EEG in Patients with Consciousness Disorder

### 6.2.1 Common Abnormal EEG Background Activity in Coma Patients

Electrophysiological methods mainly include EEG and the measuring of EPs. Electrophysiological methods can be used to check the possible causes of coma and injury sites in comatose patients and evaluate function after brain injury to predict the outcome. EEGs mainly reflect the activities of cortical neurons, which are regulated by physiological or pathological diencephalon and brainstem activity and are affected by metabolic and/or toxic factors. Many abnormal EEG patterns cannot specifically reflect primary cortical dysfunction and abnormal effects on other healthy cerebral cortical areas. The main advantage of EEG is that it can evaluate brain function noninvasively and in real time. Different from EPs, EEGs can immediately summarize the functional status of the detected brain regions to quickly detect changes in the functional status of the cortex (sleep transition, cortical response to stimuli, short-term drug effects, seizures, and interictal periods). Monitoring EEGs helps to identify changes in brain function and is of great value in predicting prognosis. Different EEG patterns can reflect the specific causes of coma and the degree of brain damage.

Common EEG configurations in coma patients mainly include α-coma, β-coma, spindle coma, TWs, FT, generalized slow waves, generalized periodic composite slow waves, and BS, etc. (see the Chap. 3 for details).

### 6.2.2 The Role of EEG-R in the Evaluation of Brain Function and the Prognosis of Patients with Severe Coma

Complete EEG-R requires the integrity of all the structures and functions of the brainstem ascending network to the hypothalamus, subthalamus, and thalamus-cortex system and is a reflection of the integrity of the overall structure and function of the cerebral cortical network. EEG-R to exogenous stimuli is an important indicator for evaluating brain function. Studies have shown that patients with EEG-R consciousness disorders have a better prognosis than those with EEG-nonresponsive consciousness disorders and that EEG-R is a predictor of acute brain injury. EEG-R is a good indicator of whether the consciousness of patients with consciousness disorder can recover. Gütling E et al. [3] compared the predictive effects of EEG-R and somatosensory evoked potential (SEP) central conduction time on the prognosis of patients with severe brain injury and coma. They evaluated 50 coma patients and tested their EEG-R. The central conduction time was followed up for one and half years. The results showed that the accuracy rate of EEG-R to distinguish between good prognosis and poor prognosis was 92%, while the accuracy rate of central conduction time was only 82%, and the accuracy rate of the GCS was 72%. When EEG-R and central conduction time were both used, the accuracy rate could reach 98%. There is much controversy about the prognostic value of α or θ coma. Some clinicians think that the prognosis of patients with unresponsive α or θ coma is poor, while patients with responsive α or θ coma have a good prognosis. Supporting the belief that EEG-R is a good indicator of long-term prognosis, Synek et al. [4] proposed the Synek grading standard by analyzing the EEGs of patients with cardiac arrest, respiratory arrest, and coma due to severe brain injury. For the first time, EEG-R was regarded as one of the main components of the grading standard. Based on the internationally recognized scale, the Synek grading is divided into five main grades. The study pointed out that using Synek grading, coma patients are first rated as grade I or reactive grade II, and their prognosis is good. Patients with small fluctuations and diffuse, irregular δ waves are rated as grade III, and patients rated as grades IV and V have poor prognosis and high mortality. The prognosis of the other intermediate grade patients is uncertain. Young proposed the Young classification on the basis of the Synek classification in 1997 [5]. Young grading is more widely used, and its reliability among observers is better. The Young classification and the Synek classification are currently widely recognized and applied EEG evaluation standards, both of which use EEG-R as an important judgment index.

### 6.2.3 The Role of Abnormal Sleep Waveforms in the Brain Function and Prognosis of Patients with Severe Coma

Sleep is an extremely common phenomenon with unique electrophysiological characteristics. The electrophysiological characteristics of sleep are mainly based on continuously alternating sleep stages, sleep cycles, and constant slow-wave regulation. Sleep spindles are the main features of the sleep cycle. The standard sleep cycle is a manifestation of the functional integrity of the brain [6]. The appearance of spindle waves in periodic sleep, stable slow-wave activity, and REM sleep periods are very reliable electrophysiological characteristics of mammalian sleep processes. The integrity of brain function can be reflected in whether a standard sleep cycle is present. Therefore, a sleep cycle, which reflects complete brain function, will change under pathological conditions such as a disturbance of consciousness.

A disturbance or disappearance of sleep structure is an independent risk factor for poor prognosis of patients with impaired consciousness, and normal sleep cycle activity on EEGs is a favorable prognostic sign for patients. Sandsmark DK et al. [7] retrospectively analyzed the EEG data of patients with severe TBI who underwent cEEG monitoring for at least 24 h within 14 days after injury. There were 64 cases in total, and the average cEEG monitoring time was 50.6 h. There were 19 patients (30%) with characteristic sleep patterns, and the study found that the presence of characteristic sleep patterns was correlated with a better prognosis (89% were discharged home or recovered quickly, $P = 0.0002$). In addition, Alekseeva EV et al. [8] performed PSG on 64 patients in VS and found that 26 patients lacked sleep patterns and had a poor prognosis. Arnaldi D et al. [9] used PSG to understand the value of sleep patterns for the prognosis of patients with subacute disturbance of consciousness. A total of 27 patients 3.5 ± 2 months after head injury were selected for PSG and clinical evaluation. Visual and quantitative indicators were used to analyze the PSG record results. Visual analysis found that those with a complete sleep pattern ($p = 0.0006$) had a better prognosis, suggesting that the appearance of a complete sleep structure is related to previous predictive indicators (such as age and basic clinical conditions). Impaired consciousness in the subacute phase can better predict a good prognosis. de Biase S et al. [10] and others performed studies to assess whether there is a correlation between sleep records and EPs, and their clinical evaluations of patients with prolonged disorders of consciousness included a total of 27 patients in VS and 5 patients in a MCS. All patients were clinically and neurophysiologically evaluated. The clinical assessment included the Coma Recovery Scale-Revised (CRS-R), Disability Rating Scale (DRS), and GCS. Neurophysiological assessment included 24-h PSG and the monitoring of SEPs, brainstem auditory evoked potentials (BAEPs), and visual evoked potentials (VEPs). The results of the study found that patients with the retention of each sleep component (sleep-wake cycle, sleep spindles, K complex waves, and REM sleep) had better clinical scores than patients without sleep component retention. Only REM sleep was significantly different among patient groups. Multivariate analysis showed that the co-occurrence of sleep spindles and REM sleep was associated with a higher CRS-R score (positive interaction, $P < 0.0001$). Therefore, it is believed that the use of PSG for patients with long-term impaired consciousness can more fully judge the patient's level of consciousness and that PSG is a reliable tool. Alekseeva EV et al. [8] also found similar findings. The researchers performed PSG on 64 patients in VS. The study found that 27 (96%) of 28 patients with good prognosis had sleep pattern retention. By contrast, only 11 (31%) of the 36 patients with poor prognosis had visible sleep patterns.

### 6.2.4 The Application of EPs in the Judgment of Brain Function and the Prognosis of Patients with Severe Coma

Cerebral cortical neurons are the most vulnerable part of the brain. SEPs are not affected by CNS inhibitors or patient consciousness. The monitoring of SEPs can accurately, reliably, and objectively determine the condition and prognosis of patients with brain injury and coma (Fig. 6.1). After stimulating the median nerve, the reaction in the sensory cortex can be used to determine the SEP. For patients with brain injury, the monitoring of SEPs can provide more disease information than the monitoring of BAEPs, and SEPs are the best evaluation indexes for severe brain injury. Rothstein T L [11] verified the role of median nerve SEPs in predicting the prognosis of coma patients; 54 CPR coma patients were enrolled, and 23 patients with bilateral disappearance of cortical EPs did not wake up and died. Of the remaining 27 patients, patients with normal central conduction times had a good prognosis, while patients with slower central conduction

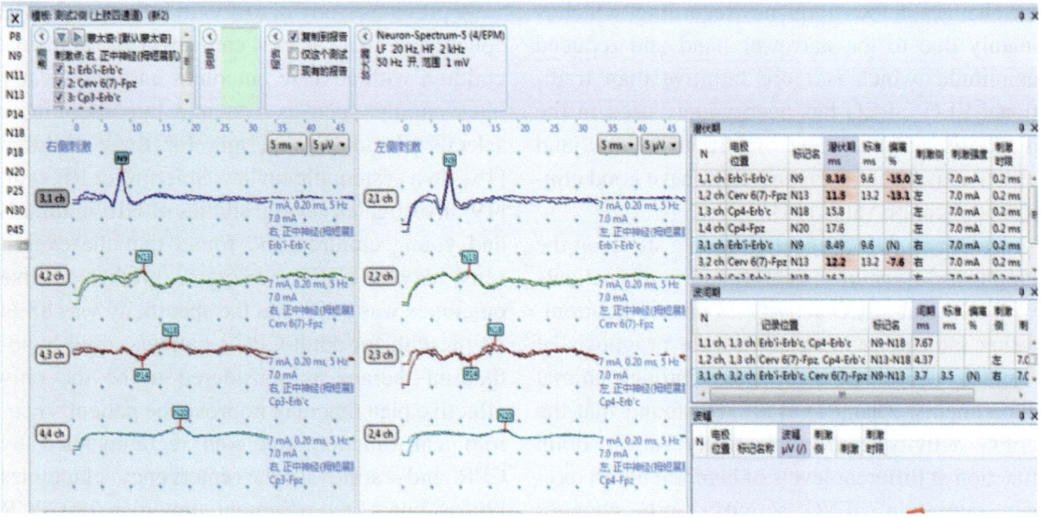

**Fig. 6.1** Female, 28 years old, with HIE. Seventy-two hours after CPR, N20 was seen on both sides of the SEP. The patient was fully awake 10 days later and had a good prognosis

times had an uncertain prognosis, and some patients transitioned to VS. A meta-analysis compared the value of exercise response, SEPs, and EEGs in predicting the prognosis of patients with hypoxic coma. A total of 25 studies were included. The results showed that SEPs were better than other items in predicting the prognosis of patients with coma, suggesting that SEPs are more predictive than clinical signs [12]. To optimize the detection time of SEPs, Zandbergen et al. [13] conducted a prospective study in conjunction with 32 ICUs. A total of 407 patients in a coma 24 h after CPR were included, of whom 356 had a poor prognosis. A total of 136 patients showed bilateral disappearance of SEPs, and the prognosis was poor. It was suggested that SEPs can stably predict the adverse outcome of patients who are unconscious 24 hours after CPR.

### 6.2.5 aEEG

As a newer brain function monitoring index, aEEG is a derivative of EEG. aEEG selectively records the neurophysiological state of the cortex through electrodes set in different parts of the brain, and aEEG activity is expressed in the form of amplitude after integration, which has simple and easy-to-understand characteristics. In addition, the decrease in brain function is revealed by the changes in low-frequency recording, which is mainly due to the narrower band and reduced amplitude, which is more intuitive than traditional EEG. aEEG has been widely used in the diagnosis and treatment of HIE in infants, and aEEG activity has been proven to have good clinical application value [14].

El-Dib et al. [15] mentioned in a study on the prognosis of neurological function in patients with HIE that aEEG activity, as one of the monitoring indicators, is related to the prognosis of patients' neurological function. Through animal experiments, Zhang D et al. [16] found that the aEEG activity could objectively reflect brain function at different levels of cerebral blood oxygen saturation. aEEG activity rarely changes when the brain is mildly hypoxic, and the aEEG band decreases during moderate hypoxia, but it is reversible. aEEG activity is continuously low and irreversible during severe hypoxia, indicating that aEEG activity can directly and continuously reflect the severity of brain injury.

A study found that aEEG activity was better than the GCS score in predicting the prognosis of brain function in coma patients [17]. Through logistic regression analysis of the value of aEEG activity and the GCS score in predicting the prognosis of brain function, it was found that aEEG activity had an independent effect on the prognosis of early brain function. The receiver operating characteristic (ROC) curve analysis of the ability of the two to evaluate the prognosis of brain function found that the AUC of aEEG activity in evaluating the prognosis of brain function in cardiopulmonary cerebral resuscitation (CPCR) patients was 0.913, and the optimal cutoff point was 1.5. aEEG activity had high sensitivity (95.7%) and specificity (75.0%). The GCS score was used to evaluate the brain function of CPCR patients. The prognostic AUC was 0.851, and when the optimal cutoff point was 1.5, it had a high sensitivity (91.3%). However, the specificity was not high (62.5%). aEEG activity was better than the GCS score in predicting the prognosis of brain function in CPCR patients.

A previous study of aEEG in infants with HIE concluded that aEEG can identify high-risk children with adverse outcomes and allow early interventions such as systemic hypothermia or selective head hypothermia for these children [18]. In a systematic review, Spitzmiller RE et al. [19] investigated several studies of HIE in infants and young children and found that the overall sensitivity of aEEG activity to predict adverse outcomes was 91%, and the specificity was 88%. At present, for adult CPCR patients, mild hypothermia therapy is considered to be the only effective plan that may improve the patient's neurological function and was recommended by CPR and cardiovascular emergency guidelines [20] as one of the treatment strategies for CPCR coma patients in 2010, but its treatment remains unclear. Studies have shown that mild hypothermia treatment can improve the neurological function of CPCR patients by reducing brain cell metabolism, inhibiting brain cell apoptosis pathways, and protecting the role of the blood-brain barrier after brain injury [21].

### 6.2.6 BIS

BIS monitoring is an electrophysiological technology widely used in monitoring the depth of anesthesia. Through the principle of FFT, this technology can transform the original EEG signal of the time–amplitude relationship into the frequency–power relationship, supplemented by the dual spectrum analysis method. On the basis of power spectrum analysis, correlation function spectrum analysis is added, and the original EEG waveform is processed, which can simultaneously realize the determination of the linear component of the EEG and the analysis of the nonlinear relationship between the EEG component waves, thereby obtaining simple quantitative indicators, that is, the BIS value [22]. The monitoring of the BIS value has the advantages of convenience, noninvasiveness, intuitiveness, and continuity. The BIS value also integrates the characteristics of frequency, power, phase, and harmonics in EEGs and can provide a comprehensive reference for the judgment of cerebral cortical function and the analysis of cerebral perfusion [23, 24].

A study compared the results of BIS monitoring after admission for patients with and without the recovery of consciousness. The results showed that, compared with patients with unrecovered consciousness, BISmax, BISmin, and BISmean were higher in patients with recovered consciousness after admission. The BIS value mainly reflected brain electrical activity and the degree of brain awakeness. A higher BIS value at admission meant that the cerebral cortex was less inhibited, and the prognosis of such patients was often better [25]. In addition, studies have shown that changes in BIS values are related to the oxygen consumption level of cerebral cortical cells and can reflect the degree of brain cell damage [26]. Therefore, the lower BIS value of the unrecovered group meant that the cerebral cortical cells were low in oxygen consumption and the brain cells were seriously damaged; therefore, these patients were more likely to transition to VS or even die.

Studies have pointed out that both BISmin and BISmean can provide a reliable reference for predicting the recovery of consciousness within 30 days of coma onset, while BISmax has low discrimination ability in predicting the prognosis of patients. Considering that BISmax reflects a patient's maximum state of consciousness, it may be related to the deviation of judgment results. Patients are often in the lowest state of consciousness when BISmean fluctuates in the range of 70–80, and when BISmean reaches the range of 50–65, patients are generally in a VS [27, 28]. Therefore, continuous monitoring of BIS to distinguish between the lowest state of consciousness and VS also has important reference value for the formulation of treatment measures for comatose patients.

**Case**

The patient went to the local people's hospital for palpitations and chest tightness 14 days prior. The ECG showed sinus tachycardia and complete right bundle branch block, and the patient was admitted to the hospital. During hospitalization, the patient suddenly lost consciousness and suffered cardiac arrest. CPR was performed immediately. Approximately 30 min after electric defibrillation rescue, spontaneous heartbeat and breathing recovered, but there was still a disturbance of consciousness. Figure 6.2 shows the head computed tomography (CT) at admission. Eight days prior, he detached the ventilator and pulled out the tracheal intubation tube. The patient was in a coma with eyes open.

The first evaluation of brain function suggested that brain function was severely damaged,

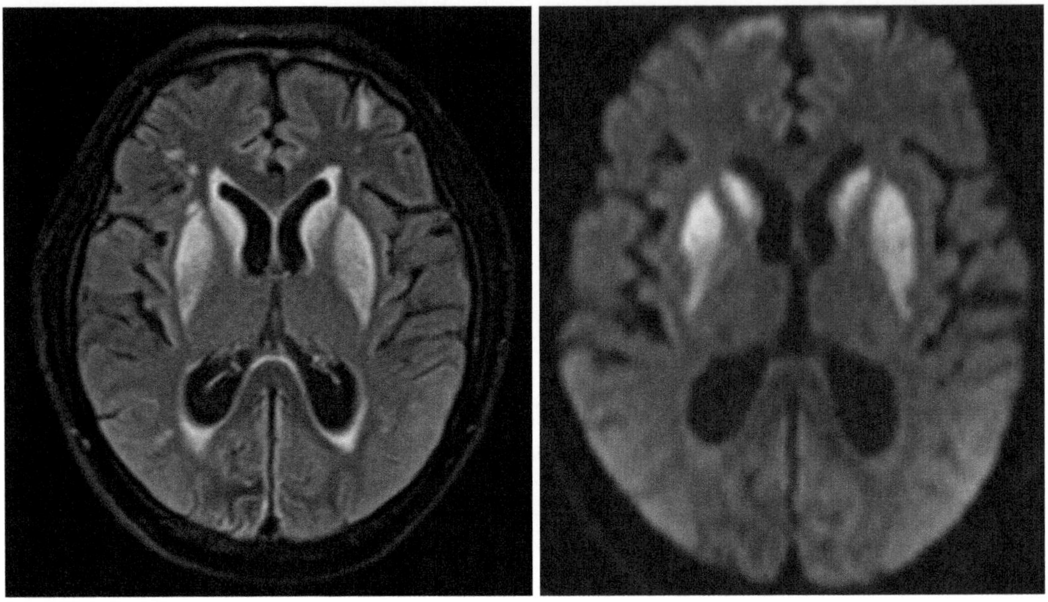

**Fig. 6.2** Head CT at admission, revealing ischemic and hypoxic changes

but sleep spindles were present, the EPs were bilaterally N20, and the CEGL (C: calcium, E: EEG reactivity, G: GCS, L: lactate) score was 3 points, indicating that the patient had a good prognosis (Table 6.1). Below for EEG and EP details (Figs. 6.3 and 6.4).

Quantitative brain function (Fig. 6.5a–c).

The second brain function assessment 1 month after hospitalization indicated that the brain function was restored, and the patient was completely awake and transferred to the rehabilitation department to continue physical rehabilitation. The patient had a good prognosis (Figs. 6.6, 6.7, 6.8, 6.9, and 6.10) below for details.

**Table 6.1** Professor Wang Xuefeng's team independently developed a CEGL score prediction model that can predict the 6-month prognosis of patients with HIE and coma

| Relevant factors | Types | Scores |
|---|---|---|
| Blood calcium | Low calcium | 2 |
| | Normal | 0 |
| EEG reactivity | No | 2 |
| | Yes | 0 |
| GCS score | $\leq 8$ | 1 |
| | >8 | 0 |
| Blood lactate | High lactic acid | 1 |
| | Normal | 0 |
| Total score | | 6 |

A total score of 6 points and a score ≥5 points indicate a poor prognosis. The patient's CEGL score was 3 points

a

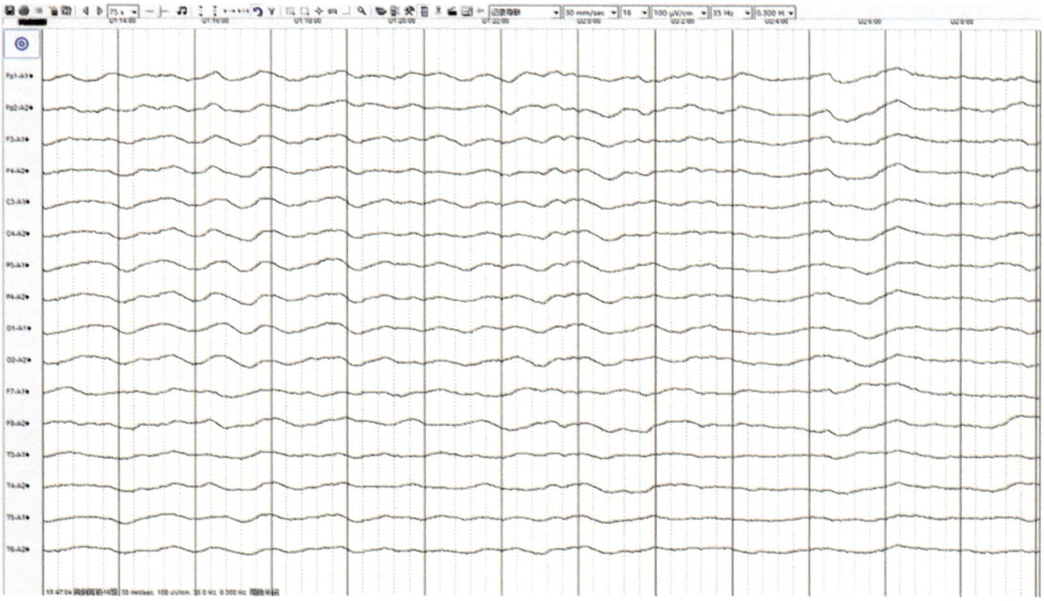

b

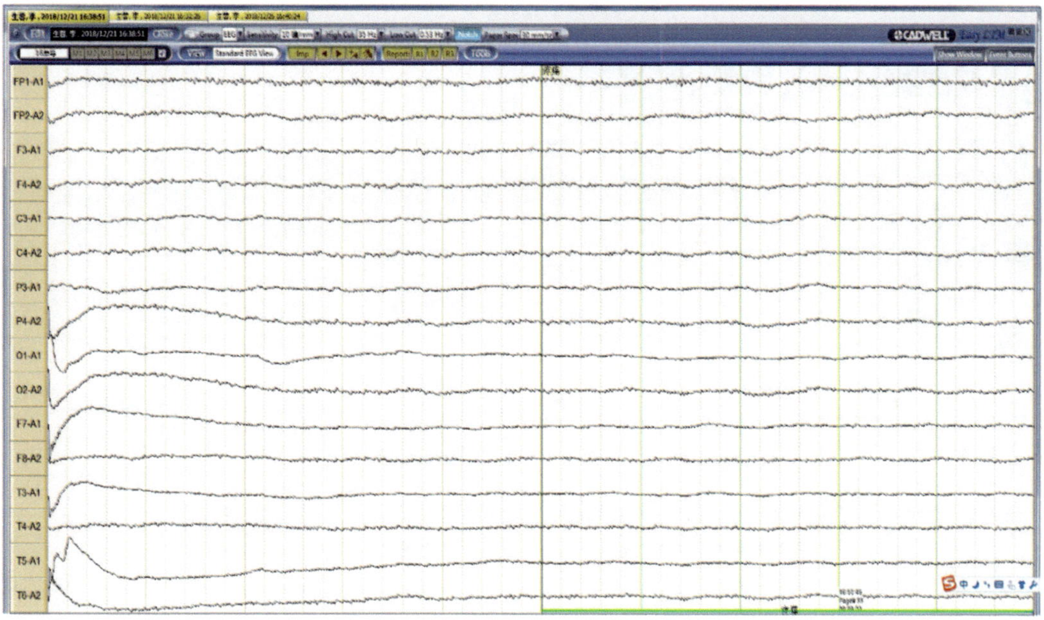


**Fig. 6.3** (**a**) EEG background activity, manifesting as a full-lead diffuse low-medium wave amplitude at approximately 1.0–2.0. (**b**) EEG showing that responsiveness had disappeared. (**c**) Sleep EEG, showing visible sleep spindles

**c**

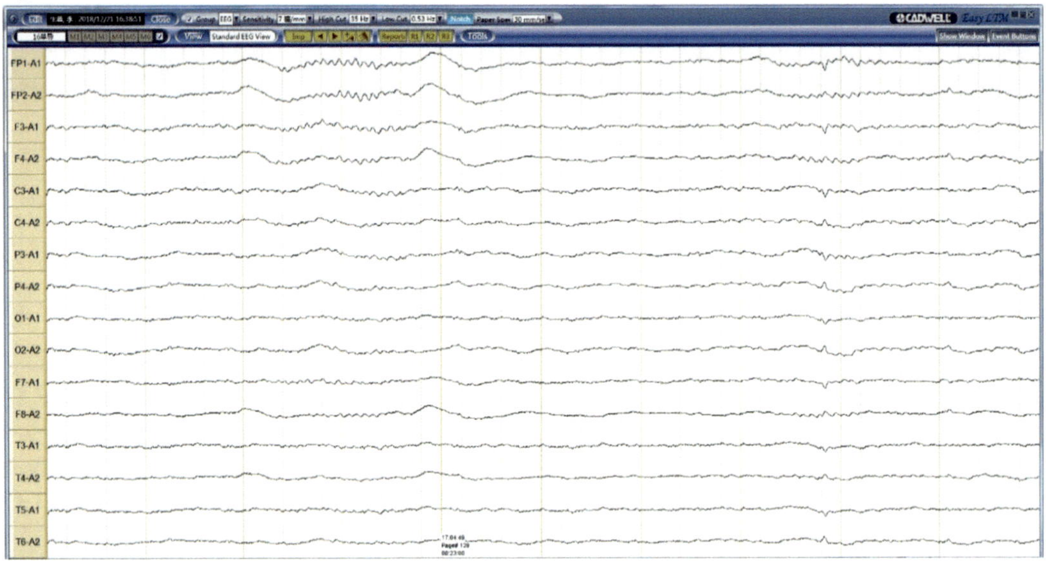


**Fig. 6.3** (continued)

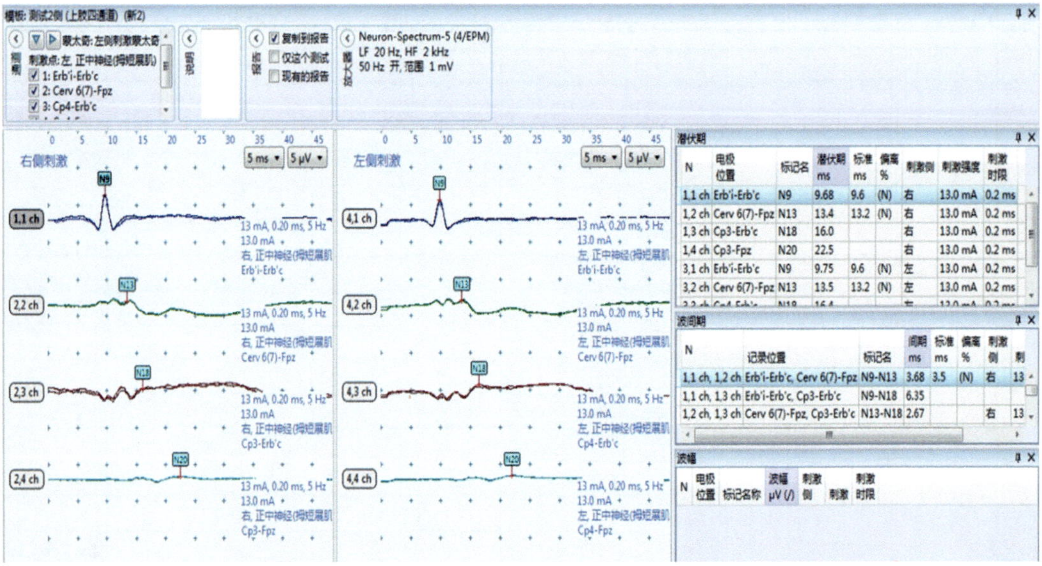


**Fig. 6.4** EPs, showing that N20 is present on both sides, the amplitude extremely low, and the latency is prolonged

a

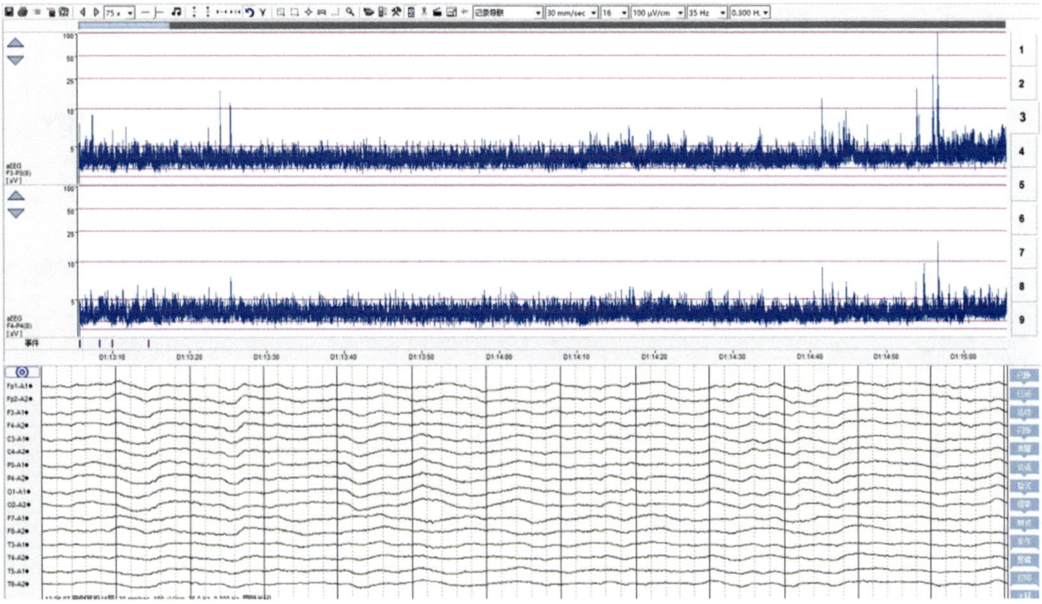

b

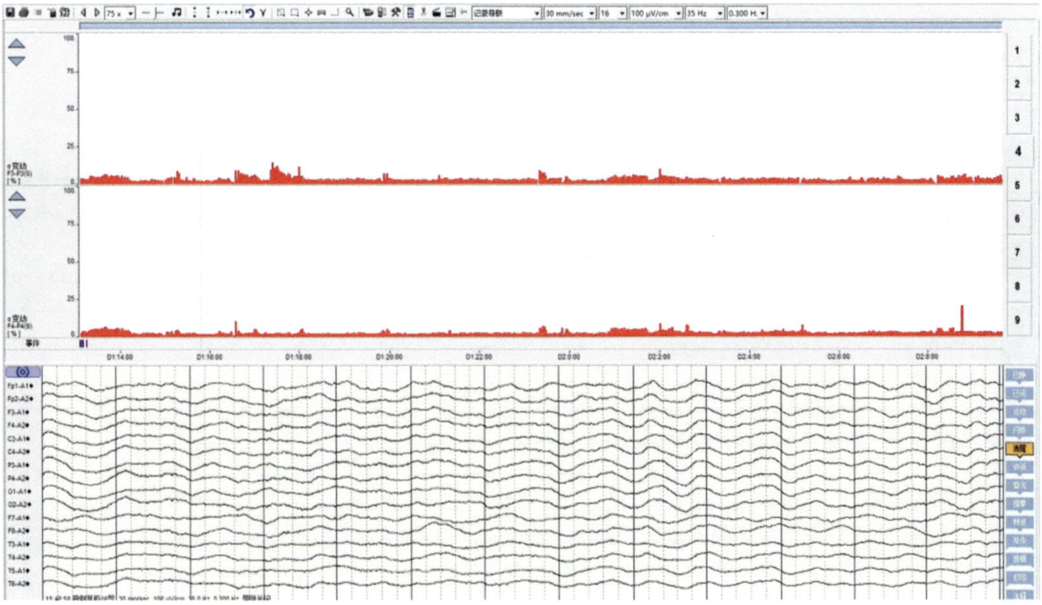

**Fig. 6.5** (**a**) aEEG shows that the upper and lower boundaries of activity are both <5 μV, indicating severe abnormality. (**b**) Two points for the variation score, indicating poor perfusion. (**c**) Spectral entropy fluctuates at approximately 40–50

c

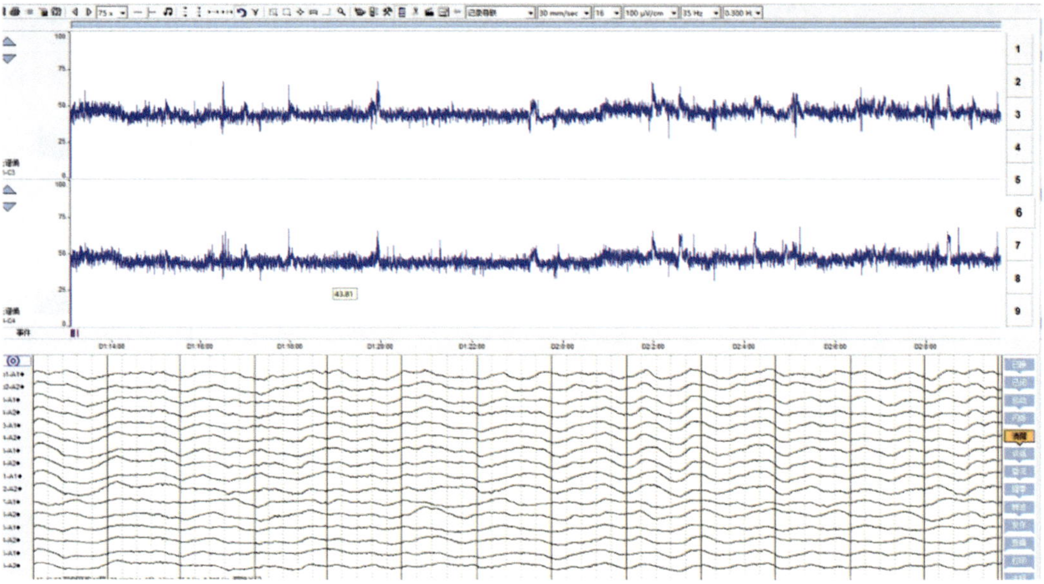

**Fig. 6.5** (continued)

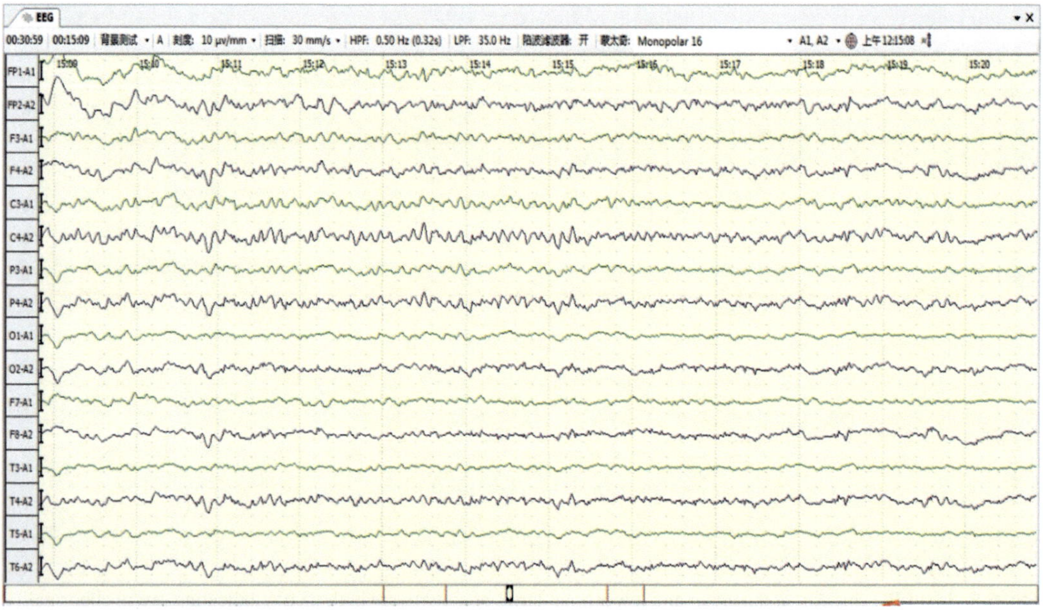


**Fig. 6.6** EEG background activity, showing that the occipital lead α rhythm is restored

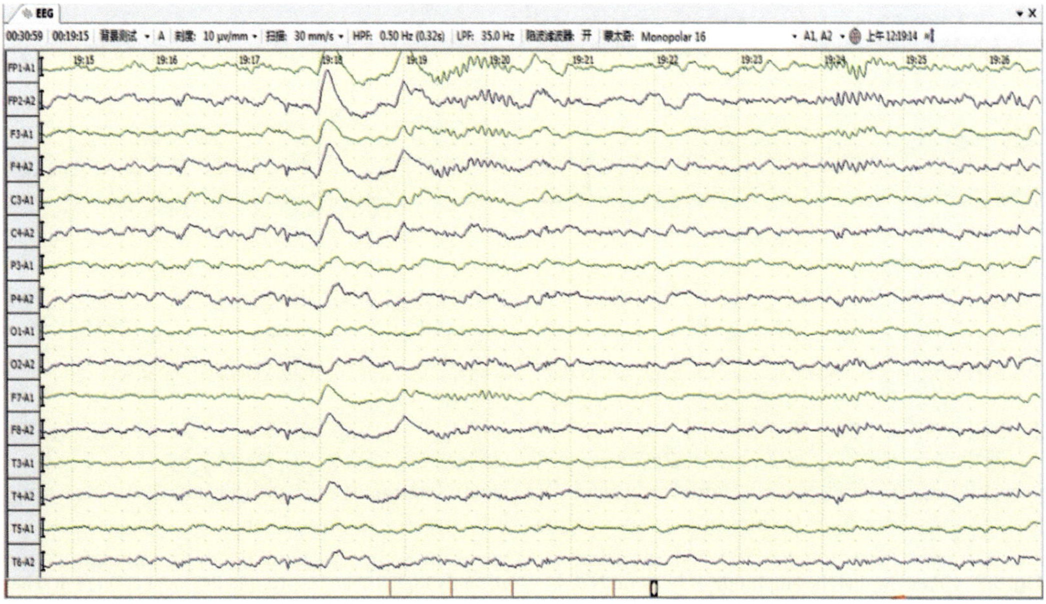

**Fig. 6.7** EEG, showing sleep phenomena

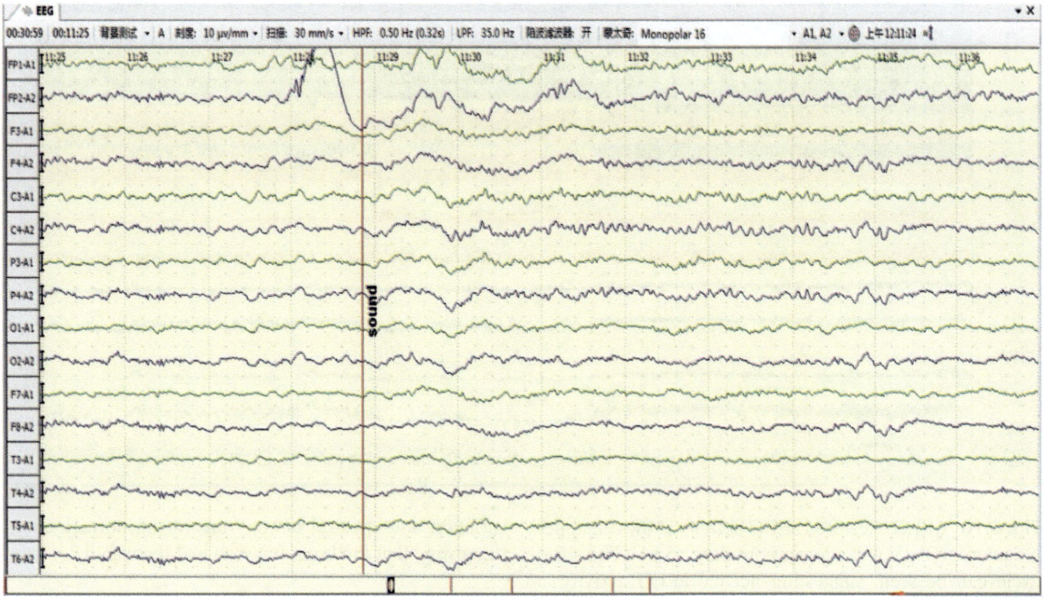

**Fig. 6.8** EEG shows responsiveness and indicating recovery

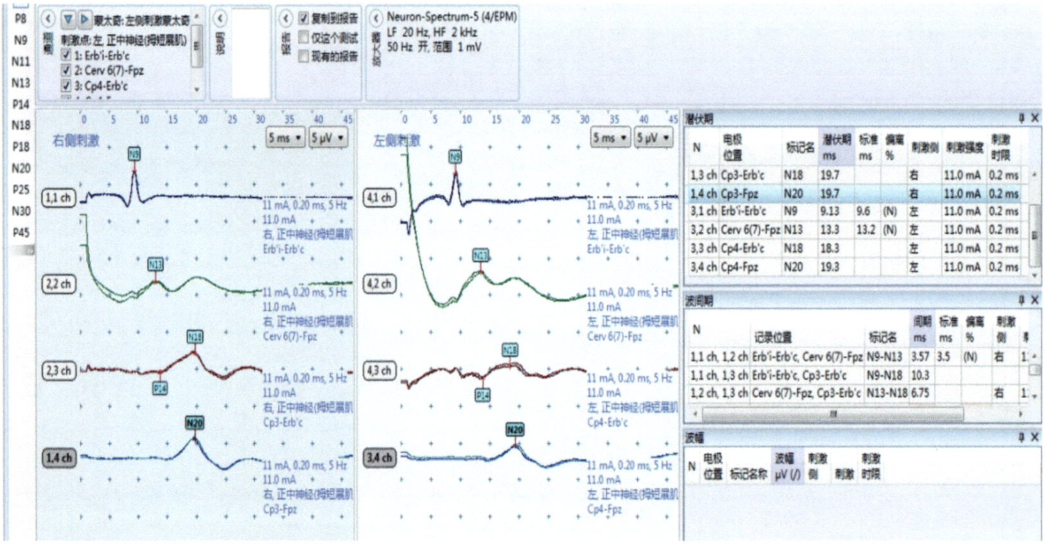


**Fig. 6.9** EPs show that the amplitude of bilateral N20 is significantly higher than before, and the incubation period has returned to the normal range

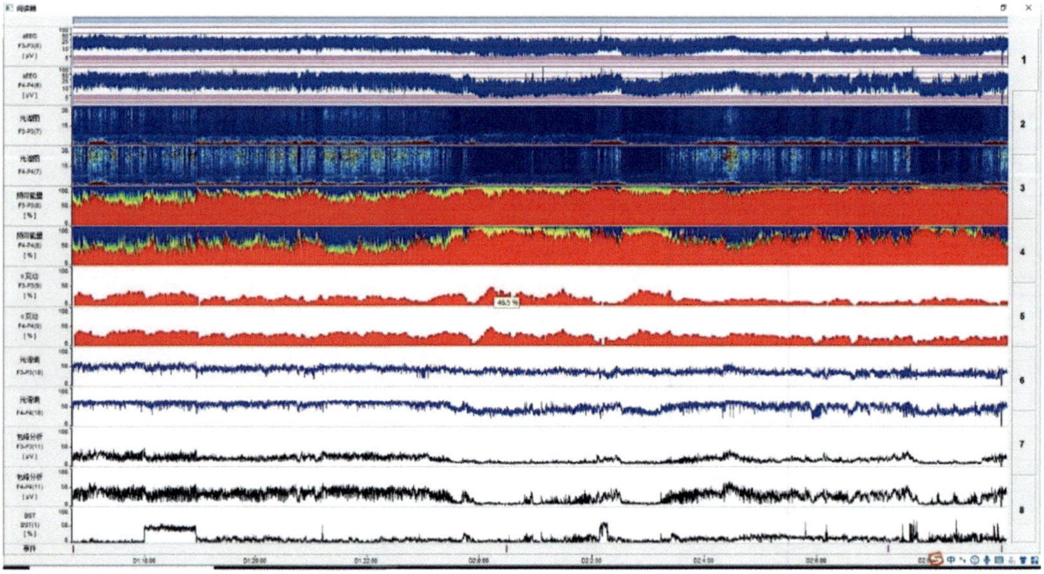

**Fig. 6.10** qEEG: Restored aEEG activity shows an upper boundary >10 μV and a lower boundary >5 μV. The sleep cycle can be seen, suggesting normal aEEG activity. a variation and spectral entropy are in the normal range, suggesting that the brain function had recovered

## References


1. Abdelmalik PA, Draghic N, Ling G. Management of moderate and severe traumatic brain injury. Transfusion. 2019;59(S2):1529–38.
2. Andriessen TM, Horn J, Franschman G, et al. Epidemiology, severity classification, and outcome of moderate and severe traumatic brain injury: a prospective multicenter study. J Neurotrauma. 2011;28(10):2019–31.
3. Gutling E, Gonser A, Imhof HG, et al. EEG reactivity in the prognosis of severe head injury. Neurology. 1995;45(5):915–8.
4. Synek VM. EEG abnormality grades and subdivisions of prognostic importance in traumatic and

anoxic coma in adults. Clin Electroencephalogr. 1988;19(3):160–6.
5. Young GB, McLachlan RS, Kreeft JH, et al. An electroencephalographic classification for coma. Can J Neurol Sci. 1997;24(4):320–5.
6. Cologan V, Drouot X, Parapatics S, et al. Sleep in the unresponsive wakefulness syndrome and minimally conscious state. J Neurotrauma. 2013;30(5):339–46.
7. Sandsmark DK, Kumar MA, Woodward CS, et al. Sleep features on continuous electroencephalography predict rehabilitation outcomes after severe traumatic brain injury. J Head Trauma Rehabil. 2016;31(2):101–7.
8. Alekseeva EV, Alasheev AM, Belkin AA, et al. Prognostic evaluation of sleep in patients in a vegetative state. Anesteziol Reanimatol. 2010;4:38–42.
9. Arnaldi D, Terzaghi M, Cremascoli R, et al. The prognostic value of sleep patterns in disorders of consciousness in the sub-acute phase. Clin Neurophysiol. 2016;127(2):1445–51.
10. de Biase S, Gigli GL, Lorenzut S, et al. The importance of polysomnography in the evaluation of prolonged disorders of consciousness: sleep recordings more adequately correlate than stimulus-related evoked potentials with patients' clinical status. Sleep Med. 2014;15(4):393–400.
11. Rothstein TL. The utility of median somatosensory evoked potentials in anoxic-ischemic coma. Rev Neurosci. 2009;20(3–4):221–33.
12. Lee YC, Phan TG, Jolley DJ, et al. Accuracy of clinical signs, SEP, and EEG in predicting outcome of hypoxic coma: a meta-analysis. Neurology. 2010;74(7):572–80.
13. Zandbergen EG, Hijdra A, Koelman JH, et al. Prediction of poor outcome within the first 3 days of postanoxic coma. Neurology. 2006;66(1):62–8.
14. Del RR, Ochoa C, Alarcon A, et al. Amplitude integrated electroencephalogram as a prognostic tool in neonates with hypoxic-ischemic encephalopathy: a systematic review. PLoS One. 2016;11(11):e165744.
15. El-Dib M, Inder TE, Chalak LF, et al. Should therapeutic hypothermia be offered to babies with mild neonatal encephalopathy in the first 6 h after birth? Pediatr Res. 2019;85(4):442–8.
16. Zhang D, Ding H, Hou X, et al. Cerebral hypoxic ischemia at different cerebral oxygen saturations in piglets: amplitude-integrated EEG study. Conf Proc IEEE Eng Med Biol Soc. 2008;2008:4712–5.
17. Dong X, Shao H, Yang Y, et al. Early evaluation of patients with amplitude-integrated electroencephalogram on brain function prognosis after cardiopulmonary cerebral resuscitation. Zhonghua Wei Zhong Bing Ji Jiu Yi Xue. 2017;29(10):887–92.
18. Feng G, Jiang G, Li Z, et al. Prognostic value of electroencephalography (EEG) for brain injury after cardiopulmonary resuscitation. Neurol Sci. 2016;37(6):843–9.
19. Spitzmiller RE, Phillips T, Meinzen-Derr J, et al. Amplitude-integrated EEG is useful in predicting neurodevelopmental outcome in full-term infants with hypoxic-ischemic encephalopathy: a meta-analysis. J Child Neurol. 2007;22(9):1069–78.
20. Koster RW, Sayre MR, Botha M, et al. Part 5: Adult basic life support: 2010 International consensus on cardiopulmonary resuscitation and emergency cardiovascular care science with treatment recommendations. Resuscitation. 2010(81 Suppl 1):e48–70.
21. Nagao K, Hayashi N, Kanmatsuse K, et al. Cardiopulmonary cerebral resuscitation using emergency cardiopulmonary bypass, coronary reperfusion therapy and mild hypothermia in patients with cardiac arrest outside the hospital. J Am Coll Cardiol. 2000;36(3):776–83.
22. Xu Y. The latest developments of monitoring techniques. Zhongguo Yi Liao Qi Xie Za Zhi. 2006;30(6):441–3.
23. Estruch-Perez MJ, Ausina-Aguilar A, Barbera-Alacreu M, et al. Bispectral index changes in carotid surgery. Ann Vasc Surg. 2010;24(3):393–9.
24. Quraishi SA, Blosser SA, Cherry RA. Bispectral index monitoring in the management of sedation in an intensive care unit patient with locked-in syndrome. Am J Crit Care. 2011;20(6):487–90.
25. Cho JH, Cheong SH, Kim HS, et al. Bispectral index monitoring to assess the level of consciousness in patients with brain injury. Korean J Anesthesiol. 2009;57(2):185–9.
26. Dias R, Dave N, Agrawal B, et al. Correlation between bispectral index, end-tidal anaesthetic gas concentration and difference in inspired-end-tidal oxygen concentration as measures of anaesthetic depth in paediatric patients posted for short surgical procedures. Indian J Anaesth. 2019;63(4):277–83.
27. Dou L, Gao HM, Lu L, et al. Bispectral index in predicting the prognosis of patients with coma in intensive care unit. World J Emerg Med. 2014;5(1):53–6.
28. Yang YL, Zhang L, He X, et al. Use of the bispectral index to predict recovery of consciousness in patients with spontaneous intracerebral hemorrhage after surgical hematoma evacuation: a prospective cohort study. Med Sci Monit. 2019;25:3446–53.

# Application of Multimodal EEG in HIE

**7**

Feng Li and Lihong Huang

## Contents



**Abstract**

HIE is one of the serious complications in patients after successful CPR. It has the characteristics of high incidence, high mortality, and high disability rate. With the improvement of CPR emergency strategies and the continuous development of early advanced life support technology, the successful resuscitation rate in HIE patients has greatly increased, and the survival time in patients has also been prolonged. Some patients gradually wake up through active treatment with only very minor sequelae. However, most patients with severe injuries still develop permanent neurological deficits, exhibiting obvious disturbances in consciousness and other abnormalities of the nervous system, which is an important cause of disability and death in HIE patients and represents an enormous challenge for clinicians. Therefore, an objective and comprehensive assessment of the severity and prognosis of patients with brain

F. Li (✉) · L. Huang
Department of Neurology, The First Affiliated Hospital of Chongqing Medical University, Chongqing, China


X. Wang et al. (eds.), *Multi-Modal EEG Monitoring of Severely Neurologically Ill Patients*,
https://doi.org/10.1007/978-981-16-4493-1_7

injury at an early stage will help clinicians and their families jointly choose a reasonable medical plan that is conducive to the harmony of the family and society and is conducive to the rational use of medical resources. This chapter briefly describes the clinical features, pathogenesis, and prognosis of HIE and proposes the importance of early and accurate judgment of the neurological prognosis of HIE patients and its diagnosis and treatment. Multimodal EEG is a brain function monitoring method developed in recent years for critically ill patients that is helpful for the early detection of HIE and its severity. This chapter further describes common brain function evaluation methods, focusing on multimodal EEG and its important role in the diagnosis, treatment and prognosis of HIE, providing references for early, systematic, objective, and accurate evaluation of brain function and clinical diagnosis and treatment of HIE patients.

**Keywords**

HIE · EEG · EEG-R · Sleep spindle · aEEG · RAV · BIS

## 7.1 Clinical Features of HIE

Although there are many causes, the main cause of HIE is the remaining brain damage after spontaneous circulation is restored after CPR. The clinical manifestations are varying degrees of a disturbance of consciousness, which may be accompanied by respiratory and circulatory system failure and focal or diffuse brain injury. HIE is an important cause of disability and death in patients.

## 7.2 The Pathogenesis of HIE

The brain damage caused by hypoxia or ischemia, especially the pathophysiological changes of the brain after CPR, can be divided into three stages: (**a**) Primary cell injury stage. After spontaneous circulation is restored, brain oxygenation and perfusion are restored, and the early brain cell edema caused by hypoxia is temporarily reduced [1–3]. As a result, neurons that are damaged by ischemia and hypoxia but are still alive recover their function. However, these cells cannot all survive after the blood supply is restored because secondary energy failure will occur hours or even days after the onset of the disease, and neuronal death will still occur at that time (secondary cell death); (**b**) energy recovery stage during resuscitation; (**c**) delayed cell damage stage.

## 7.3 The Prognosis of HIE

The prognosis of HIE is related to the time of cerebral ischemic injury. The brain tissue has poor tolerance to hypoxia. If the heart stops beating for 5–10 s, there will be disturbances in consciousness; for more than 15 s, fainting and convulsions may occur; and for more than 20 s, coma will occur. If the heart stops for more than 5 min, it will cause severe and irreversible brain injury or death. Even if CPR is successful, there will be various sequelae. The prognosis of HIE varies greatly in the clinic and can be divided into four categories: (**a**) complete recovery without sequelae; (**b**) recovery with sequelae of varying degrees; (**c**) VS or MCS; (**d**) death [4, 5].

Correctly judging the prognosis of patients with HIE is a major challenge for clinicians. If the patient's prognosis can be objectively and comprehensively assessed to predict the patient's risk of death, it will help clinicians and their families jointly choose a medical treatment scheme, which is conducive to the harmony of the family and society and the rational use of medical resources. Therefore, early and accurate judgment of the neurological prognosis of patients undergoing CPCR is of great significance to both diagnosis and treatment.

## 7.4 Common Brain Function Assessment Methods in HIE

In the past 20 years, many researchers have studied methods for reliably evaluating brain damage and predicting neurological function in patients after CPR. At present, the methods used to assess the severity of brain injury and predict the prognosis of neurological function after resuscitation mainly include assessing the symptoms and signs of neurological injury, neuroelectrophysiological monitoring, prognostic biomarker monitoring, biochemical indicator monitoring, and neuroimaging. Scale examinations based on clinical behavioral assessments (such as the GCS) are simple and easy to perform, and they can quickly determine the degree of coma. However, because the evaluator is affected by the experience and training, the evaluation is subjective. There may be differences in the judgments of different evaluators. Scale examinations based on behavioral assessments have the shortcoming of being easily affected by hypothermia treatment and sedative drugs. Biomarkers are usually recommended as predictors of prognosis after cardiac arrest. In recent years, there have been an increasing number of studies on the role of physiological index variation in brain injury assessment. Blood biomarkers and biochemical monitoring of physiological indices can easily be used as routine laboratory tests and are not affected by sedative drugs. However, the experimental results are affected by many factors and require successive dynamic monitoring. Neuroimaging examination, especially MRI, has the advantage of high spatial resolution. Neuroimaging can provide a deeper understanding of the degree and mechanism of ischemic brain injury and can be better used to predict neurological outcomes. However, the specificity of neuroimaging is poor, and the sensitivity is not sufficient. The best time to use MRI to predict neurological function is 2–5 days after cardiac arrest. After that time, other prediction methods are needed to improve the sensitivity of prediction.

The recording of the activity of brain neurons by EEG is the most direct way to reflect the physiological functions of the brain. EEG offers high time resolution and is noninvasive and reusable. It is one of the most commonly used methods for early continuous bedside monitoring of coma patients after cardiac arrest. It can provide continuous, real-time, noninvasive brain function monitoring results for the clinician; and it has certain advantages in condition judgment, therapeutic monitoring, and short-term prognosis. Existing studies have confirmed that in the middle period after CPR (6–72 h after resuscitation), the characteristics of EEGs can predict neurological prognosis [6–8].

## 7.5 Multidimensional EEG Predicts the Prognosis of Patients with HIE

### 7.5.1 Common EEG Manifestations of HIE After CPR

The EEG after CPR can reflect the brain electrical activity of cerebral cortex synapses. Since the synaptic activity of the cerebral cortex is very sensitive to the effects of hypoxia-induced brain injury, EEG is a sensitive method for detecting hypoxic brain injury. In the process of cerebral ischemia, if the CBF decreases from the normal flow of 50 ml/100 g/min to 25–35 ml/100 g/min, the electrical activity ($\alpha/\beta$ waves) in an EEG will be affected. If ischemia reaches the critical ischemic threshold of 17–18 ml/100 g/min, the slow frequency ($\theta$ and $\delta$) produced by the thalamus and the cortical cells from layer II–VI will gradually increase [9, 10].

At present, the brain electrical activity of patients with HIE after CPR can be roughly divided into widespread large slow waves (the length of the slow-wave period is related to the degree of consciousness), $\alpha$ coma, $\beta$ coma, spindle coma, TWs, BS, epilepsy (SE) and GPD, low voltage, ECS, etc. Among them, ECS, low volt-

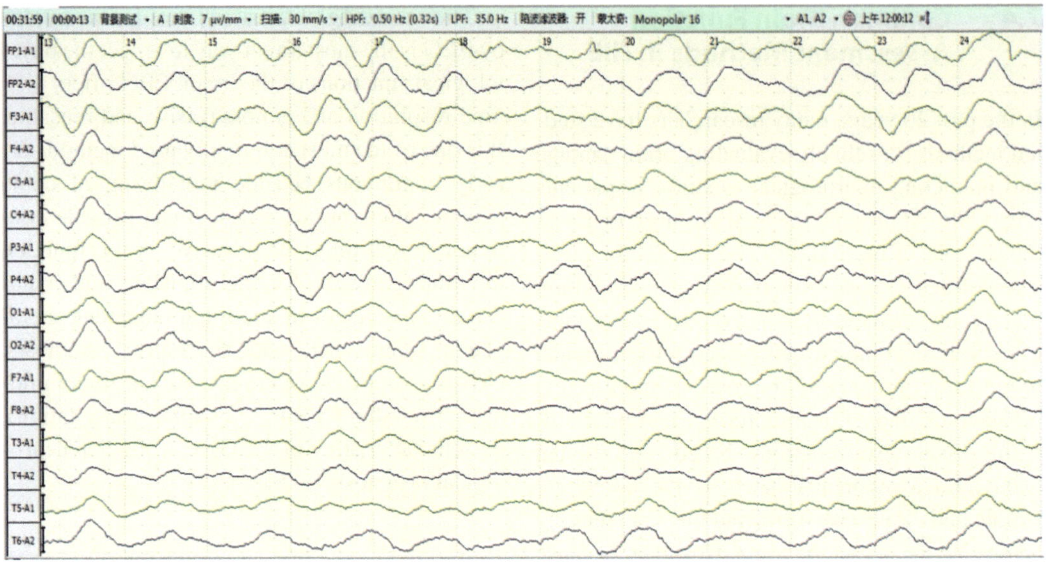


**Fig. 7.1** EEG from a 47-year-old male who suffered from cardiac arrest after myocardial infarction shows continuous δ activity after CPR

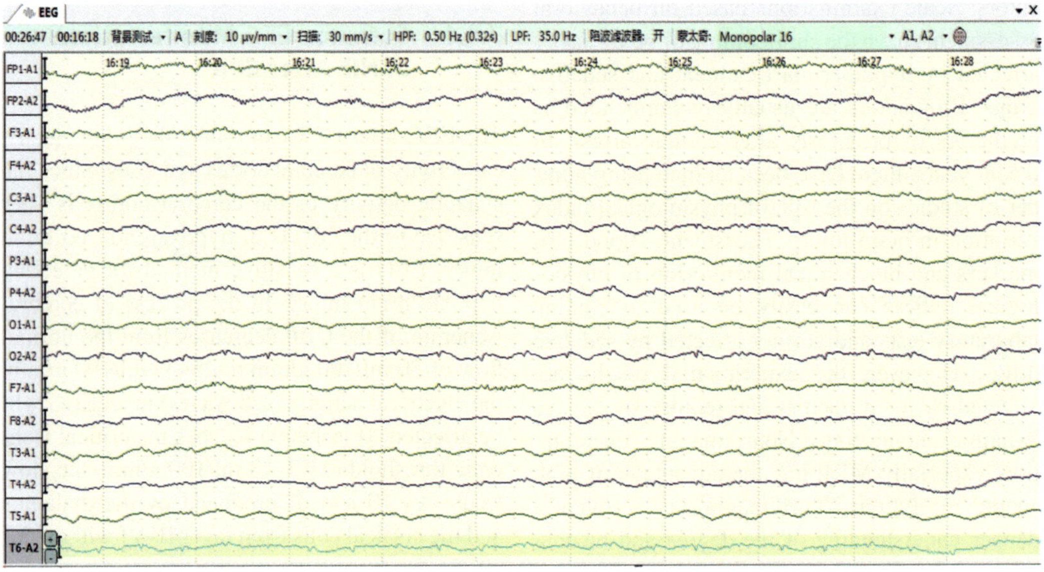


**Fig. 7.2** EEG at 24 h after CPR from an 86-year-old female patient with myocardial infarction shows unresponsive low voltage and slow activity

age, and BS patterns are usually considered to be a manifestation of a poor prognosis [9] (Figs. 7.1, 7.2, 7.3, 7.4, 7.5, 7.6, and 7.7). A recently published meta-analysis reviewed the relationship between poor EEG patterns and poor prognosis in 84 patients after CPR and found that BS and SE were predictors of adverse outcomes after rewarming [11]. It has also been suggested that the presence of a BS pattern in cardiac arrest patients within 48 h after rewarming has a specificity of 100% in predicting death or severe neurological dysfunction [9].

However, since unfavorable EEG patterns reflect ischemia of the brain tissue rather than

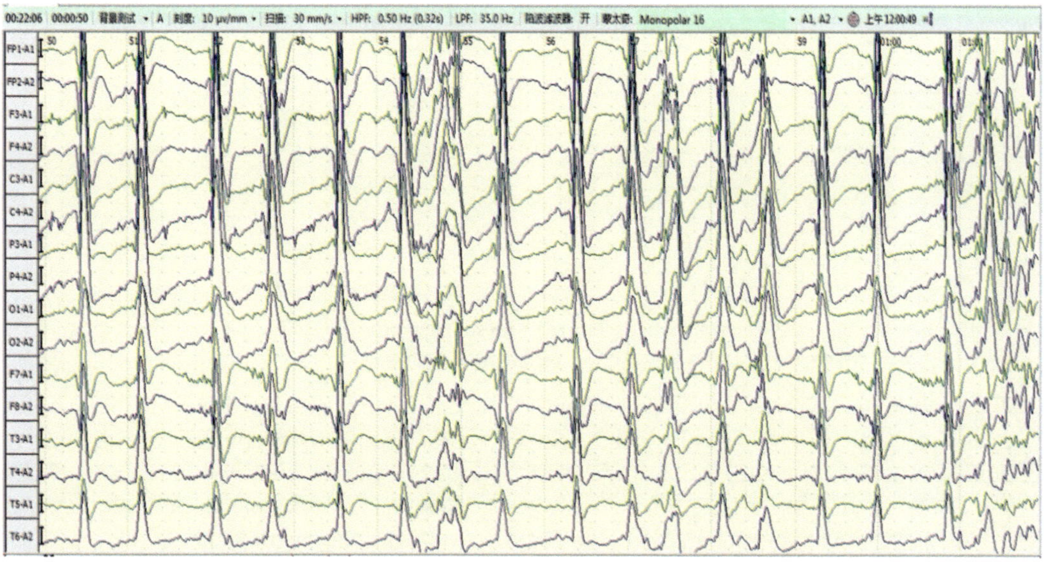

**Fig. 7.3** EEG from a 66-year-old man with HIE and NCSE in a moderate coma shows GPDs

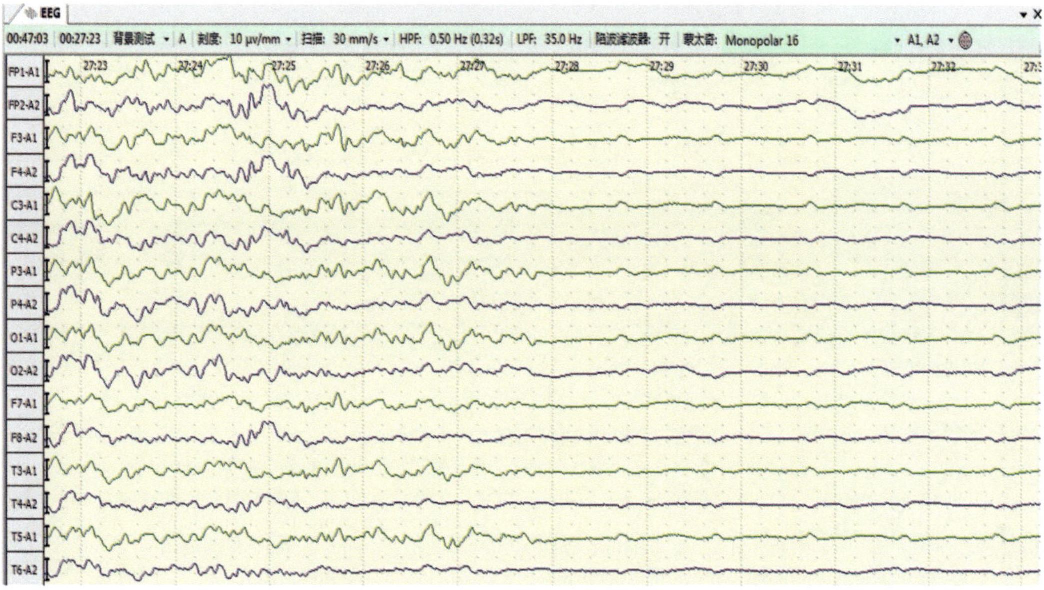

**Fig. 7.4** EEG at 48 h after CPR from an 86-year-old woman with heart failure and ventricular fibrillation shows BS

permanent brain damage, it is not enough to use a fixed pattern to determine whether the patient will have an adverse outcome (death or severe neurological dysfunction). Especially during hypothermia treatment after resuscitation, the use of sedative drugs will affect the EEG pattern [12]. Therefore, it is necessary to use multiple methods to reflect the function of the brain from different aspects. This is the greatest advantage of multimodal EEG in clinical applications.

### 7.5.2 EEG-R

EEG-R refers to the changes in the frequency or amplitude of the background waves that

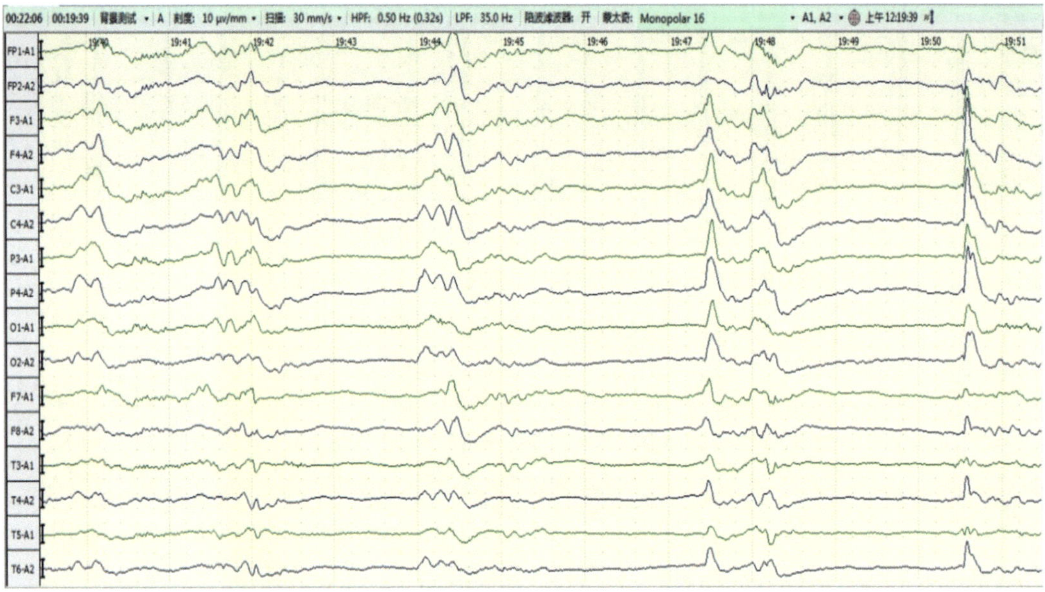

**Fig. 7.5** EEG at 72 h after CPR from a 78-year-old man with a moderate coma due to cardiac arrest shows BS

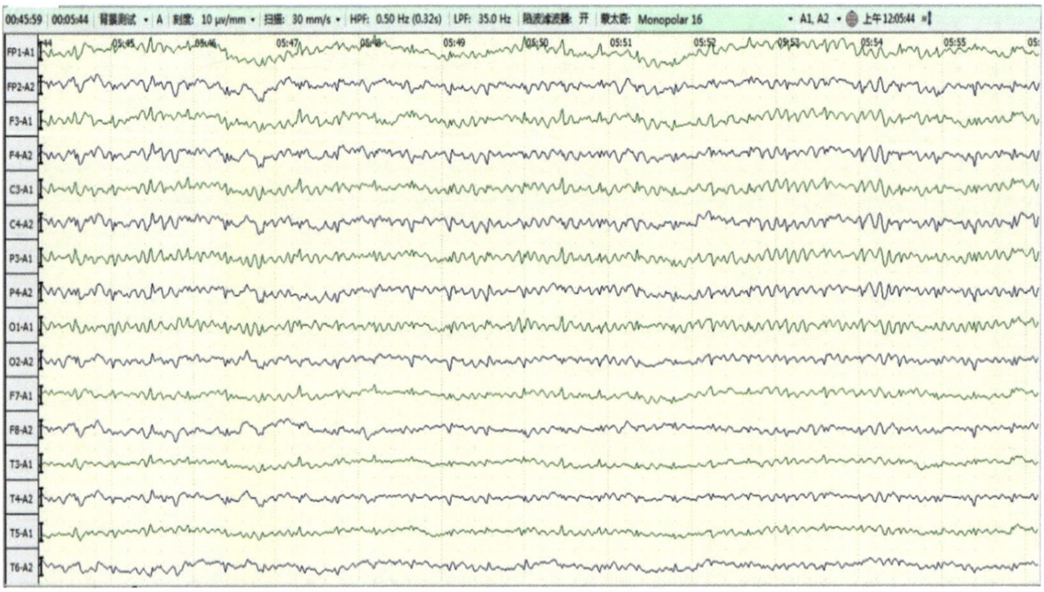

**Fig. 7.6** EEG from a 37-year-old man in a moderate coma after CPR shows α coma

occur after the human body receives external stimuli (such as sound, light, or pain), and it has a strict time-dependent relationship with the stimulus (Figs. 7.8 and 7.9). The anatomical basis of EEG-R depends on the completeness of all structures and functions from the brainstem network to the base of the thalamus, hypothalamus, and thalamus cortex, reflecting the integrity of the overall function of the cerebral cortical network. EEG-R is a good indicator for predicting the recovery of consciousness in patients with a disorder of consciousness following acute brain injury. Claassen J et al. [13] compared the predictive effects of EEG-R

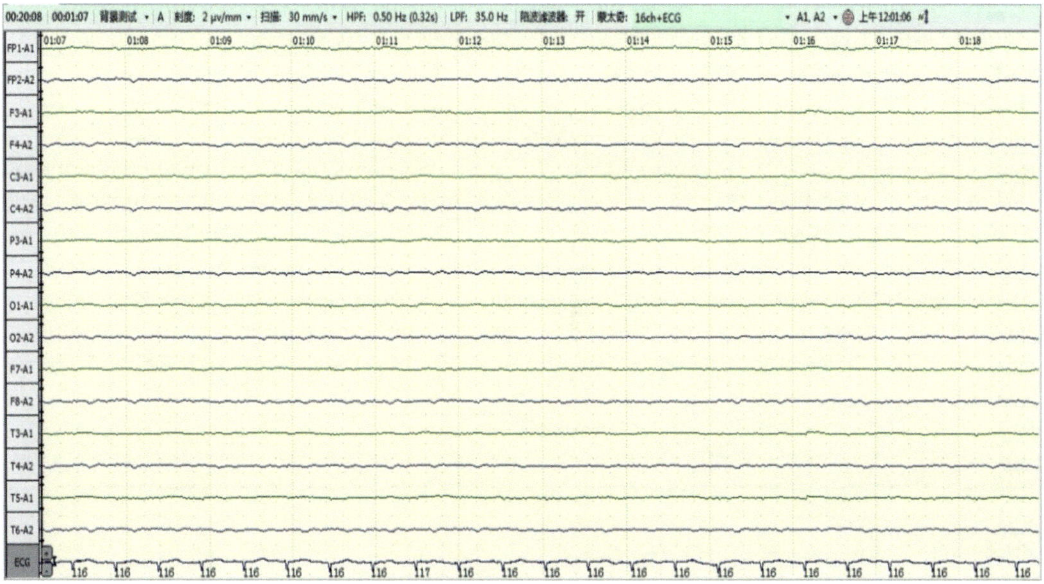


**Fig. 7.7** EEG after CPR of a 13-year-old woman in a deep coma from a lightning strike shows ECS (brain death) (sensitivity: 2 μV)

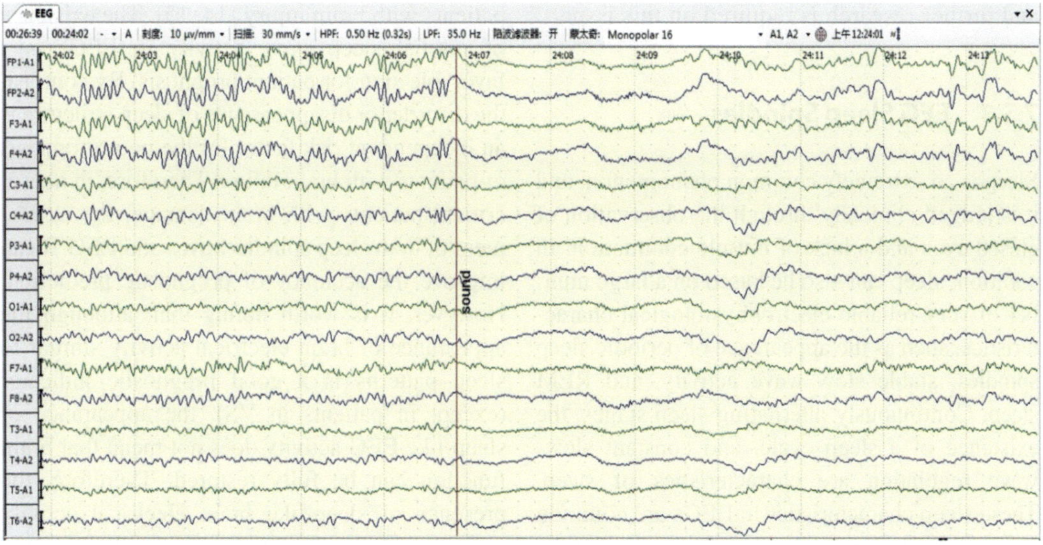


**Fig. 7.8** EEG at 48 h after CPR from a 46-year-old male patient with myocardial infarction shows reactivity

and central conduction time of SEPs on the prognosis of patients with severe brain injury and coma. After 1.5 years of follow-up, it was found that the accuracy rate of EEG-R to distinguish between good prognosis and poor prognosis was 92%, while the accuracy rate of central conduction time of S EPs was only 82%, but the accuracy rate reached 98% after combination. Therefore, EEG-R is a good indicator of long-term prognosis. Measurements of EEG-R are simple to perform and easy to interpret, and they can be effectively used in clinical practice. However, the observation of EEG-R is mostly based on visual inspection; therefore, it is not a quantitative evaluation. The use of sedative and analgesic drugs will

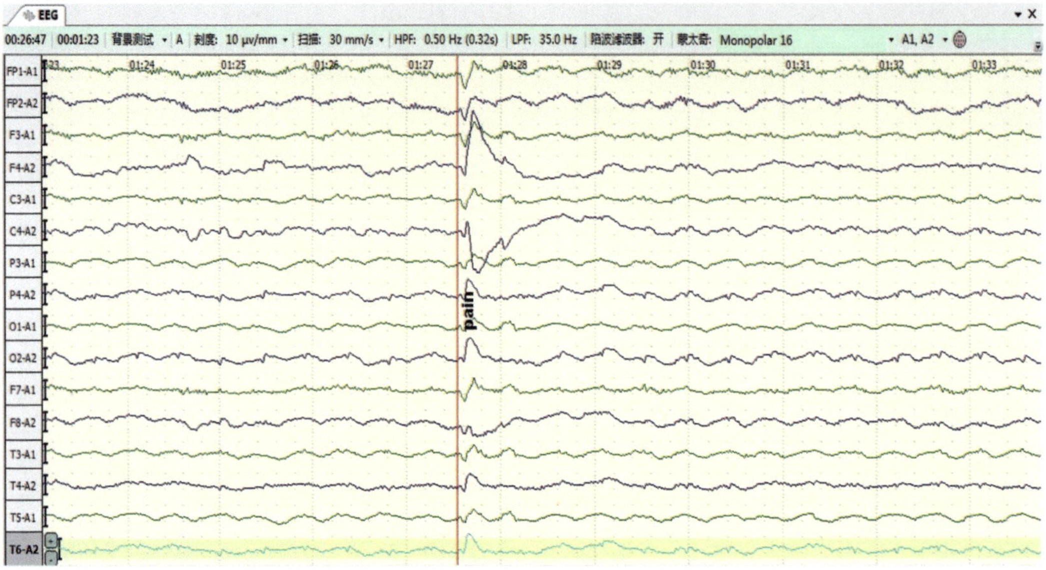


**Fig. 7.9** EEG at 32 h after CPR from a 65-year-old female shows non-reactivity

affect the accuracy of EEG-R observations, and further research is required on this issue.

### 7.5.3 EEG Sleep Spindles

Sleep is an extremely common phenomenon, and it is judged clinically through the observation of closed eyes and a lack of muscle contraction. In addition, sleep can also be based on a large number of very reliable electrophysiological characteristics, such as the appearance of periodic sleep spindles, stable slow wave activity, and REM sleep. Continuously alternating sleep stages, the existence of a sleep cycle, and constant slow-wave regulation are characteristics of sleep. These sleep characteristics in EEGs are common in healthy volunteers. The integrity of brain function can be reflected by the presence or absence of standard sleep cycle elements. In patients with severe brain injury, there is a connection between the patient's EEG sleep changes and their level of consciousness. Therefore, monitoring the electrophysiological changes during sleep and the constant slow-wave activity in EEGs can be used as an auxiliary method to evaluate the brain function of patients in VS and MCS. Studies have shown that the presence of sleep spindles can be used as the main criterion for the sleep cycle and plays an important role in the prognosis of patients with brain injury [14, 15]. The existence of normal sleep cycle activity in EEGs is a favorable sign for patient prognosis. By contrast, the disorder or disappearance of sleep structure is an independent risk factor for the poor prognosis of patients with brain injury. Therefore, in neurocritical patients with brain damage, the assessment of both sleep spindle waves and EEG-R can improve the accuracy of prognostic prediction. However, it is worth noting that, although the appearance of brain electrical activity similar to sleep patterns is a good prognostic indicator (except in patients in VS), the appearance of sleep-like EEG activity does not mean that brain function can be fully restored. Therefore, the presence of sleep-like brain electrical activity lacks specificity for prognostic prediction, and sleep-like EEG activity evaluation still needs to be combined with multiple evaluation methods.

## 7.6 The Role of Multimode EEG in the Diagnosis, Treatment, and Prognosis of HIE

The process of secondary brain injury after CPR is complex and involves multiple injury assaults, namely, secondary cerebral ischemia reperfusion injury. EEG has long been regarded as the most sensitive instrument for reflecting dynamic changes in brain function. In addition to sensitive detection of epileptic discharges, EEG can also reflect changes in the patient's depth of consciousness and cerebral ischemia and monitor the treatment effects of sedatives, vasodilators, AEDs, etc. However, due to the large amount of data generated, the traditional methods of analyzing EEGs with the naked eye are too inefficient, and various instruments and equipment in the ICU will produce strange artifacts, which will lead to difficulties in result analysis. At present, existing technologies that monitor a variety of parameters, such as CBF, cerebral oxygen saturation, and brain cell metabolism, can reflect the path of brain cell injury to a certain extent. However, no single monitoring technology can make a comprehensive and definite prediction of the prognosis of brain function. It is believed that the combination of multiple monitoring technologies will be a way to improve the efficiency of prediction [16]. Multimode monitoring is an evolving field that has been applied to some injury processes, such as head injury processes. Simultaneously, multiple brain function parameters are recorded, the pathophysiological process is monitored, and comprehensive data for targeted treatment and prognosis are provided [17]. At present, most brain function monitors are independent systems, and it is still a challenge to design an ergonomic and easy-to-interpret output format for comprehensive display. Although there are limited data on the application of multimode monitoring after CPR, it is obviously beneficial for the medical diagnosis and treatment of patients following cardiac arrest. Multimode monitoring may be a future development trend in brain monitoring after cardiac arrest. Although more research is needed, studies so far have shown that current clinical EEG monitoring technologies are helpful for medical staff to treat patients after CPR [18]. The rational use of these technologies may help doctors provide personalized brain regeneration strategies, prevent brain damage, and improve the quality of life and neurological function of patients who have experienced cardiac arrest.

Currently, commonly used qEEG techniques include aEEG and techniques monitoring the BIS, spectral entropy, RBP, RAV, etc. These technologies are increasingly widely used in the observation and evaluation of neurologically critically ill patients and directly reflect the pathophysiological characteristics of different brain functional activities. A proper understanding of these key technologies and early assessment of the brain function of patients with brain injury are of great significance for guiding early clinical intervention to improve prognosis.

### 7.6.1 Application of aEEG in HIE

aEEG is a method of continuously monitoring brain neuron activity, and it is increasingly used in neonatal ICUs. After being processed with amplitude correction and semilogarithmic compression technology, an aEEG is slowly displayed on the recording paper at a paper speed of 6 cm/h. What an aEEG shows is not the original EEG signal but the trend graph of brain electrical activity after integration; therefore, this technique is called aEEG. aEEG overcomes the limitations of expertise and technology regarding the traditional analysis of EEG results and is convenient for clinicians to make real-time judgments on the brain function of patients based on dynamic EEG results. aEEG can monitor brain activity in real time. In the 1980s, this technology was used to monitor the brain activity of newborns (mainly asphyxiated babies) [19]. However, its application in adults with HIE is still in its infancy. The technology has developed over time, but it is consistent with the basic principles of traditional EEG. Studies have shown that there is good agreement between aEEGs and conventional EEGs [20]. All these results show that the use of aEEG for long-term brain function monitoring is feasible, and the results are true and reliable.

aEEG is similar to conventional EEG in that it is also classified according to EEG waveforms. There are currently two classification methods that are widely recognized and used in clinical practice. The first method classifies waveforms into three levels according to the waveform amplitude: level I is a normal waveform (upper limit of aEEG >10 μV, lower limit >5 μV); level II is a mildly abnormal waveform (upper limit of aEEG >10 μV, lower limit ≤5 μV, or upper limit ≤10 μV, and lower limit >5 μV); and level III is a severely abnormal waveform (upper limit of aEEG <10 μV, lower limit <5 μV) [21]. The second method was proposed by Hellström-Westas et al. [22], and it classifies background electrical activity as follows: (**a**) continuous background mode with sleep-wake cycle: upper limit is 10–50 μV, lower limit is 5–10 μV, and the bandwidth is normal; (**b**) discontinuous background mode: upper limit is >10 μV, lower limit is <5 μV, and the bandwidth is wider; (**c**) BS mode: upper limit is >25 μV, lower limit is ≤10 μV, and the bandwidth is comb-shaped; (**d**) CLV: upper limit is ≤5 μV, and the bandwidth becomes narrower; (**e**) isoelectric line or parallel bands: the upper limit is <5 μV, even<2 μV, and the bandwidth is very narrow. The current research shows that the classifications of the first method more closely resemble the waveforms that are observed clinically, and they are more scientific and practical, so this method is commonly used in clinical classification [23].

A study has shown that there is a clear relationship between the severity of neonatal-HIE and the classification of aEEGs [24] (Table 7.1 and Figs. 7.10 and 7.11). In a systematic review, Spitzmiller et al. [25] investigated several studies of HIE in infants and young children and reported that the overall sensitivity of aEEGs to predict adverse outcomes was 91%, and the specificity was 88%. In a retrospective study [20] of 25 patients with HIE after CPR, according to previous research, the aEEG score was quantified and graded as follows: 5 points for normal EEG, 4 points for mild-to-moderate abnormalities, 3 points for severe abnormalities, 1 point for ECI, and 2 points for others (including SE, α coma, β coma, and other aEEG patterns that could not be classified by the above). The results showed that the aEEG score had a significant correlation with the prognosis evaluation of patients' brain function. In particular, the aEEG scores at 72 h and 1 week were most closely related to the prognosis of brain function. Patients with aEEG scores ≥3 points or a change of more than 2 points within 1 week had a better prognosis. After 13 months of follow-up observation, a small number of patients recovered their ability to take care of themselves. Burnsed et al. [26] pointed out that the aEEG classification changes with the severity of HIE. The changes in brain cell electrical activity and metabolism caused by hypoxia-ischemia are the key to different aEEG classifications in different results. Among the 31 post-CPR patients in the previous retrospective study, 7 patients with normal aEEGs were alive, 6 patients had good prognosis of brain function, and 1 patient had a poor prognosis. There were 13 patients with mild aEEG abnormalities, of whom 10 were alive and 3 died. Among the surviving patients, 2 showed good brain function, and 8 had a poor prognosis. There were 11 patients with severe aEEG abnormalities, of whom 9 died, and the 2 surviving patients had a poor prognosis of brain function. Studies have found that the ability of aEEGs to predict the prognosis of brain function in CPCR patients is better than that of the GCS score [21]. Through logistic regression analysis of the efficiency of aEEGs and GCS scores in predicting

**Table 7.1** The relationship between aEEG and prognosis

| Background electrical activity (Hellström-Westas and Rosén) | Voltage definition (Al Naqeeb) | Lower limit (in μV) | Upper limit (in μV) | Cerebral function injury |
|---|---|---|---|---|
| Continuous | Normal (Type 1) | 5–10 | 10–50 | Reversible and good prognosis |
| Discontinuous | Mildly abnormal (Type 2) | <5 | >10 | Reversible and good prognosis |
| BS | Severely abnormal (Type 3) | ≤10 | >25 (Voltage during burst) | Seen in severe brain damage<br>Irreversible and poor prognosis |
| CLV | Severely abnormal (Type 3) | | ≤5 | |
| ECS | Severely abnormal (Type 3) | | ≤2 | |

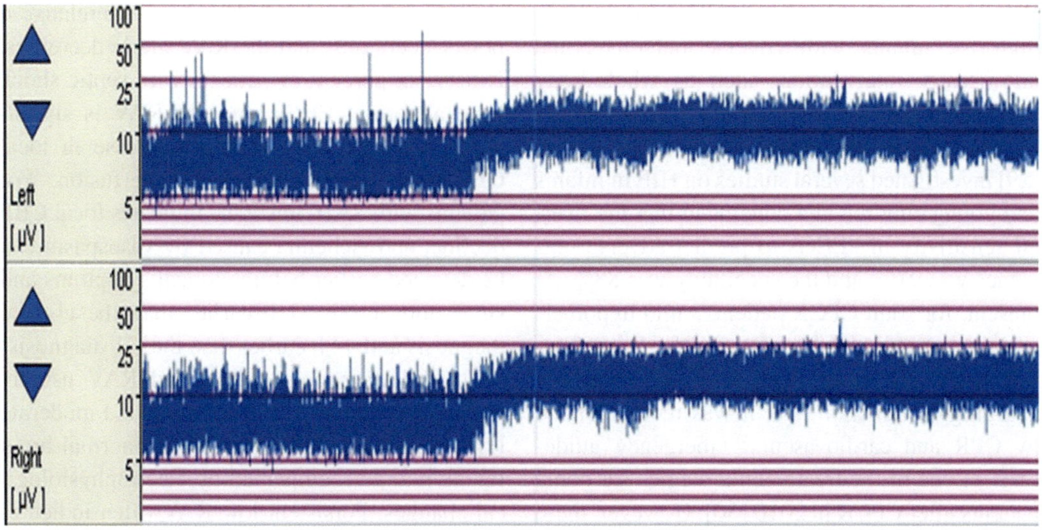

**Fig. 7.10** In the presence of a sleep-wake cycle, the aEEG shows that the upper and lower limits were lowered during the awake period, the upper and lower limits were raised during the sleep period, and the bandwidth was similar

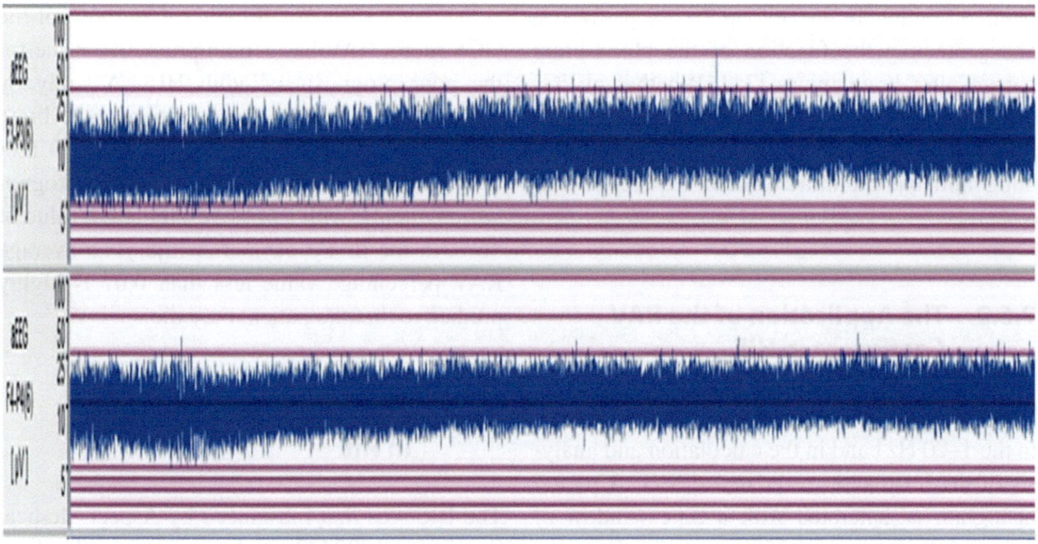

**Fig. 7.11** In the absence of a sleep-wake cycle, the aEEG shows no periodic changes in the upper and lower limits, which is seen in patients with severe brain function impairment

the prognosis of brain function, it was found that aEEGs had an independent effect on the early prognosis of brain function. ROC curve analysis of the ability of the two to evaluate the prognosis of brain function found that the AUC of aEEGs in evaluating the prognosis of brain function in CPCR patients was 0.913. When the optimal cut-off point was 1.5, aEEGs had high sensitivity (95.7%) and specificity (75.0%). The AUC of the GCS score in evaluating the prognosis of brain function in CPCR patients was 0.851. When the optimal cutoff point was 1.5, the GCS score had a high sensitivity (91.3%), but the specificity was not high (62.5%). aEEGs were better than GCS scores in predicting the prognosis of brain function in CPCR patients [27]. For adult CPCR patients, it is currently believed that mild hypothermia therapy is the only effective option that may improve the patient's neurological function. Past studies on the sus of aEEGs in infants with

HIE have concluded that aEEGs can identify high-risk infants with adverse outcomes and allow early intervention, such as whole-body hypothermia or selective cerebral hypothermia [28]. In a systematic review, ter Horst H J et al. [29] investigated several studies on HIE in infants and young children and concluded that the overall sensitivity of aEEGs to predict adverse outcomes was 91%, and the specificity was 88%. At present, for adult CPCR patients, mild hypothermia treatment is considered to be the only effective plan that may improve the patient's neurological function, and it was recommended by CPR and cardiovascular emergency guidelines as one of the treatment strategies for coma patients after CPCR in 2010 [30]. However, there are still objections to its therapeutic effect. Studies have shown that mild hypothermia treatment can improve the neurological function of CPCR patients by reducing brain cell metabolism, inhibiting brain cell apoptosis pathways, and protecting the function of the blood-brain barrier after brain injury [31]. Whether aEEGs can be used to judge the efficacy of mild hypothermia treatment and one of the criteria for initiating mild hypothermia treatment requires further research.

### 7.6.2 The Application of the RAV Coefficient in HIE

RAV refers to the proportion of 6–14 Hz activity in the 1–20 Hz band in the calculation and analysis of the relative α power in a qEEG. A period histogram is generated with a time window of 2 min. A fluctuation of 15% per hour above the median value is recorded as excellent (4 points), a fluctuation of at least 10% every 4 h is recorded as good (3 points), 4 h less than 10% is recorded as fair (2 points), and fluctuations not exceeding 2% are recorded as poor (1 point).

As CBF decreases, the fast waves in the EEG gradually diminish, and the slow waves gradually increase. When CBF continues to decrease to 10–12 ml per 100 g of brain tissue per minute, EEG activity will become low, and brain cell damage will become irreversible. Therefore, when cerebral ischemia worsens, an EEG will show that the fast wave decreases, the relative α power decreases, and the RAV grade decreases. Ninety-six percent of patients with septic shock have abnormal EEGs, and the RAV is significantly reduced, suggesting a decrease in local CBF and insufficient cerebral perfusion. For patients with SAH, low RAV indicates focal CBF decline, and ischemia caused by vasospasm can be detected earlier before clinical symptoms and signs appear (i.e., 7 h earlier than the clinical diagnosis and 44 h earlier than the CT diagnosis) [32]. In HIE patients, decreased RAV usually indicates a decrease in blood flow to a moderate level, which is considered to be abnormal brain function and accompanied by electrophysiological changes. Persistent low RAV often indicates poor neurological prognosis in patients with brain injury. In the prediction of poor prognosis of adult HIE by RAV, the sensitivity, positive-predictive value, negative-predictive value, and coincidence rate are all higher than those of the GCS score. RAV has certain predictive value for the poor prognosis of adult HIE. A study by Vespa et al. [33] showed that patients with brain injury with a GCS $\leq 8$ have an RAV of 0.1 or lower, which is highly predictive of poor prognosis in patients, with a positive-predictive value of 86%. In the first 3 days after injury, an average RAV percentage value less than 0.07 is highly predictive that the patient may die.

### 7.6.3 The Application of the BIS in HIE

The BIS was first introduced by Aspect Medical Systems in 1992 [34], and it is a statistical indicator based on a combination of time, the frequency domain, and high-order spectra. The BIS is calculated in two steps: (**a**) the discrete Fourier transform (DFT) coefficients are found; and (**b**) the equation $B(f1, f2) = X(f1) \times X(f2) \times X \times (f1 + f2)$ is used to calculate the BIS, where $B(f1, f2)$ is the complex bispectrum and $X(f)$ is the complex Fourier transform at the frequency $f$ of the EEG signal $X(n)$. Using the dual phase to obtain an EEG signal with two frequencies, $f1$ and $f2$, the bicoherence degree can be calculated separately for each electrode. The EEG measurements applied to the BIS include the BS ratio, $\alpha/\beta$ band power ratio (where $\alpha$ is the 8–13 Hz frequency band and $\beta$ is the 13–30 Hz frequency band), and bicoherence (coupling of phase measurement between two frequencies in a single EEG channel). The BS ratio is a time-domain feature that describes the relative degree of ECS compared with slow waves [35]. The measurement of the BIS usually consists of scalp EEG electrodes (3 are used in the BIS system and 4 are used in the BIS-XP system) attached to the forehead through a self-adhesive tape to obtain a mathematical combination of EEG measurements to obtain a numerical index. The range is from 0 to 100. This index is based on the empirical correlation established between EEG characteristics and patient alertness. It is generally believed that a BIS value of 85–100 is a normal value, where 100 indicates a state of cortical electrical activity during the waking period, 65–85 indicates a state of sedation, 40–65 indicates a state of general anesthesia, a value below 40 indicates sudden inhibition, and a value of 0 indicates no cerebral electrical activity. Initially, the BIS was mainly used for anesthesia monitoring. Because it can energetically, continuously, and dynamically monitor EEG signals, the BIS has the advantages of relatively simple interpretation and noninvasiveness and can be popularized and applied in ICUs.

The change in the BIS has a certain relationship with the change in oxygen consumption of the cerebral cortical cells of the patient, and it can assist in the assessment of the degree of brain damage in patients with ischemia and hypoxia after CPR. The research of Coleman et al. [36] found that the level of consciousness and the BIS are two expressions obtained from different brain regions. BIS monitoring records the electrical activity of the frontal cortex and is calibrated for neurologically intact, anesthetized patients, not for brain injury patients. BIS monitoring provides information about the interaction between the cerebral cortex and the subcortical areas. Consciousness is maintained by the upper brainstem and thalamic neurons, the reticular activating system, and its extensive connections to the cerebral hemispheres. In patients with severe brain injury, the electrical activity of the brain may vary due to brain perfusion, brain metabolism, hypoxia, sedative drugs, and seizures, which lead to changes in the BIS value of patients with constant levels of consciousness and GCS scores. A prospective study by Dunham C M et al. [37] evaluated 18 patients with severe brain injury and concluded that the survival and good prognosis of patients with severe brain injury were related to a BIS≥60, $StcO_2$ (cerebral tissue oxygen saturation) ≥70 and ICP index ≤20 ($P < 0.0001$). A retrospective study included 122 patients with acute brain injury in a coma. The mean BIS of the direct injury group was significantly lower than that of the indirect injury group. The fatality rate and neurological adverse outcome rate of the BIS <60 group were significantly higher than those of the BIS >60 group. For brain damage with different pathogenic factors, the BIS can better judge the prognosis of the disease and the neurological outcome [38]. Another study retrospectively analyzed 208 critically ill patients with coma. The BIS value and the prognostic status of coma were analyzed using Spearman's grade and obtained according to the ROC curve. The BIS value had a good correlation with the prognosis of ICU patients with coma. A BIS >42.5 had high sensitivity and specificity for the prognostic assessment of the awake coma state [39]. Similar studies have shown that the BIS value is closely related to the prognosis of patients with brain injury, but the BIS is affected by many factors and cannot be independently used as a criterion for judging the prognosis of the nervous system. The BIS may be more accurate in predicting the prognosis of patients when combined with the GCS and Acute Physiology and Chronic Health Evaluation II (APACHE-II) score.

**Case**

A 65-year-old woman was admitted to the hospital for "9 days after lumbar posterior surgery, low back pain and fever for 2 days."

Admission diagnosis: (1) postoperative lumbar intervertebral disc protrusion, (2) type 2 diabetes mellitus, and (3) fatty liver. On the fifth day after admission, she experienced sudden cardiac arrest when she went to the toilet. Her spontaneous heartbeat immediately resumed after 15 min of CPR, followed by another cardiac arrest after

1 min, and then three recurrences of cardiac arrest. The cumulative CPR time was 42 min. The patient underwent brain function monitoring 24, 48, and 72 h after CPR. The cerebral electrical activity trend changed from a BS, discontinuous background to a continuous background. The BS trend first increased, then decreased, and then disappeared. Finally, the EEG tended to be stable and showed a fully inhibited state. Reactivity and the sleep waveform disappeared. The patient had a poor prognosis and died 72 h after CPR (Figs. 7.12, 7.13, 7.14, 7.15, 7.16, 7.17, 7.18, and 7.19).

1. 24 h after CPR
2. 48 h after CPR
3. 72 h after CPR

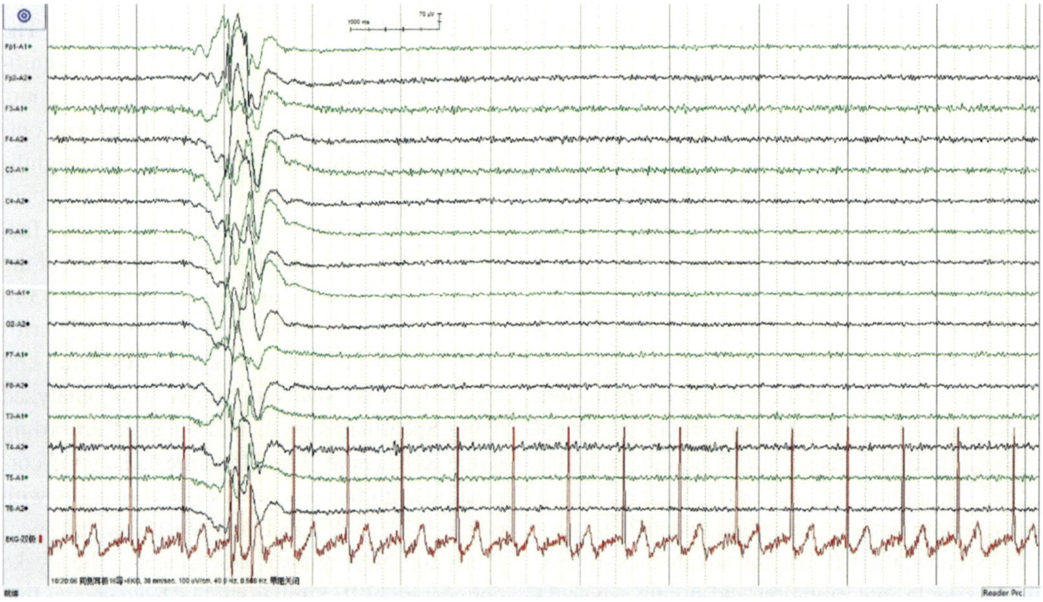

**Fig. 7.12** Early stage of recording: the EEG background is discontinuous, showing BS

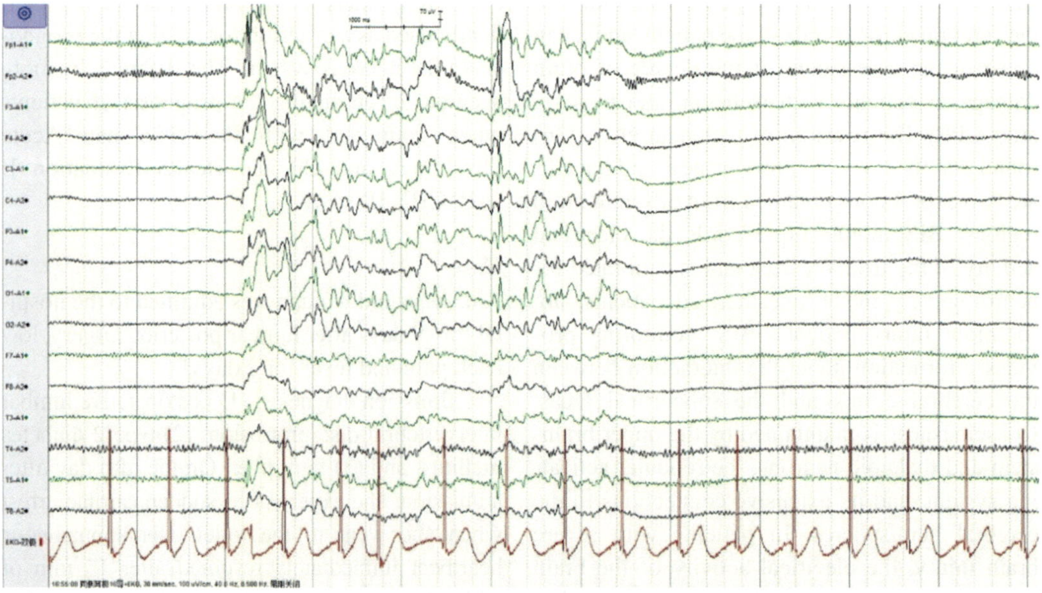

**Fig. 7.13** Late stage of recording: the number of bursts increases, and the duration of bursts is prolonged

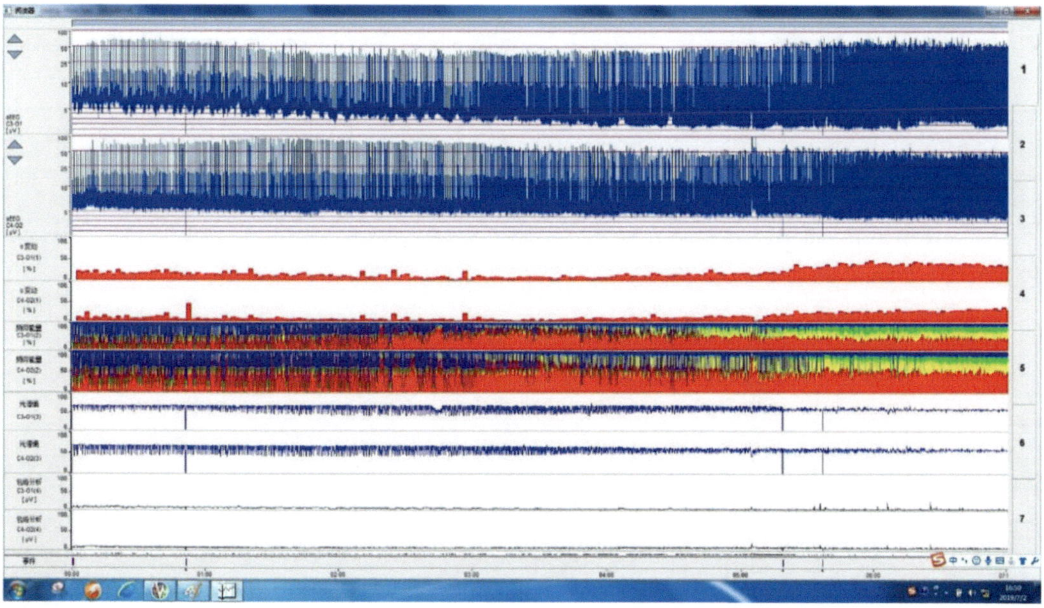

**Fig. 7.14** 24-h full-scale display: the background is discontinuous, showing BS, and the burst trend is increasing

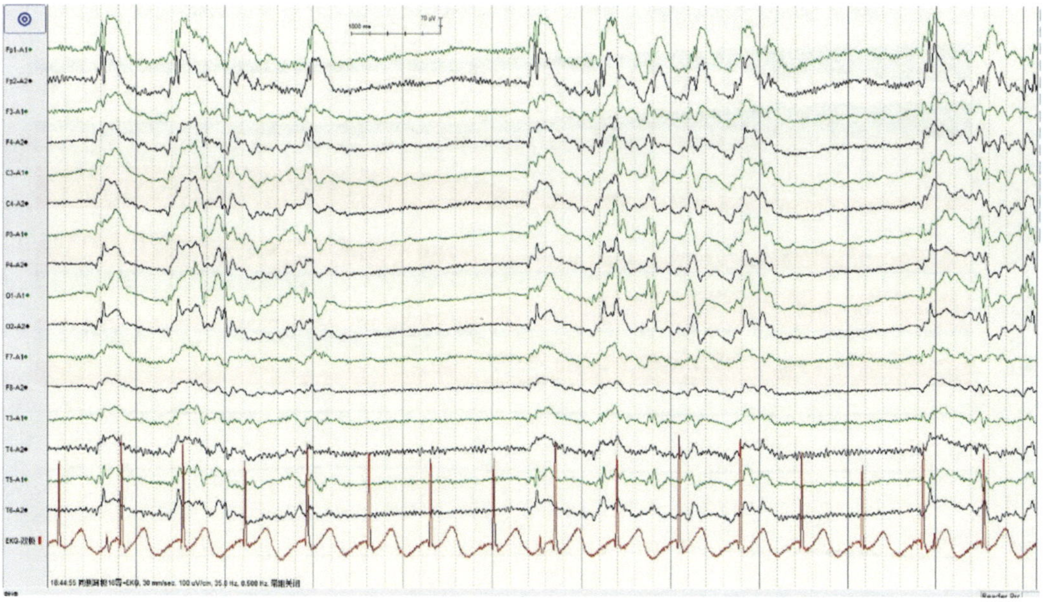


**Fig. 7.15** Early stage of recording: the number of outbreaks has further increased, the time has been extended, and the suppression ratio and the time have been reduced

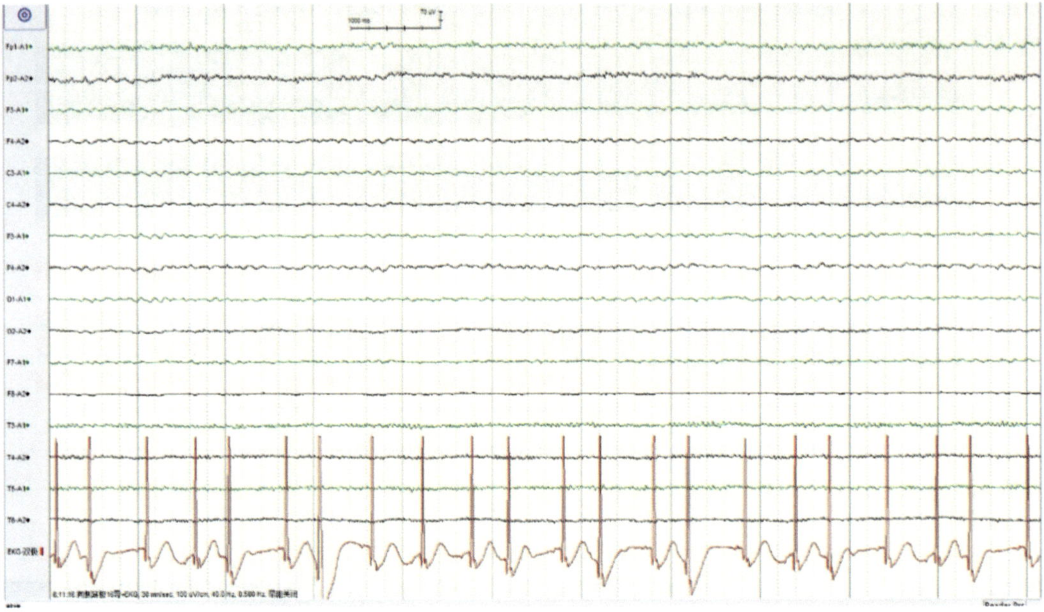

Fig. 7.16 Late stage of recording: the burst is gradually reduced to eventually disappear, and the EEG is fully suppressed

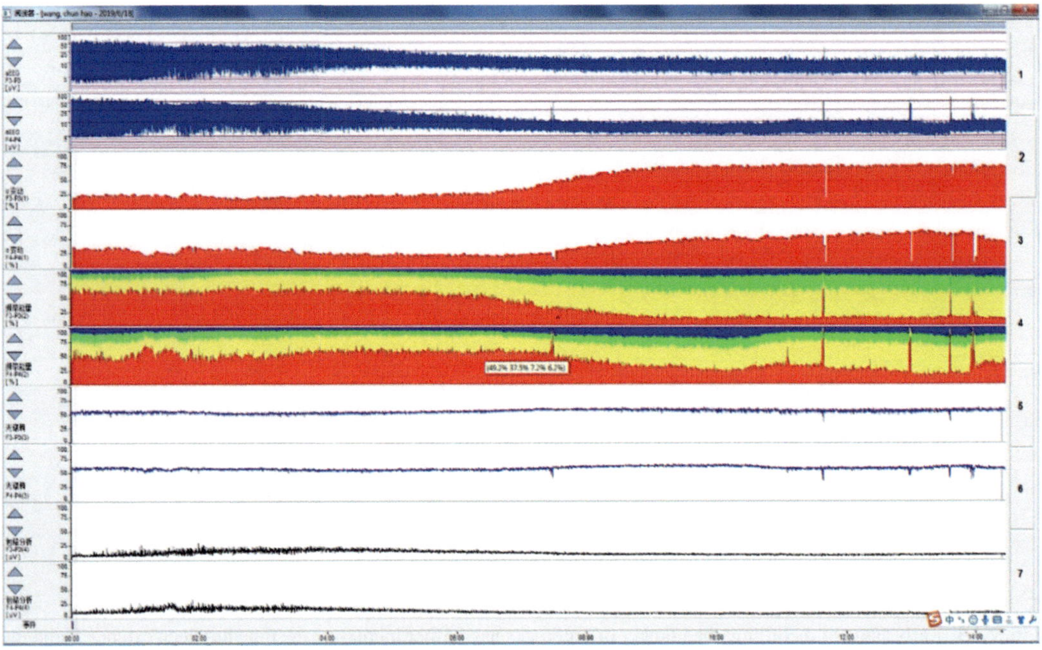

Fig. 7.17 Full-scale display at 48 h: the background changes from discontinuous to continuous, and the burst trend first increases and then decreases to eventually disappear

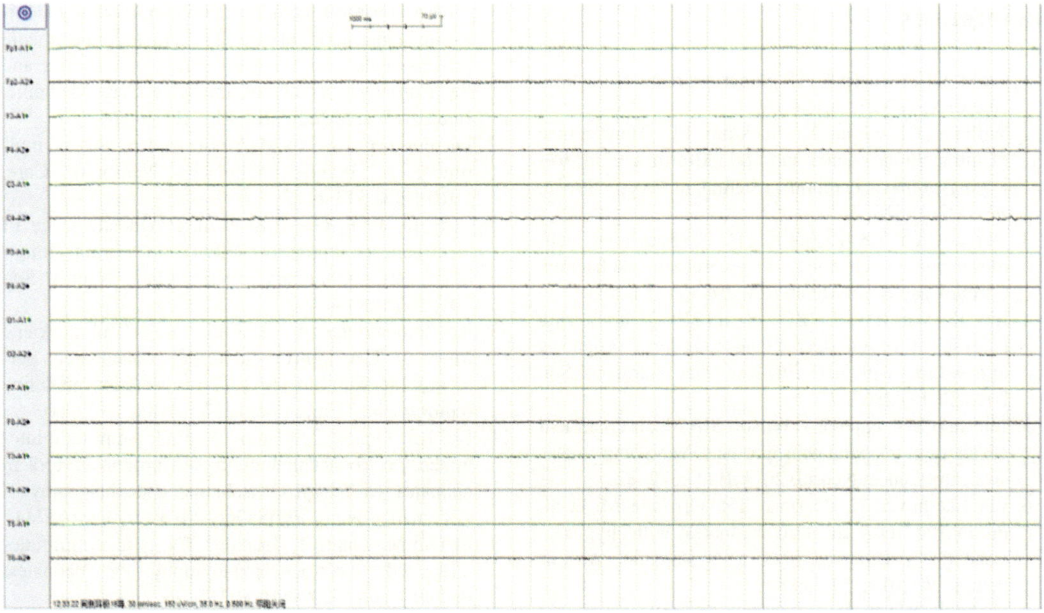

**Fig. 7.18** Cerebral electricity tends to be stable, showing a state of full suppression. The reactivity and the sleep waveform disappear

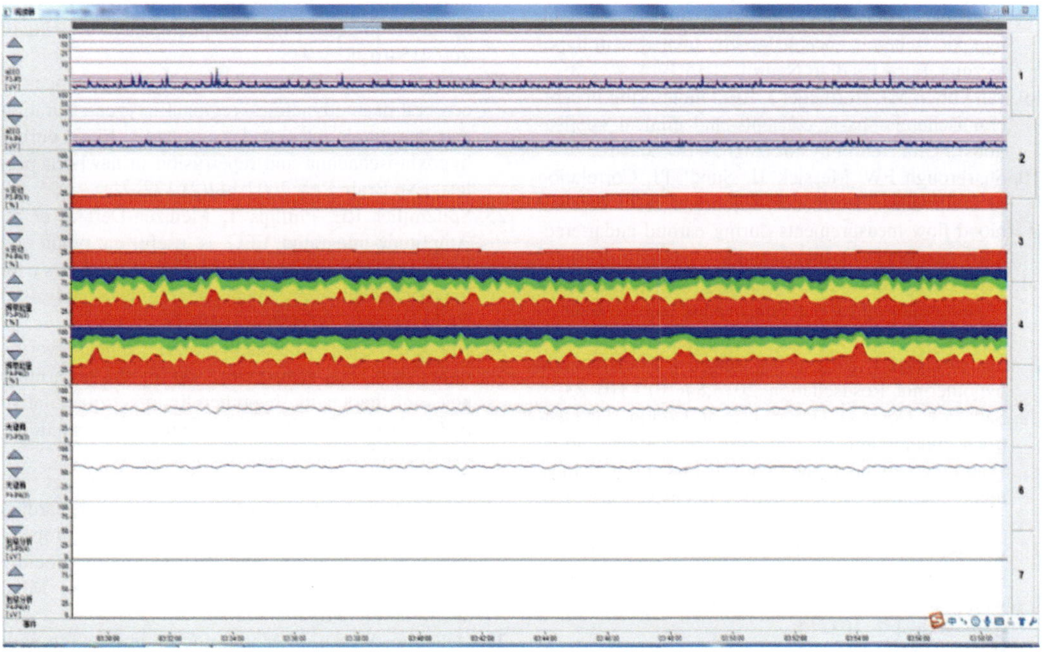

**Fig. 7.19** 72-h full-scale display: upper and lower limits of the aEEG are both <5 μV, showing a severely abnormal EEG

## References


1. Gunn AJ, Thoresen M. Hypothermic neuroprotection. NeuroRx. 2006;3(2):154–69.
2. Williams CE, Gunn A, Gluckman PD. Time course of intracellular edema and epileptiform activity following prenatal cerebral ischemia in sheep. Stroke. 1991;22(4):516–21.
3. Obrenovitch TP, Richards DA. Extracellular neurotransmitter changes in cerebral ischaemia. Cerebrovasc Brain Metab Rev. 1995;7(1):1–54.
4. Liu JF, Wu HW, Li ZG, et al. aEEG monitoring analysis of lesion degree and long-term prognosis in newborns with HIE. Eur Rev Med Pharmacol Sci. 2016;20(13):2863–7.
5. Johnston MV, Fatemi A, Wilson MA, et al. Treatment advances in neonatal neuroprotection and neurointensive care. Lancet Neurol. 2011;10(4):372–82.
6. van Laerhoven H, de Haan TR, Offringa M, et al. Prognostic tests in term neonates with hypoxic-ischemic encephalopathy: a systematic review. Pediatrics. 2013;131(1):88–98.
7. Shah DK, Wusthoff CJ, Clarke P, et al. Electrographic seizures are associated with brain injury in newborns undergoing therapeutic hypothermia. Arch Dis Child Fetal Neonatal Ed. 2014;99(3):F219–24.
8. Garfinkle J, Sant'Anna GM, Rosenblatt B, et al. Somatosensory evoked potentials in neonates with hypoxic-ischemic encephalopathy treated with hypothermia. Eur J Paediatr Neurol. 2015;19(4):423–8.
9. van Putten MJ, Hofmeijer J. EEG monitoring in cerebral ischemia: basic concepts and clinical applications. J Clin Neurophysiol. 2016;33(3):203–10.
10. Sharbrough FW, Messick JJ, Sundt TJ. Correlation of continuous electroencephalograms with cerebral blood flow measurements during carotid endarterectomy. Stroke. 1973;4(4):674–83.
11. Sandroni C, Cavallaro F, Callaway CW, et al. Predictors of poor neurological outcome in adult comatose survivors of cardiac arrest: a systematic review and meta-analysis. Part 1: patients not treated with therapeutic hypothermia. Resuscitation. 2013;84(10):1310–23.
12. Sadaka F, Doerr D, Hindia J, et al. Continuous electroencephalogram in comatose postcardiac arrest syndrome patients treated with therapeutic hypothermia: outcome prediction study. J Intensive Care Med. 2015;30(5):292–6.
13. Claassen J, Hirsch LJ, Frontera JA, et al. Prognostic significance of continuous EEG monitoring in patients with poor-grade subarachnoid hemorrhage. Neurocrit Care. 2006;4(2):103–12.
14. Knauert MP, Gilmore EJ, Murphy TE, et al. Association between death and loss of stage N2 sleep features among critically ill patients with delirium. J Crit Care. 2018;48:124–9.
15. Fernandez L, Luthi A. Sleep spindles: mechanisms and functions. Physiol Rev. 2020;100(2):805–68.
16. Le Roux P, Menon DK, Citerio G, et al. Consensus summary statement of the international multidisciplinary consensus conference on multimodality monitoring in neurocritical care : a statement for healthcare professionals from the neurocritical care society and the European Society of Intensive Care Medicine. Intensive Care Med. 2014;40(9):1189–209.
17. Diedler J, Czosnyka M. Merits and pitfalls of multimodality brain monitoring. Neurocrit Care. 2010;12(3):313–6.
18. Feng G, Jiang G, Li Z, et al. Prognostic value of electroencephalography (EEG) for brain injury after cardiopulmonary resuscitation. Neurol Sci. 2016;37(6):843–9.
19. Krikscionaitiene A, Stasaitis K, Dambrauskiene M, et al. Can lightweight rescuers adequately perform CPR according to 2010 resuscitation guideline requirements? Emerg Med J. 2013;30(2):159–60.
20. Del RR, Ochoa C, Alarcon A, et al. Amplitude integrated electroencephalogram as a prognostic tool in neonates with hypoxic-ischemic encephalopathy: a systematic review. PLoS One. 2016;11(11):e165744.
21. El-Dib M, Chang T, Tsuchida TN, et al. Amplitude-integrated electroencephalography in neonates. Pediatr Neurol. 2009;41(5):315–26.
22. Hellstrom-Westas L, Rosen I. Continuous brain-function monitoring: state of the art in clinical practice. Semin Fetal Neonatal Med. 2006;11(6):503–11.
23. Lawrence R, Mathur A, Nguyen TTS, et al. A pilot study of continuous limited-channel aEEG in term infants with encephalopathy. J Pediatr. 2009;154(6):835–41.
24. Ioroi T, Peeters-Scholte C, Post I, et al. Changes in cerebral haemodynamics, regional oxygen saturation and amplitude-integrated continuous EEG during hypoxia-ischaemia and reperfusion in newborn piglets. Exp Brain Res. 2002;144(2):172–7.
25. Spitzmiller RE, Phillips T, Meinzen-Derr J, et al. Amplitude-integrated EEG is useful in predicting neurodevelopmental outcome in full-term infants with hypoxic-ischemic encephalopathy: a meta-analysis. J Child Neurol. 2007;22(9):1069–78.
26. Burnsed J, Quigg M, Zanelli S, et al. Clinical severity, rather than body temperature, during the rewarming phase of therapeutic hypothermia affect quantitative EEG in neonates with hypoxic ischemic encephalopathy. J Clin Neurophysiol. 2011;28(1):10–4.
27. Sandroni C, Cariou A, Cavallaro F, et al. Prognostication in comatose survivors of cardiac arrest: an advisory statement from the European resuscitation council and the European Society of Intensive Care Medicine. Intensive Care Med. 2014;40(12):1816–31.
28. Hellstrom-Westas L. Monitoring brain function with aEEG in term asphyxiated infants before and during cooling. Acta Paediatr. 2013;102(7):678–9.
29. ter Horst HJ, Sommer C, Bergman KA, et al. Prognostic significance of amplitude-integrated EEG during the first 72 hours after birth in severely asphyxiated neonates. Pediatr Res. 2004;55(6):1026–33.
30. Peberdy MA, Callaway CW, Neumar RW, et al. Part 9: post-cardiac arrest care: 2010 American Heart

Association guidelines for cardiopulmonary resuscitation and emergency cardiovascular care. Circulation. 2010;122(18 Suppl 3):S768–86.
31. Chandrasekaran M, Chaban B, Montaldo P, et al. Predictive value of amplitude-integrated EEG (aEEG) after rescue hypothermic neuroprotection for hypoxic ischemic encephalopathy: a meta-analysis. J Perinatol. 2017;37(6):684–9.
32. Rots ML, van Putten MJ, Hoedemaekers CW, et al. Continuous EEG monitoring for early detection of delayed cerebral ischemia in subarachnoid hemorrhage: a pilot study. Neurocrit Care. 2016;24(2):207–16.
33. Vespa PM, Boscardin WJ, Hovda DA, et al. Early and persistent impaired percent alpha variability on continuous electroencephalography monitoring as predictive of poor outcome after traumatic brain injury. J Neurosurg. 2002;97(1):84–92.
34. Al-Kadi MI, Reaz MB, Ali MA. Evolution of electroencephalogram signal analysis techniques during anesthesia. Sensors (Basel). 2013;13(5):6605–35.
35. Bewernitz M, Derendorf H. Electroencephalogram-based pharmacodynamic measures: a review. Int J Clin Pharmacol Ther. 2012;50(3):162–84.
36. Coleman RM, Tousignant-Laflamme Y, Gelinas C, et al. Changes in the bispectral index in response to experimental noxious stimuli in adults under general anesthesia. ISRN Pain. 2013;2013:583920.
37. Dunham CM, Ransom KJ, McAuley CE, et al. Severe brain injury ICU outcomes are associated with cranial-arterial pressure index and noninvasive bispectral index and transcranial oxygen saturation: a prospective, preliminary study. Crit Care. 2006;10(6):R159.
38. Thakur S, Kaur T, Kaur S, et al. Awareness of bispectral index monitoring system among the critical care nursing personnel in a tertiary care hospital of India. Indian J Anaesth. 2011;55(6):563–6.
39. Deng R, Xiong W, Jia X. Electrophysiological monitoring of brain injury and recovery after cardiac arrest. Int J Mol Sci. 2015;16(11):25999–6018.

# Application of Multimodal EEG in SE

# 8

Xuefeng Wang, Jiyuan Li, and Wei Jing

## Contents




**Abstract**

SE is the most common critical illness in the NICU. Various system-related encephalopathies, central nervous system infections, organ transplantation, central hyponatremia, central diabetes insipidus, brain trauma, tumors, cerebrovascular diseases, and drugs can cause SE. SE patients, especially those with generalized seizures, can cause various systemic complications over time, such as cerebral edema, arrhythmia, electrolyte imbalance, acid-base imbalance, rhabdomyolysis, and pulmonary edema, which may become new



X. Wang (✉)
Department of Neurology, The First Affiliated Hospital of Chongqing Medical University, Chongqing, China

J. Li
Department of Neurology, The First Hospital of Shanxi Medical University, Taiyuan, Shanxi, China

W. Jing
Department of Neurology, Shanxi Bethune Hospital Affiliated to Shanxi Medical University, Taiyuan, Shanxi, China





X. Wang et al. (eds.), *Multi-Modal EEG Monitoring of Severely Neurologically Ill Patients*,
https://doi.org/10.1007/978-981-16-4493-1_8

causes or induce secondary epilepsy and form the pathological cycle of RSE. SE is also an important factor leading to poor patient prognosis, such as brain death or even death. This chapter briefly describes the definition and classification of SE, focusing on the performance of SE on multimodal EEG and the role of multimodal EEG in the diagnosis, treatment, and prognostic evaluation of SE patients, which provides effective references for the early discovery of SE and active and effective monitoring and prevention to improve its clinical outcome. At the same time, this chapter introduces the application of multimodal EEG in SE and new developments in combination with legends and provides valuable information for SE-related research.

**Keywords**

SE · CSE · NCSE · EEG monitoring · Multimodal EEG · aEEG · BIS · Anesthetics · RSE · Prognosis

SE is one of the most common critical illnesses in neurological diseases. There are more than 160 causes of SE recognized by the ILAE. There are 15 types of causes of SE, including cerebrovascular disease, neurodegenerative diseases, CNS infection, intracranial tumors, cortical dysplasia, head injury, alcoholism, the decrement or withdrawal of AEDs, cerebral ischemia and hypoxia, metabolic disorders, autoimmune diseases, mitochondrial disease, abnormal chromosome and genes, neurocutaneous syndrome, and others. Many patients with SE are neurocritical patients [1].

## 8.1 Definition of SE

The new definition of SE proposed by the ILAE in 2015 is based on the duration of epileptic seizures. GTCS with a single seizure of more than 5 min, partial seizures lasting more than 10 min, or absence seizures of more than 15 min are called SE [1]. However, the World Health Organization (WHO) also refers to the failure of the CNS to function normally between seizures as SE. Traditionally, it is believed that frequent seizures of epilepsy in a short period of time are also called SE, but this now tends to be called a seizure cluster [2].

## 8.2 Classification of SE

In 2015, the ILAE proposed a new classification method for SE. The ILAE advocated to divide SE into CSE and NCSE [1] (Figs. 8.1 and 8.2).

A survey of patients in the ICU showed that CSE is the most common manifestation of SE,

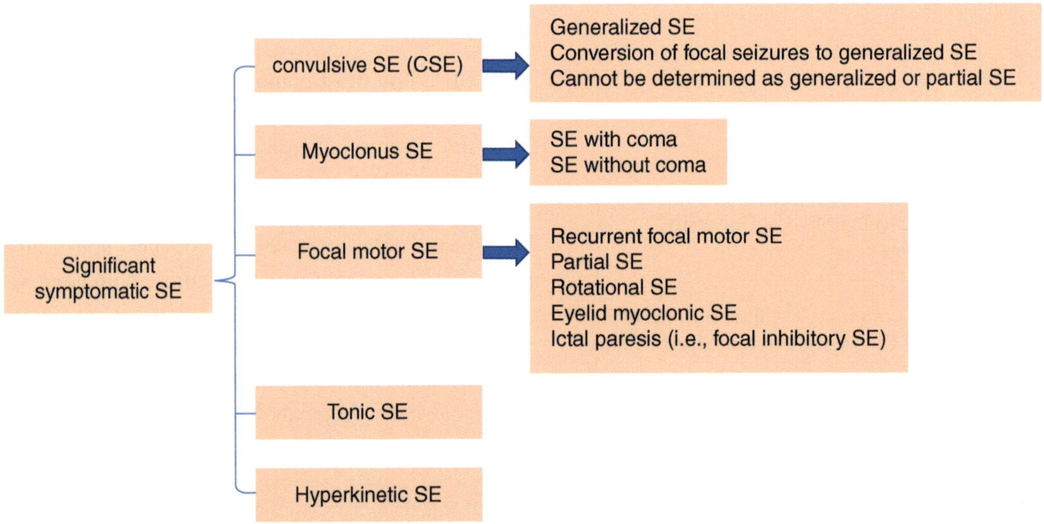


**Fig. 8.1** Generalized SE with obvious motor symptoms

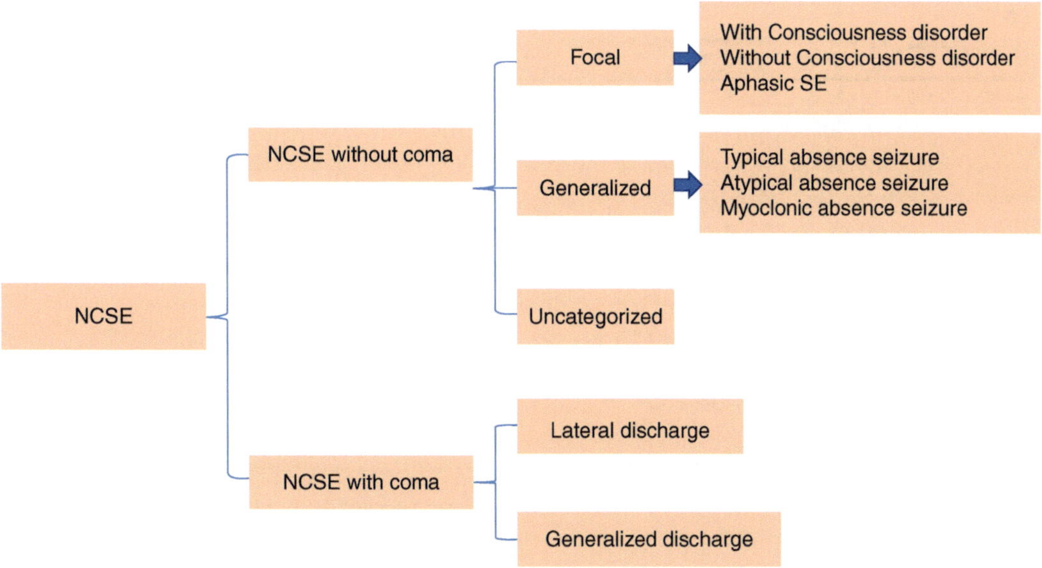


**Fig. 8.2** NCSE

followed by focal SE without consciousness disturbance and coma NCSE, accounting for approximately 7–14% of cases [3].

## 8.3 Application of Multimodal EEG in SE

### 8.3.1 Indications for EEG

EEG is mainly used in patients with SE to: (a) determine the presence of epilepsy and SE, especially NCSE (Fig. 8.3a, b); (b) identify nonepileptic seizures (Fig. 8.4a, b); (c) clarify the nature of nonspecific symptoms in the NICU, such as myoclonus, tremors, disturbances of consciousness, and mental behavior disorders; (d) assess the degree of brain damage in SE; (e) guide AED treatment of SE; and (f) judge the prognosis of patients with SE [2–8].

### 8.3.2 Manifestations of SE on EEG

#### 8.3.2.1 Traditional EEG

The EEGs of patients with SE mainly manifest continuous epileptiform discharges, which can be divided into specific and nonspecific discharges. The former includes spikes that persist on the EEG, such as spike waves, sharp waves, spike slow waves, sharp slow waves, and multispike slow waves, and the latter refers to the paroxysmal activity that highlights the background activity of the EEG, especially various periodic electrical activities and BS EEGs [2].

**Spike Waves**

Spike waves are the most characteristic manifestation of epileptic discharge. The IFSECN states that spikes are short-term and prominent background activities on the EEG, which are spike-like and last for 20–70 ms at the specified paper speed. The main components are the negative phase and variable amplitude brain waves. The traditional view is that spike waves refer to transient EEG changes with duration of 20–70 ms and varying amplitudes, but mostly at 50–150 μV, which are obviously prominent in the background activity, followed by a slow wave. In most cases, the voltage of the spike wave is very high, and it mainly refers to the amplitude of the wave that is prominent in the background activity. If the voltage of the spike wave is almost the same as the voltage of the background activity, the highlighting of the background activity mainly refers to the form, especially the frequency.

Spikes can manifest in many ways on EEGs. When spikes appear extensively in all leads,

a

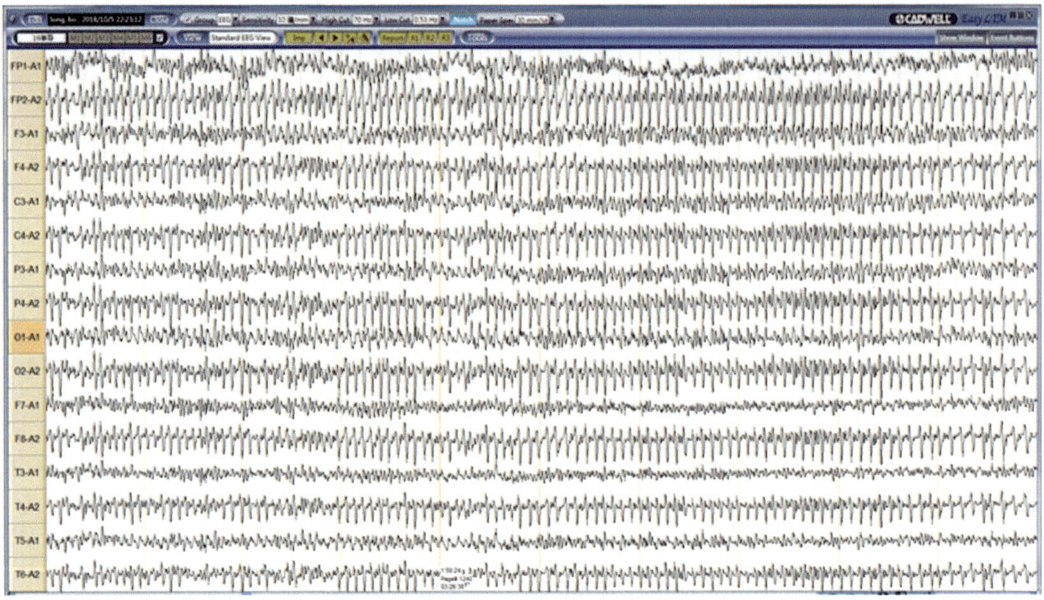

b

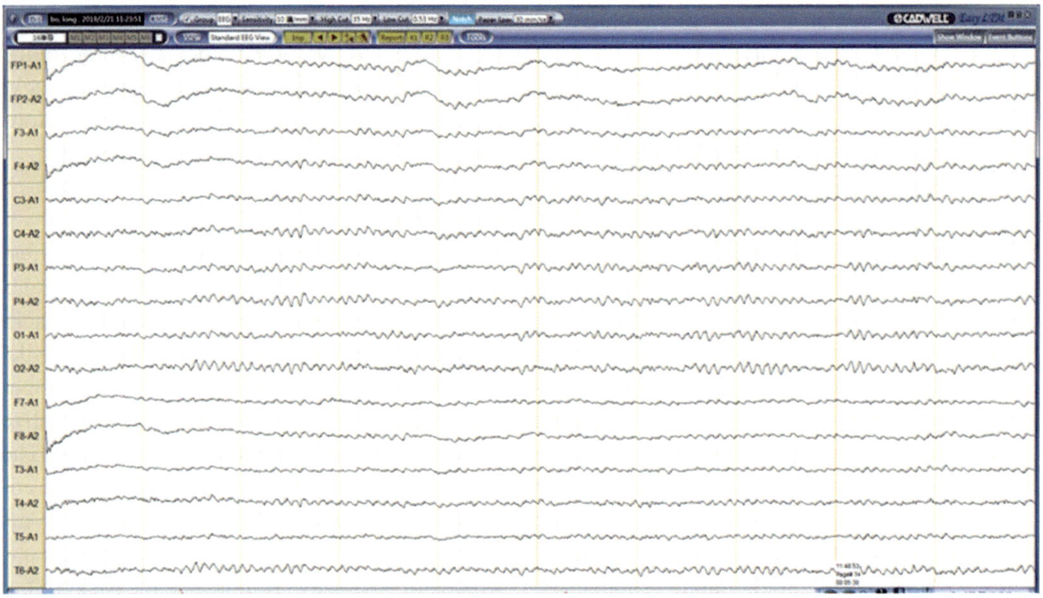

**Fig. 8.3** (**a**, **b**) EEGs from a 45-year-old male patient with NCSE with sudden mental and behavioral abnormalities. The emergency EEG results are as follows: (**a**) the background is a comprehensive spike rhythm and (**b**) 30 s after the injection of 10 mg diazepam, the α background activity recovers

they are called chronic or extensive spikes, and they are often accompanied by slower background activities (Fig. 8.5). If the spikes manifest only in a certain area or one side or one side is obviously too many and the number is small, they are called scattered spikes. Spikes have no obvious relationship with the prognosis of epilepsy. The presence of spikes does not necessarily mean that there is severe epilepsy. The epilepsy represented by some spikes may be

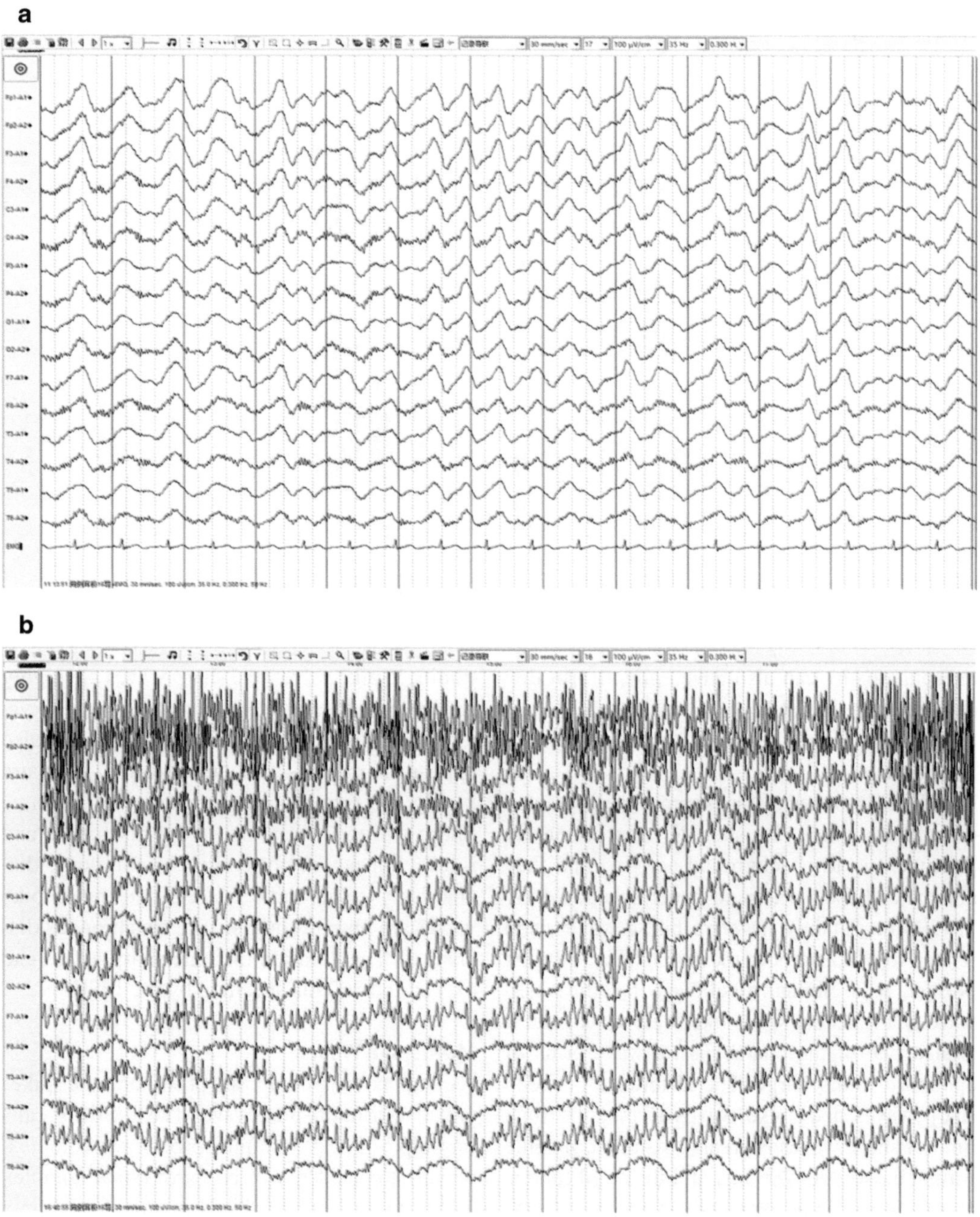

**Fig. 8.4** (**a**, **b**) EEGs from a 23-year-old woman with AE. (**a**) The EEG showed diffuse slow-wave activity. (**b**) During paroxysmal sympathetic excitement, the EEG showed hyperventilation, and the background frequency further slowed down, accompanied by a large number of myoelectric artifacts

benign. Although spikes are highly associated with epilepsy, their presence does not necessarily mean that a patient will have seizures. One percent of patients without epilepsy also have spike-like changes on EEGs, and patients without epilepsy who have visual abnormalities at the beginning of infancy can also have occipital spikes. Although patients with metabolic

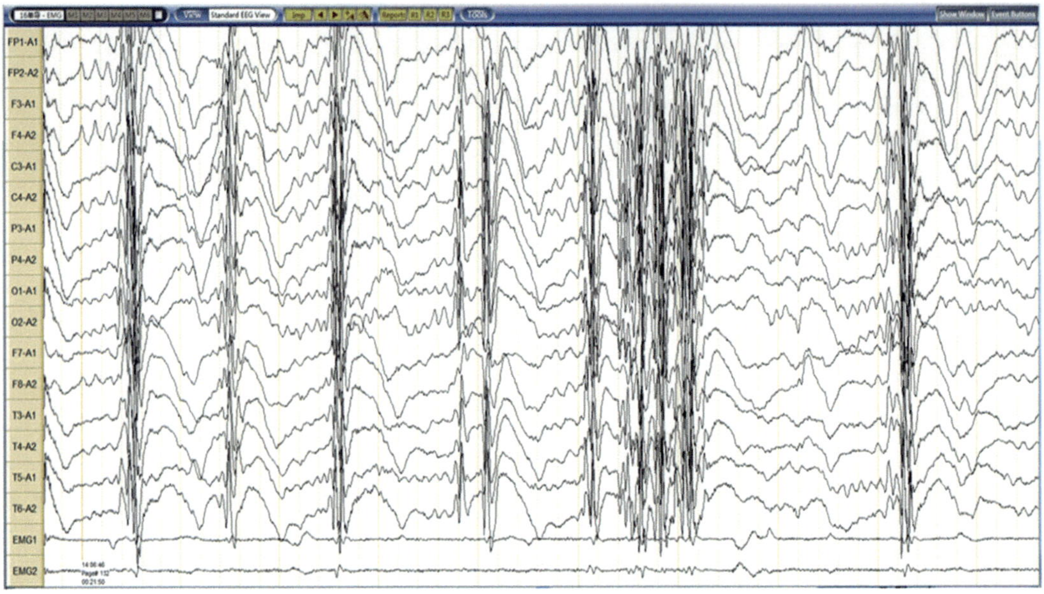


**Fig. 8.5** EEG from a 10-year-old male with myoclonic epilepsy. The interictal EEG manifested as comprehensive spike waves and multispike waves

encephalopathy can also have epileptiform discharges, they do not have epilepsy.

### Sharp Waves

The IFSECN states that a "sharp wave is electrical activity which is a short-term, prominently prominent in the background activity, and they are spike-shaped at a fixed paper speed, lasting 70–200 ms, mainly negative phase waves, and related to other parts of the brain" (Fig. 8.6). At present, it is clinically believed that the sharp wave is a transient spike-like brain wave, and it is also one of the characteristic waveforms of epileptiform discharge. The difference between sharp waves and spike waves is that the time limit of sharp waves is greater than that of spike waves, mostly 70–200 ms, and the amplitude is 100–200 μV. Some patients can reach 300 μV, which is prominent in the background activity and composed of rapidly ascending branches and slowly descending branches, with more negative phase waves. Sharp waves are mostly located on the surface of the epileptic foci, but they can also manifest on both sides or are widely distributed. Sharp waves can also be seen in isolation, which may cause false positioning. Spike waves and sharp waves are highly neurophysiologically related; both are paroxysmal discharges, and although they can also appear in patients without seizures, they are highly indicative of the presence of seizures. Sharp waves are random partial discharges and rarely appear in systemic synchronous discharges, while spike waves and multispike waves are obvious in systemic synchronous discharges. The duration of some sharp waves can exceed the 200 ms specified by the IFSECN.

### Multispike Waves

A complex wave composed of two or more spikes is called a multispike wave. The IFSECN calls this type of wave a multispike wave complex, which is considered to be paroxysmal complex waves with two or more spikes, manifesting in a more or less rhythmic manner, with different durations (Fig. 8.7). Generally, the volatility is large.

### Spike Slow Waves

The spike-and-slow wave complex is the name given by the IFSECN to all complex waves composed of a spike wave and a subsequent

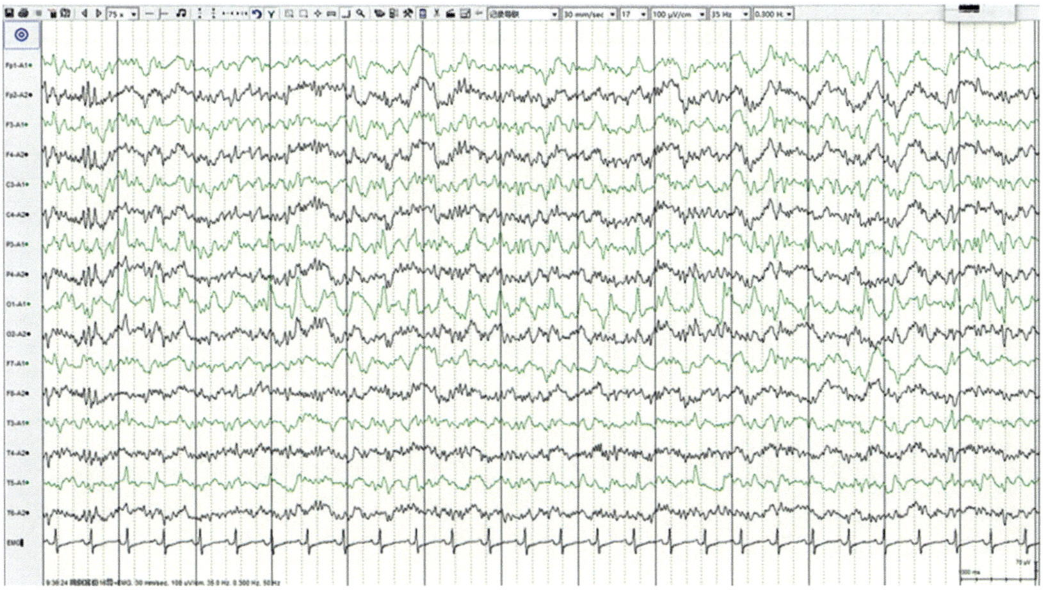

**Fig. 8.6** EEG from a 67-year-old male patient with hypertensive encephalopathy, showing continuous sharp waves on the left

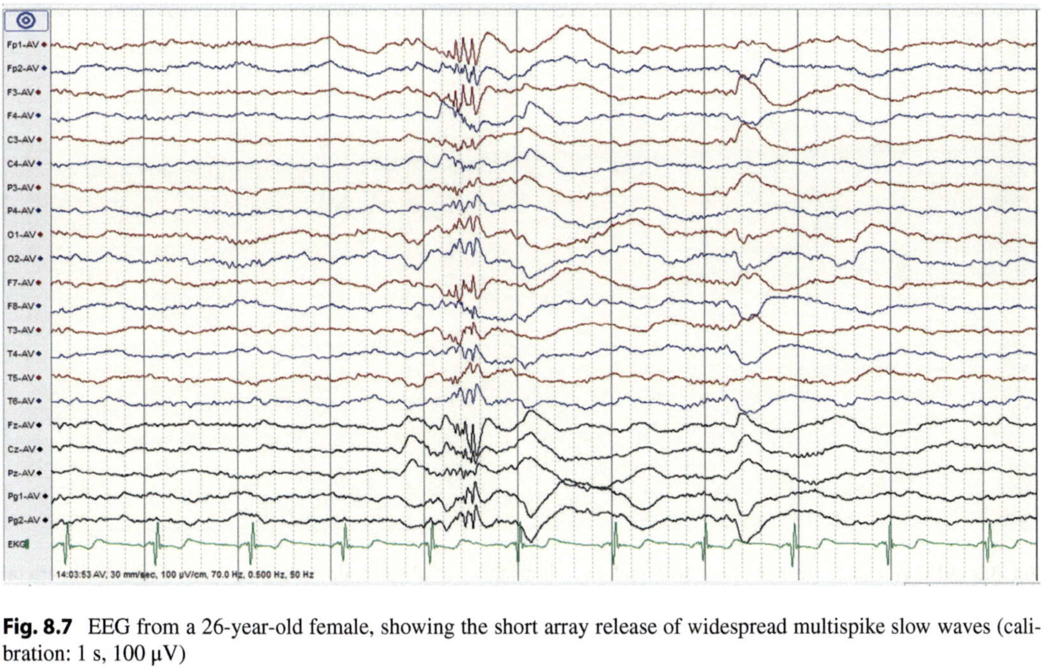


**Fig. 8.7** EEG from a 26-year-old female, showing the short array release of widespread multispike slow waves (calibration: 1 s, 100 μV)

slow wave (Figs. 8.8 and 8.9). The slow wave is the main component, and the amplitude is between 150 and 500 μV. The slow wave is relatively regular and rhythmic. Spikes can manifest in front of the slow wave or in the ascending or descending branch of the slow wave. The amplitude of the wave varies, generally not exceeding that of the slow wave. Waves usually appear on both sides at the same time, most notably in the frontal area.

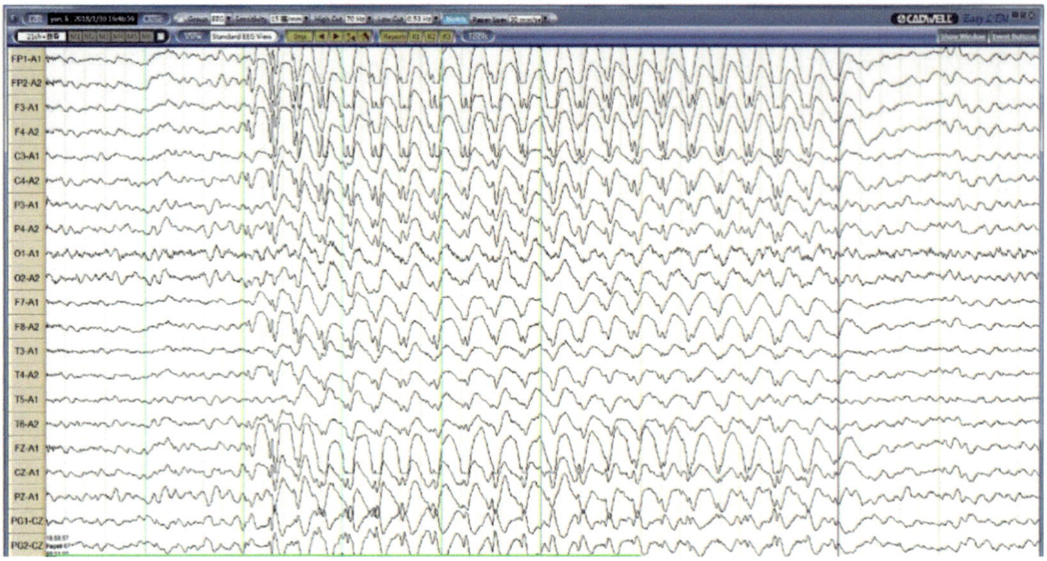

**Fig. 8.8** EEG from a 6-year-old patient with absence SE, showing fully symmetrical and synchronized 3.0–3.5 Hz spike slow waves

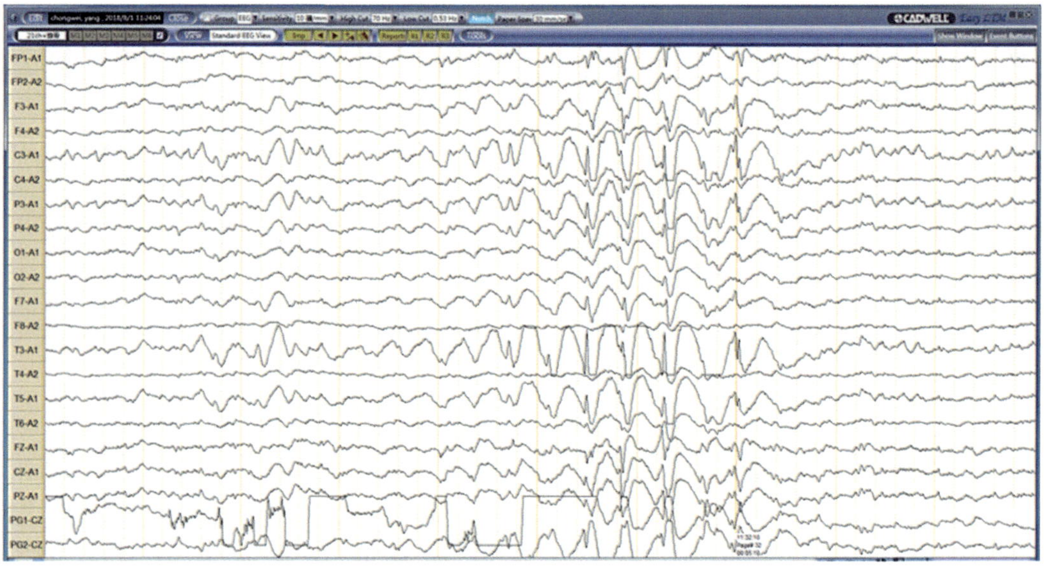

**Fig. 8.9** EEG from a 23-year-old male with epilepsy, showing a partial spike-slow wave complex during the interictal phase

### Sharp Slow Waves

A sharp-and-slow wave complex means that a slow wave appears immediately after the sharp wave, which together form a 1.5–2.5 Hz complex wave or a 4–6 Hz sharp-slow complex wave (Fig. 8.10a, b), with various manifestations, many irregular synchronous bursts, common intractable seizures, or temporal lobe epilepsy [2].

### Nonspecific Epileptiform Discharges

Nonspecific epileptiform discharges mostly occur between the epileptic period and the interictal period, which may be related to brain metab-

a

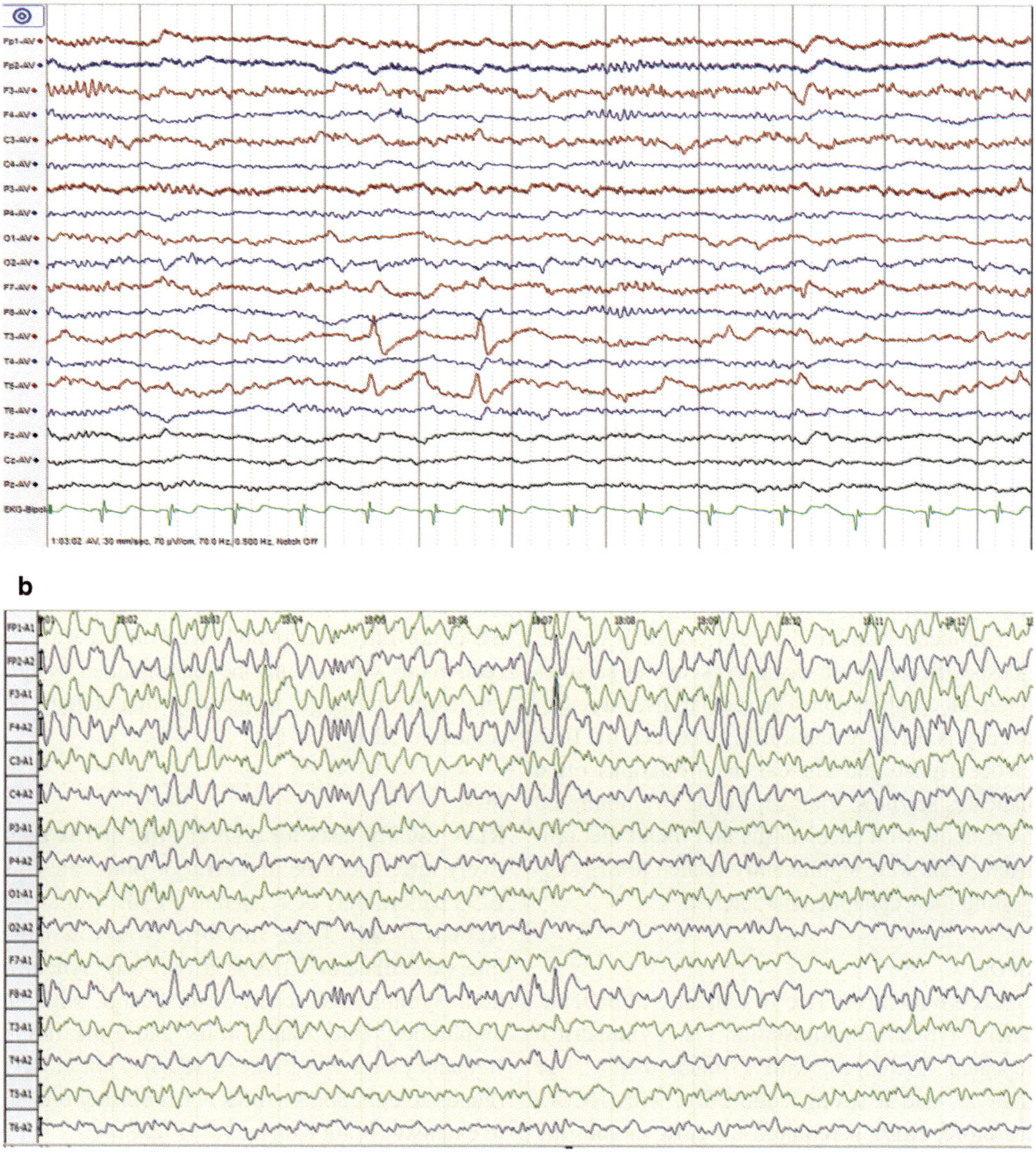

Fig. 8.10 (a) EEG from a 24-year-old male, showing sharp slow waves emanating from the left middle and posterior temporal regions (calibration: 1 s, 70 μV). (b) EEG from a 31-year-old female with LGI1 encephalitis who had sleep disturbance for 1 month and abnormal mental behavior for 7 days. The EEG shows focal sharp slow waves

olism at this time, and there may be potential neuronal damage. Nonspecific epileptiform discharges mainly include PDs, rhythmic spike slow waves, and sharp waves [2, 3]. Although these are related to epileptic seizures in neurocritical patients, they also manifest in other diseases.

PDs

PDs are regular, intermittent, repetitive, and stereotyped discharges, usually 0.5–1 Hz, which are highly correlated with epileptic activity but are also seen in acute cerebrovascular diseases, tumors, and CNS infections [3] (Fig. 8.11).

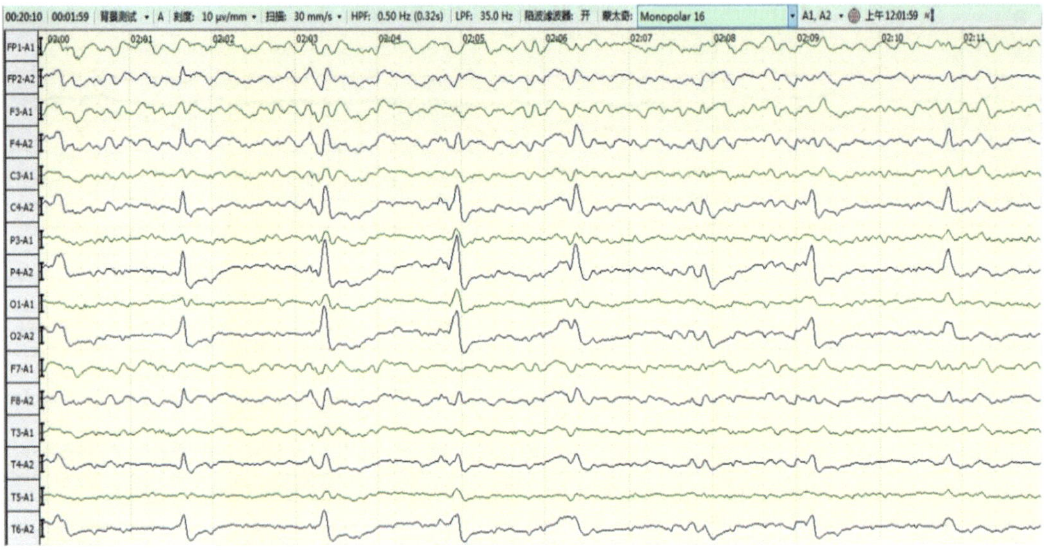


**Fig. 8.11** EEG from a 71-year-old male patient with a deep coma who suffered massive cerebral hemorrhage in the right basal ganglia that broke into the ventricle. The EEG shows unilateral periodic sharp waves

Unilateral PDs are the most common type of nonspecific epileptic discharges in the seizure-interictal combination. The regular discharge frequency is 3 Hz. A relationship between the time of occurrence and clinical manifestations often indicates seizures. Viarasilpa et al. [4] monitored 54 patients with encephalitis and found that unilateral PDs were significantly related to SE, suggesting their epileptic characteristics.

GPDs

GPDs are relatively rare in critically ill patients. Their typical manifestation is symmetrical repeated discharges, with a standard discharge interval, and a strong connection with NCSE; therefore, cEEG is required for close monitoring (Fig. 8.12). Punia et al. [5] monitored the EEGs of 200 critically ill patients and found that patients with PDs on their EEGs had seizures after being transferred from the ICU, suggesting that PDs are related to epilepsy.

BS

BS is a periodic high-voltage pattern with spikes and multispike activity followed by a period of suppression or isoelectric activity. The burst usually lasts 1–10s, and the duration of suppression may vary. The relationship between BS and SE is not fully understood. When a BS wave is seen in the NICU, it may be accompanied by epileptiform discharge, suggesting that it may be related to SE (Fig. 8.13).

RDA

RDA usually lasts for a short time and is relatively rare. It can be unilateral or bilateral. This EEG pattern may be related to NCSE. Unilateral RDA is mostly 3 Hz, and there is no discharge interval. Bilateral RDA is a two-way synchronous symmetrical repetitive discharge with an amplitude greater than 100 μV and a maximum frequency of 3 Hz. Bilateral RDA is not closely related to epileptic seizures but is closely related to extensive brain damage [3] (Fig. 8.14).

#### 8.3.2.2 aEEG

SE appears as a sharply rising and steeply falling waveform on an aEEG (Fig. 8.15).

### 8.3.3 The Role of Multimodal EEG in the Diagnosis of SE

#### 8.3.3.1 EEG Monitoring Indications

There is no consensus in the industry for EEG monitoring indications. At present, the main

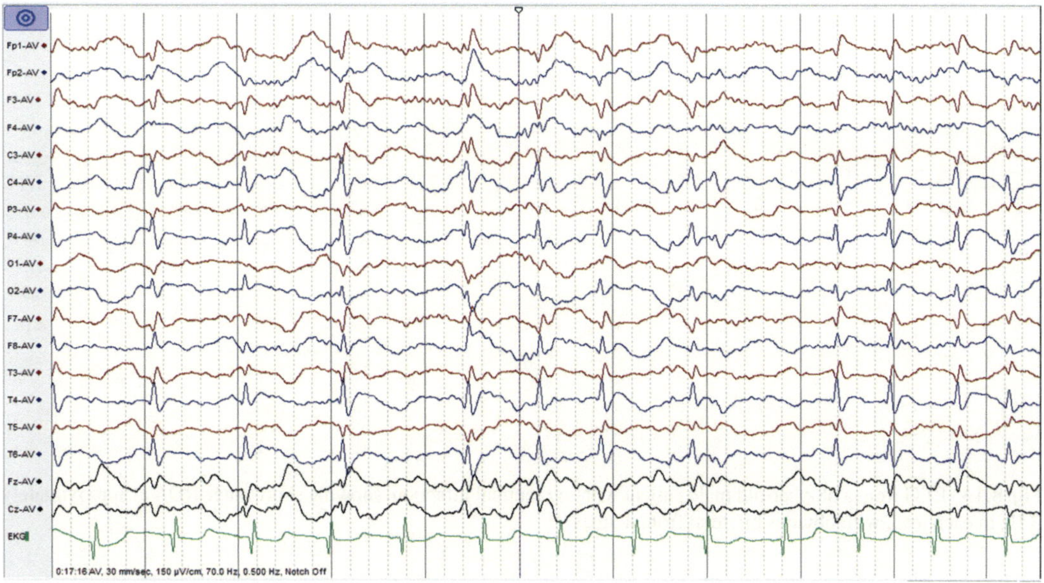


**Fig. 8.12** EEG from a 12-year-old female, showing widespread periodical spike waves and spike slow waves (calibration: 1 s, 100 μV)

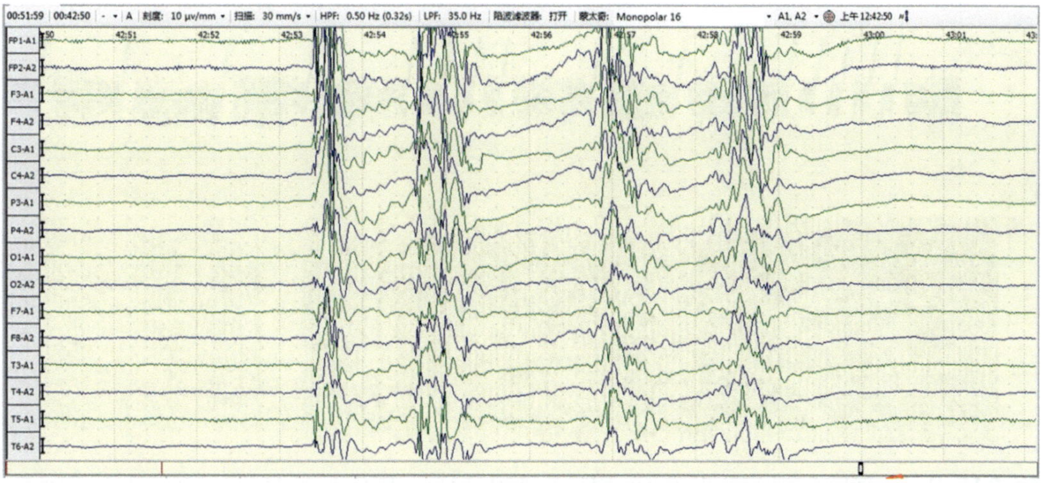


**Fig. 8.13** EEG from a 78-year-old man who was in intermediate coma after CPR due to cardiac arrest. The EEG shows a BS pattern

basis is reports from large clinical case studies. The monitoring indications advocated now are: (a) previous examination determined the presence of disorders that may cause epilepsy or SE (Table 8.1); (b) the presence of systemic diseases with impaired consciousness, such as postoperative sepsis and sepsis; and (c) CNS function does not return to normal after the onset of CSE [1].

#### Start Time of EEG Monitoring

The ACNS recommends that epileptic seizures should be ruled out at least within 24 h, while the guidelines of the Society of Neurology and

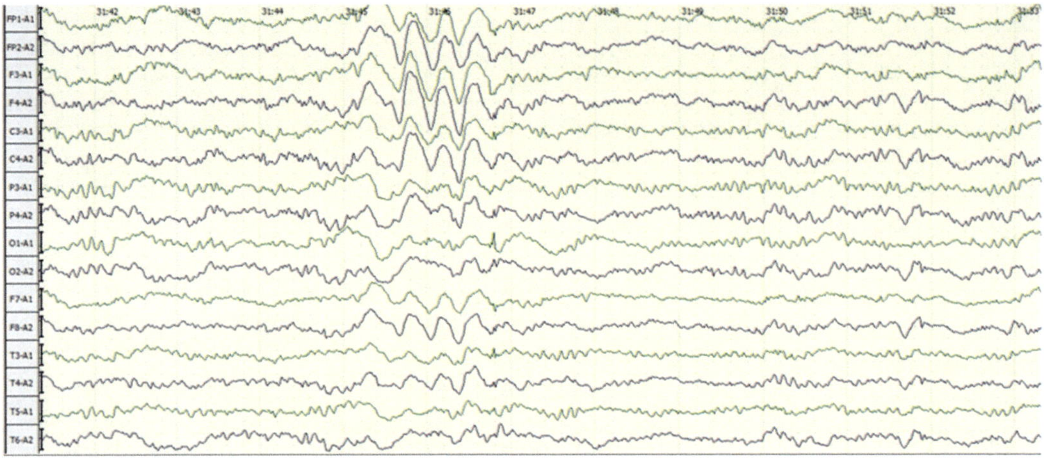

**Fig. 8.14** EEG from a 68-year-old male patient with intracranial infection, showing short-range RDA at approximately 3 Hz in each lead, with obvious bilateral frontal areas

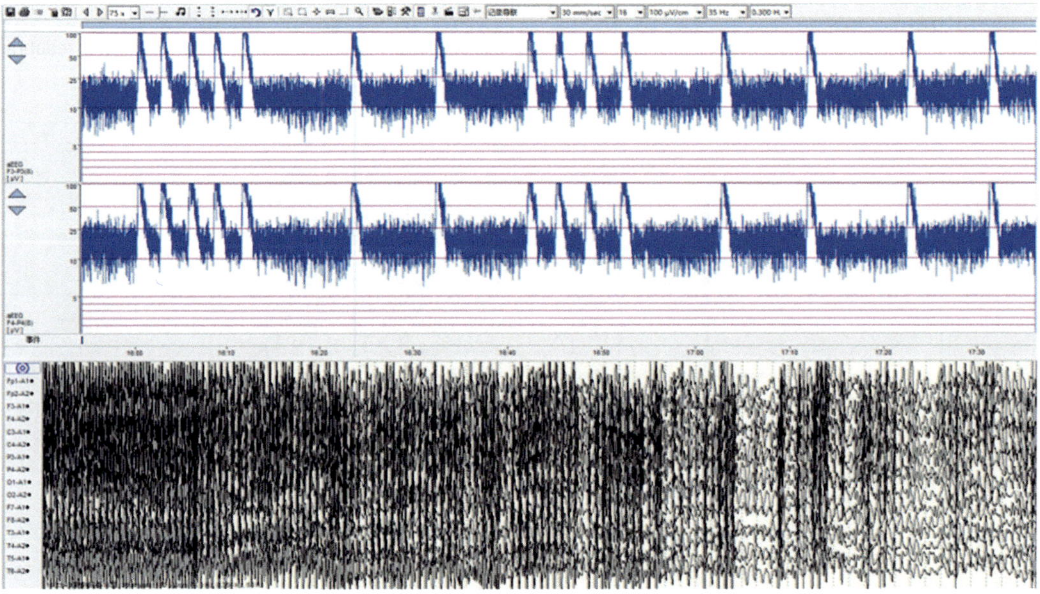

**Fig. 8.15** During epileptic seizures, the upper and lower borders of an aEEG rise and fall sharply, with a sudden rise and narrow gaps, which appear repeatedly

Critical Care recommend that the monitoring of comatose patients should start within 48 h of coma onset [6].

### Monitoring Duration

Sansevere et al. [7] monitored the EEGs (median monitoring time of 21 (16–42.2) hours) of 414 patients aged 4.2 (0.75–11.3) years and found that 25% of them had epilepsy or SE. At the same time, it was found that no epileptiform discharge was found within the first 4–6 h of monitoring, and the possibility of epileptic discharge in the future was lower. It was proposed that 4–6 h may be the appropriate monitoring duration in the pediatric intensive care unit (PICU). EEG monitoring can be

**Table 8.1** Disorders that may cause epilepsy or SE

| Classification | Diseases |
|---|---|
| Encephalopathy | |
| Hormone-sensitive encephalopathy | Hashimoto's encephalopathy<br>AE<br>Viral encephalitis<br>Lymphoma of the CNS<br>Systemic lupus erythematosus<br>Antineutrophil cytoplasmic autoantibody vasculitis |
| Metabolic encephalopathy | Uremic encephalopathy<br>Dialysis encephalopathy<br>Pulmonary encephalopathy<br>Hepatic encephalopathy<br>Pancreatic encephalopathy<br>Valproic-acid-associated encephalopathy<br>Organ-transplantation-associated encephalopathy |
| Cerebrovascular diseases | HIE<br>Severe cerebral hemorrhage<br>Massive cerebral infarction<br>Hypertensive encephalopathy<br>Subarachnoid hemorrhage<br>Subdural hematoma<br>Epidural hematoma<br>Intracranial venous sinus thrombosis<br>Reversible leukoencephalopathy<br>Vascular dementia |
| CNS infections | Tuberculous meningoencephalitis<br>Japanese encephalitis<br>Purulent meningoencephalitis<br>Chronic bacterial meningitis<br>Herpes simplex encephalitis<br>Herpes zoster encephalitis<br>Toxoplasmosis<br>Cerebral cysticercosis<br>Cerebral paragonimiasis<br>Cerebral malaria<br>Human immunodeficiency virus<br>Creutzfeldt-Jakob disease<br>Cryptococcal infection<br>Fungal brain infection<br>Subacute sclerosing panencephalitis |
| Intracranial tumors | Primary intracranial tumors (such as glioma, meningioma, ependymoma)<br>Metastatic tumors<br>Paraneoplastic-associated encephalopathy |
| Head injuries | Brain contusion<br>Diffuse axonal injury (DAI)<br>Intracranial hematoma |

stopped if the EEG background is normal or there is no epileptiform discharge in the first 24 h of recording. Another scholar reported that qEEG can capture 56% of epileptic seizures within 1 h of monitoring and 88% of epileptic seizures within 24 h. Another study compared repeated intermittent 30-min EEG recordings with cEEG recordings. In detecting NCS, it was found that the detection rate of epileptic seizures increased from 58% within the first 30 min of EEG monitoring to 67% with repeat EEG monitoring 24 h later. The positive rate of repeat EEG monitoring at 12 h increased to 71%, at 6 h increased to 87% and at 3 h increased to 92%. The researchers determined that if more than 6 seizures occurred during the cEEG recording, EEG monitoring every 6 h and 30 min might detect this seizure burden. If EEG monitoring was repeated for 30 min only at 12 or 24 h, 6% of NCSE cases would be missed. The researchers summarized that patients with NCSE generally need to be monitored for approximately 24 h, and patients in coma or patients with epileptiform discharges on EEGs usually need to be monitored for approximately 48 h [3].

### The Positive Rate of Monitoring

Scholars performed 48-h EEG monitoring of 136 infants and found that 20% of them had SE. After cardiac surgery, 48-h EEG monitoring was performed on 183 children; among them, 12% developed NCSE. A retrospective analysis of 93 infants with congenital heart disease (CHD) surgery found that 6% of patients had SE. Viarasilpa et al. [4] performed at least 12 h of EEG monitoring on 1735 patients. The monitored patients were analyzed, and 22 of 54 patients with encephalitis (41%) had epileptic discharges on EEGs. Abend et al. [8] investigated 200 critically ill children undergoing EEG examinations due to EEG changes and acute neurological problems, and they found that 84 children had epileptic seizures, 41% of which were transformed into SE, and 43% of which manifested as SE.

#### 8.3.3.2 Standards for the Diagnosis of SE by EEG

Seizures and SE may exist in neurocritical patients. According to the standards of the ILAE [1], the diagnostic criteria for SE are a single convulsive seizure that lasts more than 5 min, a focal seizure that lasts more than 10 min, and an absence seizure that lasts 15 min. Both the American Epilepsy Society and the WHO consider frequent seizures to be a manifestation of SE. The EEG standard for this type of SE is that the time of epileptiform discharge exceeds 30 min within 1 h.

#### 8.3.3.3 The Role of Conventional EEG in the Diagnosis of NCSE

NCSE is an electrical-clinical syndrome that mainly manifests as abnormal mental behavior, changes in consciousness, or autonomic dysfunction. Although there may be minor movements, most patients have no obvious motor symptoms. These manifestations are also common in neurocritical patients without SE, which makes clinical diagnosis challenging, but NCSE can be seen on EEGs with persistent or recurrent episode epileptiform discharges; therefore, this electrical seizure performance can be used to diagnose the presence of NCSE (Fig. 8.16a–e).

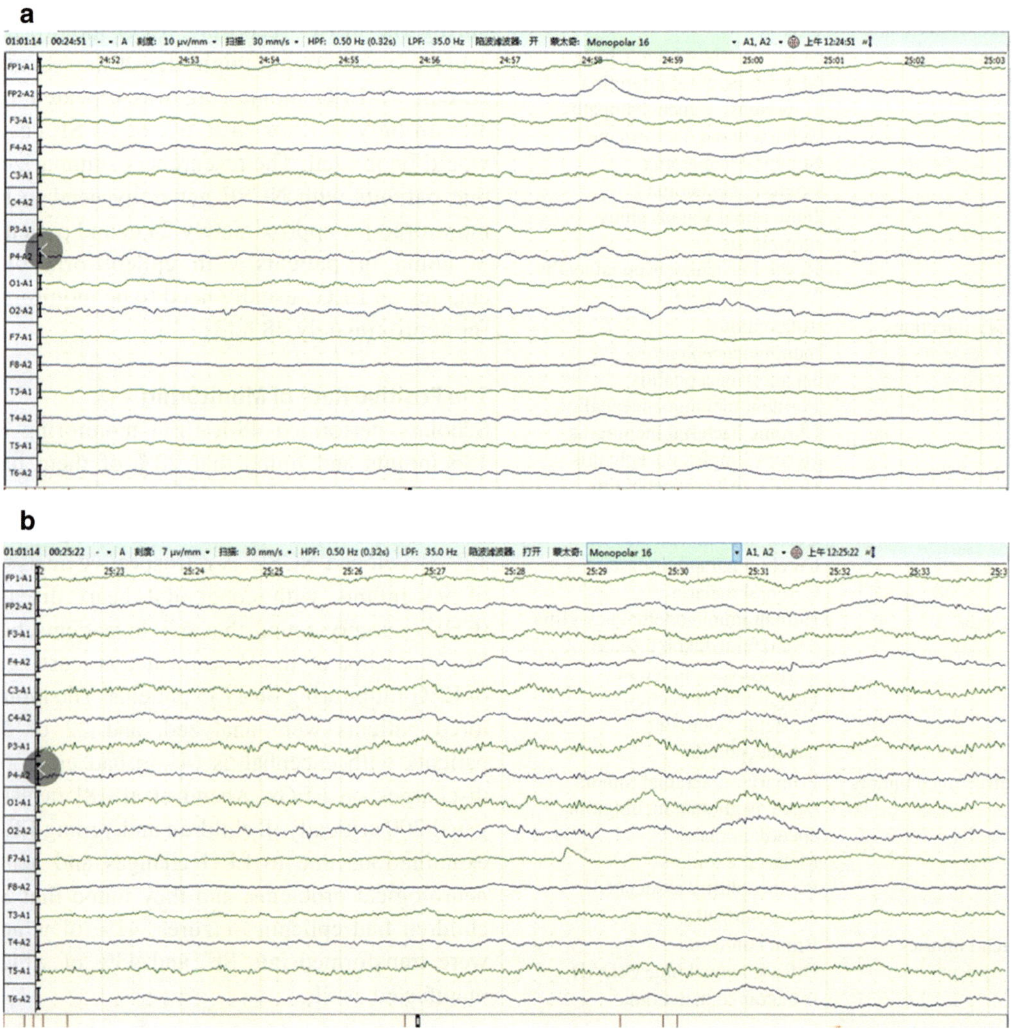


**Fig. 8.16** (**a–e**) EEGs from a 55-year-old male patient with HIE in NCSE. The EEG manifestations are as follows: (**a**) low-amplitude and unresponsive EEG background; (**b**) low-amplitude fast activity starting on the left; (**c**) the recruitment rhythm spreading to each lead; (**d**) the spike rhythm of each lead; and (**e**) frequency reduction in late episodes

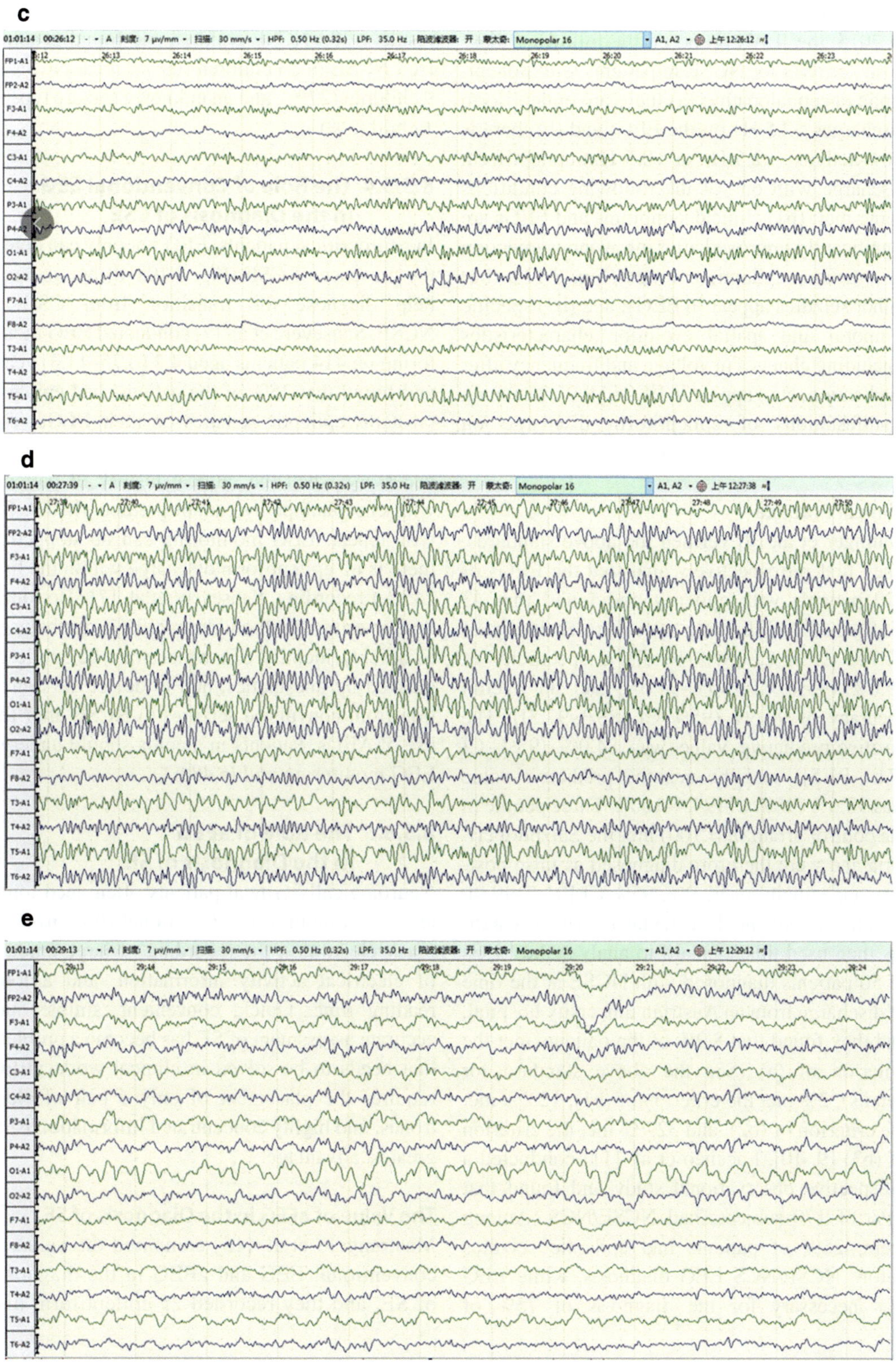


**Fig. 8.16** (continued)

#### EEG Diagnostic Criteria for NCSE

In 2015, the ILAE proposed the following diagnostic criteria for NCSE in patients with nonepileptic encephalopathy: (a) there are epileptiform discharges >2.5 Hz on the EEG; and (b) there is slow-activity (<2.5 Hz or >0.5 Hz) epileptiform discharge with one of the following conditions being met: (b1) clinical symptoms and EEGs are significantly improved after intravenous injection of antistatus epilepticus drugs (Fig. 8.17); (b2) minor seizures appear in EEGs; and (b3) specific temporal and spatial evolution characteristics (including changes in voltage and frequency after medication, etc.) appear in EEGs [1, 2]. The main manifestations of epileptiform discharge on EEGs are shown in Fig. 8.18.

#### Clinical Practice

Leitinger et al. [9] verified the above standards. They first retrospectively analyzed the EEGs of 220 patients with epilepsy and found that 43 (36%) had NCSE, with a cohort sensitivity of 97.7% (95% CI [87.9–99.6]), a specificity of 89.6% (95% CI [80.8–94.6]), and an overall accuracy of 92.5% (95% CI [88.3–97.5]). The positive-predictive value was 84.0% (95% CI [74.1–91.5]), and the negative-predictive value was 98.6% (95% CI [94.4–100]). Three people in the control group ($n = 100$) met the Salzburg criteria and were therefore diagnosed as false positives (specificity of 97.0%, 95% CI [91.5–99.0], sensitivity could not be calculated). The researchers then used this standard to analyze the EEGs of 50 patients diagnosed with NCSE at the time of discharge from an Austrian university hospital, and they found that 8.2% of the patients met the criterion of (a) (See the above standard for details), 2% met the criterion of (b1), 12.2% met the criterion of (b2), and 32.7% met the criterion of (b3) [9, 10]. Laccheo et al. [11] conducted a prospective observational study and found that 21% of 170 subjects had NCSE/NCS. Among them, 25% of patients had epileptic seizures before NCSE/NCS EEG diagnosis, while EEG was necessary for the diagnosis of 75% of patients. Fatema et al. [12] studied the EEG results of 33 NCSE children and found generalized NCSE in 23 children (69%), focal NCSE in 9 children (27%), and an unknown seizure type in 1 child (3%).

### 8.3.3.4 The Role of Conventional EEG in the Diagnosis of CSE

In neurocritical patients, EEG not only can detect the presence of CSE (Fig. 8.19a–d) but also can help diagnose the transition from CSE to NCSE. Sansevere et al. [7] conducted EEG monitoring on 414 patients aged 4.2 (0.75–11.3) years and found that 25% of the patients had epilepsy or status epileptic seizures on their EEGs. The authors considered acute EEG monitoring to be necessary when the clinical history of patients with encephalopathy cannot predict whether SE will appear. EEG monitoring can be stopped if there is no epileptiform discharge within the first 24 h of recording. Sansevere et al. [7] also found that, in critically ill children, cEEGs can be used to quickly identify SE, which may be subtle or masked by anesthetics, and to detect the transition from convulsive seizures to NCSE after the use of AEDs. Patients in a coma should undergo EEG monitoring within 48 h.

### 8.3.3.5 The Role of aEEG in the Diagnosis of SE

Neurologically critical patients often need long-term EEG monitoring. Traditional EEG involves many electrodes, the recording of large amount of electrical activity information, and a long reading time. Quick, convenient, simple, and accurate assessment of SE has become a problem that needs to be solved in clinical work. aEEG requires the placement of only a pair of electrodes, and highly concentrated information is its greatest advantage.

#### The Value of aEEG in the Diagnosis of SE

Mastrangelo et al. [13] compared the value of conventional EEG and aEEG in the diagnosis of SE, and they recorded 25 epileptiform dis-

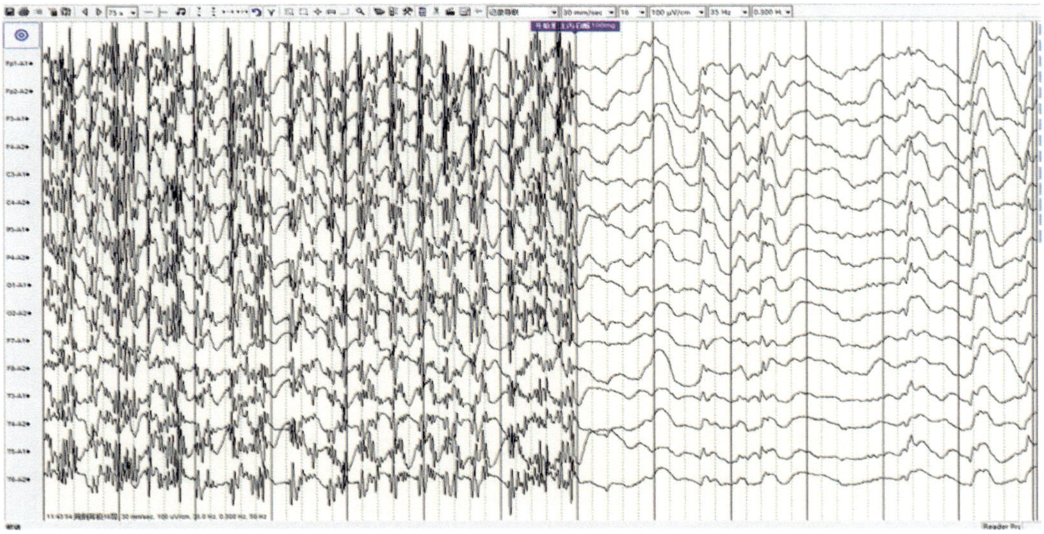

**Fig. 8.17** EEG from a 32-year-old female patient with NCSE who suffered from a sudden disturbance of consciousness. The seizure terminated after a 100 mg intravenous bolus of propofol. The patient was awakened, and the clinical symptoms and EEG showed significant improvement after intravenous injection of antistatus epilepticus drugs

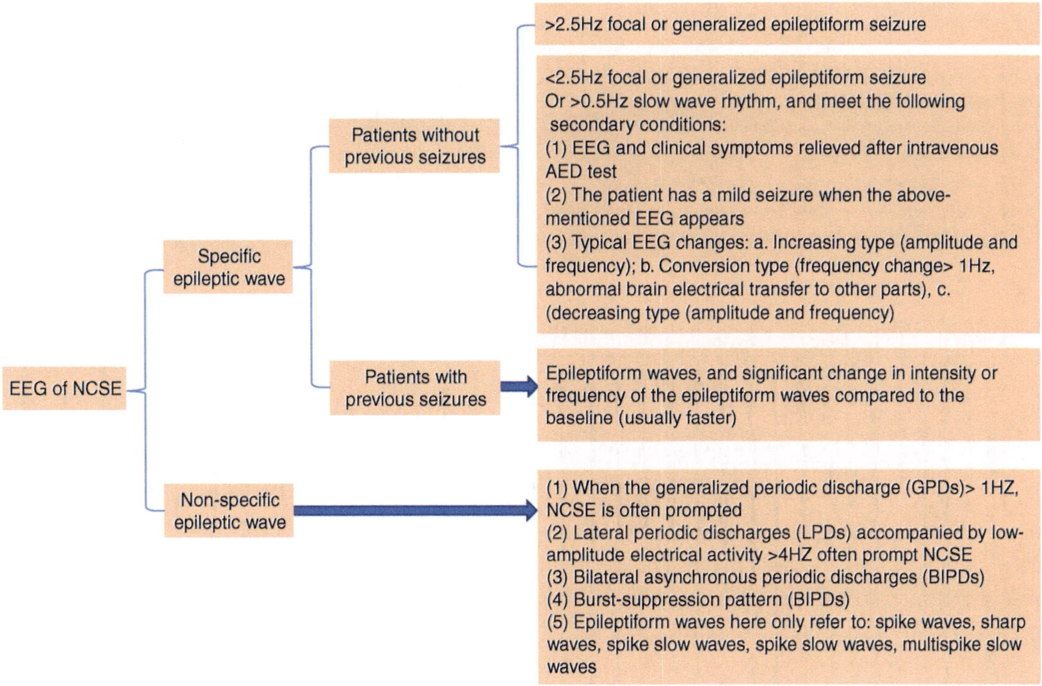


**Fig. 8.18** EEG manifestations of NCSE

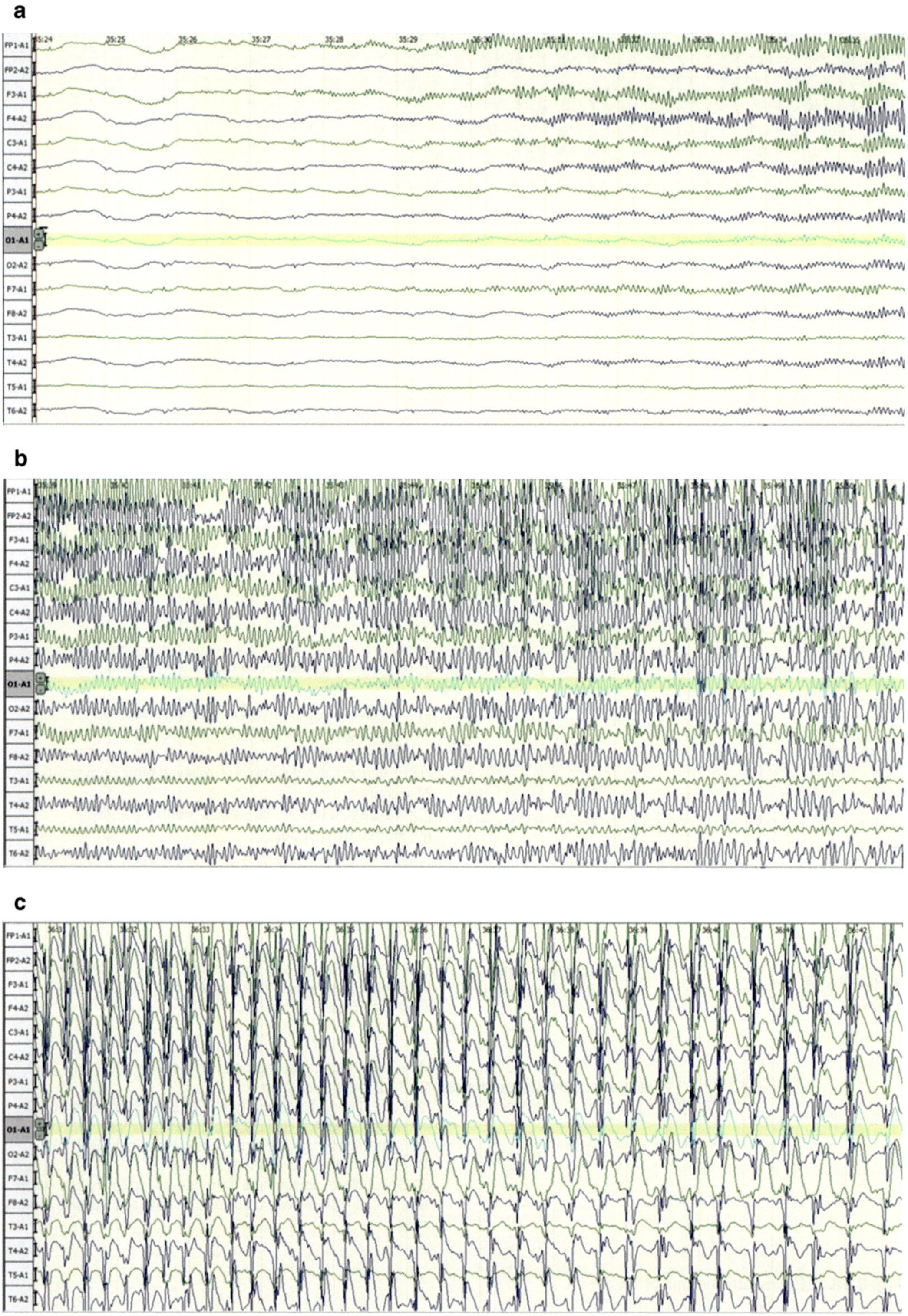

**Fig. 8.19** (**a–d**) EEGs from a patient with GTCS. (**a**) In the preseizure stage, the EEG shows the diffusion of the recruiting rhythm to each lead; (**b**) In the rigid phase, the EEG manifests as the spike rhythm of each lead; (**c**) In the clonic phase, the EEG manifests as spike slow waves and multispike slow waves of each lead; (**d**) In the late stage, the EEG is fully suppressed

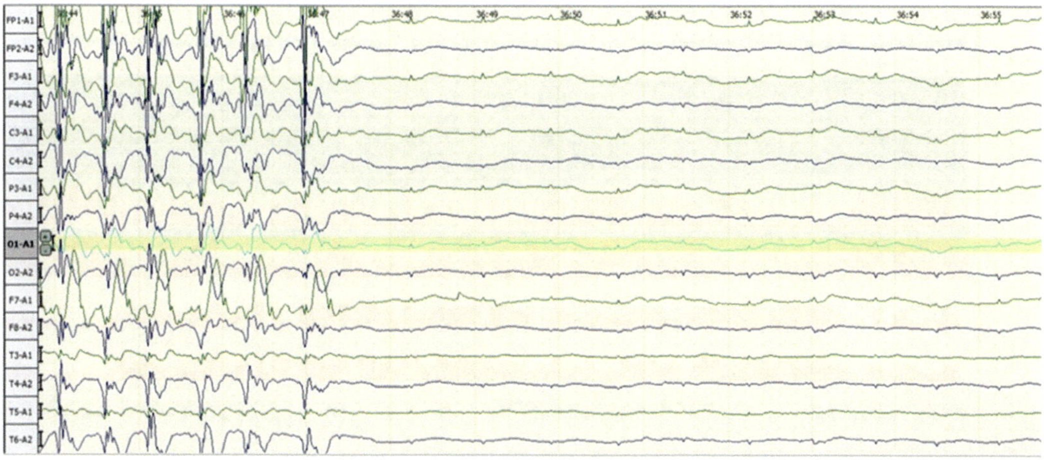


**Fig. 8.19** (continued)

charges on 31 EEGs. Two pediatric neurologists and a neonatologist used only aEEGs to confirm the existence of SE with an accuracy of 100%. Therefore, they believe that aEEG may be a useful tool for detecting SE in the ICU.

#### The Performance of SE on aEEG

An aEEG is a graph that reflects the trend in high and low EEG amplitudes. The upper boundary represents the high amplitude, the lower boundary represents the low amplitude, and the difference between the upper and lower boundaries is the bandwidth, which represents the difference between the high and low amplitudes. aEEGs can be used to visualize the amplitude changes in long-term brain electrical activity.

During the onset of SE, there is a continuous high-voltage discharge, the amplitude of which far exceeds the activity of normal neurons, the duration is very long, and it is easily captured by aEEG, making it the most useful tool for diagnosing SE. aEEG has been widely used clinically in recent years. The main manifestation of SE on an aEEG is the steep rise and fall of the band (Fig. 8.20).

#### Clinical Practice

van Rooij et al. [14] used aEEG to monitor 56 critically ill patients and found that 18% of the patients had SE. The relations between patients' prognosis and SE duration, background pattern before and after SE, and successful control of SE with AEDs were studied. It was found that the duration of SE on an aEEG was effective for identifying infants with HIE, and the aEEG background pattern was related to the overall prognosis of the disease. Mastrangelo et al. [13] asked two pediatric neurologists and a neonatologist to read 31 long-term aEEG recordings from 38 newborns independently, and the study results showed that three doctors identified 100% of the occurrences of SE found in the conventional EEGs by only the aEEG recordings, and the author believes that aEEG is a useful tool for detecting SE in the ICU.

### 8.3.3.6 The Role of Sleep EEG in the Diagnosis of SE

Sleep is closely related to SE. Fröscher et al. [15] summarized the EEG manifestations of SE during sleep. They found that absence seizures can appear in sleep and are manifested as a 3 Hz spike-slow wave complex, but this discharge can be integrated with synchronized sleep patterns, thereby destroying the continuous discharge in the absence state. At this time, the continuous discharge will be replaced by the isolated multispike wave or multispike-slow wave complex. Abnormal EEG activity in the absence state can last all night and can also recur at night or when waking up in the morning. Simple partial SE can

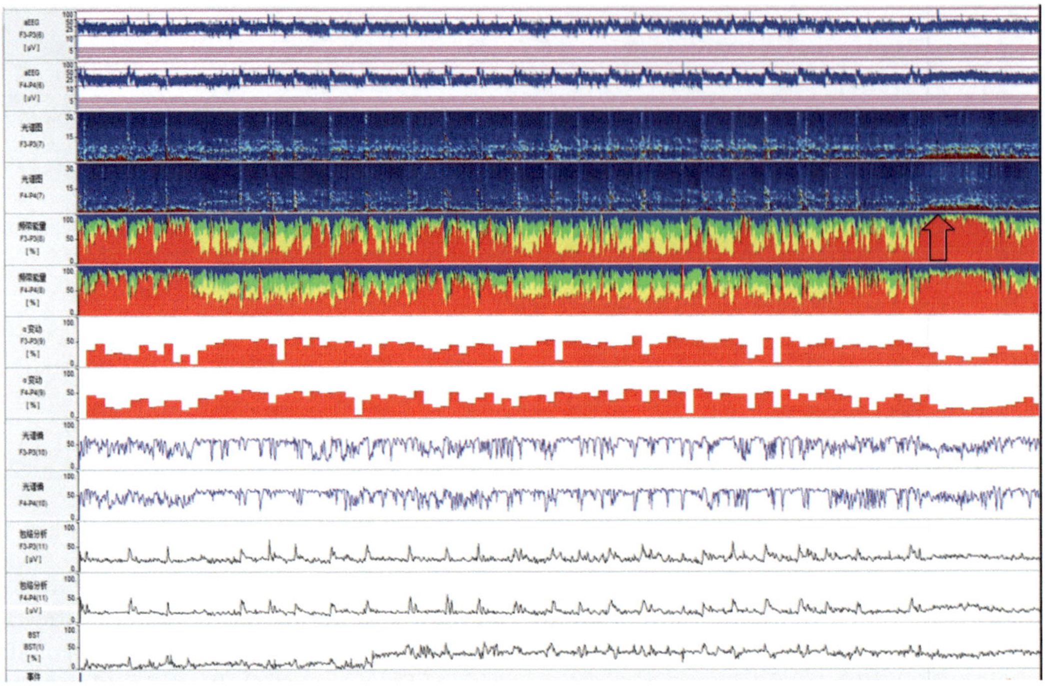

**Fig. 8.20** SE on an aEEG

appear throughout sleep, but sleep can improve the motor seizures of this type of SE. Patients with Lennox-Gastaut syndrome often have frequent tonic convulsions during the NREM phase of sleep.

Electrical SE during sleep is a special epilepsy syndrome. It manifests as a continuous epileptiform discharge during slow wave sleep, often accompanied by abnormalities in high-level neural activity. Caraballo et al. [16]. analyzed the characteristics of 117 patients with electrical SE syndrome and found that the age of disease onset was 2–21 years. The EEGs of patients with electrical SE during sleep are characterized by a persistent spike-slow wave complex that exceeds 85% of its waveform during NREM sleep.

### 8.3.4 The Role of Multimodal EEG in the Treatment of SE

The clinical manifestations of critically ill patients are diverse, and in many cases, it is difficult to distinguish whether their manifestations are paroxysmal or nonseizure related. The manifestations of NCSE, such as mental abnormalities and disturbances of consciousness, are not specific. Motor symptoms of CSE also need to be differentiated from nonepileptic myoclonus and paroxysmal convulsions. Subtle seizures or the transition from convulsive seizures to NCSE after the use of AEDs are not possible to identify through clinical observation. As a result, the treatment of SE is not realized, and subsequent treatment of the condition is challenging. EEG, especially qEEG, which allows quick viewing and interpretation of EEG data, can help clinicians solve these treatment problems. At the same time, EEG also helps to rule out psychotic nonepileptic states and avoid misdiagnosis and treatment.

#### 8.3.4.1 Treatment Goals

The ILAE emphasized that the treatment of SE must not only terminate clinical seizures but also completely terminate epileptiform discharge on EEGs. Especially when CSE transforms into NCSE after medication, the termination of epileptiform discharge on EEGs is the key to successful treatment.

#### 8.3.4.2 Efficacy Criterion

The termination of epileptiform discharge on EEGs for at least 12–24 h is the most commonly used treatment standard. For RSE, BS on EEGs may be required.

#### 8.3.4.3 The Role of aEEG in the Treatment of SE

qEEG involves a special algorithm to compress the original EEG components for several hours onto a display and reduces the number of electrodes required for recording. This technology allows neurobiologists to quickly perform EEG analysis, as the trends in EEGs will be displayed over time; therefore, it is also called digital trend analysis EEG.

The qEEG currently used clinically mainly includes aEEG, color density spectral array (CDSA), and envelope trend (ET). Because epileptic seizures usually contain higher frequencies and amplitudes than background activities, seizures on aEEGs are clearly shown as steep rises and falls in the trace, which are easy to identify and can be used not only for subclinical evaluation of SE but also to guide the treatment of SE.

Fatema et al. [12] used qEEG to evaluate the curative effect of treatment in 33 children with NCSE, and they found that of 18 patients receiving midazolam treatment, one patient had complete EEG remission, six patients had >80% remission, five patients had >50% remission, and five patients had a mild or no response. Thirteen patients received methylprednisolone treatment, of whom two patients had complete remission, four had >80% remission, four had >50% remission, and three had no response. Sansevere et al. [7] analyzed the diagnosis and treatment of SE in children with severe diseases. They believe that qEEG is very important for the diagnosis and treatment of SE. Hellstrom-Westas et al. [17] believe that aEEG can reveal the existence of subclinical seizures and that it can be used to evaluate the effects of antiepileptic treatment by studying the aEEGs of newborns.

### 8.3.5 The Role of Multimodal EEG in Judging the Prognosis of SE

The manifestation of SE in neurocritical patients often indicates a poor prognosis. Therefore, it is an important task to evaluate the patient's prognosis after receiving the expected treatment for SE. The key factor that reflects the prognosis of patients is whether their physiological functions are damaged.

#### 8.3.5.1 The Use of aEEG to Judge the Prognosis of Patients with SE

##### The Role of aEEG in Judging Prognosis

An aEEG is a trend map of brain function changes. Under normal circumstances, an aEEG upper boundary voltage >10 μV, a lower boundary >5 μV, and continuous background activity accompanied by a sleep-waking cycle represent the integrity of brain function. When this integrity is destroyed, it indicates a poor prognosis for the patient.

##### Clinical Practice

In the study of 56 infants with SE, van Rooij et al. [14] found that 42 infants (75%) had poor prognosis, of which 50% had abnormal aEEGs before SE, and 71% had abnormal aEEGs after SE. Among infants with good outcomes, the percentages of infants with abnormalities in aEEGs before and after SE were 14% and 7%, respectively. In a subgroup study of 48 infants with HIE, it was found that 48% of infants with poor prognosis had abnormal aEEGs before and after SE, while 25% and 13% of infants with good prognosis had abnormal aEEGs before and after SE, respectively. In a study of the aEEGs of 160 severely ill neonatal patients, 65 children were found to have severe abnormalities in the aEEG amplitude, and 25 showed BS. During follow-up, they found that the amplitude of the aEEGs of six children recovered to a CNV within 24 h. All six babies survived. In the BS group, the EEGs of 12 patients improved significantly within 24 h. Of these infants, one died, four returned to normal, and seven survived but were disabled.

Newborns who fail to recover within 24 h will likely die, and they will be severely disabled if they do survive. The researchers believe that infants with severely abnormal aEEGs within 6 h after birth return to a continuous normal background within the first 24 h, and 61% of infants survive without disability or with only mild disabilities. They believe that the background pattern of EEGs before and after the onset of SE is an important predictor of disease prognosis [3]. Patients with HIE almost always have seizures, and many patients suffer from SE. The overall prognosis can be divided into four types: (a) complete recovery without functional damage; (b) recovery but functional damage; (c) death; (d) VS. aEEG can help predict the prognosis of patients. Spitzmiller et al. [18] conducted a literature meta-analysis on the value of aEEGs in judging the prognosis of patients with HIE. They found that the sensitivity of aEEGs in judging the prognosis of such patients was 91% (95% CI [87–95]). It is believed that aEEG is a useful tool for identifying patients with HIE and determining which patients with HIE are most likely to respond to treatment.

#### 8.3.5.2 The Role of BIS in Judging the Prognosis of Patients with SE

BIS is a tool for judging the depth of anesthesia. The BIS is usually over 80–100 for consciousness, 60–80 for mildly impaired consciousness, and 40–60 for severely impaired consciousness. When the BIS is lower than 40, the prognosis is usually poor. The accuracy of the BIS in judging the poor prognosis of patients can exceed 80%, when it is with a critical value lower than 40 (see the Sect. 16.4 for details).

#### 8.3.5.3 Video-EEG to Judge the Prognosis of Patients with SE

- *EEG-R*: EEG-R is an inspection method that has been used with wide application in qEEG in clinical practice. EEG-R refers to the changes in EEG amplitude or frequency after standardized stimulation. Clinical studies have found that the prognosis of those who do not show EEG-R is very poor (see the Sect. 4.3 for details).
- *EEG BS ratio*: The BS ratio refers to the percentage of suppression activity accounting for brain electrical activity within the selected range. When the BS ratio on the EEGs of neurocritical patients exceeds 0.239, the mortality of the patient is significantly increased, with a sensitivity of 97.1% and a specificity of 73.3%.
- *Sleep EEG*: Sleep is the most primitive structure of humans, and the various metabolites produced during the day can be excreted into the CSF and discharged through the veins to maintain brain metabolism only during sleep.

When disease damages sleep structure or function, the patient's prognosis will be significantly affected. Existing studies have shown that a patient's prognosis is poor when the sleep-waking cycle disappears and the sleep structure is disturbed, and sleep EEG can provide information on whether a sleep-waking cycle is present (Figs. 8.21 and 8.22) and whether the sleep structure is abnormal to help medical staff judge the patient's prognosis (see the Chap. 5 for details).

## 8.4 New Developments in Multimodal EEG

### 8.4.1 Improvement of EEG Electrodes

The condition of neurocritical patients is complex and requires monitoring multiple physiological indicators, thereby reducing the space available for placing EEG electrodes. To overcome this difficulty, Westover et al. [19] conducted an interesting experiment, and they retrospectively collected 212 adult EEGs, which were reviewed by two epilepsy experts. They

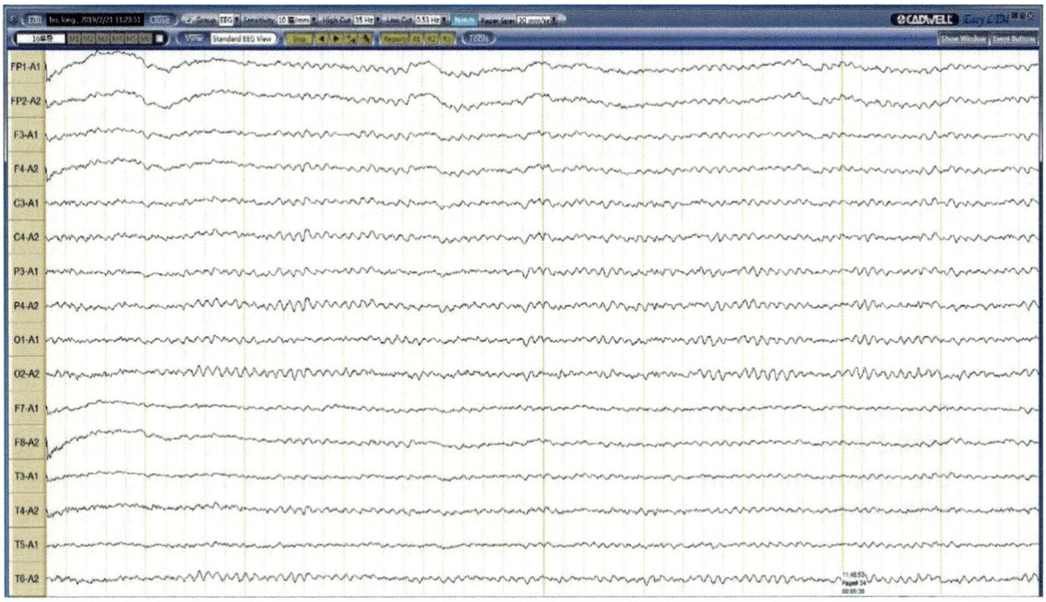

**Fig. 8.21** EEG showing alpha background activity during the awake period

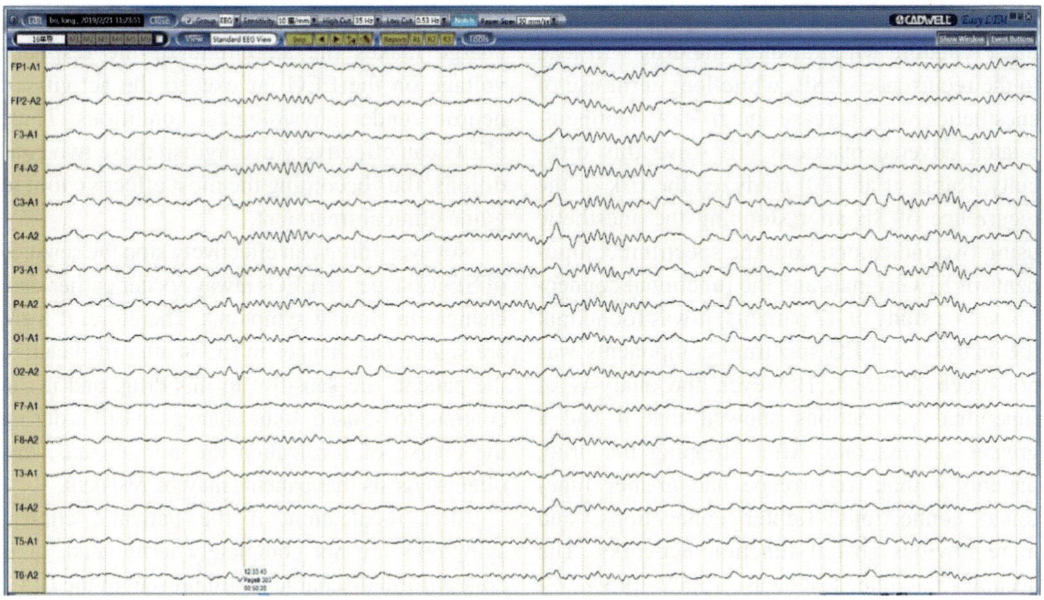

**Fig. 8.22** EEG showing the apex, spindles, and the K-complex wave during sleep

could obtain clinical, trend, and video information and then reconfigure the EEG of the first 4 h with ten electrodes. New readers were asked to explain the EEG without obtaining any other auxiliary information. As a result, they found that in the selected 95 EEGs without seizures, readers found that 92 (97%) had no seizures. Of the 117 EEGs with "seizures", none of them were marked on the EEG. Normally, in the pathological activity reported by readers, 77 cases were marked as epileptic seizures, 24 cases as rhythmic or periodic patterns, 7 cases as epileptiform discharge and 6 cases as exposure suppression. The authors believe that the placement of ten electrodes in a circular configuration can both retain the key functions of the traditional EEG system and reduce the electrode placement space.

### 8.4.2 Predicting the Recurrence of RSE After the Discontinuation of Anesthetics

RSE often requires the use of anesthetics. After successfully controlling SE, the anesthetic needs to be stopped. However, until now, there have been almost no data to guide the withdrawal of anesthetics for patients with SE. Premature withdrawal of the drug will lead to the recurrence of SE, while long-term use of anesthetics will increase the risk of treatment-related adverse reactions. To solve this difficulty, Rubin et al. [20] analyzed the risk of the recurrence of SE after stopping the anesthetic using two indicators, both the spectrum components of EEG signals and the functional connections. In a study of 47 patients, it was found that the analysis of EEG spectrum components was not much different. However, the analysis of functional connections showed that it had a greater success rate. After stopping the drug, patients without recurrence had greater functional connections, tighter connections, and more obvious spatial function networks. The accuracy of the test was 75.5% (95% CI [73.1–77.8]).

## 8.5 Discussion

Almost all patients with HIE develop seizures that easily convert to SE. The ILAE advocates the classification of SE into two categories: CSE and NCSE. The former has obvious motor symptoms, and the latter is mainly characterized by mental behavior abnormalities and consciousness disorders. After the seizure, the consciousness disorders in this patient may have been NCSE or a consciousness disorder caused by HIE, or both. The most important method for definitive diagnosis is EEG. EEG monitoring at admission showed sustained epileptiform discharges, suggesting that she may have had NCSE and that treatment was needed to terminate its onset.

The treatment of SE requires not only the termination of the patient's clinical seizures but also the termination of epileptiform discharges on the EEG. Without EEG guidance, treatment is difficult to complete. Unlike pure seizures, traditional seizures are transient, and it is difficult to capture the presence of epileptiform discharges with EEG. SE lasts for a long time and is easily found by EEG. Simultaneously, SE is caused by the highly synchronized abnormal discharge of thousands of neurons. This discharge makes the amplitude of the response voltage on the EEG far exceed the activity of neurons under physiological conditions. Thus, aEEG can effectively distinguish these two conditions, thus becoming the most effective tool to guide clinical treatment.

Not every drug can effectively stop the seizures of SE. Changes in EEGs always occur earlier than changes in clinical symptoms. Therefore, if there are significant changes in EEGs after medication, the patients are sensitive to this drug, and it can continue to be used. If the changes in EEGs during the course of medication are not obvious, this often suggests that patients may be resistant.

After medication, if the patient's clinical symptoms are not completely terminated, or if epileptiform discharge is still present in the EEG, this suggests either that the drug dose is insufficient or that the patient is resistant to the drug. The former necessitates an increase in the dose of the drug, and the latter requires a change in the drug; the index EEG can help judge which choice is correct. When the index EEG reaches 40–50%, the drug dose has reached its maximum (Fig. 8.23a, b). Then, if we continually increase

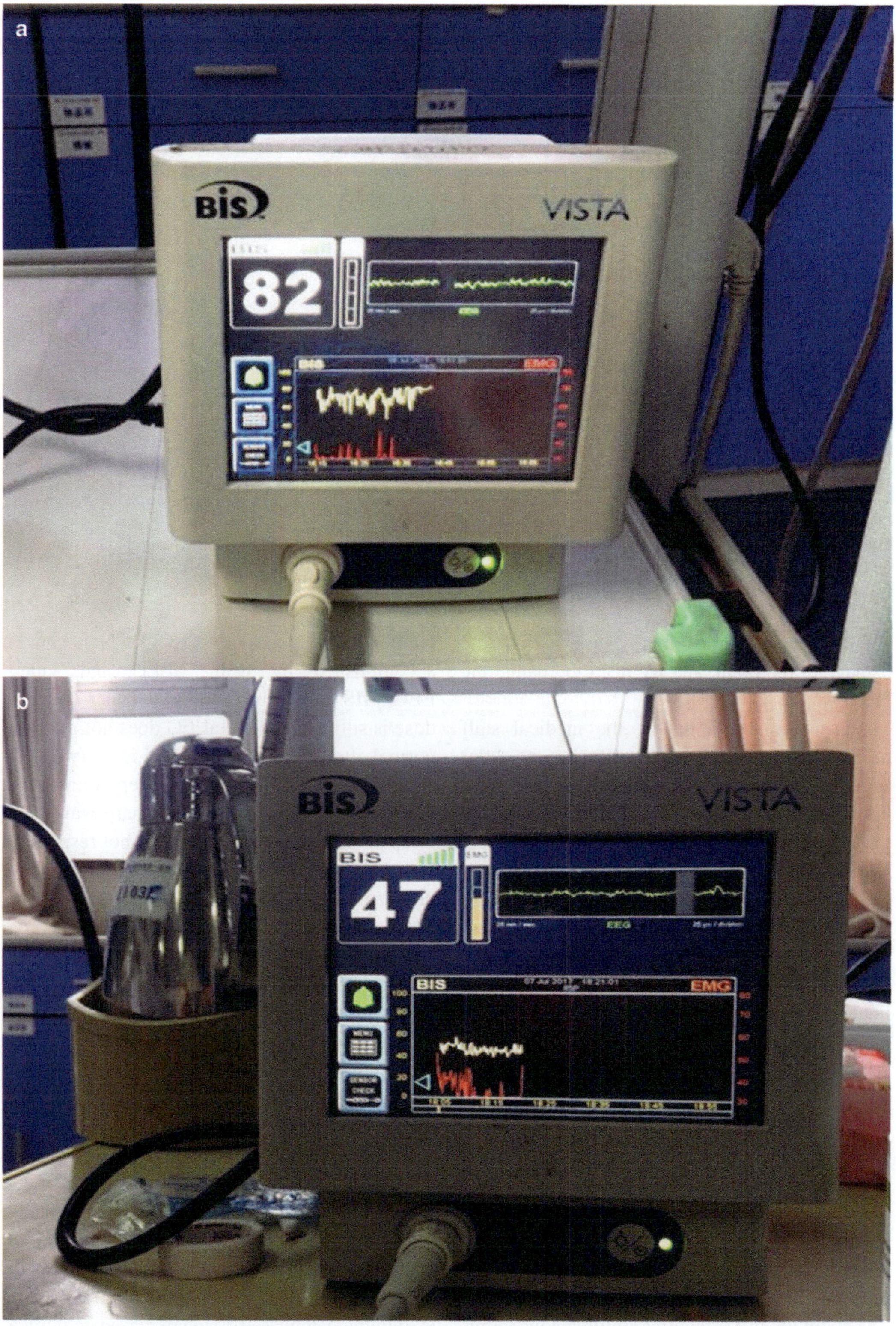


**Fig. 8.23** (**a**) The BIS value before medication is 82. (**b**) The BIS decreased after propofol injection, and the index value was 47

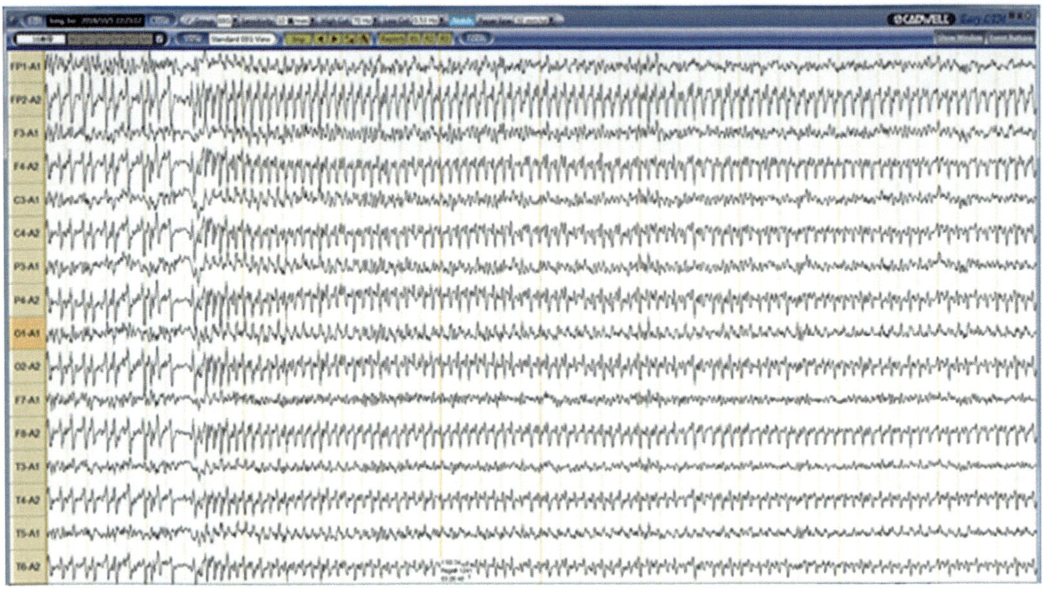

**Fig. 8.24** EEG showing NCSEs: a spike rhythm can be found in all channels. In addition, the right channels are more obvious

the dosage, the drugs may cause irreversible damage to the brain, and we need to change the medicine.

When SE is terminated, the medical staff needs to judge the prognosis of the patient. After HIE, the aEEG, which can reflect comprehensive brain function, returns to normal within 24 h, and the patient's consciousness can often recover with almost no sequelae. If the aEEG does not recover after more than 72 h, this suggests a very poor prognosis. If the sleep cycle is disordered, vertex sharp waves disappear, sleep spindles are unclear, and the EEG does not respond to sound, light, or pain stimulation, this often suggests a poor prognosis.

**Case**

EEGs indicate that when a sudden cessation of cardiopulmonary function causes brain ischemia, and even if the heart and lung function recover quickly, the patient will have difficulty regaining consciousness. Almost all patients with HIE develop SE, especially NCSE, and EEG is the most reliable tool for understanding its etiology. The treatment of SE requires simultaneous termination of the patient's clinical seizures and epileptiform discharges on EEGs, which can be accomplished by using aEEG and video-EEG. BIS can help us judge whether the drug dose is sufficient. If the aEEG does not return to normal after 72 h, sleep EEG can identify a sleep rhythm disorder. If important sleep components are not present, such as vertex sharp waves and sleep spindles, and the EEG does not respond to sound, light, or pain stimulation, this often suggests a poor prognosis.

Case X was a formerly healthy 28-year-old woman. On February 21, 2017, the patient went to the local hospital to prepare for abdominal surgery. After 5 min of anesthesia, the patient experienced cardiac arrest for unknown reasons before her breathing stopped, and CPR was immediately initiated. After 20 min, the patient's heart rhythm and spontaneous respirations recovered, but she did not regain consciousness. After 5 min, the patient developed frequent epileptic seizures that lasted 6–10 min, characterized by a sudden binocular gaze, tight jaw bite, and stiff limbs. Repeated attacks followed, and the symptoms were similar. This condition was diagnosed as SE. The medical staff immediately used 20 mg of diazepam intravenously, but to no effect. They repeated the dose

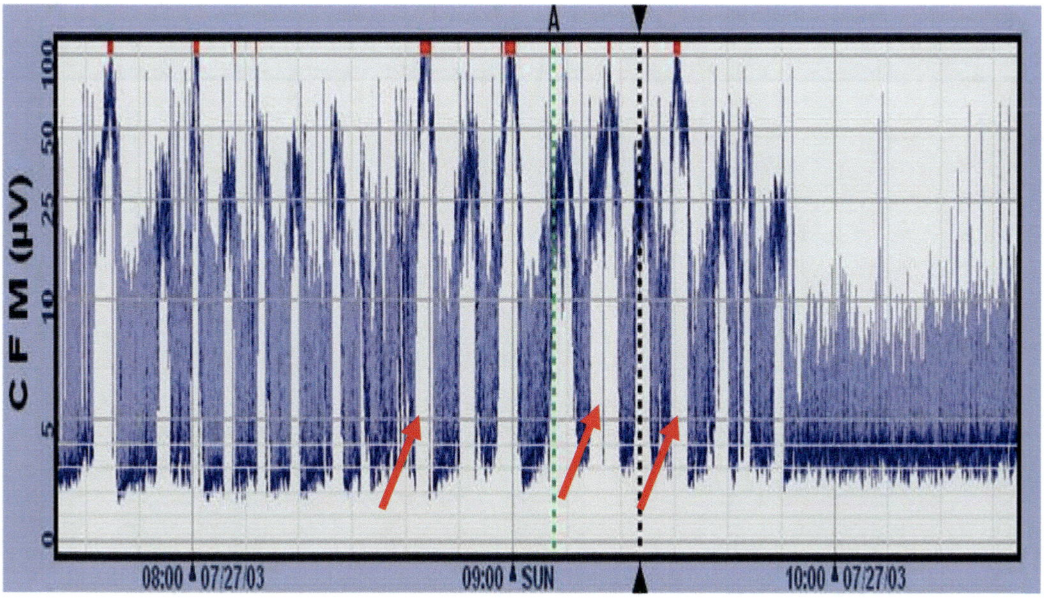


**Fig. 8.25** EEG showing NCSE: the red arrow points to the spike rhythm

once, but it was still ineffective. Then, they switched to 10 mg of midazolam intravenously, but this was also ineffective. They replaced the drug with 0.6 g of phenobarbital administered intravenously at a slow speed, and the clinical seizures stopped, but the patient did not regain consciousness. To make a definitive diagnosis, the patient was transferred to our hospital. Physical examination on admission found that the patient's consciousness was unclear, and she had no response to voice commands. The patient had spontaneous breathing of 10–12 tpm and a heart rate of 100–120 bpm. Her pupils were 0.3 cm in diameter. The size and shape of the bilateral pupils were identical, and there was no pupillary light reflex. The bilateral pathological reflex was positive. Venous blood examination was performed, including examinations of routine blood, electrolyte, liver and kidney function, and blood biochemical parameters. Arterial blood was drawn for blood gas analysis, and a multiconductive physiological tester was immediately placed. The results of the EEG examination are shown in Fig. 8.24, and they suggested the presence of NCSE. Under aEEG and EEG monitoring (Figs. 8.24 and 8.25), a 100 mg propofol intravenous bolus was given, and the EEG was unchanged from an intermittent generalized tonic seizure. The BIS was 82. Then, we pushed 50 mg of propofol. The BIS was 47 (Fig. 8.23a, b), and the seizure was slightly reduced. We stopped the injection and replaced it with 100 mg of ketamine administered intravenously at a slow speed (Fig. 8.26a, b). When injected at 50 mg, the epileptiform discharge on the EEG was significantly reduced. The BIS was 74. Ketamine was continued with a bolus of 100 mg, the clinical seizure stopped, and the video-EEG showed BS (Fig. 8.27). The bolus was stopped, and the dose was maintained intravenously at 100 mg/h, while 125 ml of 20% mannitol was given Q8h, in addition to an IV bolus being added. Simultaneously, life function support was strengthened. The EEG was continuously monitored for 7 h, during which no epileptiform discharges occurred (Fig. 8.28). Then, the ketamine was reduced to 10 mg/h. After 6 h, ketamine was stopped and switched to 1200 mg/d intravenous valproic acid, which was maintained. At this time, the patient's consciousness was still unclear, the cardiopulmonary function was basically normal, and head CT indicated diffuse mild cerebral edema.

a

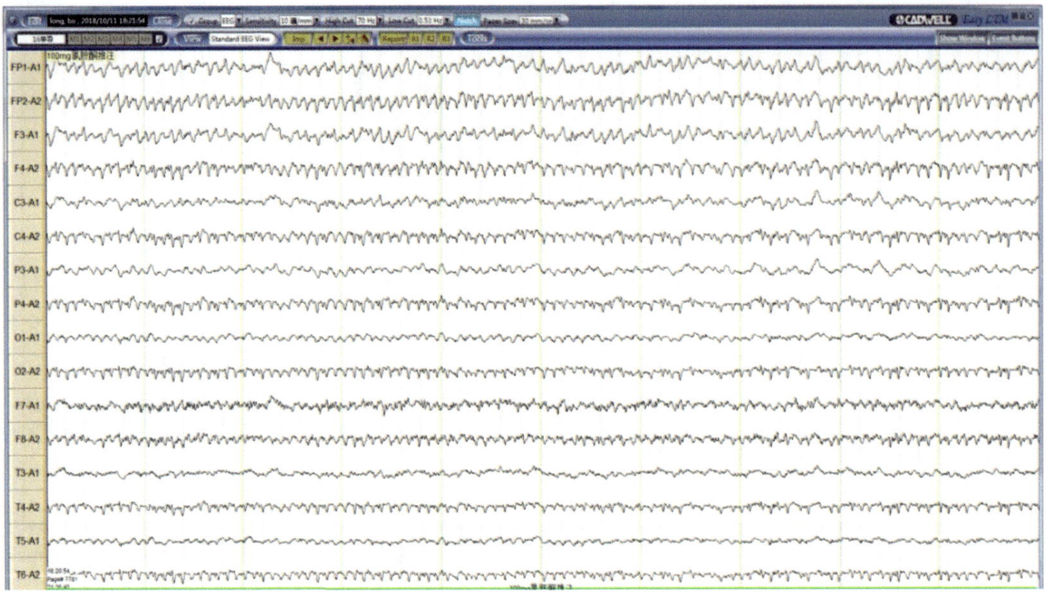


b

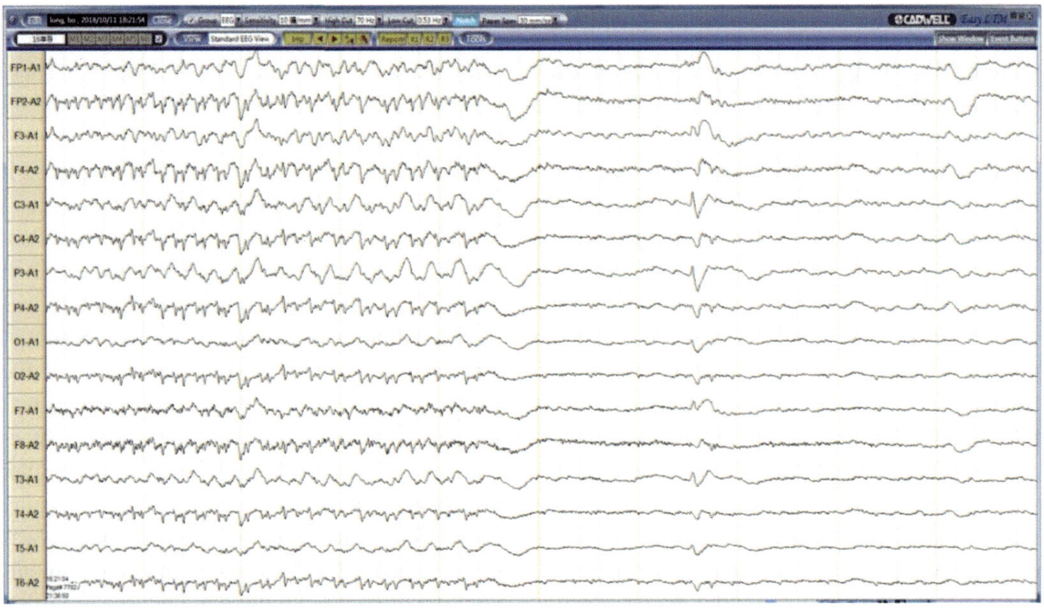


**Fig. 8.26** (**a**) EEG at the beginning of the intravenous bolus of ketamine. (**b**) EEG during ketamine push. Compared to the spike of the previous EEG, the frequency and voltage of the spike at this time are significantly reduced, indicating that epileptiform discharge is controlled

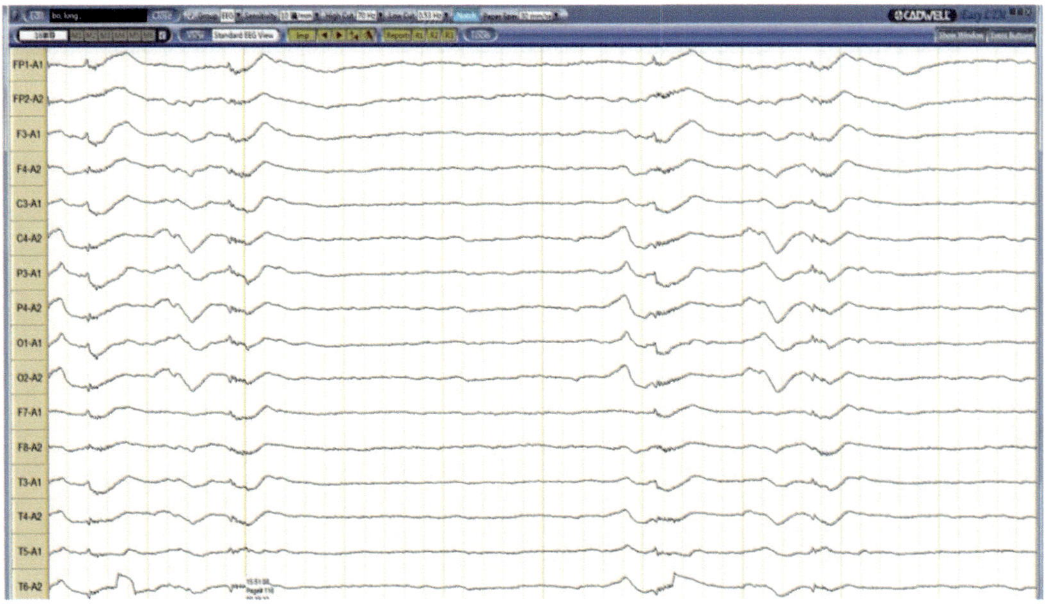

**Fig. 8.27** Ketamine was continued with a bolus of 100 mg, the clinical seizure stopped, and the video-EEG showed BS

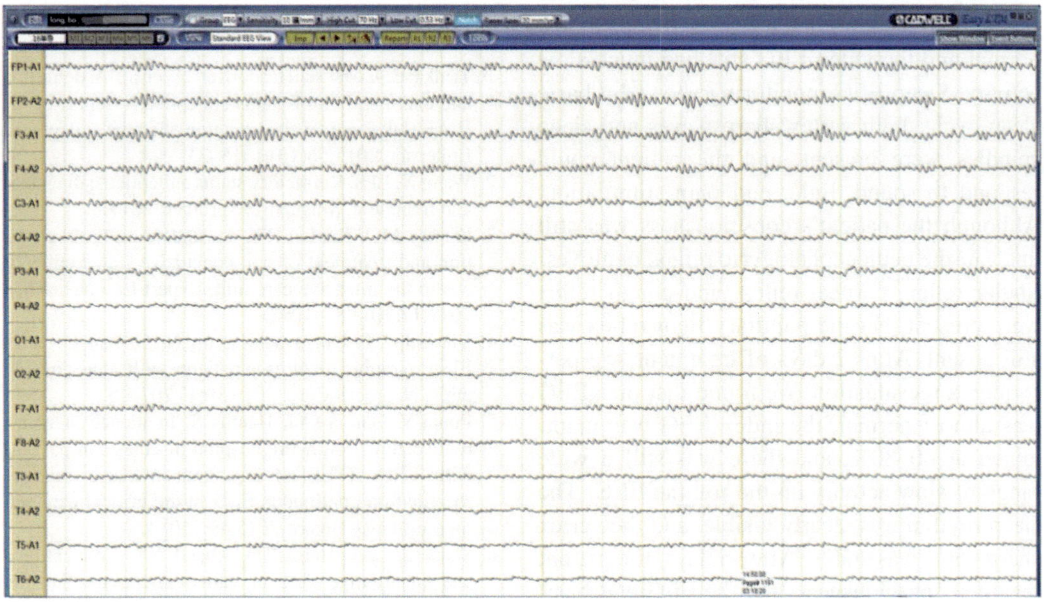

**Fig. 8.28** The EEG was continuously monitored for 7 h, during which no epileptiform discharges occurred

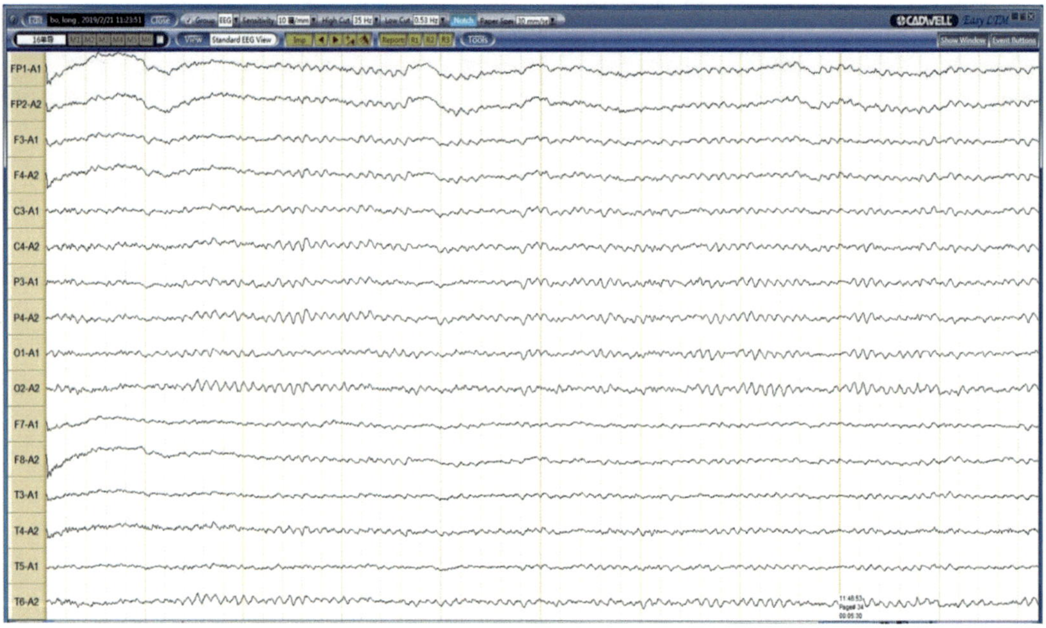

**Fig. 8.29** The video-EEG was normal after 45 days

The patient's first EEG assessment 24 h after seizure onset showed the aEEG to be almost normal and the video-EEG still had much slow activity. Sleep EEG monitoring showed a basic sleep cycle; both vertex sharp waves and sleep spindles were present, and the patient could respond to sound, light, and pain stimulation. Although the patient's consciousness was still unclear, the oculocephalogyric reflex, oculovestibular reflex, corneal reflex, and cough reflex were present, but the pupillary light reflex was still absent. After 2 days of treatment, we performed a reevaluation. We found that the aEEG was almost normal, the index EEG was maintained at 60–80%, and there was still a wide range of slow activity on the routine EEG. The sleep rhythm was clearly visible, and the vertex sharp wave was stable. After 6 days, the patient regained consciousness, and the EEG was basically normal (Fig. 8.29), but the reaction was still insensitive. After 45 days in the hospital, she was discharged. After half a year, the patient had basically returned to normal life.

## References


1. Trinka E, Cock H, Hesdorffer D, et al. A definition and classification of status epilepticus—report of the ILAE task force on classification of status epilepticus. Epilepsia. 2015;56(10):1515–23.
2. Wang X, Li S. Refractory status epilepticus: diagnosis and treatment. Singapore: Springer; 2017.
3. Kinney MO, Kaplan PW. An update on the recognition and treatment of non-convulsive status epilepticus in the intensive care unit. Expert Rev Neurother. 2017;17(10):987–1002.
4. Viarasilpa T, Panyavachiraporn N, Osman G, et al. Electrographic seizures in patients with acute encephalitis. Neurocrit Care. 2019;30(1):207–15.
5. Punia V, Garcia CG, Hantus S. Incidence of recurrent seizures following hospital discharge in patients with LPDs (PLEDs) and nonconvulsive seizures recorded on continuous EEG in the critical care setting. Epilepsy Behav. 2015;49:250–4.
6. Sansevere AJ, Hahn CD, Abend NS. Conventional and quantitative EEG in status epilepticus. Seizure. 2019;68:38–45.
7. Sansevere AJ, Duncan ED, Libenson MH, et al. Continuous EEG in pediatric critical care: yield and efficiency of seizure detection. J Clin Neurophysiol. 2017;34(5):421–6.

8. Abend NS, Chapman KE, Gallentine WB, et al. Electroencephalographic monitoring in the pediatric intensive care unit. Curr Neurol Neurosci Rep. 2013;13(3):330.
9. Leitinger M, Trinka E, Gardella E, et al. Diagnostic accuracy of the Salzburg EEG criteria for non-convulsive status epilepticus: a retrospective study. Lancet Neurol. 2016;15(10):1054–62.
10. Leitinger M, Beniczky S, Rohracher A, et al. Salzburg consensus criteria for non-convulsive status epilepticus—approach to clinical application. Epilepsy Behav. 2015;49:158–63.
11. Laccheo I, Sonmezturk H, Bhatt AB, et al. Non-convulsive status epilepticus and non-convulsive seizures in neurological ICU patients. Neurocrit Care. 2015;22(2):202–11.
12. Fatema K, Rahman MM, Akhter S, et al. Non-convulsive status epilepticus in children: clinical profile, EEG characteristics and treatment. Mymensingh Med J. 2018;27(1):185–92.
13. Mastrangelo M, Fiocchi I, Fontana P, et al. Acute neonatal encephalopathy and seizures recurrence: a combined aEEG/EEG study. Seizure. 2013;22(9):703–7.
14. van Rooij LG, de Vries LS, Handryastuti S, et al. Neurodevelopmental outcome in term infants with status epilepticus detected with amplitude-integrated electroencephalography. Pediatrics. 2007;120(2):e354–63.
15. Froscher W. Sleep and prolonged epileptic activity (status epilepticus). Epilepsy Res Suppl. 1991;2:165–76.
16. Caraballo RH, Veggiotti P, Kaltenmeier MC, et al. Encephalopathy with status epilepticus during sleep or continuous spikes and waves during slow sleep syndrome: a multicenter, long-term follow-up study of 117 patients. Epilepsy Res. 2013;105(1–2):164–73.
17. Hellstrom-Westas L, Rosen I. Continuous brain-function monitoring: state of the art in clinical practice. Semin Fetal Neonatal Med. 2006;11(6):503–11.
18. Spitzmiller RE, Phillips T, Meinzen-Derr J, et al. Amplitude-integrated EEG is useful in predicting neurodevelopmental outcome in full-term infants with hypoxic-ischemic encephalopathy: a meta-analysis. J Child Neurol. 2007;22(9):1069–78.
19. Westover MB, Gururangan K, Markert MS, et al. Diagnostic value of electroencephalography with ten electrodes in critically ill patients. Neurocrit Care. 2020;33(2):479–90.
20. Rubin DB, Angelini B, Shoukat M, et al. Electrographic predictors of successful weaning from anaesthetics in refractory status epilepticus. Brain. 2020;143(4):1143–57.

# Clinical Application of Multimodal EEG in Acute Ischemic Stroke

9

Shengnian Zhou and Suyue Pan

## Contents



**Abstract**

Acute ischemic stroke conveys high disability and high mortality and has created huge medical care and economic burdens to the world. The focus of acute ischemic stroke includes the ischemic central area and the surrounding ischemic penumbra. Because there are still a large number of surviving neurons in the brain tissue of the ischemic penumbra, quickly restoring blood flow in this region can effectively save nerve cell function in the ischemic area and restore brain tissue function, which is very important for reducing disability and mortality in ischemic stroke. Since nerve cells can rapidly change their potential after ischemia and hypoxia, electroencephalogram (EEG) can be used as a sensitive indicator that reflects the electrical activity of brain tissue, cerebral blood flow, and brain function. EEG has characteristic manifestations for different levels of ischemia, different ischemic locations, and different ischemic ranges of brain tissue. Therefore, cEEG monitoring can assist clinicians in the early judgment of patients' brain function and in making clinical decisions. In this chapter, based on the pathophysiological basis of EEG changes in patients with ischemic stroke, we introduce the characteristics of multimodal EEG and related parameters of qEEG in ischemic stroke. At the same time, the relationship between multimodal EEG and the brain function and prognosis of patients is explained to provide an effective reference for the early prognostic judgment

S. Zhou
Department of Neurology, Qilu Hospital of Shandong University and Brain Science Research Institute, Shandong University, Jinan, Shandong, China
e-mail: zhoushengnian@sdu.edu.cn

S. Pan (✉)
Department of Neurology, Nanfang Hospital of Southern Medical University, Guangzhou, Guangdong, China
e-mail: pansuyue@smu.edu.cn



X. Wang et al. (eds.), *Multi-Modal EEG Monitoring of Severely Neurologically Ill Patients*,
https://doi.org/10.1007/978-981-16-4493-1_9

and clinical decision-making in patients with acute ischemic stroke.

**Keywords**

Acute ischemic stroke · Multimodal EEG · Ischemic penumbra · Slow-wave activity · ADR · RBP · Brain symmetry index (BSI) · Prognosis

Acute ischemic stroke is a general term for insufficient blood supply to the brain due to stenosis, occlusion or embolism in the arteries supplying blood to the brain. The focal symptoms and nervous system signs caused by ischemic stroke are consistent with the blood supply area of the affected cerebrovascular. Acute ischemic stroke is the disease with the highest disability rate in the world. Up to 70% of patients have residual moderate or severe disease. Functional impairment is common in acute ischemic stroke patients, and acute ischemic stroke has a very high mortality rate [1]. According to the Trial of ORG 10172 in Acute Stroke Treatment (TOAST) classification, acute ischemic stroke is divided into five types: large-artery atherosclerosis, cardiogenic embolism, arteriolar embolism, stroke with other clear etiology, and stroke with an unknown cause. The most common type is aortic atherosclerosis [2]. Owing to vascular wall disease caused by atherosclerosis or other reasons, the lumen of arteries is narrowed and occluded, or thrombosis occurs, resulting in ischemia and a lack of local PbtO2 due to the interruption of the blood supply. The resulting necrosis causes corresponding neurological symptoms and signs.

The focus of acute ischemic stroke is composed of the ischemic central area and the surrounding ischemic penumbra. The CBF threshold of the ischemic central area is 10 ml/(100 g.min), energy metabolism fails, and the brain tissue is irreversibly damaged. The blood flow in the ischemic penumbra is between electrical failure (20 ml)/(100 g.min) and energy metabolism failure [at a blood flow of 10 ml/(100 g.min)], and there is residual blood flow in the large arteries and collateral circulation in the local brain tissue, and a large number of surviving neurons. If the blood flow in the ischemic penumbra can be quickly restored in a short period of time, the function of brain tissue in this area is restorable, and nerve cells can survive and their function can be restored [3]. Therefore, it is very important to restore the blood supply to the ischemic penumbra as soon as possible and to apply effective brain protection drugs to reduce the disability rate of ischemic stroke.

## 9.1 Pathophysiological Basis of EEG Changes in Ischemic Stroke

Nerve cells have potential changes more than 10 s after complete ischemia and hypoxia. After 20–30 s, the bioelectrical activity of the cerebral cortex disappears, and the bioelectrical activity of the cerebellum and medulla oblongata also disappears after 30–90 s. When cerebral artery blood flow is interrupted for 5 min, nerve cells will be irreversibly damaged. The energy of severely ischemic brain tissue is quickly exhausted, and the function of energy-dependent nerve cell membranes fails, causing membrane depolarization and a massive release of presynaptic excitatory transmitters (mainly glutamate and aspartate). Ca2+ in the extracellular fluid enters human cells through voltage-gated channels. Due to insufficient ATP supply and lactic acidosis in the cells, a large amount of combined calcium in the cells is released. The imbalance in intracellular Ca2+ homeostasis starts with ischemic damage to nerve cells, with an important role of intracellular calcium overload. A variety of enzymes regulated by Ca2+ are activated, leading to membrane phospholipid decomposition and cytoskeletal destruction, generating a large number of free radicals and resulting in irreversible damage to cells. In the above process, transcription factors, as well as the synthesis and production of inflammatory mediators, are involved [4, 5].

## 9.2 EEG Manifestations of Ischemic Stroke

Because pyramidal cells are very sensitive to decreased cerebral blood flow (CBF) and hypoxia, some researchers have introduced the monitoring of conventional EEGs to the early evaluation of patients with acute ischemic stroke [6]. There is a good correlation between the degree of abnormality in EEGs and the degree of local CBF decline. The EEG waveforms from the center of the infarct focus to the surrounding normal brain tissue are FT, low flat slow waves, large slow waves, θ waves, and slow α waves [7]. The blood supply area of the involved blood vessel determines the location of the brain injury and the corresponding clinical manifestations, and EEGs can reflect the location and degree of the brain injury. The larger the infarct size and the shallower the site, the more obvious the EEG abnormalities; damage to the deep blood vessels (such as in brainstem and cerebellar vascular disease) is farther from the cortex [8]. It is worth noting that a large area of cerebral infarction can cause secondary extensive cerebral edema (Fig. 9.1) and increased ICP, leading to diffuse abnormalities in EEGs, which mask the focal abnormalities. Abnormalities may be difficult to find in scalp EEGs. In acute ischemic stroke, in addition to focal or extensive slow-wave activities, various physiological brain electrical activities can also be weakened to varying degrees, such as a decrease in the occipital lobe α rhythm (Fig. 9.2), a disappearance of one side of the sleep spindle wave (Fig. 9.3), or an attenuation of the top wave (Fig. 9.4). The presence of local electrical suppression of background activity has significance for the localization of the lesion, and the retention of background fast-wave activity indicates that a considerable number of neurons still

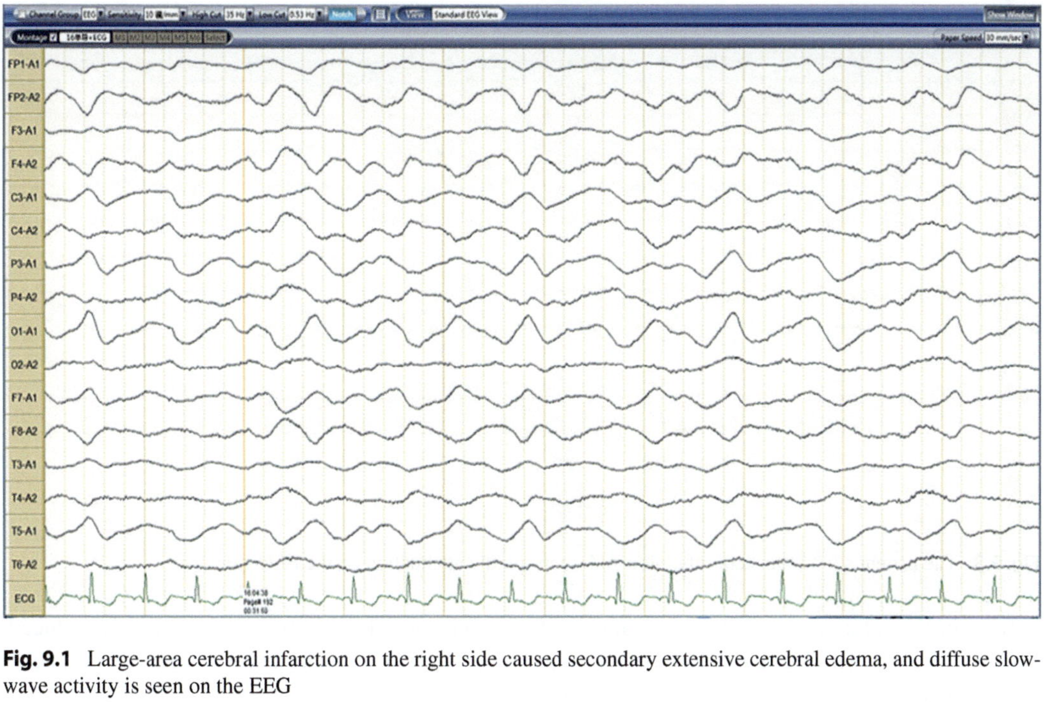


**Fig. 9.1** Large-area cerebral infarction on the right side caused secondary extensive cerebral edema, and diffuse slow-wave activity is seen on the EEG

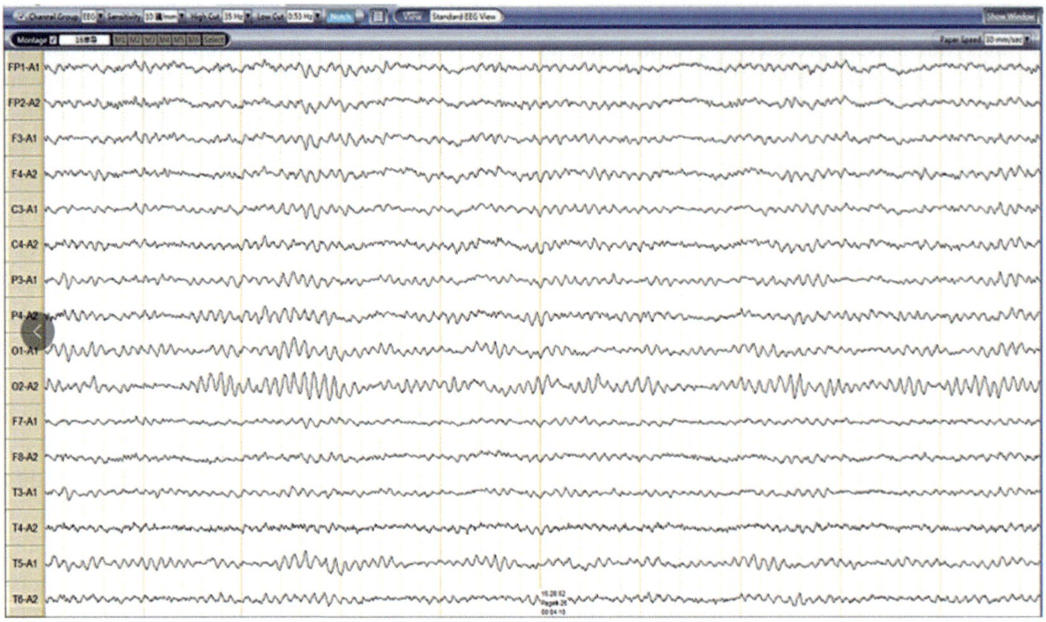


**Fig. 9.2** Cerebral vasospasm occurred, and α rhythm decreased in the back of the head

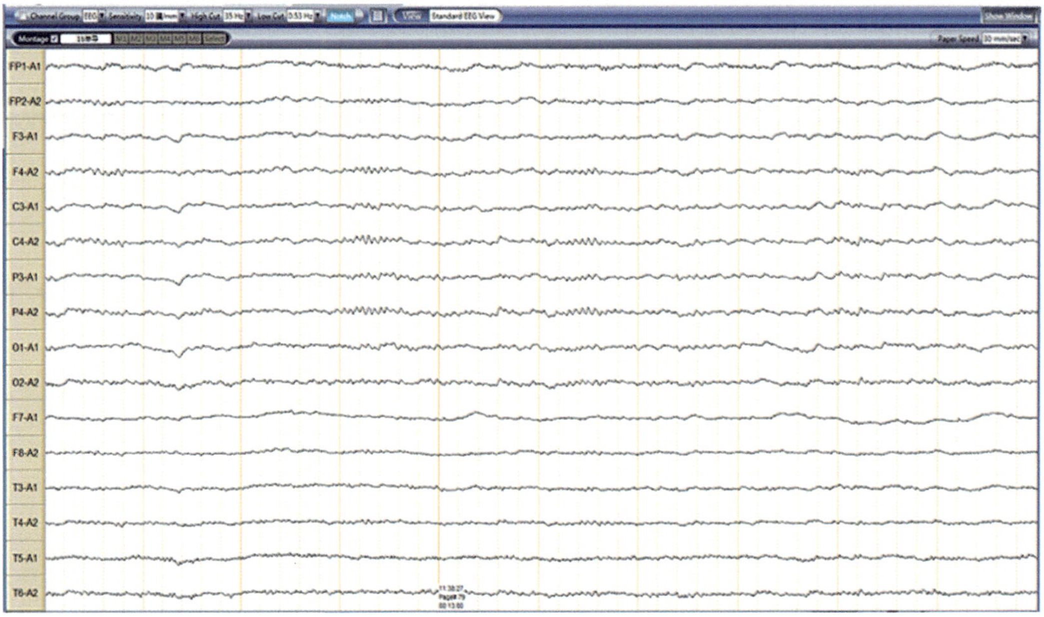


**Fig. 9.3** The patient's left brainstem infarction and sleep spindle attenuation on the EEG side

survive in the infarcted area. A large number of studies have shown that the EEG background activity on the damaged cerebral hemisphere side is dominated by slow activity, continuous pleomorphic δ activity is significantly increased, α activity and β activity are significantly reduced, and EEG background activity appears asymmetrical.

Compared with neuroimaging (head CT, MRI, and cerebrovascular angiography), EEG is

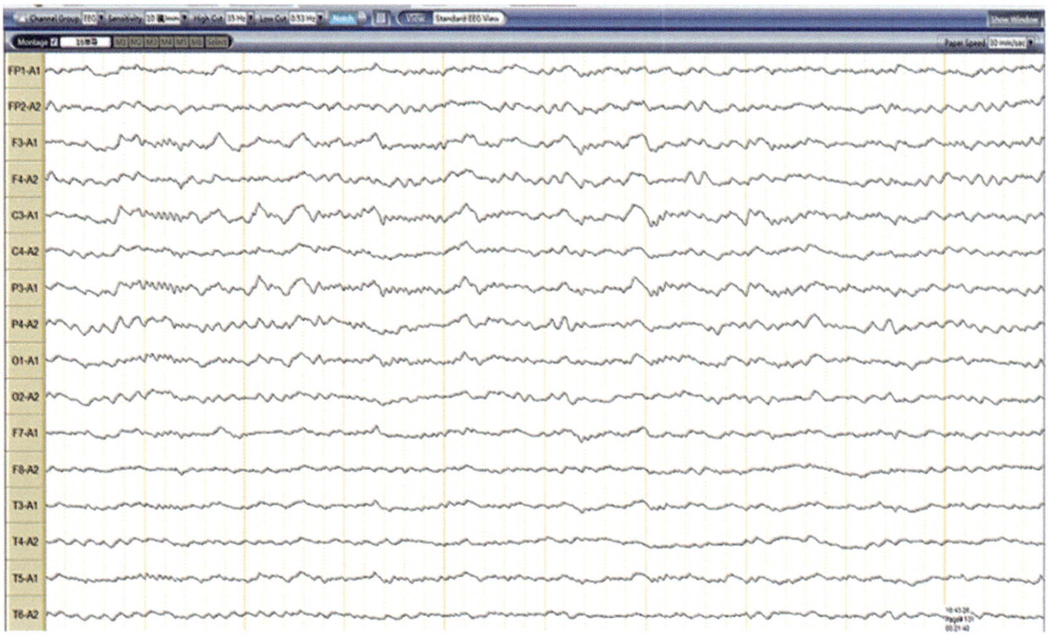


**Fig. 9.4** The patient's right brainstem infarction, sleep spindle and apex wave attenuation on the EEG side

very sensitive to cortical ischemia and brain dysfunction, and focal or extensive brain dysfunction can be found in the early stages. About 30 s after CBF is blocked, EEGs show abnormal changes. When the CBF drops to 25–30 ml/(100 g.min), EEGs show that the fast wave disappears quickly, and the slow-wave background appears. A decrease in CBF to 8–10 ml/(100 g. min) will cause irreversible cell death, and all brain electrical activity will be inhibited. It takes 2–6 h for MRI and 1–5 days for CT to reflect a change following stroke [9]. Therefore, cEEG monitoring can be used as a supplement to neuroimaging, as this helps to detect reversible damage early and guide clinical intervention in a timely manner.

Ischemia in different parts has different characteristics on EEGs. Studies [10–12] pointed out that all frequencies are attenuated without corresponding δ waves. This is a typical EEG characteristic of patients with acute severe focal cerebral ischemia, and it suggests malignant cerebral edema (Fig. 9.5); patients with cerebral infarction in a large portion of the middle cerebral artery supply area have asymmetrical background activity, the pleomorphic δ activity of the affected cerebral hemispheres increases, particularly in the temporal and frontotemporal areas. The ipsilateral α and β activities and sleep spindle wave weaken or disappear, and the synchronization of α and θ activities is enhanced. In patients with extensive cerebral hemisphere infarction, all brain electrical activities in the affected cerebral hemisphere are significantly inhibited due to the space-occupying effect and the shift in the midline, there may be δ activity and intermittent paroxysmal δ rhythm in the contralateral frontal area, and the above changes are obvious in the acute phase of ischemia. Jordan et al. [3] found that if 45% of cerebral ischemia deteriorated within 24 h of onset, the EEG features showed increased focal slow-wave activity, spike-like discharge or widespread slow waves, and as the condition improved, 50% changes in these EEG parameters preceded clinical changes, manifesting as partial or complete disappearance of focal slow waves.

EEGs have value for predicting the prognosis of patients with acute ischemic stroke. Patients with slow activity on the damaged cerebral hemisphere side often have a poor prognosis (Fig. 9.6). In contrast, patients with insignificant changes in

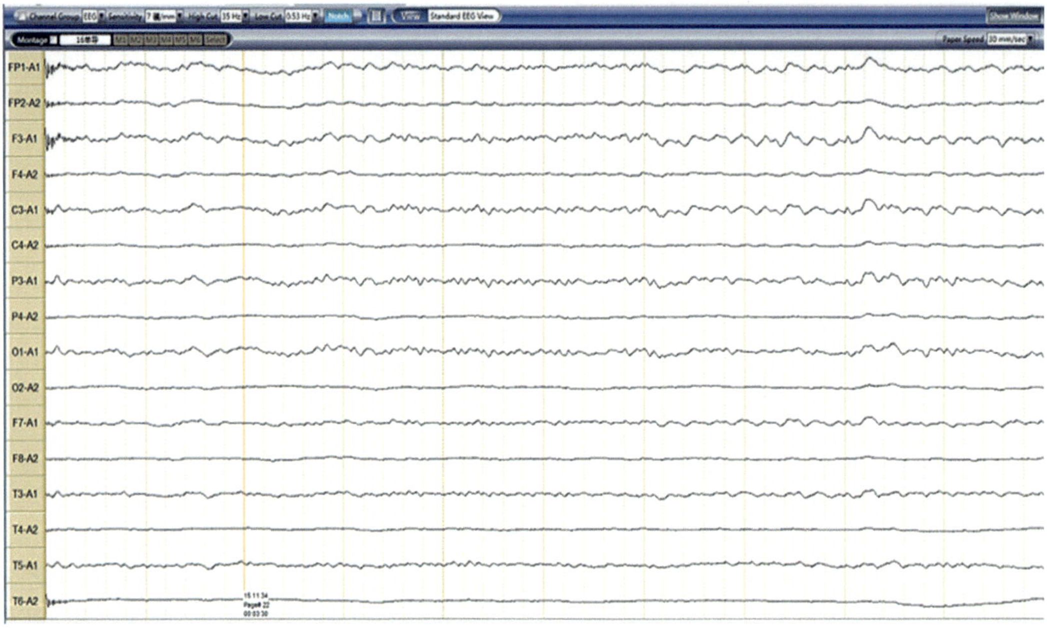


**Fig. 9.5** A large area of cerebral infarction is shown on the right, and a suppression of EEG activity is shown on the right

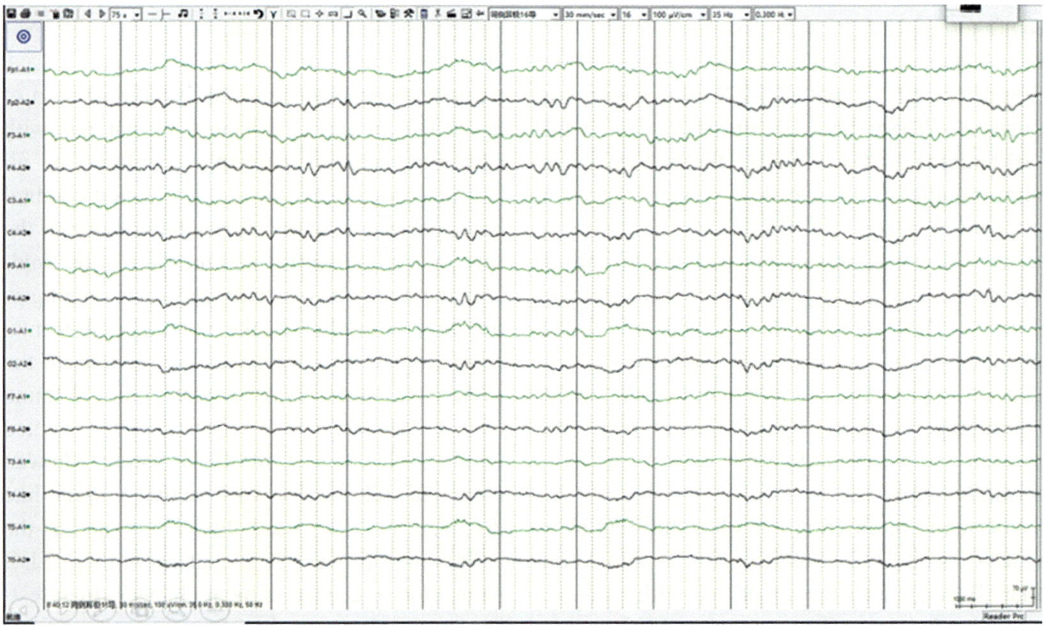

**Fig. 9.6** Left brainstem infarction. The EEG slow-wave activity on the left cerebral hemisphere is increased, and the patient had a poor prognosis

background activity tend to have a good prognosis (Fig. 9.7). Carla Bentes et al. [13] compared the early EEG results and long-term (1 year) prognosis of patients with acute cerebral infarction and found that early EEGs showed the activity of patients with less slow activity and fast

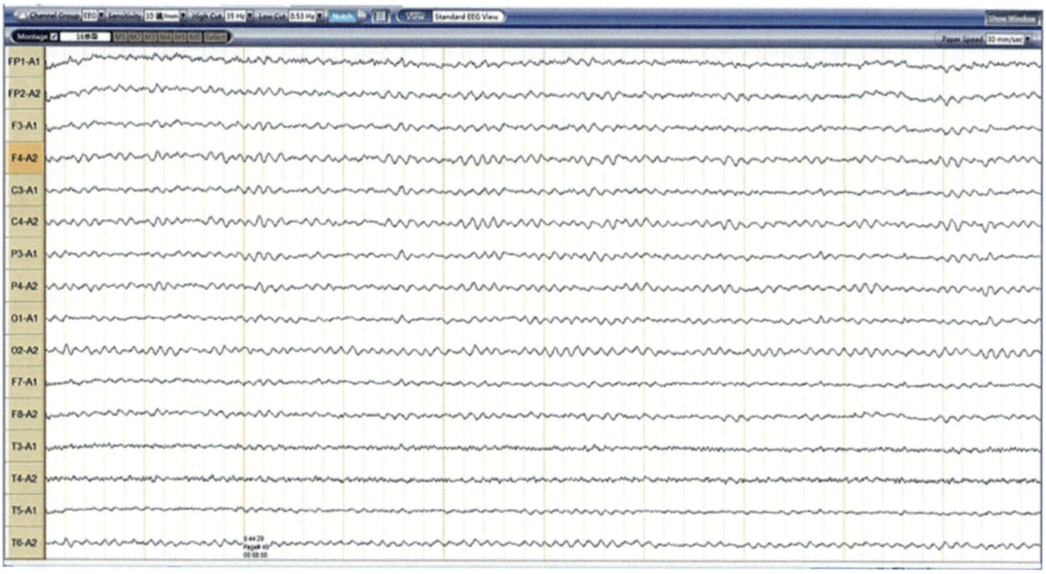

**Fig. 9.7** For cerebral infarction in the left basal ganglia area, the frequency on the left side slowed slightly, the background activity changes little, and the patient had a good prognosis

activity was not inhibited, and the long-term prognosis was good. Early EEGs also showed that when the activity of patients was inhibited and accompanied by continuous slow activity, the long-term prognosis was poor.

## 9.3 qEEG Changes in Acute Ischemic Stroke

Research on qEEGs in acute ischemic stroke mostly focuses on frequency parameters, including the total power, RBP, RAV, ADR, and BSI (Fig. 9.8). Van Putten and Tavy [14] analyzed the correlation between the power spectrum in the qEEGs of patients with anterior circulation infarction and the clinical neurological function score and found that the average power spectra of the left and right cerebral hemispheres in the qEEGs were different, as was the National Institutes of Health Stroke Scale (NIHSS) score. In addition, the researchers monitored the qEEGs of patients undergoing r-tPA thrombolytic therapy and recorded the NIHSS scores before and after thrombolysis. They also found that the power spectra of the qEEGs changed after thrombolysis. The qEEGs were significantly related to the parts of the clinical changes of the patients [15].

The qEEGs of patients with brain injury mainly manifest an increase in slow-wave frequency bands such as θ activity and δ activity, with or without a decrease in fast-wave frequency bands such as α activity and β activity. Fernandez Bouzas et al. [16] believe that δ activity and θ activity are produced from different sources. The brain electrical activity of infarcts is often expressed as δ activity, while edema around the infarction is often characterized by θ activity; δ activity is considered to be related to afferent nerve block of electrical activity in necrotic tissue. The absolute frequency band energies of δ activity and θ activity can be used as indicators for short-term prognosis evaluation, and δ activity can be used as the best choice for a long-term prognosis evaluation indicator. Finnigan et al. [17] found that in acute cerebral infarction, the change in the absolute frequency band energy of the δ activity in qEEGs was closely related to the NIHSS score 30 days after the onset of stroke, and its prognostic value was the same as the average within the lesion tissue shown by perfusion-weighted imaging (PWI) at the onset of stroke. The prognostic value was evaluated at the same

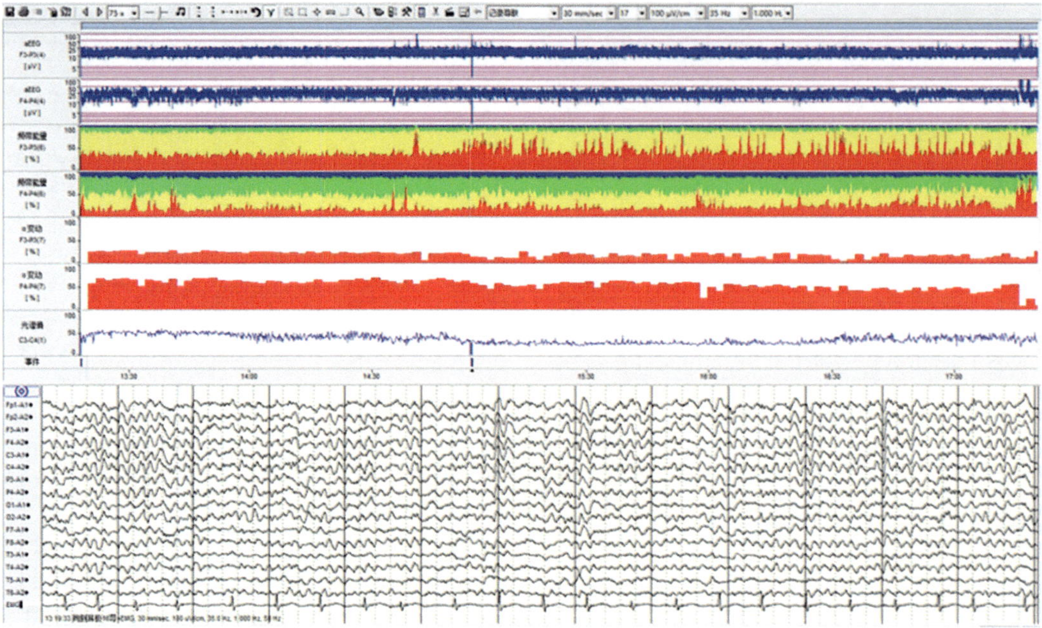

**Fig. 9.8** Frequency parameters of qEEG (RBP, RAV, etc.)

time and was greater than when the lesion volume was displayed by DWI. In addition, the subacute stroke δ/α power ratio (δ-α power ratio) and the NIHSS score had a higher correlation than the δ absolute frequency band energy.

Compared with the absolute frequency band energy, the RBP is more sensitive and intuitive in judging brain tissue ischemia. A related study found that large-area cerebral infarction manifests as asymmetrical frequency band energy between cerebral hemispheres. Among the absolute frequency band energy on the side of the lesion, only the absolute frequency band energy of the δ wave was significantly larger than that of the healthy side, and there was no significant difference in the remaining α wave, β wave, or θ wave. However, in the analysis of the RBP, the RBP of each band was significantly different between the lesion side and the healthy side. The absolute frequency band energy and RBP of the δ wave on the lesion side were significantly larger than those on the healthy side. The absolute frequency band energy was reduced, but the difference was not statistically significant, and its RBP was significantly reduced; the RBP of the θ wave was also significantly reduced. Compared with the control group, the absolute frequency band energy difference and RBP difference of δ wave in the left and right cerebral hemispheres of the infarction group were significant [18].

The BSI is a set of quantitative values obtained by FFT of the EEG. The value range of the BSI is 0–1. When the BSI is closer to 0, the brain waves in each frequency band of both hemispheres, the difference in the distribution range, and the magnitude of the amplitude are not obvious. When the BSI is closer to 1, there is a bilateral significant difference in the hemispheres, which can also be used to predict changes in brain function [19]. To further improve the sensitivity and accuracy of the index, Van Putten [20, 21] proposed a temporary BSI and a revised BSI. Sheorajpanday and De Deyn [22] proposed a paired BSI, and a large amount of research work went into the paired BSI. The correlation coefficient between the index and the area of new infarct lesions was 0.54, and the index was relatively stable.

Comparative analysis with imaging found that the paired BSI could more accurately indicate new lesions than the NIHSS score with an accuracy rate of 80%, and the paired BSI could predict the deterioration of neurological function with an accuracy rate of 95%. De Vos et al. [23] studied 16 patients who received thrombolytic therapy and found that the change in the BSI was significantly related to the NIHSS score. The ability of the BSI is stronger than that of the $\delta + \theta/\alpha + \beta$ ratio (DTABR) and NIHSS scores to predict changes in brain function after thrombolysis. In related studies on prognosis, Myles and Cairo [24] found that the prognosis of patients with cerebral infarction was related to the BSI, and the BSIs of patients with good prognosis were significantly higher than those of patients with poor prognosis. Therefore, the BSI can effectively reflect changes in acute ischemic stroke and predict the early prognosis.

**Case**

Female patient, 65 years old, with acute cerebral infarction (Fig. 9.9).

a

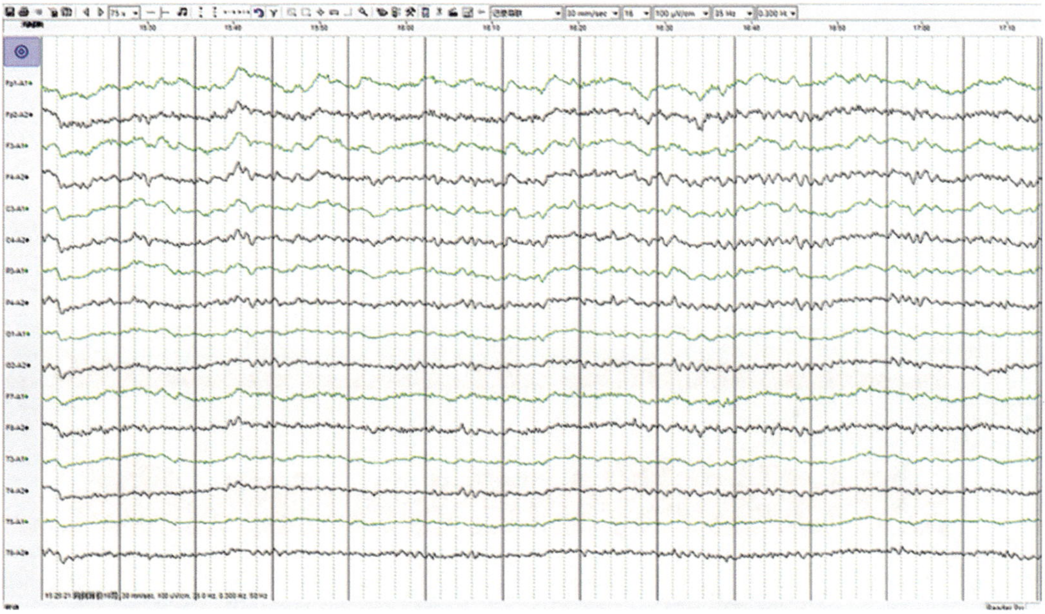

**Fig. 9.9** (**a–c**) shows the results of multimodal evaluation when the patient was admitted to the hospital. (**a**) There is much slow-wave (δ activity dominated) activity in the left lead of the EEG and α rhythm in the right lead, and there is obvious asymmetrical activity between the left and right cerebral hemispheres. Infarct focus on the left side; (**b**) The left side of the aEEG shows a discontinuous background of 10–25 μV, with widened bandwidth and asymmetry between the left and right sides. (**c**) The RAV on the left is less than 10%, and cerebral blood perfusion is insufficient. (**d–g**) is after 1 week of comprehensive treatment. (**d**) The activity in the left lead of the original EEG with a low-medium amplitude of 6–7 Hz is increased compared with before treatment, and there is slightly asymmetrical activity between the left and right hemispheres; (**e**) The upper and lower boundaries on the left and right sides of the aEEG are higher than in the front, which shows continuous background activity of 10–50 μV, and the asymmetry between the left and right sides is smaller than in the front; (**f**) The RAV on the left side is more than 10%, and cerebral blood perfusion is significantly improved; (**g**) The RBP shows that the θ activity in the left lead is greater than before treatment, and the δ activity is less than before treatment. The results of multimodal evaluation show that the treatment was effective and that brain function was well restored

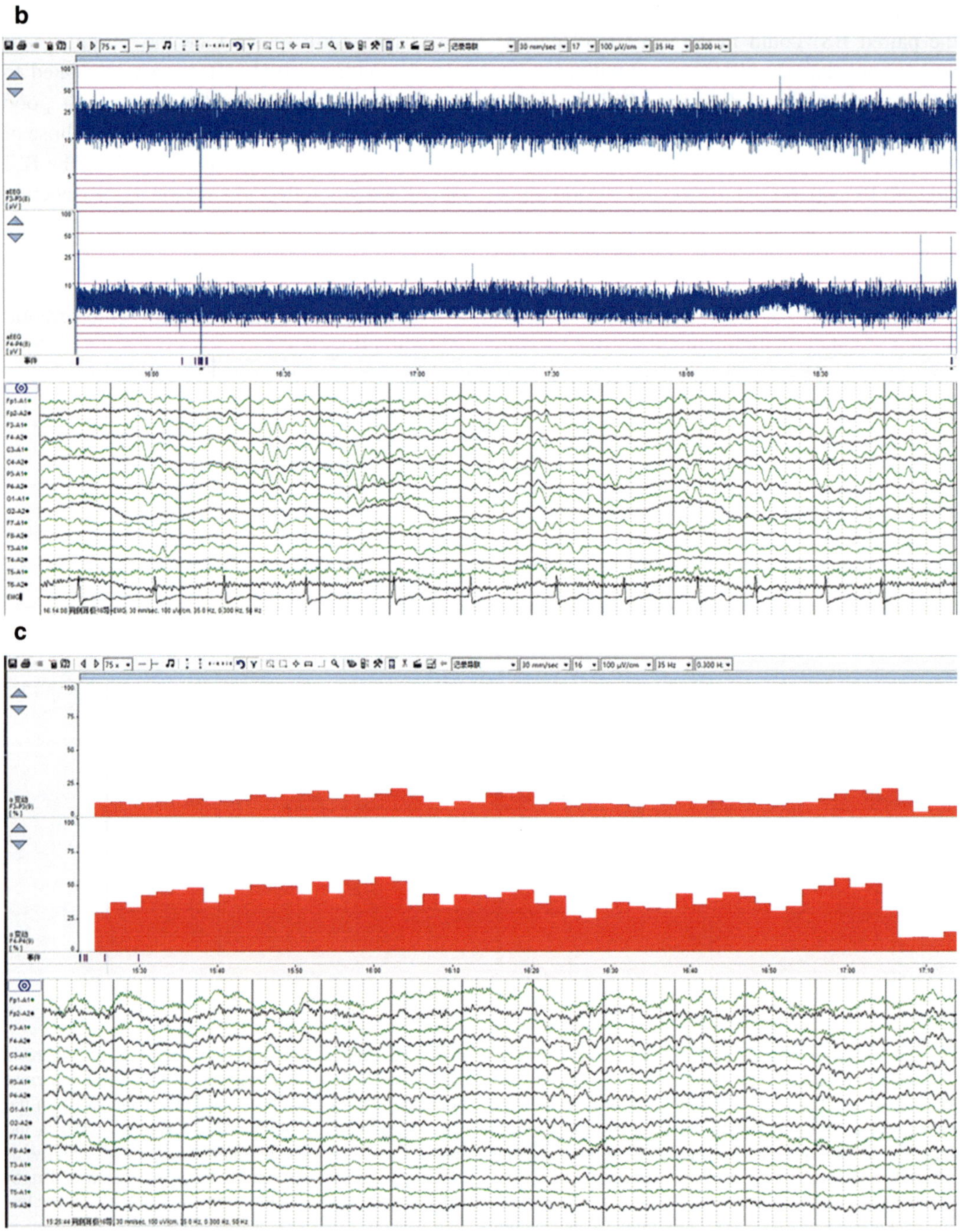


**Fig. 9.9** (continued)

**d**

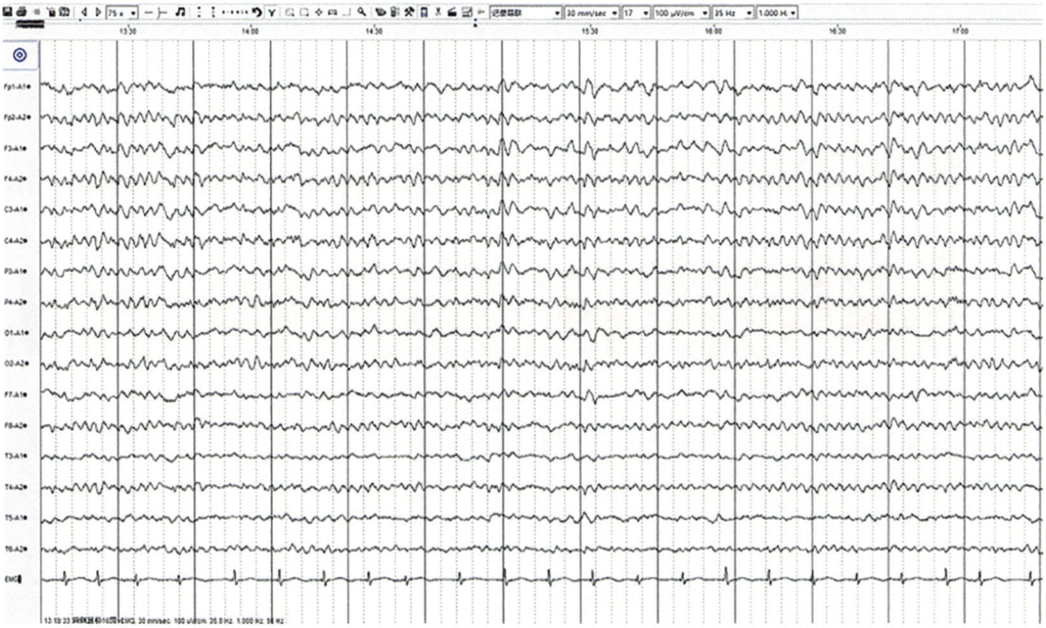

**e**

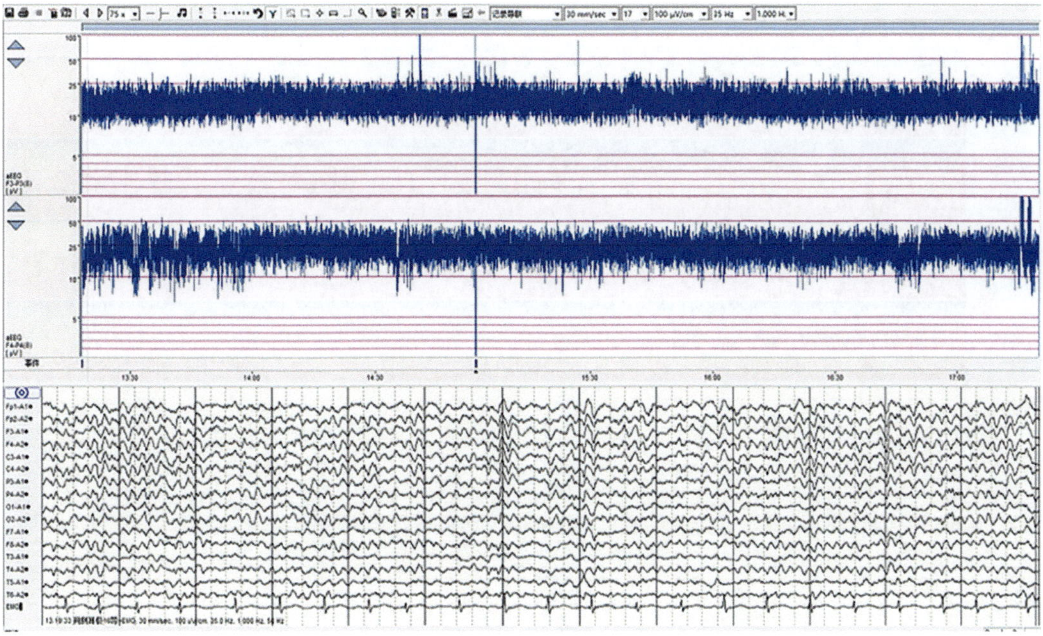

**Fig. 9.9** (continued)

f

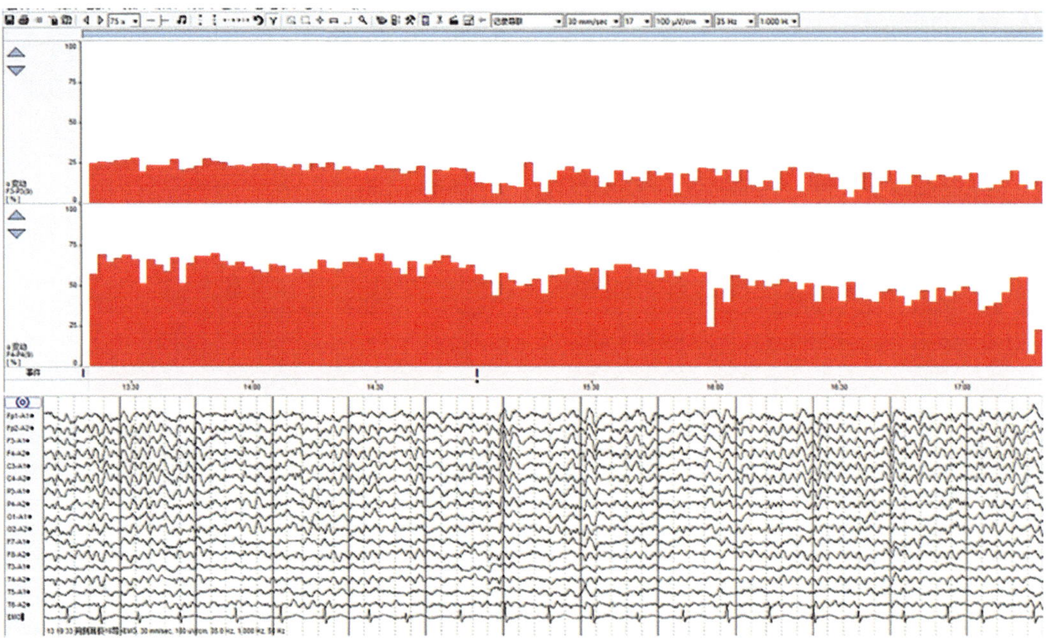

g

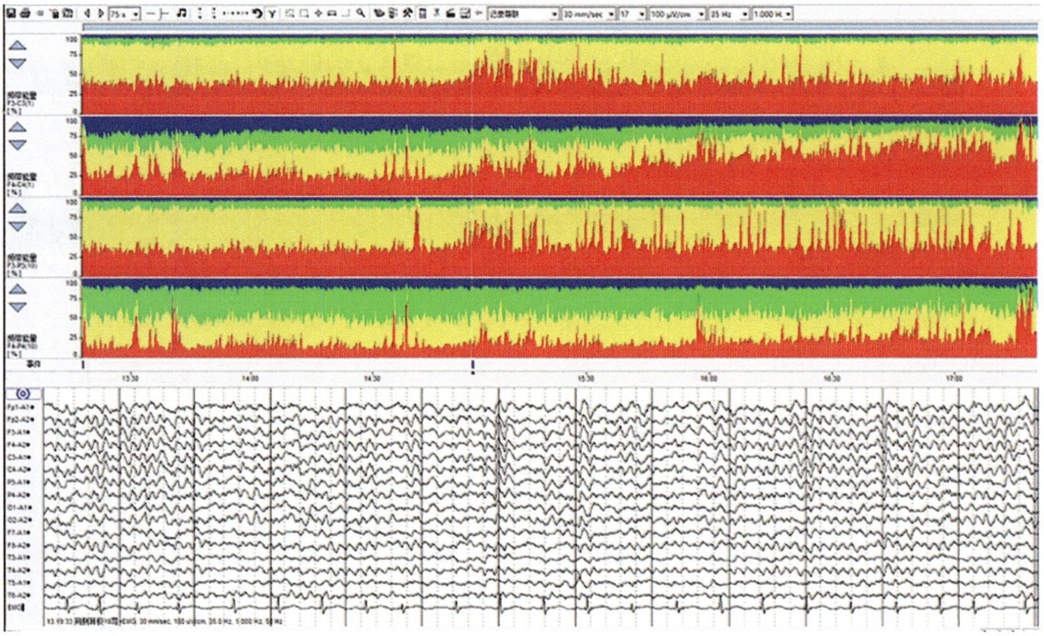

Fig. 9.9 (continued)

## References

1. Gadidi V, Katz-Leurer M, Carmeli E, et al. Long-term outcome poststroke: predictors of activity limitation and participation restriction. Arch Phys Med Rehabil. 2011;92(11):1802–8.
2. Adams HJ, Bendixen BH, Kappelle LJ, et al. Classification of subtype of acute ischemic stroke. Definitions for use in a multicenter clinical trial. TOAST. Trial of Org 10172 in Acute Stroke Treatment. Stroke. 1993;24(1):35–41.
3. Jordan KG. Emergency EEG and continuous EEG monitoring in acute ischemic stroke. J Clin Neurophysiol. 2004;21(5):341–52.
4. Dohmen C, Sakowitz OW, Fabricius M, et al. Spreading depolarizations occur in human ischemic stroke with high incidence. Ann Neurol. 2008;63(6):720–8.
5. Nedergaard M. Mechanisms of brain damage in focal cerebral ischemia. Acta Neurol Scand. 1988;77(2):81–101.
6. Finocchi C, Gandolfo C, Gasparetto B, et al. Value of early variables as predictors of short-term outcome in patients with acute focal cerebral ischemia. Ital J Neurol Sci. 1996;17(5):341–6.
7. Fernandez-Bouzas A, Harmony T, Fernandez T, et al. Sources of abnormal EEG activity in brain infarctions. Clin Electroencephalogr. 2000;31(4):165–9.
8. Liu S, Guo J, Meng J, et al. Abnormal EEG complexity and functional connectivity of brain in patients with acute thalamic ischemic stroke. Comput Math Methods Med. 2016;2016:2582478.
9. Bateman RM, et al. 36th international symposium on intensive care and emergency medicine: Brussels, Belgium. 15–18 March 2016. Crit Care. 2016;20(Suppl 2):94.
10. Azabou E, Navarro V, Kubis N, et al. Value and mechanisms of EEG reactivity in the prognosis of patients with impaired consciousness: a systematic review. Crit Care. 2018;22(1):184.
11. Su YY, Wang M, Chen WB, et al. Early prediction of poor outcome in severe hemispheric stroke by EEG patterns and gradings. Neurol Res. 2013;35(5):512–6.
12. Hirsch LJ. Brain monitoring: the next frontier of ICU monitoring. J Clin Neurophysiol. 2004;21(5):305–6.
13. Bentes C, Peralta AR, Viana P, et al. Quantitative EEG and functional outcome following acute ischemic stroke. Clin Neurophysiol. 2018;129(8):1680–7.
14. van Putten MJ, Tavy DL. Continuous quantitative EEG monitoring in hemispheric stroke patients using the brain symmetry index. Stroke. 2004;35(11):2489–92.
15. Finnigan S, van Putten MJ. EEG in ischaemic stroke: quantitative EEG can uniquely inform (sub-)acute prognoses and clinical management. Clin Neurophysiol. 2013;124(1):10–9.
16. Fernandez-Bouzas A, Harmony T, Fernandez T, et al. Cerebral blood flow and sources of abnormal EEG activity (VARETA) in neurocysticercosis. Clin Neurophysiol. 2001;112(12):2281–7.
17. Finnigan SP, Rose SE, Walsh M, et al. Correlation of quantitative EEG in acute ischemic stroke with 30-day NIHSS score: comparison with diffusion and perfusion MRI. Stroke. 2004;35(4):899–903.
18. Foreman B, Claassen J. Quantitative EEG for the detection of brain ischemia. Crit Care. 2012;16(2):216.
19. Xin X, Chang J, Gao Y, et al. Correlation between the revised brain symmetry index, an EEG feature index, and short-term prognosis in acute ischemic stroke. J Clin Neurophysiol. 2017;34(2):162–7.
20. van Putten MJ. Extended BSI for continuous EEG monitoring in carotid endarterectomy. Clin Neurophysiol. 2006;117(12):2661–6.
21. van Putten MJ, Peters JM, Mulder SM, et al. A brain symmetry index (BSI) for online EEG monitoring in carotid endarterectomy. Clin Neurophysiol. 2004;115(5):1189–94.
22. Sheorajpanday RV, De Deyn PP. Epileptic fits and epilepsy in the elderly: general reflections, specific issues and therapeutic implications. Clin Neurol Neurosurg. 2007;109(9):727–43.
23. de Vos CC, van Maarseveen SM, Brouwers PJ, et al. Continuous EEG monitoring during thrombolysis in acute hemispheric stroke patients using the brain symmetry index. J Clin Neurophysiol. 2008;25(2):77–82.
24. Myles PS, Cairo S. Artifact in the bispectral index in a patient with severe ischemic brain injury. Anesth Analg. 2004;98(3):706–7.

# Application of Multimodal EEG in TBI

# 10

Wei Dan and Xuefeng Wang

## Contents



**Abstract**

TBI is a common neurological disease, especially moderate to severe brain injury, and has a high fatality and disability rate. It remains as a focus and challenge in neurology research. After TBI, in addition to the brain damage caused by the primary injury that cannot be reversed, the secondary pathophysiological changes initiated thereafter are the primary causes of brain damage and can even lead to the death of the patient. Therefore, after TBI, early multimodal monitoring, timely detection of early secondary brain damage in patients, and timely adoption of corresponding treatment measures are undoubtedly the keys to reducing the mortality and disability rate. This chapter introduces the pathophysiological mechanism of secondary brain damage caused by the electrical activity of nerve cells after TBI from the perspective of electrophysiology, focusing on cortical spreading depolarization (CSD), ictal epileptic field potential (IEFP), the mechanism of secondary pathological changes, invasive cortical EEG and noninvasive scalp EEG monitoring methods in the NICU, multimodal EEG monitoring technology, the relationship between different

W. Dan (✉)
Department of Neurosurgery, The First Affiliated Hospital of Chongqing Medical University, Chongqing, China

X. Wang
Department of Neurology, The First Affiliated Hospital of Chongqing Medical University, Chongqing, China





X. Wang et al. (eds.), *Multi-Modal EEG Monitoring of Severely Neurologically Ill Patients*,
https://doi.org/10.1007/978-981-16-4493-1_10

EEG patterns and the degree of brain injury, and prognosis to provide electrophysiological guidance for clinical treatment after TBI.

**Keywords**

TBI · CSD · Spreading depression (SD) · IEFP · Traumatic axonal injury · Multimodal EEG monitoring

## 10.1 Overview

TBI refers to organic injury to the brain caused by a violent blow to the head. TBI can exist independently or in combination with other injuries, and its incidence accounts for approximately 20% of systemic injuries. The mortality and disability rate of TBI rank first in systemic traumas, and TBI is still the main cause of death and disability worldwide. According to statistics in 2015, 69 million people (95% CI [64–74 million]) suffered brain trauma each year worldwide. The proportion of TBI caused by road-traffic collisions in Africa and Southeast Asia was the largest, 56%, and that in North America was the lowest, 25% [1]. In 2017, according to statistics of road injuries in 92 countries and regions, there were approximately 540 million new cases of TBI, and 1.3 million of these individuals died. TBI has become the ninth leading cause of death in the world and the number one cause of death among young people aged 15–29; therefore, some people call TBI a silent epidemic [2].

TBI consists of two stages. The first stage is primary injury, which is the tissue damage that occurs when the brain is hit by trauma, such as concussion, brain contusion, DAI, and primary brainstem injury. The severity of the injury is related to the situation at the time of the injury and cannot be prevented clinically; the second stage is secondary injury, which is the cell and related cascade reactive damage that occurs after the primary injury, including the destruction of the blood-brain barrier, the development of brain edema, the increase in various excitatory amino acids, calcium overload, the generation of free radicals, mitochondrial dysfunction, oxidative stress, inflammation, and coagulation dysfunction, which in turn lead to secondary cerebral hemorrhage, increased ICP, and neuronal death. This secondary injury can start immediately after the injury, or it can occur several hours later, but it can continue for several days. This provides a time window for clinical intervention of secondary brain injury after TBI; therefore, early monitoring of this pathological change is the key to clinical treatment [3].

The ideal method for timely monitoring of brain function would have the following characteristics: (a) real-time intervention at the bedside before tissue damage occurs; (b) high sensitivity and specificity, with little interference from other signals; (c) noninvasiveness or limited invasiveness to reduce the risk of side effects; (d) a simple and durable implementation procedure, minimizing the possibility of patient movement or operation failure; (e) automatic analysis to minimize human workload and allow a prespecified diagnosis standard trigger alarm; and (f) rapid response to treatment, with real-time reflection of the treatment effect.

There are many modern brain monitoring techniques, such as CT, MRI, and other imaging examinations, as well as ICP monitoring, PbtO2 monitoring, CBF monitoring, brain temperature monitoring, and microdialysis monitoring of interstitial fluid. These techniques provide objective indicators for observing whether intracranial hemorrhage and edema are aggravated after TBI, the changes in ICP and cerebral perfusion pressure, and whether there is ischemia and hypoxia in the brain tissue. However, each of these techniques has certain limitations, including that they may be invasive, the patient may need to be moved, or the examination results lag and do not reflect the dynamic changes in nerve function in a timely manner. An EEG directly records the electrical activity changes in neurons with millisecond-level time resolution, and it is inexpensive and convenient. EEGs can be monitored repeatedly or continuously at the bedside, especially digital EEGs, which are interpreted by non-neural electrophysiologists in a simple mode. Multimodal EEG monitoring is increasingly widely used in the NICU [4, 5].

For decades, research on the relationship between EEG and brain function after head injury has developed rapidly. After the twenty-first century, cEEGs are indispensable for patients with moderate and severe head injury in the acute phase to monitor their neurological changes and seizures, especially subclinical or NCSs, and to assess prognosis [6]. Therefore, this chapter will discuss the relationship between pathophysiological changes of TBI and EEG changes, the clinical significance of common EEG patterns, and the value of prognostic judgment.

## 10.2 Mechanisms of EEG Changes Related to the Pathophysiology of TBI

EEG mainly detects the synchronization of dendritic synaptic potentials (EPSPs and IPSPs) at the top of cortical pyramidal neurons [7]. The membrane potential of these apical dendrites has a tendency to oscillate, and the physiological basis of their oscillation comprises the inherent characteristics of neurons (ion conduction) and unique network connections. Under physiological conditions, neurons and their neural networks oscillate repeatedly according to their own inherent laws every second. The normal classic frequency bands include (0.5–4 Hz), (4–7 Hz), (8–13 Hz), (14–30 Hz), and (30–100 Hz), which have unique underlying physiological mechanisms, cortical topology, and function. Different frequency oscillations are mainly controlled by the cortex-cortex connection and the thalamus-cortex connection. Different combinations of different numbers of frequency bands constitute different background patterns of the brain, reflecting its different functional states (for example, wakefulness, lethargy, and different stages of sleep). TBI may break the inherent physiological balance and destroy the ion flow of nerve cells and neural network connections in terms of structure and function, thereby affecting their normal electrical activities.

The following describes several common mechanisms of EEG changes related to the pathophysiology of TBI.

### 10.2.1 Cortical Spreading Depolarization (CSD) or Cortical Spreading Depression (CSD)

The modern view believes that the core mechanism of a series of pathophysiological changes caused by TBI is SD in neurons and glial cells. Because SD mainly occurs in the cerebral cortex, it is also called CSD by some scholars. At present, it is known that SD and the common pathological changes of secondary brain injury, such as cerebral edema, cerebral ischemia, and hypoxia, nerve cell necrosis, and hemorrhagic progression of contusions, are mutually causal [7–13].

#### 10.2.1.1 Discovery and Definition

In 1944, Brazilian physiologist Leão et al. [14, 15] observed in an animal model of epilepsy that when an electric current was stimulated in the cerebral cortex of a rabbit, the spontaneous brain electrical activity of the cortex was inhibited, and this inhibition spread between adjacent electrodes. He called this electrical activity SD. Later, a direct-current amplifier was used to observe the slow biphasic direct-current drift, which could also spread between adjacent electrodes. Further research found that when SD occurred, the extracellular fluid K+ increased abnormally, and they believed that this was a kind of depolarization phenomenon. It is believed that this wave can cause continuous vasoconstriction and brain tissue ischemia.

Although SD was discovered as early as the 1940s, many scientists believe that SD is just a man-made product that mainly occurs in the brains of rodents and under experimental conditions. Because of the high impedance of the dura and skull, it takes 10–20 $cm^2$ of cortex for electrical activity to be observed on a scalp EEG, and it is impossible to record the SD waves in the relatively narrow cortex area. The clinical understanding of it is vague, and opposing opinions exist. With the development of new imaging technology, Hadjikhani et al. [16] used MRI on migraine patients and found that the cortical blood flow velocity change wave at migraine aura is similar to the SD wave observed in experimental animals. It is believed that SD waves are related to the occurrence of migraine.

In 2002, Strong et al. [17] placed a 6-lead strip electrode (electrocorticography, ECoG) under the dura in patients with brain trauma after surgical removal of hematoma or decompressive craniectomy, and the SD wave was found in clinical monitoring for the first time. It is believed that SD waves occur in injured human brains and appear more frequently than previously reported in animal models. They also proposed that depolarization around the infarction may indeed occur in the border area of the ischemic human cerebral cortex, which led to the establishment of multiple Cooperative Studies on Brain Injury Depolarization (COSBID) centers worldwide in 2003 [18]. Since then, COSBID has conducted a large number of prospective, multicenter pathological comparative studies on SD waves and acute TBI, and COSBID researchers believe that SD is a new indicator to guide personalized and precise targeted treatment plans after acute brain injury.

SD is defined as when the cerebral cortex is stimulated, large and continuous depolarization of neurons or glial cells occurs suddenly, causing almost complete destruction of the transmembrane ion gradient and temporary inhibition of synaptic activity. SD is a general term for nerve electrical activity that propagates from the source at 1.5–9.5 mm/min in the form of waves to the surroundings and causes a series of hemodynamic and pathophysiological changes. Diffusion depolarization and diffusive inhibition are two poles of the same pathological process. Generally, diffusive depolarization can cause spreading inhibition or not. Diffusive depolarization can occur in active nerve tissue or inactive nerve tissue; that is, SD waves can also be monitored by electrodes placed where spontaneous activity is inhibited. This SD is called equipotential SD [19–22].

#### 10.2.1.2 The Relationship Between SD and Pathophysiological Changes in TBI

When the head is hit, the cortical shear stress caused by various biological forces acting on the head increases, causing microvascular damage, cell death, and damage to local functions. Once a certain threshold is exceeded, neurons in the damaged area will be polarized; if a sufficient number of neurons depolarize, SD or CSD will be triggered [17]. The modern view believes that SD is the core mechanism of secondary brain injury in TBI [22], and its common pathophysiological changes include the following:

1. *SD causes the loss of ion homeostasis and leads to malignant edema in cells.* Nilsson et al. [23] found that extracellular [K+] (3.0 ~ 40 mm) increased and [Ca2+] (1.1 ~ 0.1 mM) decreased immediately after rat cortex contusion, which corresponds to a negative direct-current drift. Ca2+ influx causes cell-derived edema. These changes lasted for 5–15 min in the diseased area but lasted only a few minutes in the surviving adjacent tissues. The normal gradients of other ions, such as Na+, H+, Cl−, and HCO3−, were also destroyed.
2. *Hemodynamic changes.* When SD occurs, there are two hemodynamic reactions. One is that, in healthy tissues, there is a short-term dilation and congestion of blood vessels, followed by a mild contraction of blood vessels and a lasting decrease in blood volume. When neurovascular coupling is normal, SD will neither cause significant cell energy shortages in fully perfused tissue nor cause any histologically significant cell damage. The second is that when neurovascular coupling is damaged, it will cause initial and severe microvascular constriction in tissues with moderate ischemia or even full perfusion. As long as the tissue remains depolarized, vasodilation will continue. Focal ischemia can propagate along with neuronal depolarization waves, causing widespread ischemia and ultimately leading to extensive cortical infarction [22].
3. *Energy metabolism crisis.* Rogers et al. [12] used microdialysis technology and ECoG simultaneous monitoring and found that when SD occurred, extracellular K+ ions increased, lactic acid increased, and glucose decreased. An increased lactic acid-to-pyruvate ratio

(LPR) is a sign of ischemia and/or diffuse hypoxia, which can lead to anaerobic glycolysis or mitochondrial failure under normal oxygen conditions (such as intracellular calcium overload). An increased LPR also affects the energy supply of nerve cell membrane pumps, making cells unable to repolarize, leading to continuous depolarization and inhibiting spontaneous activity.

4. *Increased release of excitatory substances and other inflammatory substances*. Glutamate is released, and sodium and calcium channels are activated through NMDARs, which cause a large amount of cations to flow rapidly along the concentration gradient, causing cell edema. Others, such as the release of tumor necrosis factor-α (TNF-α), affect oxidative stress response metabolic disorders and increase cytotoxicity [11, 24, 25].

## 10.2.2 IEFPs and Spreading Convulsions (SCs)

### 10.2.2.1 Discovery and Definition

Another electrophysiological phenomenon of TBI that has been widely studied is IEFPs and SCs. The phenomena of IEFPs and SCs were discovered by Leao in 1944 and by Harreveld and Stamm in 1953, respectively [14, 26]. They found in animal experiments that after SD, not only there is suppression of the spontaneous electrical activity of brain cells but also continuous high-potential activity, which propagates between adjacent electrodes with diffuse depolarization waves, which causes highly synchronized firing of neurons and is related to clinical epileptic seizures. For the discharge of IEFPs, there are many manifestations in scalp EEGs.

### 10.2.2.2 The Relationship Between the Pathophysiology of TBI and IEFPs and SCs

IEFPs, SCs, and SD cause energy metabolism disorders by affecting the ion pathways of nerve cells and reversing hemodynamic reactions, which ultimately lead to secondary brain damage. IEFPs, SCs, and SD can influence and cause each other. In a study of acute epilepsy models, it was found that there are several common induction pathways for IEFPs and CSD, such as an increase in extracellular potassium, a decrease in magnesium, a blockade of sodium pumps, and an inhibition of GABA receptors [27, 28]. In 1991, the surgical epilepsy group at Yale University used deep electrodes combined with microdialysis analysis and found that epileptic seizures caused a large increase in local extracellular lactic acid and a decrease in glucose, leading to energy metabolism crisis, damage to the blood-brain barrier and brain edema [29, 30]. These pathological changes may aggravate brain injury. Therefore, it is not difficult to understand that epileptiform activities, such as SD, are involved in the pathological process of brain injury and can also aggravate secondary brain damage.

### 10.2.2.3 The Relationship Between IEFPs and SD

Both SD and IEFPs are related to secondary brain injury. Both are related and can appear independently. The relationship is described as follows:

1. In intracranial electrode monitoring, ictal epileptiform events (IEEs) and CSDs often occur at the same time and induce or interrupt each other. Fabricius et al. [31] performed ECoG monitoring on 63 patients with TBI: 32 had CSD, 11 had IEEs, and only one had clinical seizures. Among the 11 patients with epileptic activity during seizures, ten developed CSD, and CSD was significantly related to epileptic activity during seizures. They concluded there were four relationships: IEEs induced CSD; IEEs suspended CSD; CSD suspended IEEs; and IEEs induced CSD near the electrode, regardless of whether this occurred at the same electrode.
2. There are some differences between SD and IEEPs. For example, the diffusion rate is different. The diffusion rate of CSD is slow, with an average of 1.5–9.5 mm/min, while IEEs not only have the accompanying CSD spreading at a slow speed between adjacent electrodes but also their own speed in spreading to

other areas quickly. Dreier [32] believes that IEEs may have a transmission mechanism that is different from that of CSD. In their study, they also observed the rapid spread of seizure events in the independent seizure phase, which reached almost 40 mm/min, accompanied by high-frequency oscillations of IEEs and CSD spreading slowly.

3. There are some differences in the electrophysiological mechanisms of IEEPs and SD. CSD is characterized by a large amount of ion translocation of nerve cells, nearly complete and continuous depolarization with neuron and glial membrane potentials above the inactivation threshold of the AP channel, neuron swelling, and the initiation of diffuse inhibition of electrical activity. In contrast, the epileptic field potential exhibits a moderate ion shift and mild continuous depolarization, the interference of the ion steady state is not obvious, and the membrane potential is below the inactivation threshold of the AP channel. This moderately sustained depolarization allows synchronized, highly frequent neuronal firing [20, 33].
4. The differences between their waveforms and clinical practice. The difference in waveforms on ECoG and CSD is the suppression of spontaneous activity or slow high-amplitude drift. IEEs manifest as high frequency or rhythmic electrical activity. CSD mainly manifests as migraine or functional loss in clinical practice, and IEEs are related to clinical seizures. CSD is mainly prevented by the NMDA antagonist ketamine. IEEs are controlled with AEDs.

### 10.2.3 Traumatic Axonal Injury and Neural Network

In addition to electrophysiological changes, such as neuronal SD and IEFPs after TBI, another common injury is DAI [34]. Axonal injury was first described by Strich in 1956 [35], and he observed diffuse axonal degeneration during the autopsy of patients with severe TBI. Adams officially named DAI in 1984 [36]. Geschwind [37] proposed in 1965 that advanced brain functions come from decentralized brain networks. When these networks are damaged, behavioral disorders will occur, which is called "disconnection syndrome". Bigler [38] proposed that TBI is a typical example of this network dysfunction. In addition to behavioral disorders, traumatic axonal injuries can also cause changes in EEGs. Synek et al. [39] studied 90 patients with diffuse TBI and suggested that the EEG pattern after injury is related to prognosis. He believes that after DAI, the initial EEG pattern in patients is benign; if EEG maintains normal electrical activity in the first stage, the main EEG change is in the theta rhythm in the second stage, a spindle-wave coma appears on the EEG in the third stage, and most patients can survive. For patients with malignant EEGs (such as low-amplitude δ activity, a BS pattern, and α coma), the prognosis is most often death. The influence of axonal network connection on brain electrical activity can provide immediate information on brain function and has important value for prognostic judgment.

## 10.3 Common EEG Manifestations and Clinical Significance of TBI

According to the placement of EEG electrodes, the current EEG monitoring of patients with TBI is divided into noninvasive scalp EEG examination and invasive intracranial EEG examination. Intracranial EEG examination includes intracranial ECoG and depth EEG electrodes. In the former, electrodes are placed on the surface of the cerebral cortex to directly record the local brain electrical activity of the cerebral cortex. In the latter, electrodes are implanted into the brain tissue to record deep electrical activity. Scalp EEG examination is still the most widely used examination method. Scalp EEG examination is safe, convenient, noninvasive, and inexpensive; it can reflect the functional status of the whole brain; and it is widely used in neurosurgery and primary hospitals. Although intracranial EEG examination is invasive, it can find abnormalities that cannot be reflected by scalp EEG examination, such as diffuse depolarization and epileptiform discharge. The positive rate of intracranial EEG examination is significantly better than that of scalp EEG examination.

The analysis of EEG signals after TBI includes the following: (a) Changes in background activity. EEG main background frequency, symmetry, slow activity frequency distribution, sleep structure, and responsiveness can be analyzed. (b) The presence or absence of intermittent activities. For example, periodic or rhythmic discharge, epileptiform activity, and diffuse depolarization can be used to monitor and analyze EEG patterns and interpret their possible clinical significance.

### 10.3.1 Abnormal Background Activity

Background activities are the main content of EEG analysis. According to the ICU guidelines for the recording and analysis of EEGs by the IFSECN and ACNS [40, 41], a large number of studies have shown that EEG patterns are very important for the judgment and prediction of the prognosis of brain function after TBI. Features of TBI background mode are as follows:

#### 10.3.1.1 The Diversity of EEG Background Patterns

After TBI, especially in the acute phase, EEG patterns are diverse and change rapidly (Fig. 10.1a–c). Bricolo et al. [42] conducted a combined clinical and EEG examination on 1600 patients with acute post-traumatic coma and divided them into five basic groups according to the EEG pattern: borderline, variable, sleep-like, monotonous, and ECS. It is believed that the presence of the borderline, sleep-like, and changeable EEG patterns proves that the brain has the ability to articulate the circadian rhythm and change its activity in a spontaneous or stimulated manner, while slow monotonic activity indicates an extreme degree of brain damage; flattening until the EEG is silent indicates the beginning of brain death.

#### 10.3.1.2 The Main Frequency of EEG and TBI

The main frequency and changes in the EEG background after injury reflect the condition and prognosis of TBI. The patients' EEGs that are shown in Figs. 10.2 and 10.3, had different GCS scores, and their EEG background frequencies were significantly different. Beridze et al. [43] analyzed the main frequency seen in post-traumatic EEGs in 53 patients with severe head injury (GCS score of 4–8), and they found that the GCS score was positively correlated with theta frequency ($r = +0.62$; intraoperative, 0.05). δ frequency was positively correlated with death and persistent VS within 1 month ($r = +0.57$, $r = +0.16$, $p = 0.05$). δ frequency was positively correlated with the size of the brain injury area ($r = +0.3$; $p = 0.04$). Multiple logistic regression analysis indicated that the brain injury area, GCS score, and EEG patterns have an impact on the functional outcome of coma patients. The theta waveform of patients with severe traumatic coma is closely related to deep coma and can predict poor functional outcomes within 1 month. Alexander et al. [44] explored the potential value of resting-state EEGs in predicting the 6-month survival rate after brain injury in the VS and MCS clinical results, and they found that if patients had δ waves alone or δ waves in combination with slow-wave oscillations in the first EEG assessment, they had a poor prognosis within 6 months after injury, which indicated that the probability of death was higher. The probability of the presence of θ and α oscillations in the EEGs of surviving patients was higher, and the diversity and variability of nonsurvivors' EEGs were significantly lower than those of survivors' EEGs.

#### 10.3.1.3 The Sleep Structure of EEGs and TBI

Sleep structure analysis is also an important indicator for judging brain damage and prognosis (Fig. 10.4). Sandsmark Danielle et al. [45] performed cEEG examination for patients with severe head injury for 24 h or longer within 14 days after injury. The results indicated that the presence of sleep characteristics in the acute phase after brain injury suggested early participation in the treatment of rehabilitation and good functional recovery, whereas no sleep structure indicated a poor prognosis. Valente et al. [46] performed 24-h PSG on 24 patients with brain injury and coma. The predictive abilities of the presence of different stages of the sleep-wake cycle in the PSG and other possible prognostic indicators (such as neuroradiology results, age, and GCS score) were compared. The results showed that the existence of a structured sleep pattern in the PSG predicted the results better than the GCS score (odds ratio = 10.78, $p = 0.01$).

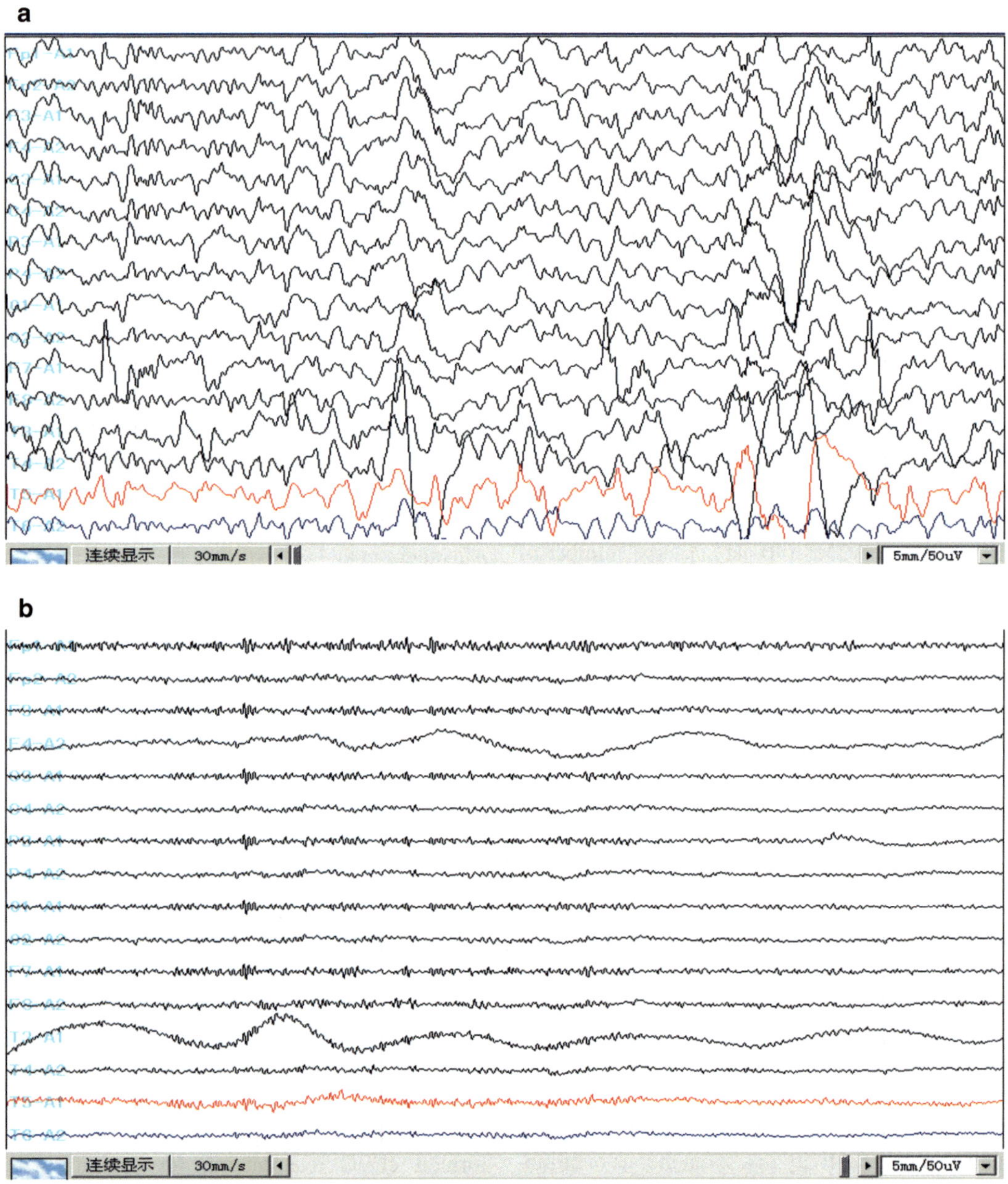


**Fig. 10.1** (**a**–**c**) A 82-year-old female with car accident injury. EEG monitoring and examination, lasted 3 h (from the time of injury to death); (**a**) shows that the main frequency is 6–7 Hz theta activity, mixed with fast activity, and limited slow waves in the left frontotemporal lead; (**b**) At 2 h and 59 min, the amplitude of each lead is low; (**c**) after 3 h and 1 min, blood oxygen saturation continued to drop, and the patient's heartbeat and breathing stopped

**c**

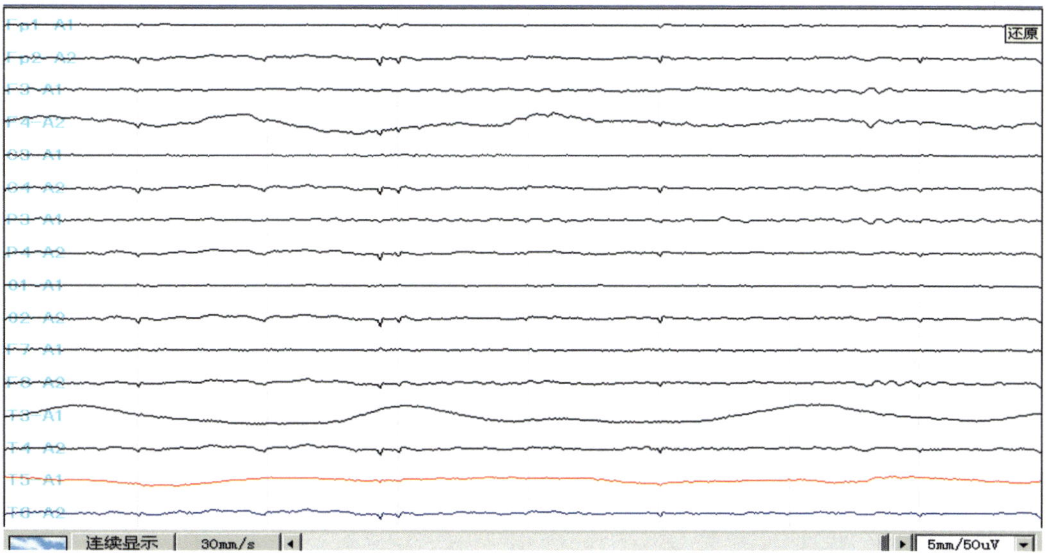


**Fig. 10.1** (continued)

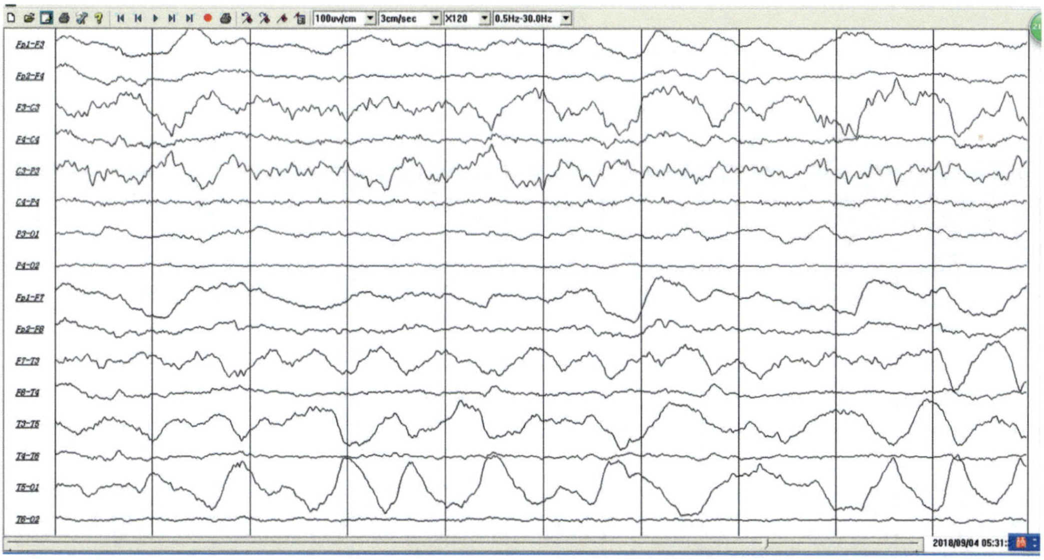


**Fig. 10.2** Zhou X, female, 24, car accident injury, GCS score 4.3 days after admission, the EEG pattern showed θ activity and fast activity in the left side

#### 10.3.1.4 The Variability and Reactivity of EEGs and TBI

The variability and reactivity of EEGs are closely related to the degree of trauma and prognosis (Fig. 10.5a, b). Azabou et al. [47] used the PubMed database to conduct a systematic search on EEG responsiveness and coma. There were 202 articles on EEG published in March 2018, and 42 articles were considered to be relevant. They found that patients with impaired consciousness with reactive EEGs had a better prognosis than patients with unresponsive EEGs regardless of the causes. Bricolo et al. [42]

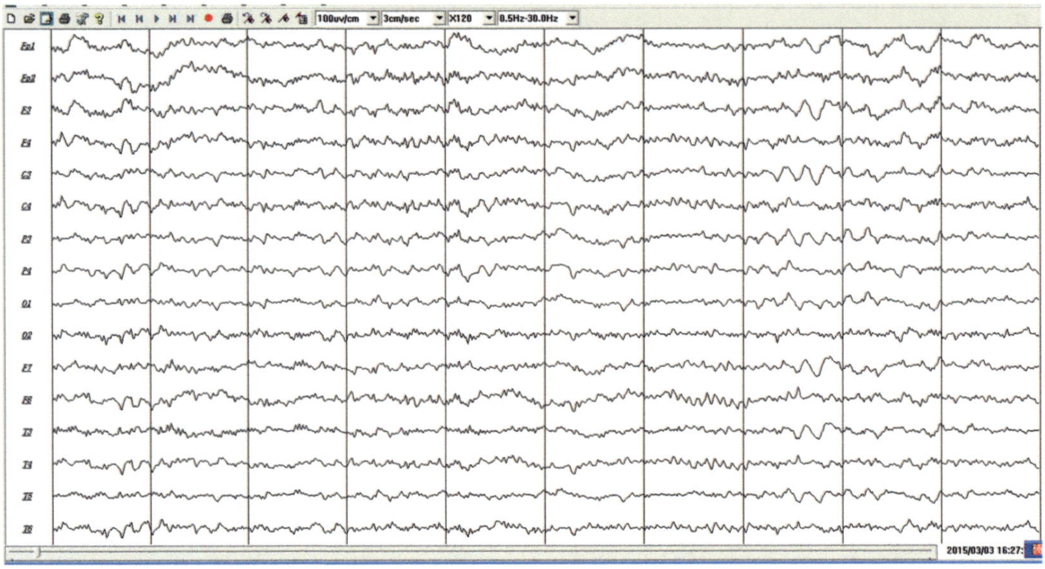

**Fig. 10.3** Xue X, who was admitted to the hospital for 3 h after a car accident, with impaired consciousness, DAI, GCS score was 8. EEG shows asymmetry, with lateral 4–6 Hz rhythmic θ activity on the left side and α rhythm on the right side

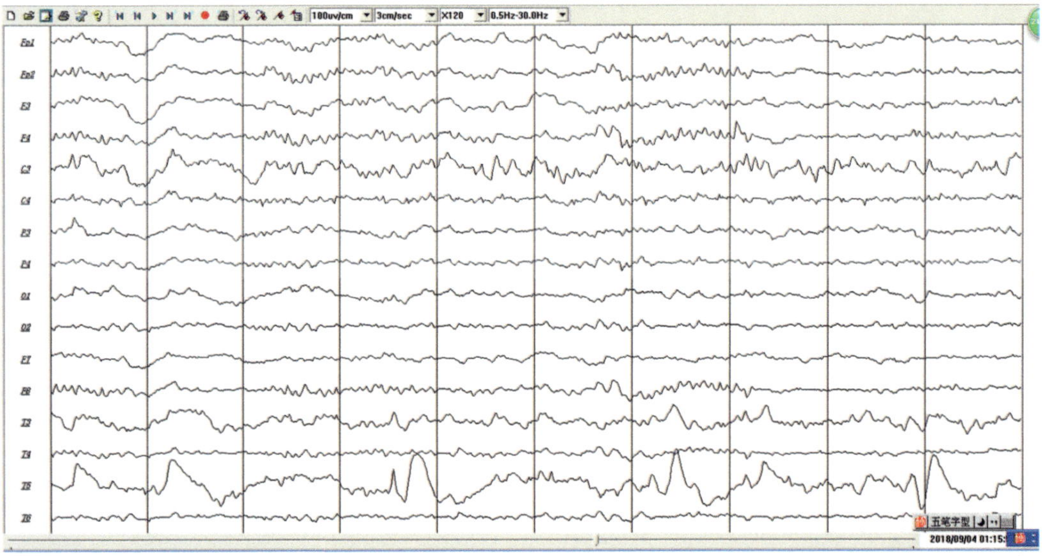

**Fig. 10.4** Zhou X, female, 24, car accident injury, GCS score was 4. EEG shows the presence of sleep cycle changes and sleep shuttle waves 3 days after admission

believe that the variable EEG model has a better prognosis than the single slow-wave model. Therefore, the variability and responsiveness of EEGs indicate that brain electrical activity has its own ability to regulate and respond to the outside world, which is a valuable prognostic parameter.

#### 10.3.1.5 The Continuity of EEG Background Activities and TBI

It is generally believed that the occurrence of discontinuity patterns in EEG background activities, including burst weakening and BS, is related to

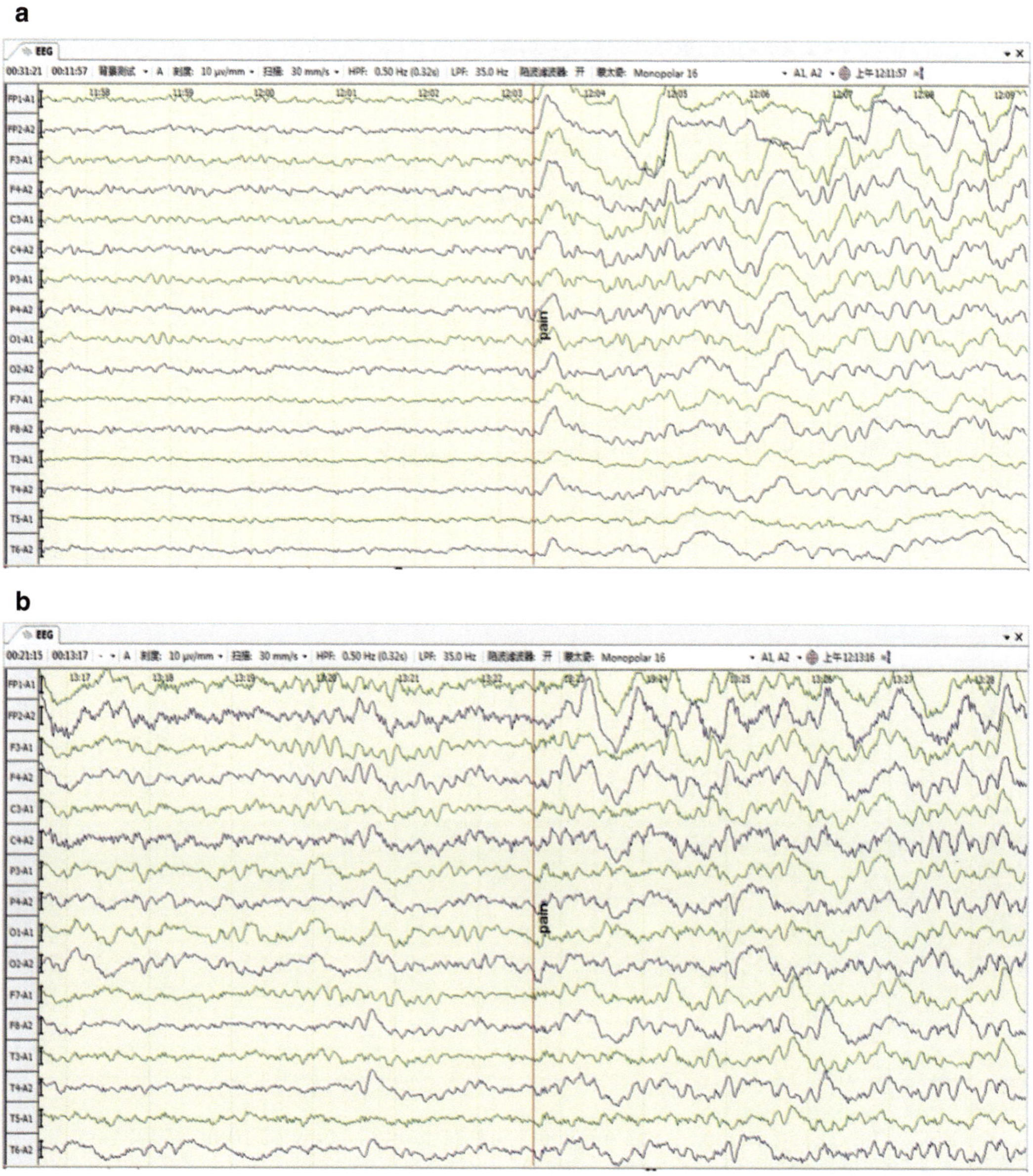


**Fig. 10.5** (**a**) The reactivity of EEGs. Liu X, female, 18 years old, injured from falling from a height. EEG shows there is responsiveness to stimuli. (**b**) After painful stimulation, the EEG wave amplitude increases and the frequency decreases slightly

more severe damage and poor prognosis (Fig. 10.6a). However, care should be taken to exclude the influence of sedative drugs, such as propofol and midazolam, and mild hypothermia treatment on BS patterns. Some scholars [48] have proposed that the shape of the BS caused by drugs is more consistent (Fig. 10.6b), while the burst waves caused by cerebral ischemia and hypoxia are inconsistent, and the presence of the latter indicates a poor prognosis.

Generally, the main frequency is α or θ band, and variable EEG patterns, the presence of sleep waves, and responsive patterns suggest a better prognosis. δ activity in the background, a single

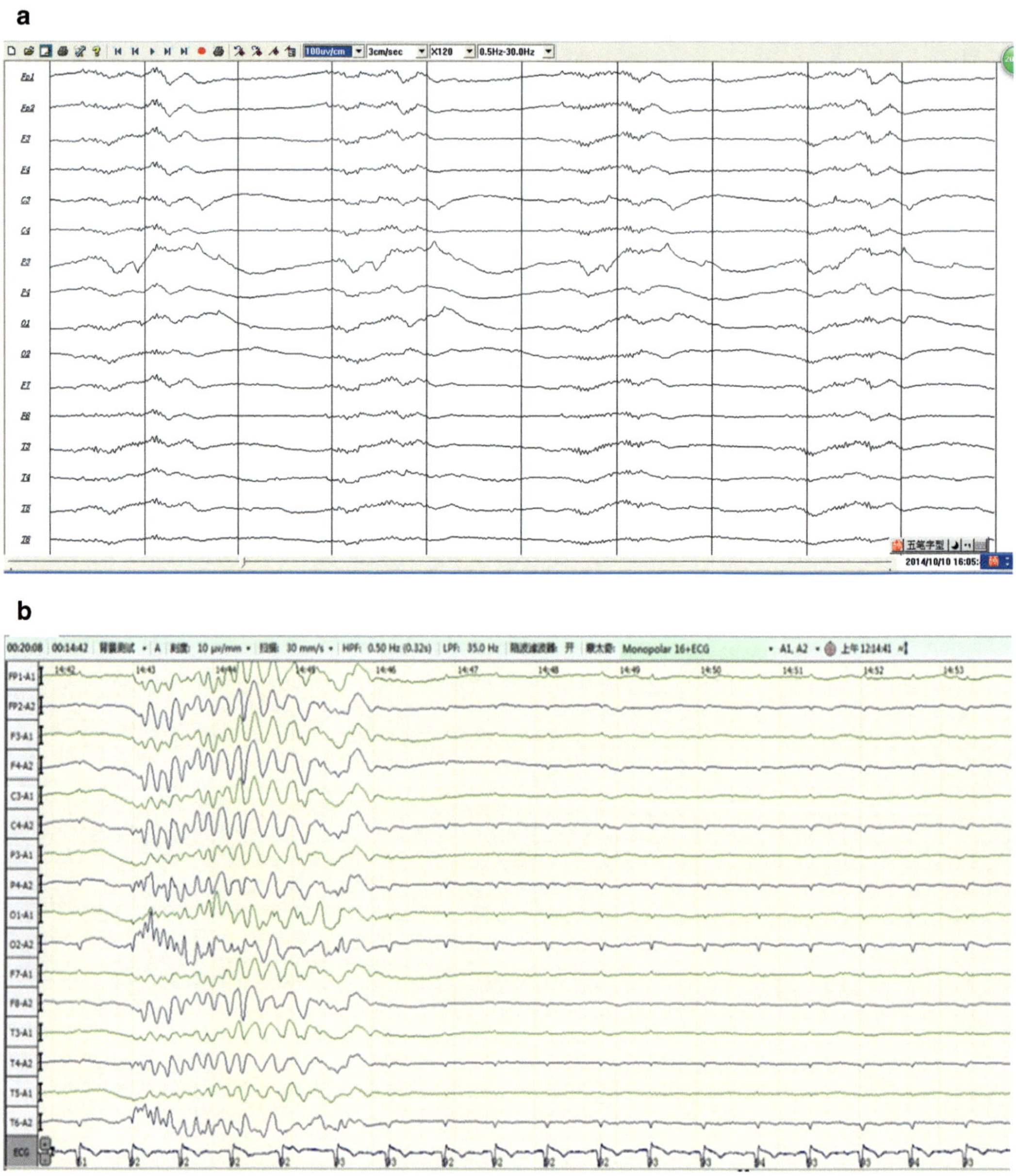


**Fig. 10.6** (**a**) Luo X, female, 76 years old, with primary brainstem injury. EEG shows a discontinuous BS pattern. (**b**) Male, 46 years old, with SE. After a 50 mg bolus of propofol, a BS pattern was seen in the EEG, and the burst content was similar

pattern, no sleep structure or responsiveness, a discontinuous EEG pattern (BS), and low voltage are poor prognostic EEG patterns [49–51]. Lee et al. [52] analyzed the results of cEEG examinations of 152 patients with moderate and severe brain injury with GCS scores of 4–12 in 20 primary trauma centers in the United States according to ACNS intensive care EEG standard terminology [41]. The EEG background activities of patients with TBI were characterized into three levels:

I. Normal or mildly abnormal: mainly from α to θ activity, NREM or basic sleep structure exists.

II. Moderate abnormality: δ activity is dominant, and NREM II sleep waves are lacking (K-complex wave, sleep shuttle wave).
III. Severe abnormality: BS, burst attenuation, and suppression.

Their research indicates that different EEG background activity patterns are related to the prognosis 3 months after injury. The prognosis of patients with level II–III EEG background activity is poor. For example, the lack of dominant frequency in the back of the head, the lack of NREM II sleep waves, δ activity as the main background activity, and the discontinuous background activity in EEGs are related to a poor prognosis. Taking the factors of post-injury time into account, it is believed that the loss of the main frequency in the back head within 24 h is more valuable for prognostic judgment than the loss within 72 h. Therefore, cEEG monitoring is recommended within 24 h after injury.

EEG monitoring after TBI can be used for visual analog signal analysis. Although digital EEG analysis has certain limitations and controversies, it is still very important as it reduces manpower, simply and intuitively displays EEG patterns, and allows continuous monitoring and rapid judgment of injury. Tolonen et al. [53] monitored cEEGs in patients with moderate and severe brain injury in the NICU, and combined with visual analysis, they extracted 59 cEEG parameters; 17 (28.8%) parameters showed significant differences based on the AUC. Most parameters measure the power of or variability in EEGs. The best cEEG parameters for predicting results were the α index (AUC = 0.87, $p < 0.01$) and the theta power of relatively fast frequency (AUC = 0.84, $p < 0.01$). Due to the heterogeneity of TBI damage (multiple pathologies coexist, such as bleeding, contusion, and axonal injury), abnormal background activities often appear as asymmetrical or focal changes (Fig. 10.7). When analyzing digital EEG signals, attention should be paid to combining the original EEG signals and imaging examination results. In short, EEG background activity observations in patients with TBI are more comprehensive in noninvasive scalp EEG examinations. According to the standard terminology of intensive care EEGs, the ACNS advocates early continuous monitoring, dynamic follow-up observation, spontaneous activity and evoked reactivity monitoring, and comprehensive analysis in the simulation of original signals, and digital multimodal monitoring to provide help for clinicians and patients' family members in treatment decisions.

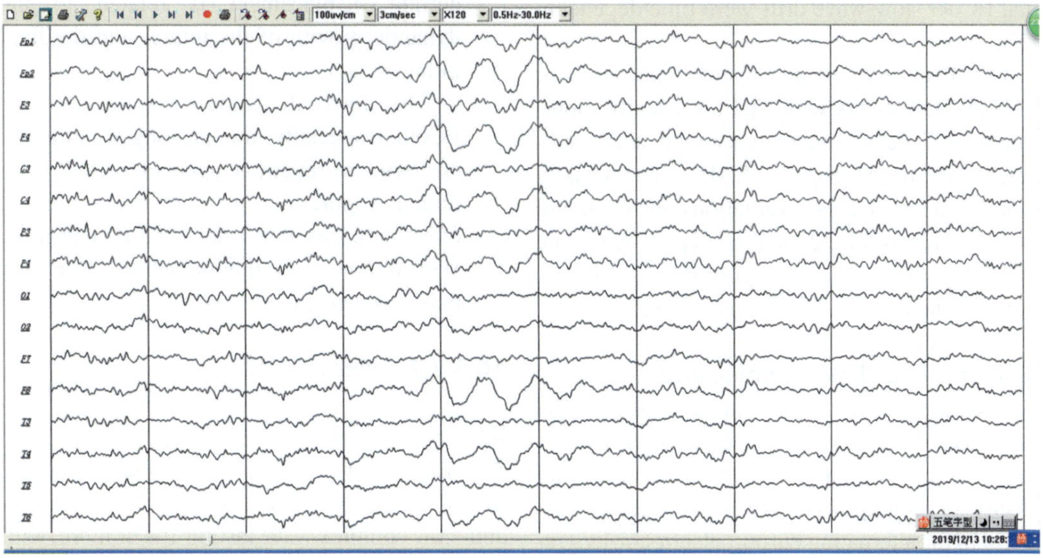


**Fig. 10.7** Patient, female, 78, hematoma in the right frontal lobe. In the background of low-amplitude α activity, the right frontotemporal leads show limited slow waves

## 10.3.2 Abnormal Paroxysmal Activity

Paroxysmal EEG activity abnormalities mainly include epileptiform activity and cortical diffuse depolarization. They are very common in TBI. In the recordings of cEEG or ECoG in the first week after TBI, the incidence of epileptiform activity is 23–50%, and the spread of cortical depolarization is 56–90% [13, 14]. Either epileptiform activity or diffuse cortical depolarization can aggravate secondary brain damage.

### 10.3.2.1 SD Wave Monitoring and Clinical Significance

#### Monitoring Methods

Since SD waves may occur in a small area of the cortex, they are not easy to find in scalp EEGs. Intracranial ECoG is the gold standard for SD examination [22]. COSBID recommends that in patients who need surgery after acute brain injury, six contact strip cortical electrodes should be placed around the bleeding or hematoma after the operation. For nonsurgical patients, electrodes can be placed in the small bone window. At present, it is reported that intracranial electrodes and scalp electrodes could be used synchronously to evaluate SD, and it was found that the inhibition of scalp EEG spontaneous activity and intracranial ECoG slow-wave drift were time dependent [22].

COSBID recommends a collection time of 7–14 days. Patients with TBI are usually monitored for 7 days, and patients with acute subarachnoid hemorrhage (aSAH) are usually monitored for 14 days. Evaluation content should include a record of the total SD suppression time every day, the number of occurrences of isoelectric SD, and the time of SD and SCs [22].

#### SD Model and Clinical Significance

To identify SD, the full frequency band on the EEG needs to be observed [22]. Low-pass filtering is 0 or less than 0.05 Hz for direct current electrocorticography (DC-ECoG) or greater than 0.05 Hz for alternating current electrocorticography (AC-ECoG) observation. Three characteristics of an SD wave: First, it appears as a slow potential wave on DC-ECoG. Second, it manifests as a suppression of self-generation activity on AC-ECoG. Third, it diffuses between at least two adjacent electrodes. The SD produced under the continuous suppression of self-generation activity is the equipotential SD.

The clinical significance of the SD wave mode is as follows:

(a) SD can appear singly or in clusters. TBI animal experiments have shown that the appearance of SD is positively correlated with the degree of concussion. Eriksen et al. [54] reported that SD is highly correlated with aSAH and subdural hemorrhage caused by TBI, and they believe that recurrent SD (>3 times within 2 h) and clustered CSD have a poor clinical prognosis.
(b) Isoelectric SD. It often suggests the presence of a new ischemic area. Even if it is not at the recording position, it also indicates that the nearby tissues have an energy metabolism disorder. A multicenter clinical study of TBI demonstrated that isoelectric SD predicts the 6-month prognosis of patients, and its adverse risk is 8 times higher than that of the nonisoelectric SD group.
(c) The duration of SD is extended. The extension of the local duration of negative direct-current displacement is related to the dynamic growth of the infarct and the final infarct size.

Therefore, the monitoring of SD on ECoG, especially the prolonged duration, clustering or repetitive appearance with continuous suppression of spontaneous activity, often indicates the occurrence of ischemia. With intervention, this pathological process may be reversed.

### 10.3.2.2 IEEs and IIC

#### IEEs

According to the definition of COSBID, an IEE refers to any spike wave, sharp wave, or sharp-and-slow complex wave lasting 10s or more, with a frequency of at least 3 Hz or at least 1 Hz but accompanied by the evolution of the wave's frequency, shape, or recording part, with or without obvious clinical manifestations [22]. In the acute phase of TBI, more than 50% of seizures are NCSs [55].

The performance of IEEs in TBI is similar to that of other seizures, but it is mainly derived from focal seizures (Figs. 10.8 and 10.9). The origin wave can show low-amplitude fast rhythm activity, a sharp-wave rhythm, or a slow-wave rhythm of various frequencies [32]. Then, the amplitude, frequency, waveform, and location evolve. When analyzing EEGs, when the background activity changes suddenly and there is a beginning-diffusion-end evolution, clinicians should be alert to the occurrence of an IEE (Fig. 10.10a–d). Especially for comatose patients in the NICU, if there is an unexplained increase in unconsciousness, the EEG should be checked immediately, and NCS and NCSE should be excluded.

In recent years, the use of intracranial electrodes to monitor electrical seizures has been more sensitive than scalp EEG electrodes. Lee et al. [55] reported 48 cases of multimodal EEG monitoring of coma patients, and found deep electrode recording and scalp electrode recording identified epileptic activity in 38% and 8% of cases, respectively. Waziri et al. [56] used mini-deep electrodes and scalp EEG electrodes simultaneously and found that intracranial electrodes could detect seizures that were not obvious on the scalp EEG. In two other patients, the cortical electrodes showed spontaneous attenuation of activity 2 h earlier than other examination methods and 8 h earlier than clinical deterioration. A study using the intracranial electrode ADR found that the ADR decreased by >25%, lasting more than 4 h, which is 1–3 days earlier than angiography in predicting cerebral vasospasm and better than the result of the calculation based on the scalp EEG [57].

The clinical significance of IEEs: Studies have shown that IEEs can cause additional harm and long-term negative consequences for TBI patients. NCSE may increase nerve damage and deterioration. In many studies in critically ill patients, even when trying to control for other factors, such as the severity of injury or comorbidities, the appearance of epileptic activity is still associated with a poor prognosis [58–60]. In patients with TBI with NCS and NCSE, during the acute attack or for several days after the seizure ceases, the ICP and the ratio of lactate/pyruvate increase [61]. De Giorgio et al. [62] reported

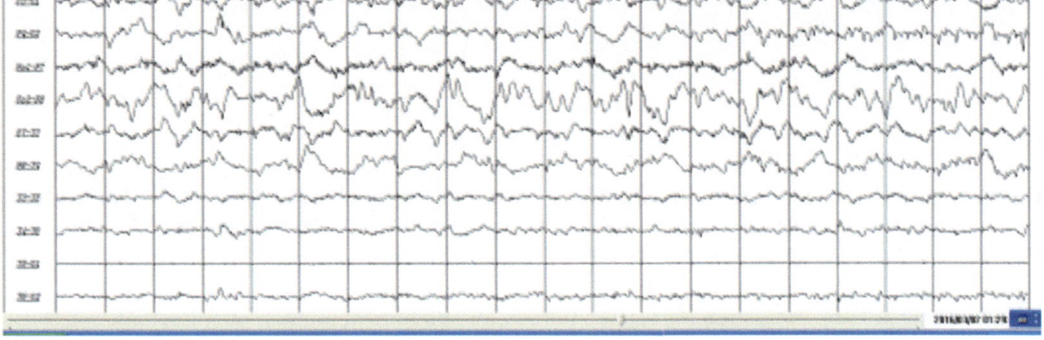

**Fig. 10.8** A patient, with TBI, EEG shows low-amplitude fast rhythm with spike-wave rhythm derived from right frontal region, which was IEE evolution pattern

**a**

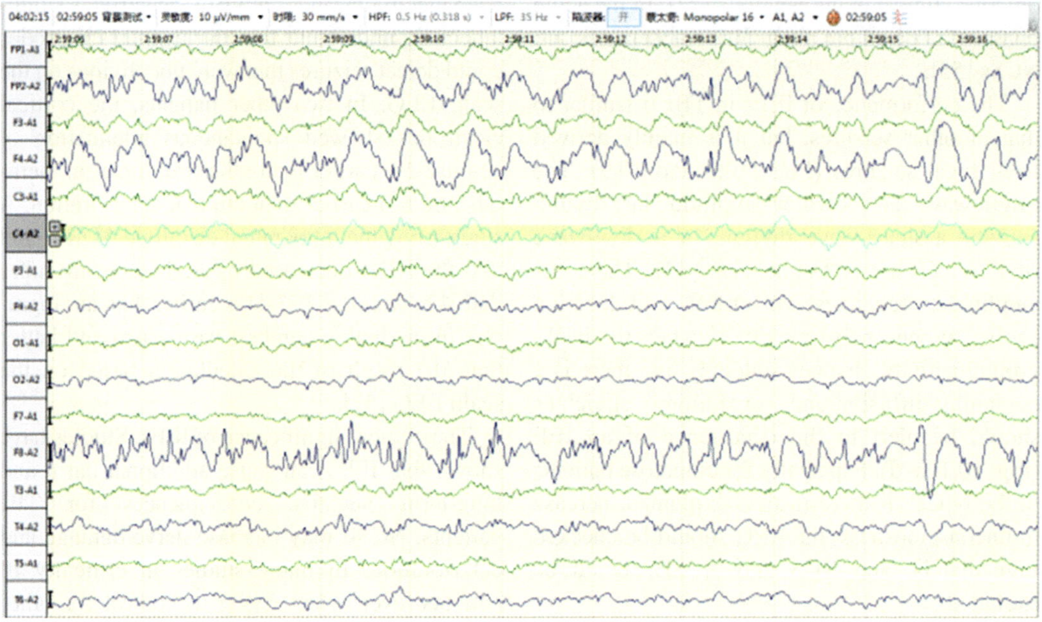

**b**

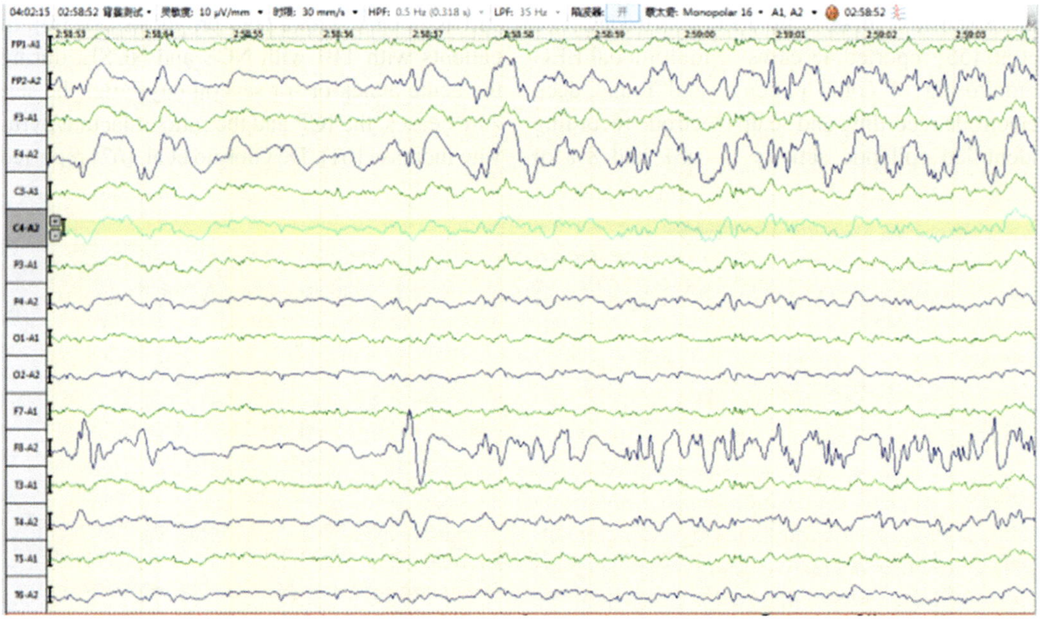

**Fig. 10.9** (**a**) Focal δ + F activity in the right frontal-related lead started. (**b**) In the late stage of focal δ + F activity, the slow wave frequency slowed and the fast wave frequency gradually decreased. (**c**) The frequency further slowed to disappear, lasting about 1–2 min

**c**

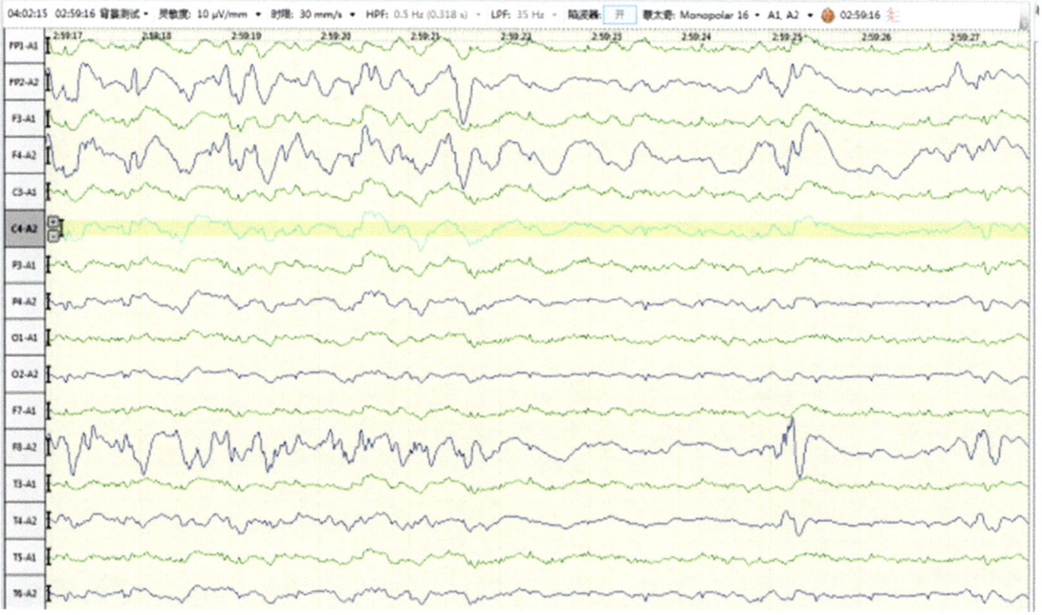

**Fig. 10.9** (continued)

that NSE is a biomarker of neuronal damage. Compared with patients without seizures, NSE in critically ill patients with NCSE or NCS is elevated. In another study, TBI patients with recurrent NCS or NCSE showed hippocampal atrophy compared with matched TBI patients who did not develop seizures, especially the hippocampus on the same side of the seizures [63]. This suggests that NCSE may cause long-term changes in the brains of patients with brain damage.

## IIC

Another common paroxysmal activity after TBI seen clinically is that the EEG does not conform to interictal discharge. In recent years, this has been called IIC in the literature [52]; that is, cycle waves, spike-wave rhythms or RDAs have no evolution in frequency, shape or location (Figs. 10.11, 10.12, 10.13, and 10.14).

IIC mode and clinical significance: Lee et al. [52] summarized the common IIC mode in patients with moderate to severe TBI with a GCS score of 4–12 and divided it into four levels:

I. Normal, no IIC
II. Mild, GRDA
III. Moderate, frequency <1.5 Hz LRDA or GPDs
IV. Severe, LPDs or GPDs or electrographic seizure.

They believe that severe IIC and electrographic seizures are related to the severity of brain injury but have nothing to do with the prognosis of brain function after 3 months. Another study on the relationship between IIC and brain metabolism demonstrated that in IIC, especially LPDs, there is a positive correlation between discharge frequency and high metabolism [55]. The author used digital EEG examination combined with intracranial multimodal monitoring to find that the frequency of LPDs increased, the PbtO2 decreased, the ICP increased, and the local CBF

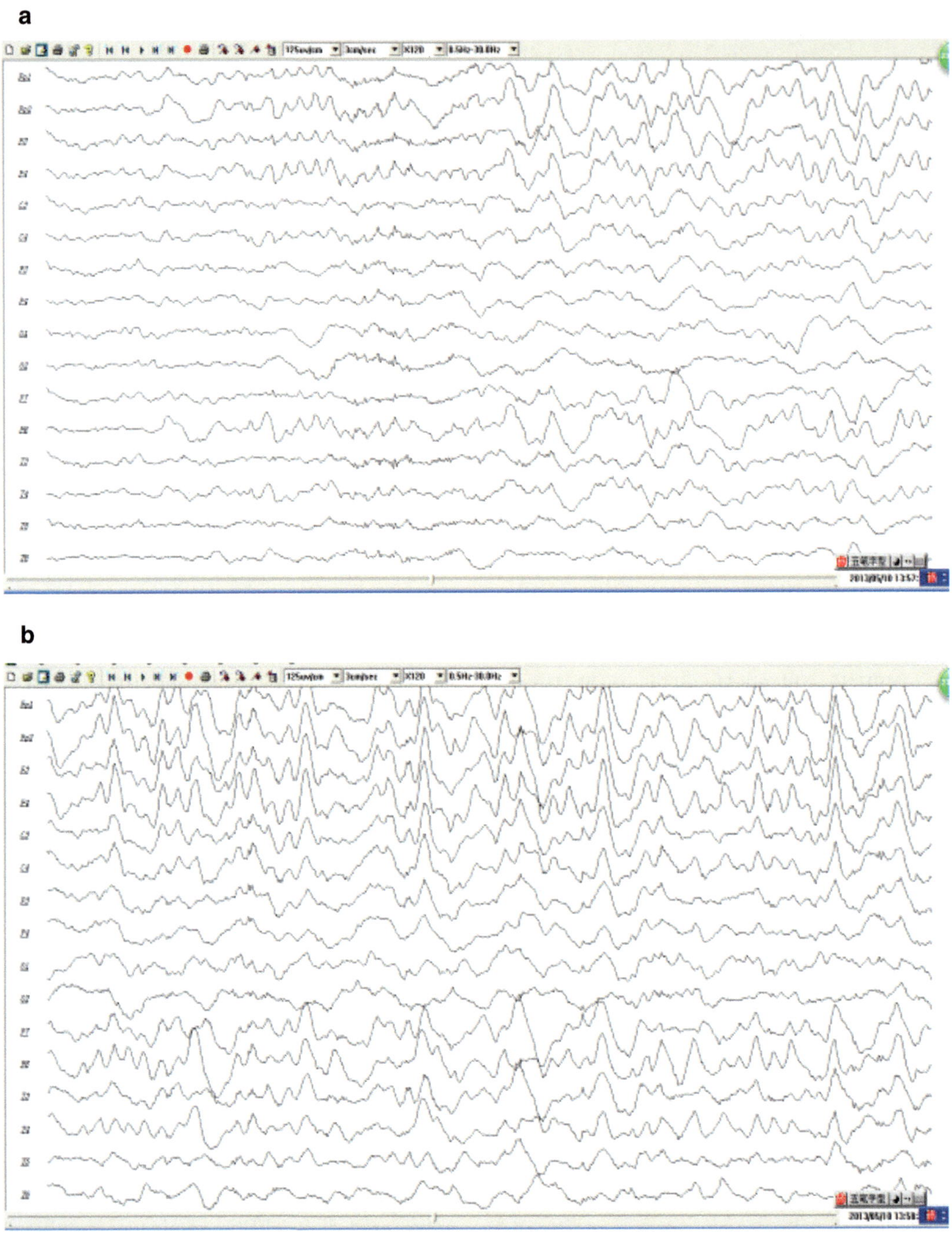

**Fig. 10.10** (**a**) In the right frontal region, the medium amplitude α-like rhythm wave about 8.0 Hz started, and then gradually inserts into the medium-high amplitude slow wave about 3.0–4.0 Hz. (**b**) The amplitude increased gradually, the frequency decreased gradually, and spread to the whole lead. In the whole lead, the slow wave activity with medium amplitude increased, accompanied by the insertion of sharp wave with high amplitude, this was obvious in the frontal region. (**c**) The frequency was further decreased to diffuse slow wave activity of 2.0–5.0 Hz in the whole lead. High amplitude sharp wave of 5 Hz was found in frontal lead. (**d**) The background activity was restored after the slow wave disappeared

c

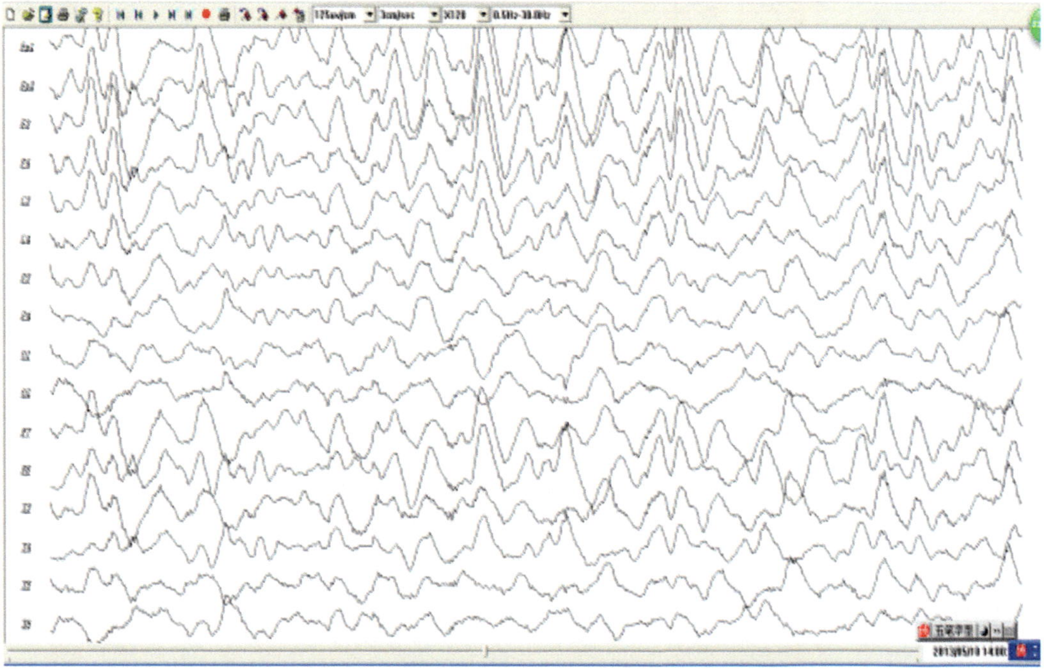

d

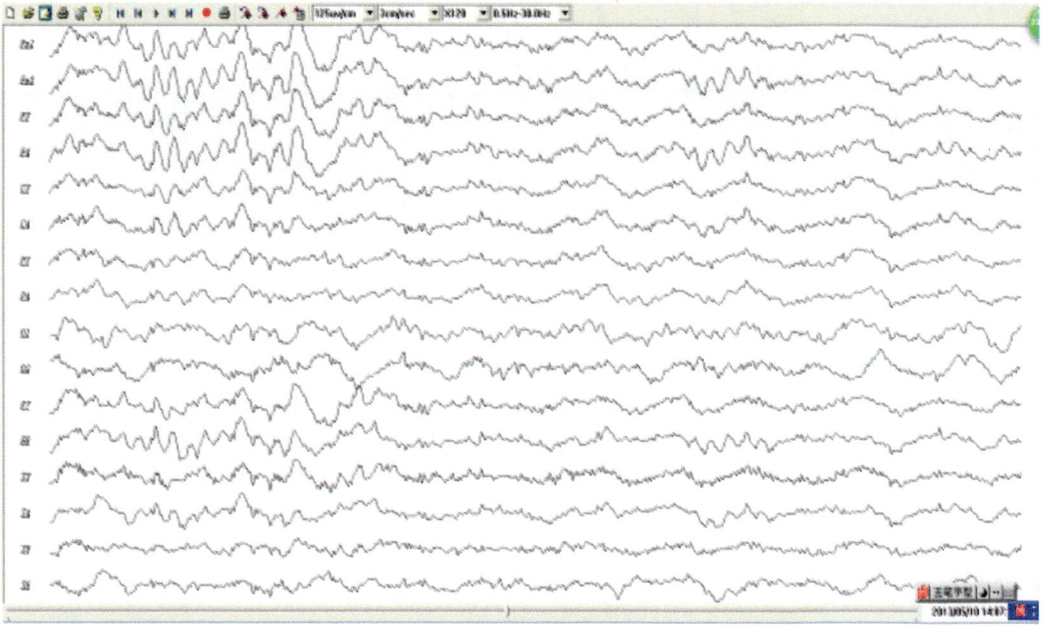

Fig. 10.10 (continued)

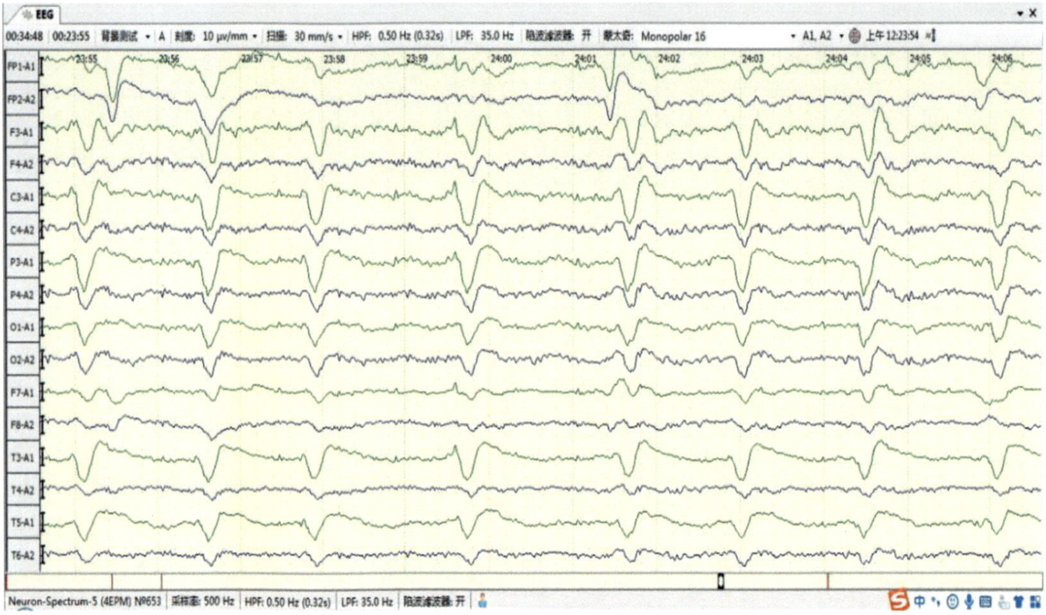

**Fig. 10.11** LPDs

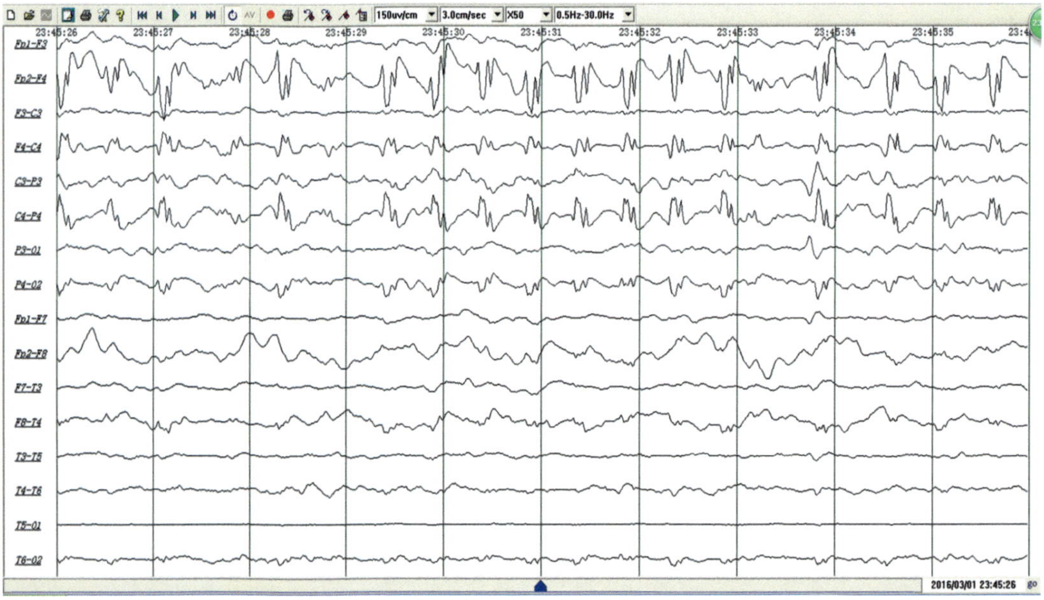

**Fig. 10.12** Asymmetric PD on both sides

increased. The increase in local CBF compensates for energy consumption. When the frequency is over 2 Hz, brain damage may result due to insufficient compensation.

**Case**

A 52-year-old male patient was admitted to the hospital for a "loss of consciousness 3 plus hours due to traffic accident injury".

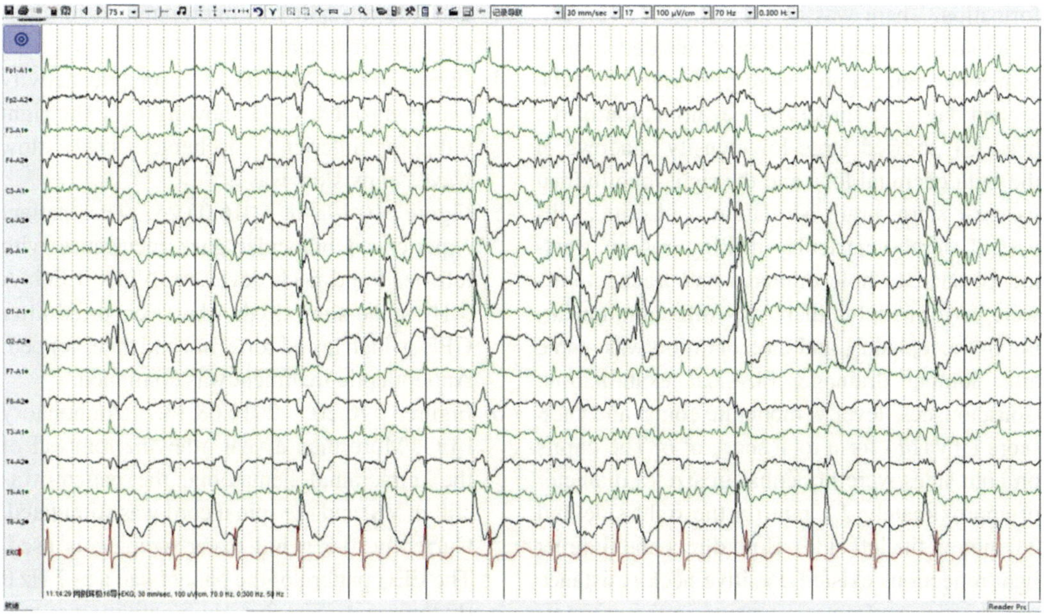

**Fig. 10.13** LPDs

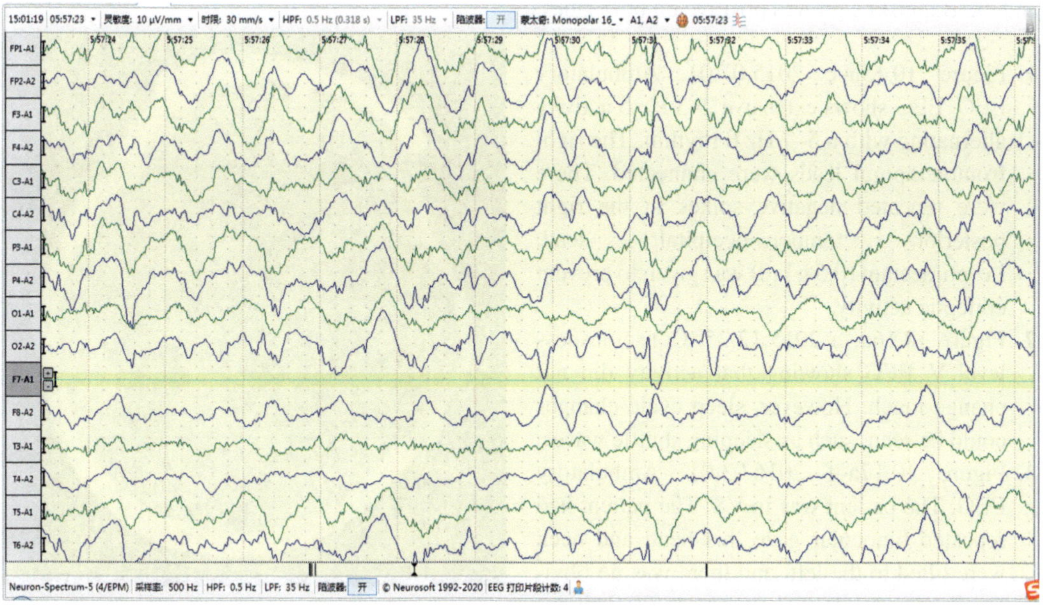


**Fig. 10.14** GRDA

Admission diagnosis: (a) Severe craniocerebral injury; (b) Contusion and laceration of the right frontal and parietal lobe with intracerebral hematoma formation; (c) Multiple injuries; (d) Hypertension grade 3 (very high risk); and (e) Type 2 diabetes.

Three hours before admission, the patient lost consciousness due to a traffic accident and suffered multiple injuries throughout the body. He was sent to the emergency department of our hospital. CT showed right frontal-parietal lobe contusion and laceration with intracerebral hematoma formation. There was an indication for surgery. Craniotomy, hematoma removal, and decompression with craniectomy were performed. On the second day after surgery, a reexamination of the head CT showed large low-density shadows in the right occipital lobe and the right longitudinal fissure cistern, brain herniation, and critical illness. Lateral ventricular drilling rescue treatments, such as hole drainage and tracheotomy, were performed, but there was still communicating hydrocephalus, and the condition was stable after lumbar drainage. Physical examination: Consciousness level V, moderate coma, and GCS score E1V1M4 for a total score of 6. The pupils on both sides were not equal in size (a diameter of approximately 2.5 mm on the right side and 2.0 mm on the left side). Both direct and indirect light reflections existed. Positive neck resistance was present, and muscle tension in the extremities was extremely high, showing paroxysmal tension. The physiological reflex was weakened, and the Babinski sign was positive on both sides.

1. Figure 10.15a–c 2015.07.01. Ambulatory EEG. EEG shows extensive 2–3 Hz δ activity alternating with a 5–7 Hz θ rhythm. The right frontotemporal leads were connected. There were repeated negative spikes in the right posterior temporo-occipital lead. Levetiracetam (0.5 g bid) was given to prevent epileptic activity.
2. Figure 10.16a, b 2015.12.25. Consciousness level V. EEG showing that activity did not change much. However, sleep cycle changes could be seen, such as sleeping shuttle waves.
3. Figure 10.17a–f 2016.03.01. Ambulatory EEG. The patient was in VS. The patient had repeated binocular gaze, his head and neck were tilted to the left, and there was no obvious limb movement. Ambulatory EEG shows the pattern of EEG changes during the onset, and the original EEG monitoring reveals the evolution of EEG from the right frontal origin. Then, 800 mg was injected intravenously, and 400 mg q8h was micropumped for antiepileptic treatment.
4. Figure 10.18 2016.03.16. Epileptic activity was controlled. EEG showing only the right temporal interictal discharge: spike slow wave, spiny slow wave.
5. Figure 10.19a–d 2016.03.24. The patient experienced binocular gaze recurrence with left head and neck deviation. Video-EEG: A 3 Hz spike-slow rhythm burst occurred after GPD, which lasted for 2 min and then stopped. Antiepileptic treatment was continued.
6. Figure 10.20 2016.08.18. Ambulatory EEG. More than a year after the removal of the intracranial hematoma, the patient was still in VS, and the spinal cord was stimulated. Currently, 0.6 g bid oxcarbazepine is used. The EEG pattern of the patient had a 5–7 Hz θ rhythm, and focal 2–3 Hz δ activity was still seen in the right temporal area. The patient receives rehabilitation treatment.

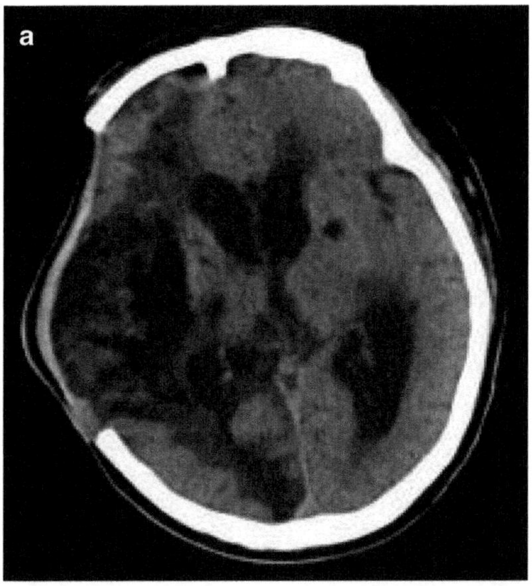


**Fig. 10.15** (**a**) CT showed large low-density shadows in the right occipital lobe and the right longitudinal fissure cistern. (**b**) Extensive δ activity of 2–3 Hz and θ rhythm of 5–7 Hz appeared alternately. This was obvious in the right frontotemporal lead. (**c**) Repeated negative spikes appeared in the right posterior temporo-occipital lead

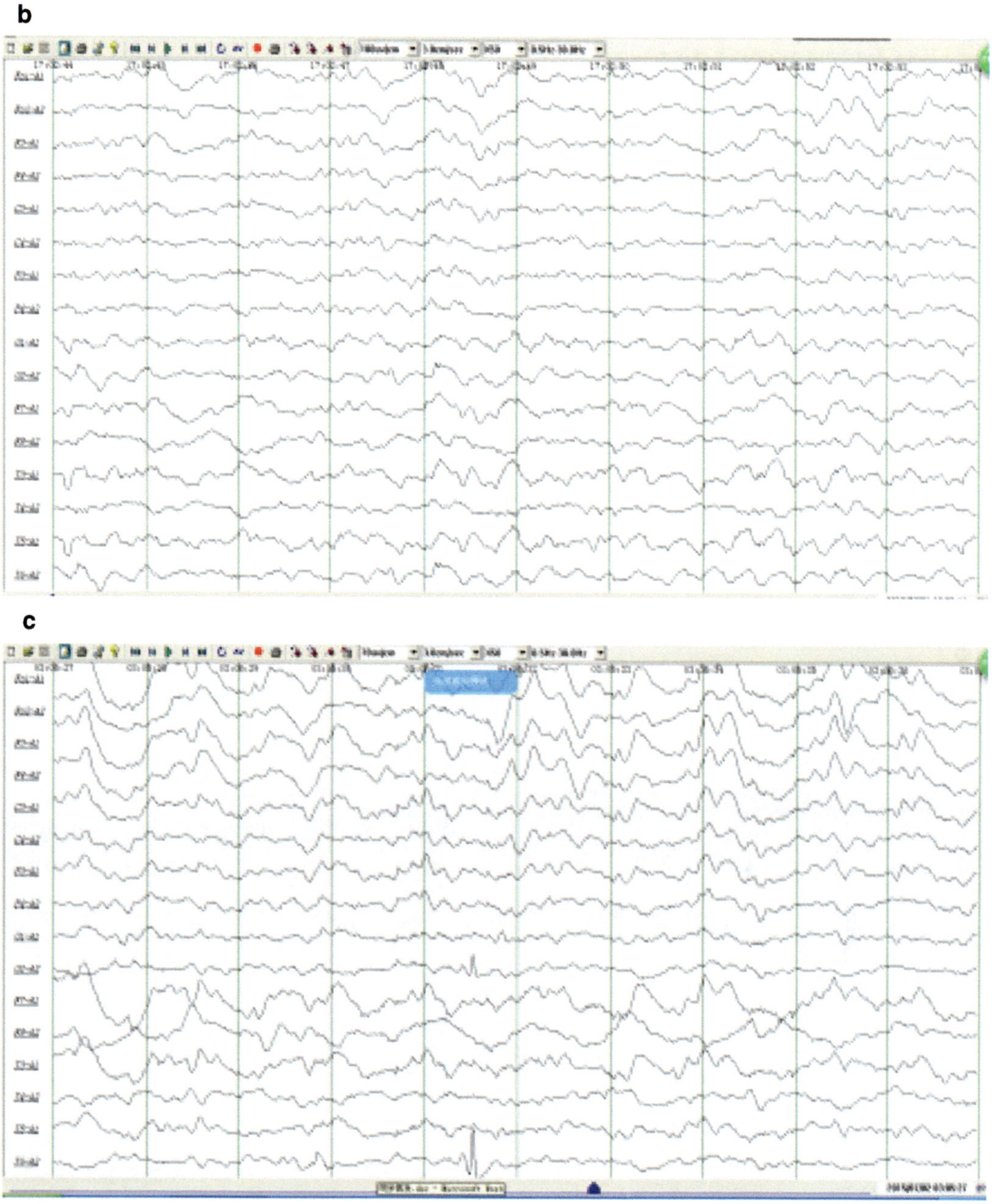

Fig. 10.15 (continued)

**a**

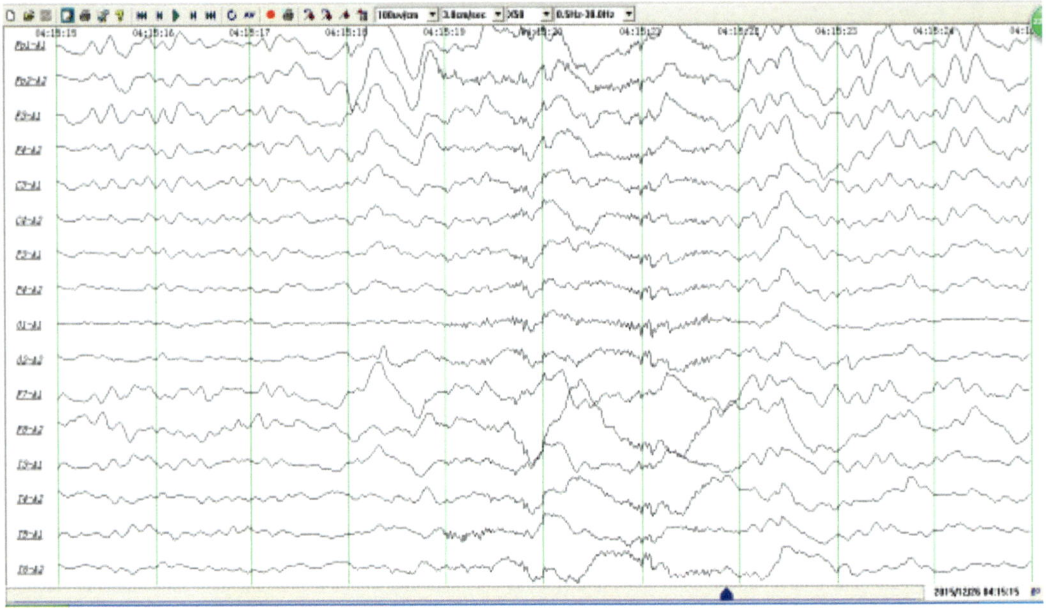

**b**

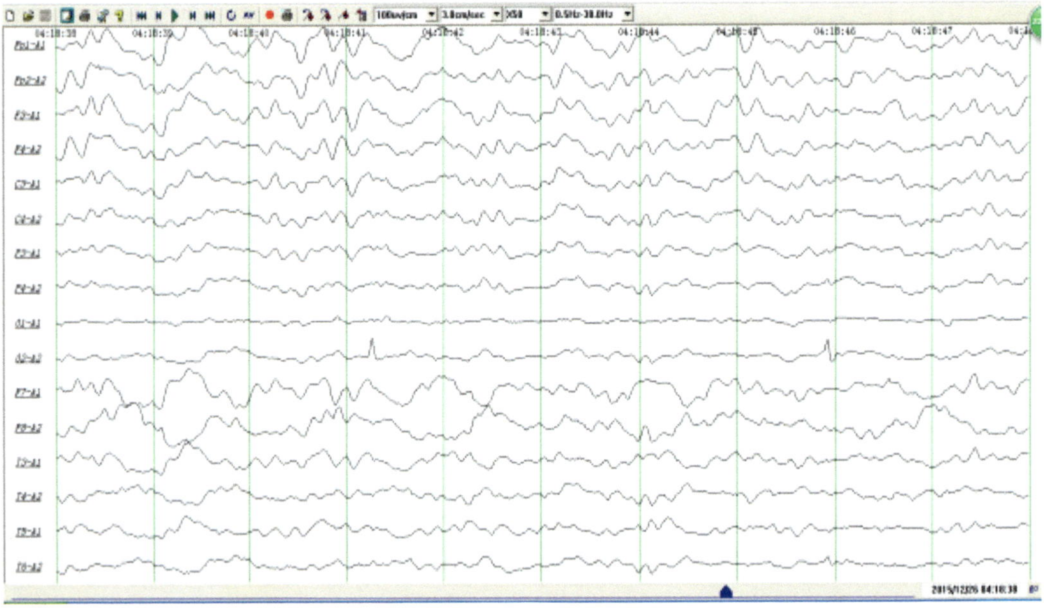

**Fig. 10.16** (**a**) EEG background activities did not change much. (**b**) Sleep cycle changes could be seen, such as sleeping shuttle waves

a

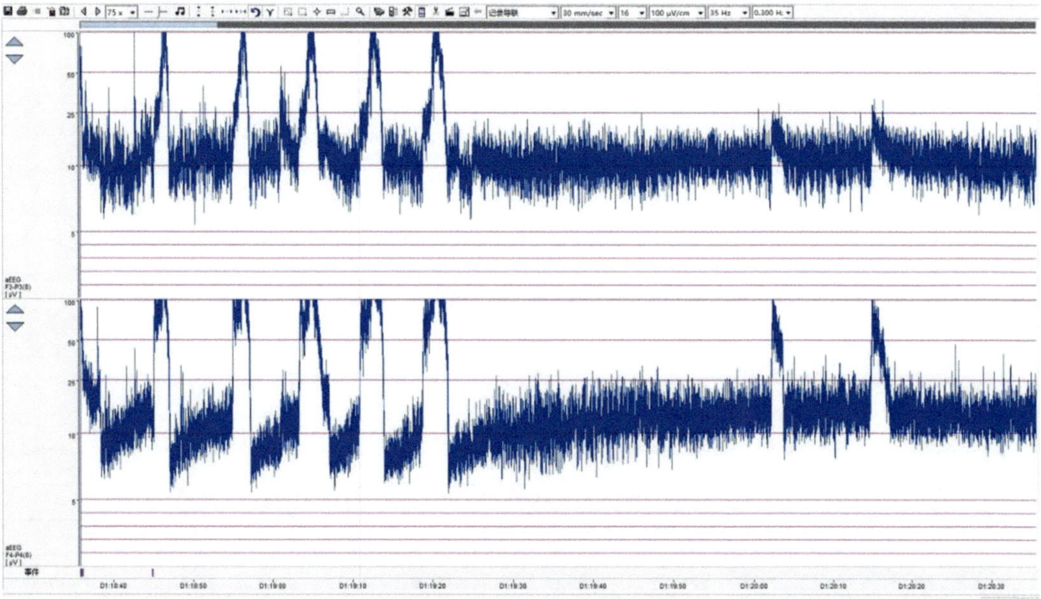

b

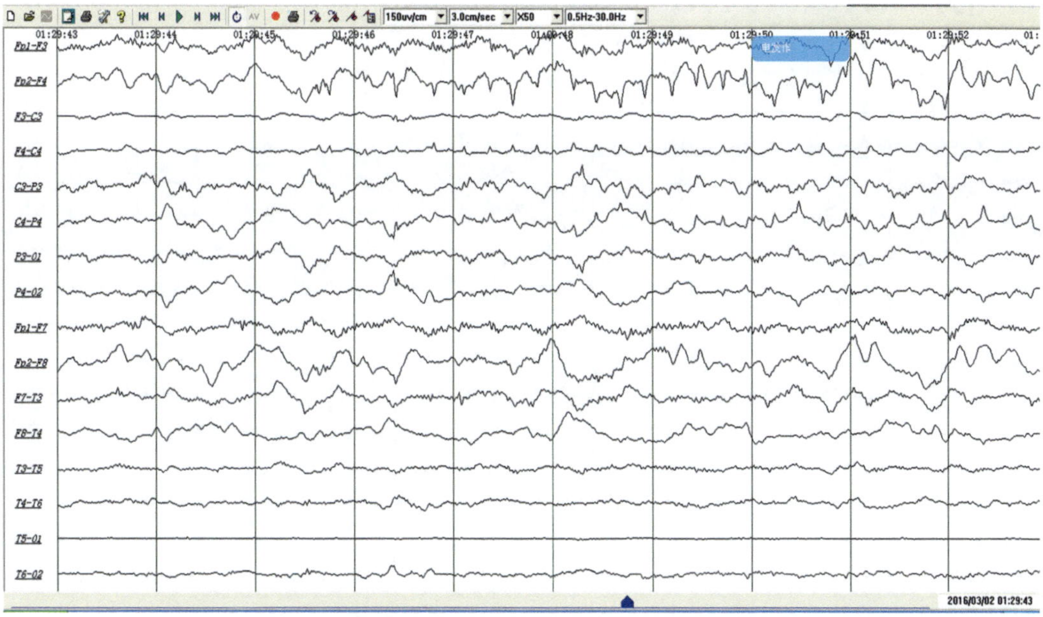

**Fig. 10.17** (**a**) aEEG showed multiple episodes. (**b**) EEG monitoring reveals the evolution of EEG from the right frontal origin. (**c**) EEG changes during seizure. (**d**) EEG changes during seizure. (**e**) EEG changes in the late stage of seizure. (**f**) The reexamination of head CT

c

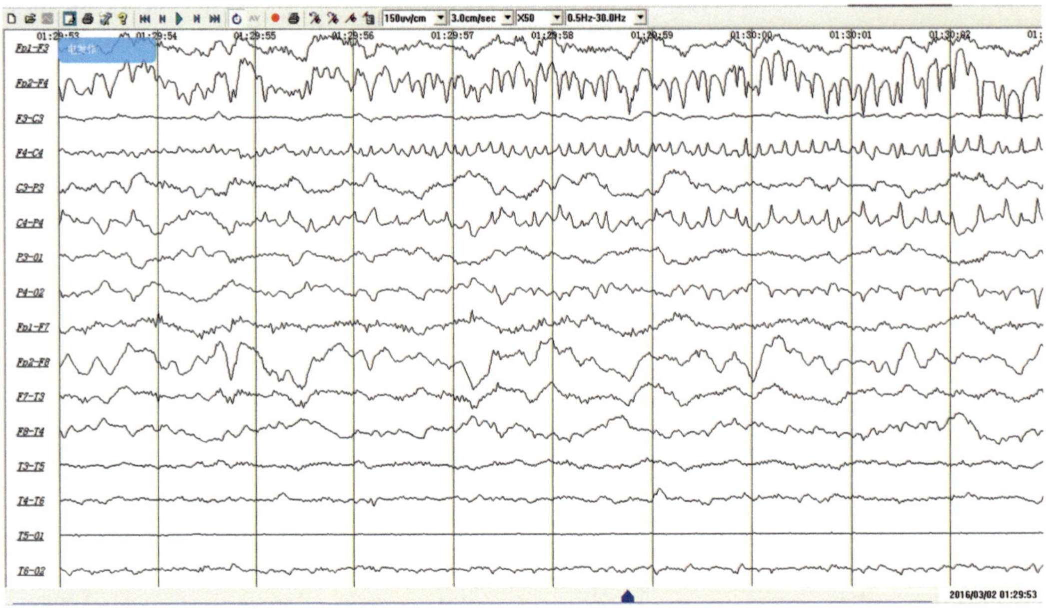


d

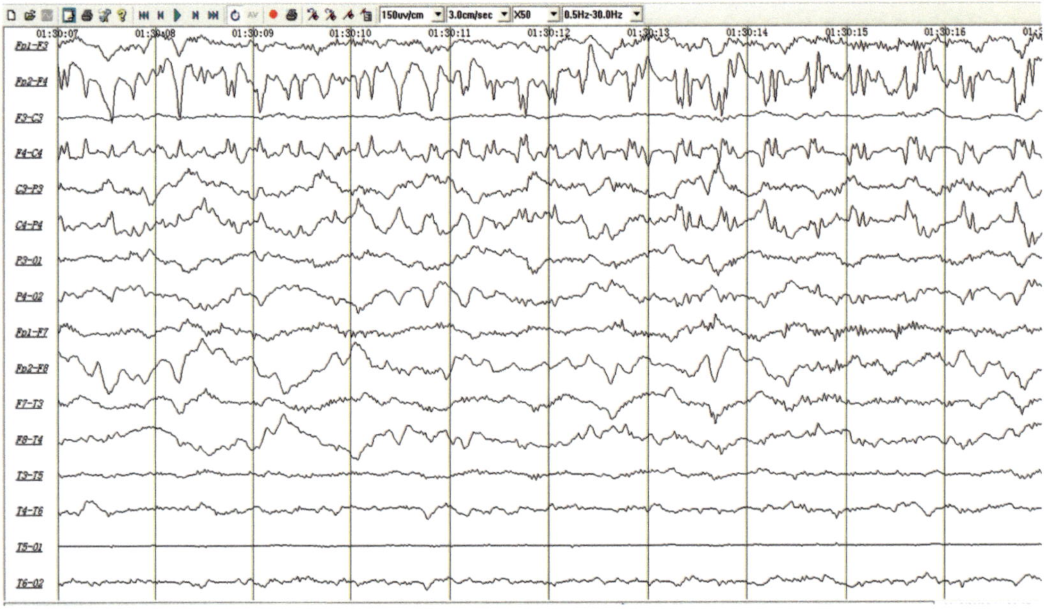


**Fig. 10.17** (continued)

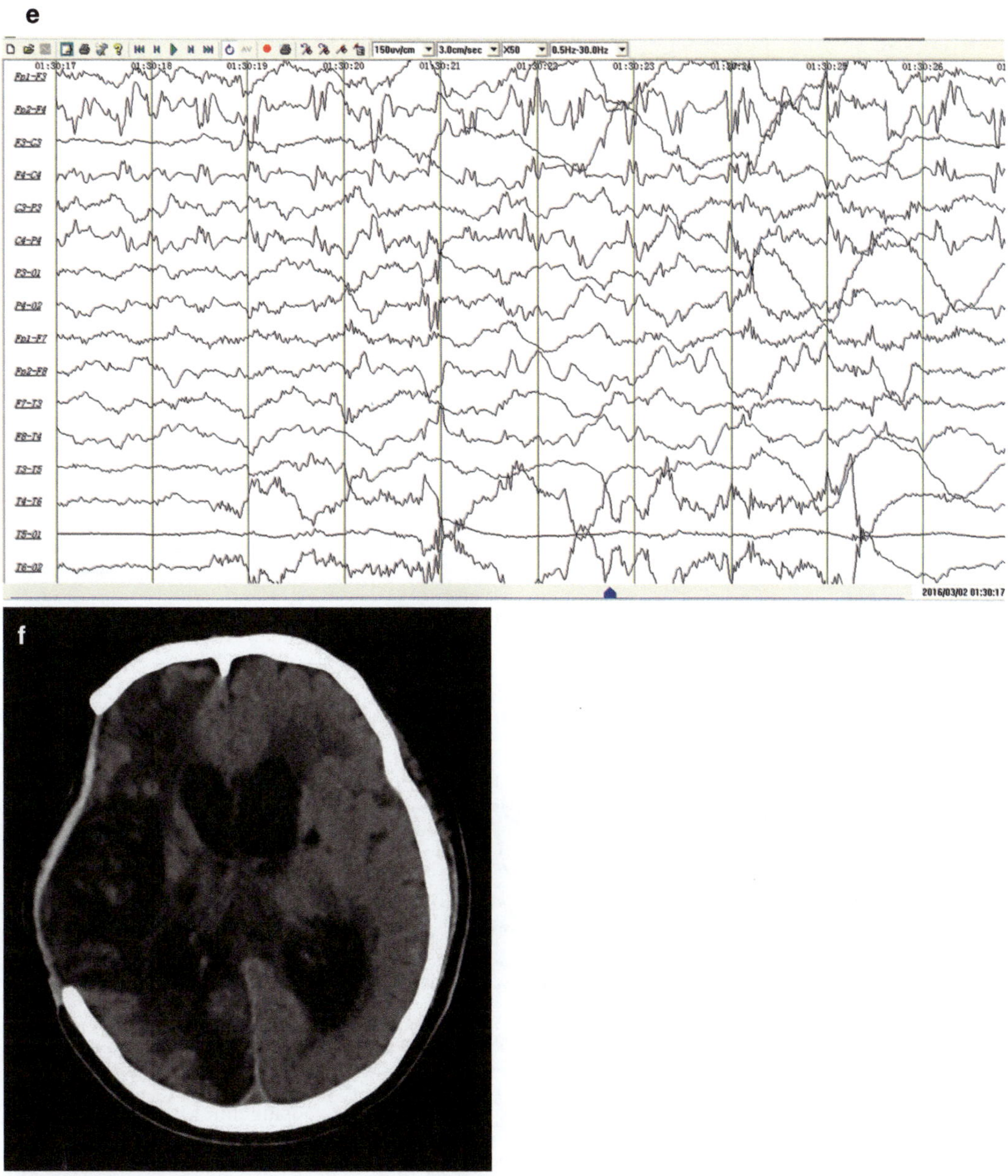


**Fig. 10.17** (continued)

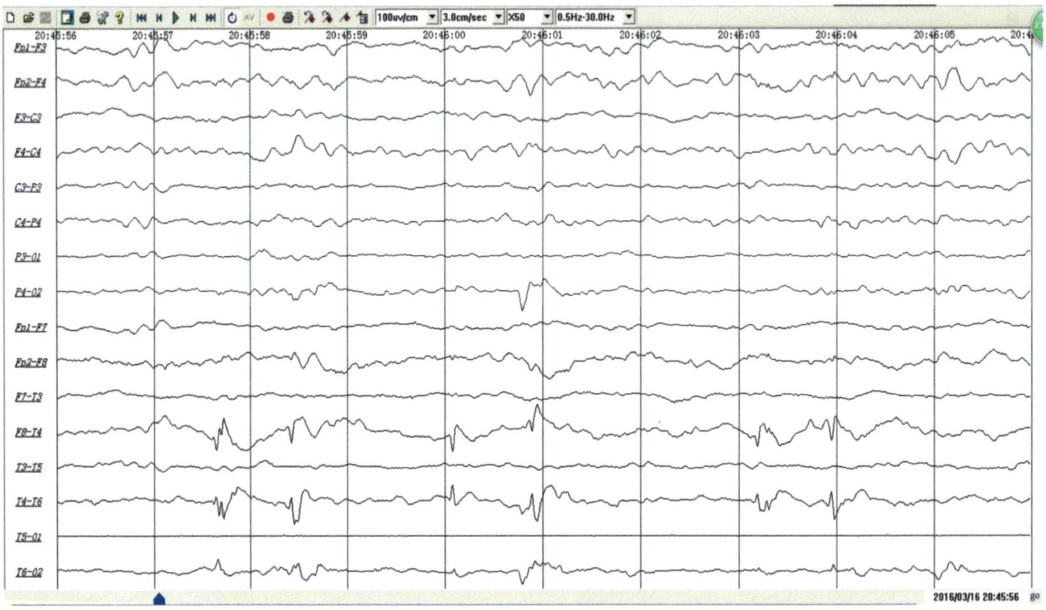

Fig. 10.18 EEG showed only the right temporal interictal discharge: spike slow wave, spiny slow wave

a

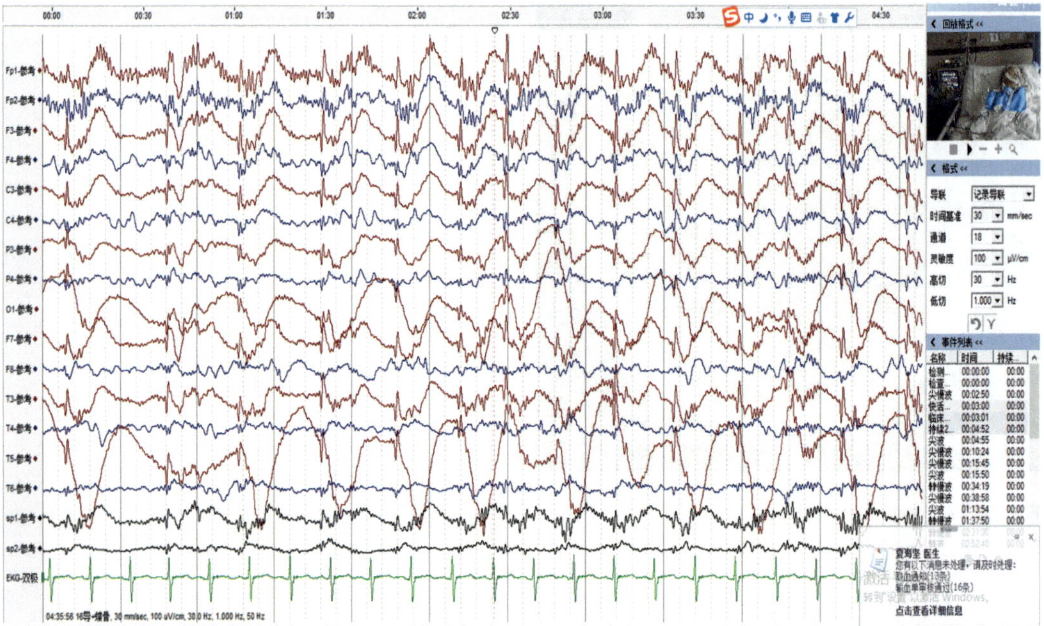

Fig. 10.19 (a) GPDs. (b) A 3 Hz spike-slow rhythm burst occurred after GPD. (c) Epileptic discharges lasted for 2 min and then stopped. (d) 2016.07.21. CT reexamination of the brain

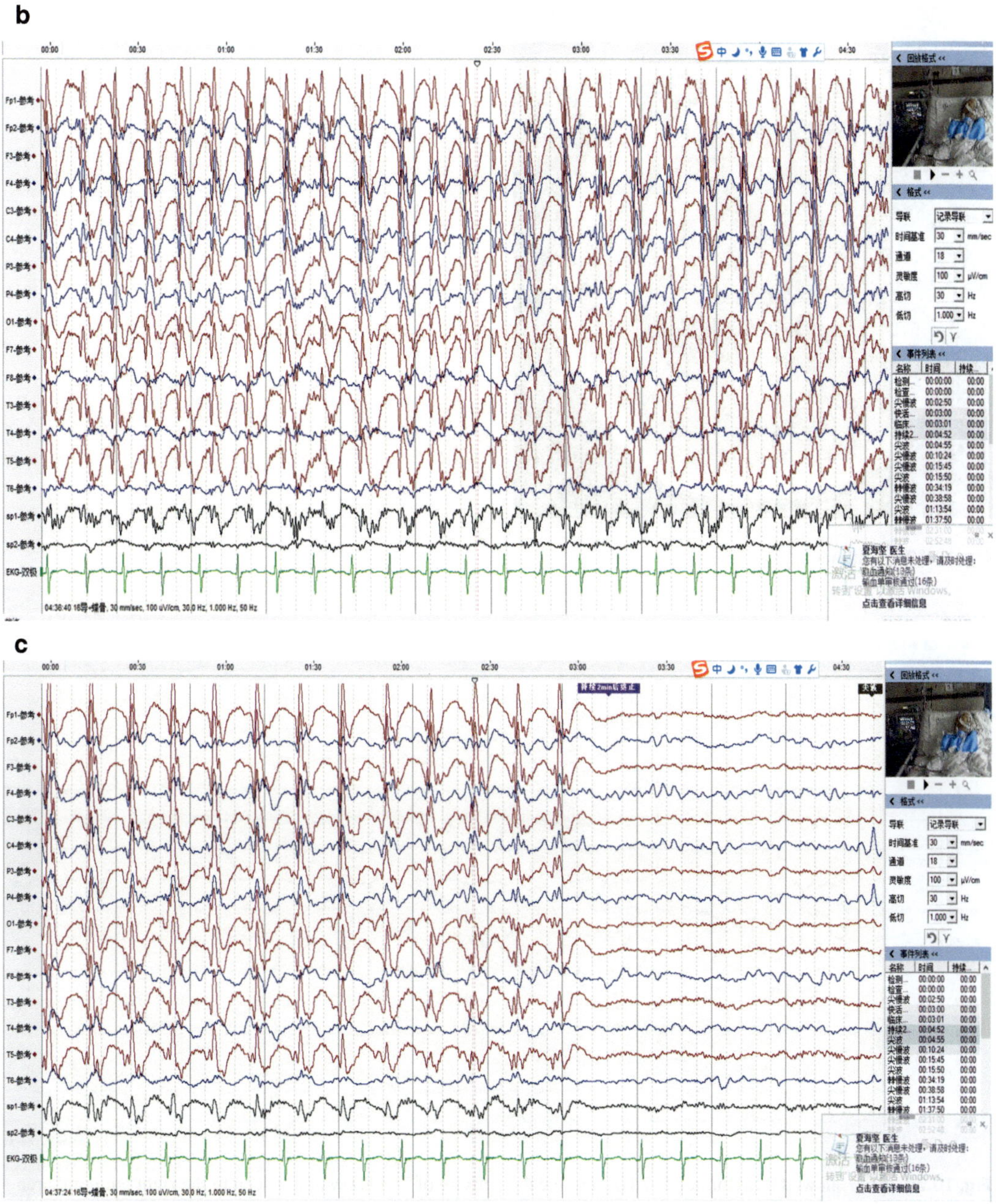

**Fig. 10.19** (continued)

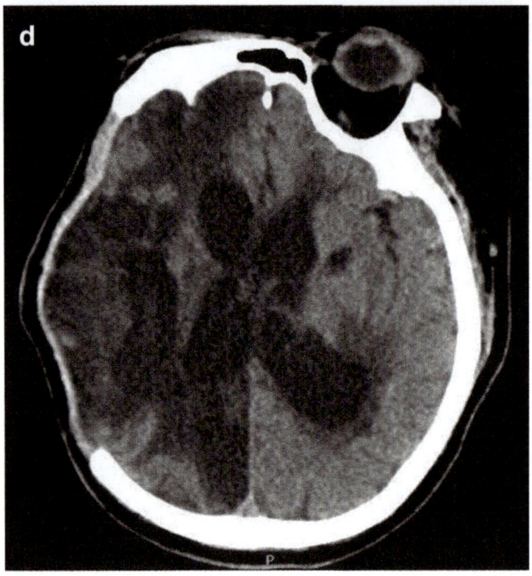


**Fig. 10.19** (continued)

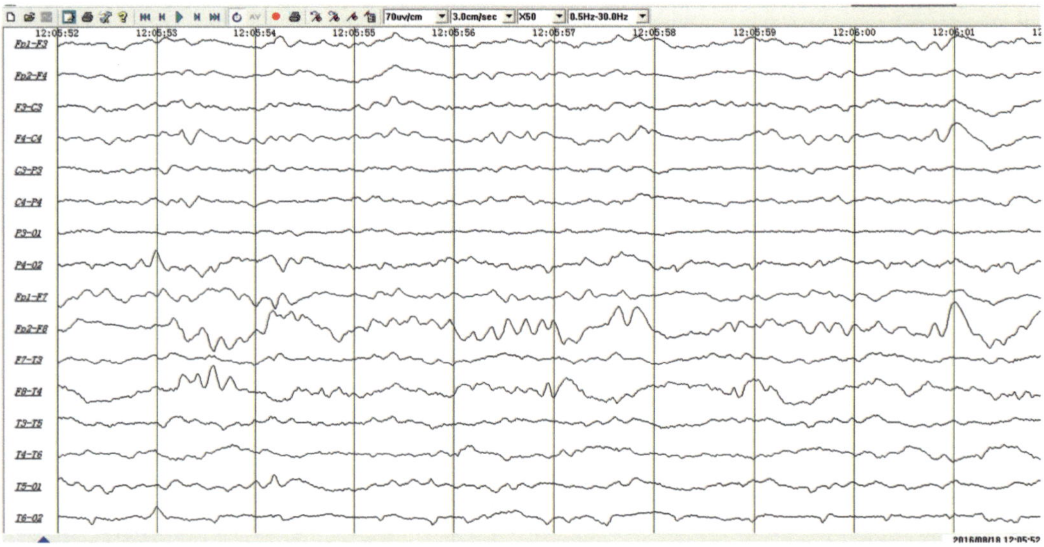


**Fig. 10.20** EEG showed θ rhythm of 5–7 Hz, and focal δ activity of 2–3 Hz was still seen in the right temporal area

## References

1. Dewan MC, Rattani A, Gupta S, et al. Estimating the global incidence of traumatic brain injury. J Neurosurg. 2018;130(4):1–18.
2. James SL, Lucchesi LR, Bisignano C, et al. Morbidity and mortality from road injuries: results from the Global Burden of Disease Study 2017. Inj Prev. 2020;26(Supp 1):i46–56.
3. Abdelmalik PA, Draghic N, Ling G. Management of moderate and severe traumatic brain injury. Transfusion. 2019;59(S2):1529–38.
4. Canac N, Jalaleddini K, Thorpe SG, et al. Review: pathophysiology of intracranial hypertension and noninvasive intracranial pressure monitoring. Fluids Barriers CNS. 2020;17(1):40.
5. Narayan V, Mohammed N, Savardekar AR, et al. Noninvasive intracranial pressure monitoring for severe traumatic brain injury in children: a con-

cise update on current methods. World Neurosurg. 2018;114:293–300.
6. Amantini A, Carrai R, Lori S, et al. Neurophysiological monitoring in adult and pediatric intensive care. Minerva Anestesiol. 2012;78(9):1067–75.
7. Rapp PE, Keyser DO, Albano A, et al. Traumatic brain injury detection using electrophysiological methods. Front Hum Neurosci. 2015;9:11.
8. Lauritzen M, Strong AJ. 'Spreading depression of Leao' and its emerging relevance to acute brain injury in humans. J Cereb Blood Flow Metab. 2017;37(5):1553–70.
9. Somjen GG. Aristides Leao's discovery of cortical spreading depression. J Neurophysiol. 2005;94(1):2–4.
10. Hartings JA, Shuttleworth CW, Kirov SA, et al. The continuum of spreading depolarizations in acute cortical lesion development: examining Leao's legacy. J Cereb Blood Flow Metab. 2017;37(5):1571–94.
11. Soldozy S, Sharifi KA, Desai B, et al. Cortical spreading depression in the setting of traumatic brain injury. World Neurosurg. 2020;134:50–7.
12. Rogers ML, Leong CL, Gowers SA, et al. Simultaneous monitoring of potassium, glucose and lactate during spreading depolarization in the injured human brain—proof of principle of a novel real-time neurochemical analysis system, continuous online microdialysis. J Cereb Blood Flow Metab. 2017;37(5):1883–95.
13. Ayata C, Lauritzen M. Spreading depression, spreading depolarizations, and the cerebral vasculature. Physiol Rev. 2015;95(3):953–93.
14. Leao AAP. Spreading depression of activity in the cerebral cortex. Neurophysiology. 1944;7(6):359–90.
15. Leao AA. Further observations on the spreading depression of activity in the cerebral cortex. J Neurophysiol. 1947;10(6):409–14.
16. Hadjikhani N, Sanchez DRM, Wu O, et al. Mechanisms of migraine aura revealed by functional MRI in human visual cortex. Proc Natl Acad Sci U S A. 2001;98(8):4687–92.
17. Strong AJ, Fabricius M, Boutelle MG, et al. Spreading and synchronous depressions of cortical activity in acutely injured human brain. Stroke. 2002;33(12):2738–43.
18. Helbok R, Hartings JA, Schiefecker A, et al. What should a clinician do when spreading depolarizations are observed in a patient? Neurocrit Care. 2020;32(1):306–10.
19. Somjen GG. Mechanisms of spreading depression and hypoxic spreading depression-like depolarization. Physiol Rev. 2001;81(3):1065–96.
20. Dreier JP. The role of spreading depression, spreading depolarization and spreading ischemia in neurological disease. Nat Med. 2011;17(4):439–47.
21. Woitzik J, Hecht N, Pinczolits A, et al. Propagation of cortical spreading depolarization in the human cortex after malignant stroke. Neurology. 2013;80(12):1095–102.
22. Dreier JP, Fabricius M, Ayata C, et al. Recording, analysis, and interpretation of spreading depolarizations in neurointensive care: review and recommendations of the COSBID research group. J Cereb Blood Flow Metab. 2017;37(5):1595–625.
23. Nilsson P, Hillered L, Olsson Y, et al. Regional changes in interstitial K+ and Ca2+ levels following cortical compression contusion trauma in rats. J Cereb Blood Flow Metab. 1993;13(2):183–92.
24. Stocker RA. Intensive care in traumatic brain injury including multi-modal monitoring and neuroprotection. Med Sci (Basel). 2019;7(3):37.
25. Van Harreveld A, Fifkova E. Glutamate release from the retina during spreading depression. J Neurobiol. 1970;2(1):13–29.
26. Van Harreveld A, JS S. Spreading cortical convulsions and depressions. J Neurophysiol. 1953;16(4):352–66.
27. Kramer DR, Fujii T, Ohiorhenuan I, et al. Cortical spreading depolarization: pathophysiology, implications, and future directions. J Clin Neurosci. 2016;24:22–7.
28. Takahashi H, Manaka S, Sano K. Changes in extracellular potassium concentration in cortex and brain stem during the acute phase of experimental closed head injury. J Neurosurg. 1981;55(5):708–17.
29. Szerb JC. Glutamate release and spreading depression in the fascia dentata in response to microdialysis with high K+: role of glia. Brain Res. 1991;542(2):259–65.
30. Somjen GG, Aitken PG, Czeh GL, et al. Mechanism of spreading depression: a review of recent findings and a hypothesis. Can J Physiol Pharmacol. 1992;70(Suppl):S248–54.
31. Fabricius M, Fuhr S, Willumsen L, et al. Association of seizures with cortical spreading depression and peri-infarct depolarisations in the acutely injured human brain. Clin Neurophysiol. 2008;119(9):1973–84.
32. Dreier JP, Major S, Pannek HW, et al. Spreading convulsions, spreading depolarization and epileptogenesis in human cerebral cortex. Brain. 2012;135(Pt 1):259–75.
33. Heinemann U, Lux HD. Ceiling of stimulus induced rises in extracellular potassium concentration in the cerebral cortex of cat. Brain Res. 1977;120(2):231–49.
34. Tsitsopoulos PP, Abu HS, Marklund N. Current opportunities for clinical monitoring of axonal pathology in traumatic brain injury. Front Neurol. 2017;8:599.
35. Strich SJ. Diffuse degeneration of the cerebral white matter in severe dementia following head injury. J Neurol Neurosurg Psychiatry. 1956;19(3):163–85.
36. Adams JH, Doyle D, Graham DI, et al. Diffuse axonal injury in head injuries caused by a fall. Lancet. 1984;2(8417–8418):1420–2.
37. Geschwind N. [The problem of language in relation to the phylogenetic development of the brain]. Sist Nerv. 1965;17(6):411–9.
38. Bigler ED. Behavioural and cognitive changes in traumatic brain injury: a spouse's perspective. Brain Inj. 1989;3(1):73–8.

39. Synek VM, Walker EB, Shaw NA, et al. Electroencephalographic abnormalities in patients with normal contrast computerised axial tomography brain scans. Clin Exp Neurol. 1987;24:159–67.
40. Guerit JM, Fischer C, Facco E, et al. Standards of clinical practice of EEG and EPs in comatose and other unresponsive states. The International Federation of Clinical Neurophysiology. Electroencephalogr Clin Neurophysiol Suppl. 1999;52:117–31.
41. Hirsch LJ, LaRoche SM, Gaspard N, et al. American Clinical Neurophysiology Society's standardized critical care EEG terminology: 2012 version. J Clin Neurophysiol. 2013;30(1):1–27.
42. Bricolo A, Faccioli F, Turazzi S. [EEG in post-traumatic coma. Diagnostic and prognostic value (author's transl)]. Rev Electroencephalogr Neurophysiol Clin. 1979;9(2):116–30.
43. Beridze M, Khaburzania M, Shakarishvili R, et al. Dominated EEG patterns and their prognostic value in coma caused by traumatic brain injury. Georgian Med News. 2010;186:28–33.
44. Fingelkurts AA, Fingelkurts AA, Bagnato S, et al. Life or death: prognostic value of a resting EEG with regards to survival in patients in vegetative and minimally conscious states. PLoS One. 2011;6(10):e25967.
45. Sandsmark DK, Kumar MA, Woodward CS, et al. Sleep features on continuous electroencephalography predict rehabilitation outcomes after severe traumatic brain injury. J Head Trauma Rehabil. 2016;31(2):101–7.
46. Valente M, Placidi F, Oliveira AJ, et al. Sleep organization pattern as a prognostic marker at the subacute stage of post-traumatic coma. Clin Neurophysiol. 2002;113(11):1798–805.
47. Azabou E, Navarro V, Kubis N, et al. Value and mechanisms of EEG reactivity in the prognosis of patients with impaired consciousness: a systematic review. Crit Care. 2018;22(1):184.
48. Benarous L, Gavaret M, Soda DM, et al. Sources of interrater variability and prognostic value of standardized EEG features in post-anoxic coma after resuscitated cardiac arrest. Clin Neurophysiol Pract. 2019;4:20–6.
49. Logi F, Pasqualetti P, Tomaiuolo F. Predict recovery of consciousness in post-acute severe brain injury: the role of EEG reactivity. Brain Inj. 2011;25(10):972–9.
50. Bauer G, Trinka E, Kaplan PW. EEG patterns in hypoxic encephalopathies (post-cardiac arrest syndrome): fluctuations, transitions, and reactions. J Clin Neurophysiol. 2013;30(5):477–89.
51. Rossetti AO, Carrera E, Oddo M. Early EEG correlates of neuronal injury after brain anoxia. Neurology. 2012;78(11):796–802.
52. Lee H, Mizrahi MA, Hartings JA, et al. Continuous electroencephalography after moderate to severe traumatic brain injury. Crit Care Med. 2019;47(4):574–82.
53. Tolonen A, Sarkela M, Takala R, et al. Quantitative EEG parameters for prediction of outcome in severe traumatic brain injury: development study. Clin EEG Neurosci. 2018;49(4):248–57.
54. Eriksen N, Pakkenberg B, Rostrup E, et al. Neurostereologic lesion volumes and spreading depolarizations in severe traumatic brain injury patients: a pilot study. Neurocrit Care. 2019;30(3):557–68.
55. Lee JW, The EEG. Ictal-interictal continuum-a metabolic roar but a whimper of a functional outcome. Epilepsy Curr. 2019;19(4):234–6.
56. Waziri A, Claassen J, Stuart RM, et al. Intracortical electroencephalography in acute brain injury. Ann Neurol. 2009;66(3):366–77.
57. Stuart RM, Waziri A, Weintraub D, et al. Intracortical EEG for the detection of vasospasm in patients with poor-grade subarachnoid hemorrhage. Neurocrit Care. 2010;13(3):355–8.
58. Young GB, Jordan KG, Doig GS. An assessment of nonconvulsive seizures in the intensive care unit using continuous EEG monitoring: an investigation of variables associated with mortality. Neurology. 1996;47(1):83–9.
59. McBride MC, Laroia N, Guillet R. Electrographic seizures in neonates correlate with poor neurodevelopmental outcome. Neurology. 2000;55(4):506–13.
60. Pisani F, Cerminara C, Fusco C, et al. Neonatal status epilepticus vs recurrent neonatal seizures: clinical findings and outcome. Neurology. 2007;69(23):2177–85.
61. Vespa PM, Miller C, McArthur D, et al. Nonconvulsive electrographic seizures after traumatic brain injury result in a delayed, prolonged increase in intracranial pressure and metabolic crisis. Crit Care Med. 2007;35(12):2830–6.
62. DeGiorgio CM, Correale JD, Gott PS, et al. Serum neuron-specific enolase in human status epilepticus. Neurology. 1995;45(6):1134–7.
63. Vespa PM, McArthur DL, Xu Y, et al. Nonconvulsive seizures after traumatic brain injury are associated with hippocampal atrophy. Neurology. 2010;75(9):792–8.

# Application of Multimodal EEG in AE

# 11

Qun Wang and Xuefeng Wang

## Contents




**Abstract**

AE generally refers to a type of encephalitis mediated by autoimmune mechanisms in which the body produces an autoimmune response to neurons. With the popularity of AE antibody determination, the incidence rate reported worldwide has increased each year. The disease often presents with an acute/subacute onset. After onset, patients quickly develop mental and behavioral abnormalities, language disorders, seizures, movement disorders, disturbances of consciousness, autonomic dysfunction, and other serious central nervous system symptoms that can threaten their lives. Because the clinical symptoms and related examinations of AE in the early stage are not specific, the disease is easily misdiagnosed. Some patients go to the psychiatric or infectious diseases department, delaying the optimal period of treatment. In addition, most AE patients enter the NICU for intensive care. The NICU typically includes a long hospital stay and high cost, which brings mental shock



Q. Wang
Department of Neurology, Beijing Tiantan Hospital, Capital Medical University, Beijing, China
e-mail: wangq@ccmu.edu.cn

X. Wang (✉)
Department of Neurology, The First Affiliated Hospital of Chongqing Medical University, Chongqing, China







X. Wang et al. (eds.), *Multi-Modal EEG Monitoring of Severely Neurologically Ill Patients*, https://doi.org/10.1007/978-981-16-4493-1_11

and huge economic pressure to the patient's family, reducing the patient's compliance and affecting further treatment with a serious impact on the recovery and prognosis of the patient. Therefore, the early diagnosis of AE is helpful to formulate individualized treatment plans for patients and reduce the incidence of residual sequelae and death. This chapter briefly describes the epidemiology of AE and related examination methods, focusing on the common EEG features of AE, such as slow waves, extreme δ brushes (EDBs), epileptiform discharges, and increased fast waves. At the same time, this chapter elaborates on the role of EEG in the early diagnosis, treatment, effective evaluation, and prognostic evaluation in AE, indicating that early, comprehensive evaluation and accurate diagnosis are important for the formulation of treatment plans and good prognosis in AE patients.

**Keywords**

AE · Anti-NMDA receptor encephalitis · GRDA · Epilepsy · SE · Excessive β activity (EBA) · EDB · Prognosis · EEG · qEEG

## 11.1 Overview

As early as the 1960s, AE, manifesting mainly as subacute progressive memory impairment, disorientation, and emotional irritability, was first described. Because imaging of AE patients mostly suggests abnormal signals of the limbic system, such as the medial temporal lobe and hippocampus, it is defined as limbic encephalitis [1]. The disease is usually related to hallucinations, seizures, and sleep disorders and is considered to be highly related to tumors due to its production of antitumor neuron intracellular antigen antibodies, such as lung cancer related to nuclear or cytoplasmic proteins such as Hu, Ma, and Ri, and testicular tumors [1–3]. In recent years, unlike paraneoplastic limbic encephalitis, which produces intracellular antigen antibodies, another group of AE mediated by synaptic receptor extracellular antigens or transsynaptic protein complex antibodies—neuron surface antibody (NSAb)-related encephalitis [1–3]—has also attracted attention. In view of its rare associated tumors, it is also called "nonparaneoplastic limbic encephalitis" [2]. Currently known pathogenic NSAb includes leucine-rich glioma inactivated 1(LGI1) antibody, contactin-associated protein-like 2 (Caspr2) antibody, NMDAR antibody, a-amino-3-hydroxy-5-methyl-1-4-isoxazolepropionic acid receptor (AMPAR) antibody, GABA (B) receptor antibody, and glycine (Gly) receptor antibody [4, 5]. Among them, AE involving NMDAR antibody and LGI1 antibody is the most common [6].

## 11.2 Epidemiology of AE and Related Inspection Methods

Studies have shown that the above mentioned NSAb-related encephalitis responds well to immunosuppressive treatment, and early initiation of treatment can significantly improve the prognosis. Therefore, early recognition and diagnosis are particularly important in clinical diagnosis and treatment [4]. As the disease progresses or if the patient is not given timely treatment, the patient's level of consciousness will gradually decrease. In clinical practice, we have found that this period often lasts for a long time. Patients with impaired consciousness need long-term observation in a hospital setting, leading to high costs and substantial emotional and economic burden for the patient's family, which leads to less patient compliance and, thus, a poor prognosis for the patient. Therefore, accurate brain function assessment and reliable prediction of awakening time and neurological function prognosis of patients with NMDAR encephalitis disorder can provide clinicians and their families with useful information.

The diagnosis of AE needs to incorporate the patient's clinical manifestations, CBF examination, neuroimaging and EEG examination results, and a positive antineuron antibody result is the main basis of the diagnosis. However, because the diversity of symptoms and antibody detection technology are not yet fully popularized, early diagnosis of AE is still a major difficulty. Overreliance on antibody detection and accurate assessment of immunotherapy response may lead to treatment delays. Among the biochemical indicators, NSE and S-100 calnexins have been widely used in the evaluation of brain damage and neuroprognosis, but there is only one relevant study on the prognostic evaluation of anti-NMDAR encephalitis. This study showed that the concentration of NSE or S100B in the CBF within 72 h of onset is significantly related to the mRS score and can be used to evaluate the prognosis of the disease [7]. However, anti-NMDAR encephalitis is often difficult to identify in the early stage; therefore, early specimens are rarely obtained, and specimens are clinically difficult to obtain. The sample size of this study was small. In the future, large samples and multicenter studies are still needed for confirmation. MRI is often used in neuroimaging examinations. Head MRI of patients with NSAb encephalitis is usually normal or shows nonspecific changes. Previous studies have shown that only 23–50% of patients with anti-NMDAR encephalitis have abnormal head MRI changes, which include frontal, parietal, and medial temporal white matter lesions [8]. The results of an imaging study on antivoltage-gated potassium channel (VGKC) complex antibody-related encephalitis showed that most patients can have an increase in the volume of the medial temporal lobe (including the hippocampus and amygdala) and high T2-FLAIR imaging signals [9]. Since the incidence of anti-NMDAR encephalitis is much higher than that of other NSAb-related encephalitides, the overall rate of abnormal head MRI is still low. Different from conventional structural MRI; EEG, as a method of neurological function detection, is widely used in the diagnosis and treatment of NSAb-related encephalitis. Compared with immunological detection and head MRI examination, EEG is more popular and economical, and its clinical application value is more practical. Previous studies have shown that EEG in the early stage of the disease has a certain prompting significance for the diagnosis of the disease, and specific EEG manifestations also indicate different severities and prognoses of the disease [10].

## 11.3 EEG Features of AE

In the early stage of anti-NMDAR encephalitis, EEG is mainly used to monitor seizures and NCSE and is used to distinguish epilepsy and abnormal movement [11]. Related research mainly focuses on a wide range of nonspecific δ slow-wave activities, mainly in the frontotemporal lobe. Some studies attribute this waveform to NCSE, but there is no detailed description or unified definition [12]. In 2012, Schmitt et al. [13] found extensive and continuous δ waves of 0.3–1.0 Hz combined with β activities of 20–30 Hz in patients with anti-NMDAR encephalitis, called EDB, which is considered to be the characteristic brain electrical activity of anti-NMDAR encephalitis and can be used for early diagnosis. Relevant studies have pointed out that AE can have four longitudinal EEG stages [14]. In the early stage (when behavioral changes and/or orofacial and limb movement disorders are the most common clinical features), the EEG background activity during wakefulness and sleep is mostly normal, with a symmetrical and reactive posterior α rhythm (8–12 Hz) and intermittent or continuous visible unilateral and/or bilateral slow waves of medium to high amplitude (1–3 Hz) that are unresponsive, especially in the frontotemporal area. Approximately 2–3 weeks after the onset of symptoms, at the peak of disease development (when the impairment of consciousness and limb movement is more severe), background activities gradually deteriorate, the posterior α rhythm disappears, and unique patterns not related to clinical changes appear, but the background activity during sleep is relatively intact. This background activity during sleep is characterized by diffuse or scattered rhythmic δ and/or θ activities that are 2–2.5 Hz and 4–5 Hz, respectively, last from a few seconds to a few hours, do not respond to stimuli, and usually disappear during sleep. These rhythmic δ and/or θ activities can occur independently or simultaneously in one area or different areas of both hemispheres. During the recovery period, the above-mentioned rhythmic δ and/or θ activities gradually decrease, the responsiveness and the posterior α rhythm gradually recover, and the background activity improves. Eventually, 2–5 months after the onset of the disease, the EEG shows complete normalization of electrical activity. In recent years, with the development of EEG monitoring technology and the increase in the number and duration of monitoring sessions, EEG research on AE has been more detailed and has identified more patterns, such as diffuse RDA, FIRDA or TIRDA, EDB, epileptiform discharges (focal, focal spread to total conduction, lateral discharge), PDs (unilateral, bilateral), TW, and an increase in fast waves [15]. The identification of these patterns has certain auxiliary significance for the early diagnosis of AE and the evaluation of the severity of the disease. The specific manifestations are as follows.

### 11.3.1 Slow Waves

A large number of studies have reported that non-specific diffuse slow waves are the most common waveform of anti-NMDAR encephalitis [16]. Compared with the EEGs of viral encephalitis, those of anti-NMDAR encephalitis have a higher proportion of diffuse slow waves. Data provided by the California Encephalitis Program in the United States showed that 80% of patients with anti-NMDAR encephalitis have diffuse slow waves, and the extent of slow-wave activity and the number of slow waves can reflect the severity of the disease [17]. Previous studies [18] on EEG changes in the initial period (equivalent to the rising period and the extreme period) and the intermediate period (equivalent to the falling period and the recovery period) have shown that the background activities in the rising period and the extreme period are mostly composed of slow waves, and the slow-wave distribution range is relatively extensive; From the falling period, the background activity is dominated by an α rhythm. The slow-wave distribution range in the recovery period is reduced, indicating that the EEG background slow wave and its distribution range are consistent with the severity of the disease; that is, it appears to increase first from the rising period to the recovery period and to reduce later. Since persistent diffuse slow waves are related to the severity of the disease, the different nature of slow waves reflects the severity of the disease. Related research [19] found that the possible cause of slow waves in AE is that the NMDAR is an ionotropic glutamate receptor that has many different structural regulatory sites and ligand-gated calcium channels throughout all brain tissues. After the NMDAR interacts with the anti-NMDAR antibody, the cell depolarization time is shortened, causing slow waves in the EEG. At the same time, encephalitis itself can cause brain tissue damage, such as damage to the cortex, white matter, basal ganglia, midbrain, or ascending reticulum activation system. Depending on the location of the injury, focal slow waves or diffuse slow waves will appear. Different studies have provided different descriptions of slow waves. Some scholars believe that slow waves occur repeatedly in anti-NMDAR encephalitis, with the same shape and duration and no changes in frequency and location [20]. Other studies have shown that there is a wide range of RDA in the waveform and frequency evolution [21]. Recently, Jeannin et al. [22] conducted a focused study on the EEG of patients with anti-NMDAR encephalitis and described this slow wave as a GRDA.

GRDA is a diffuse, synchronous, continuous rhythmic δ wave or δ complex wave, and this kind of activity is relatively single, without acceleration or recruitment [22] (Figs. 11.1, 11.2, 11.3, and 11.4). GRDA is different from epileptic discharge in that it is not altered by visual or sensitive stimuli. It persists after AED treatment, but it can be temporarily blocked by propofol. GRDA can exist throughout 30 min of EEG monitoring, and it can last from several minutes to several hours in cEEG monitoring. Sometimes GRDA will be replaced by specific irregular δ or θ waves that last for several hours, intermittently superimposed with drug-induced fast-wave activity (>20 Hz) [23]. Because GRDA is easy to observe in EEGs and has a long duration, it is easy to record and recognize, and there are relatively many clinical studies. Some scholars believe that GRDA is an EEG

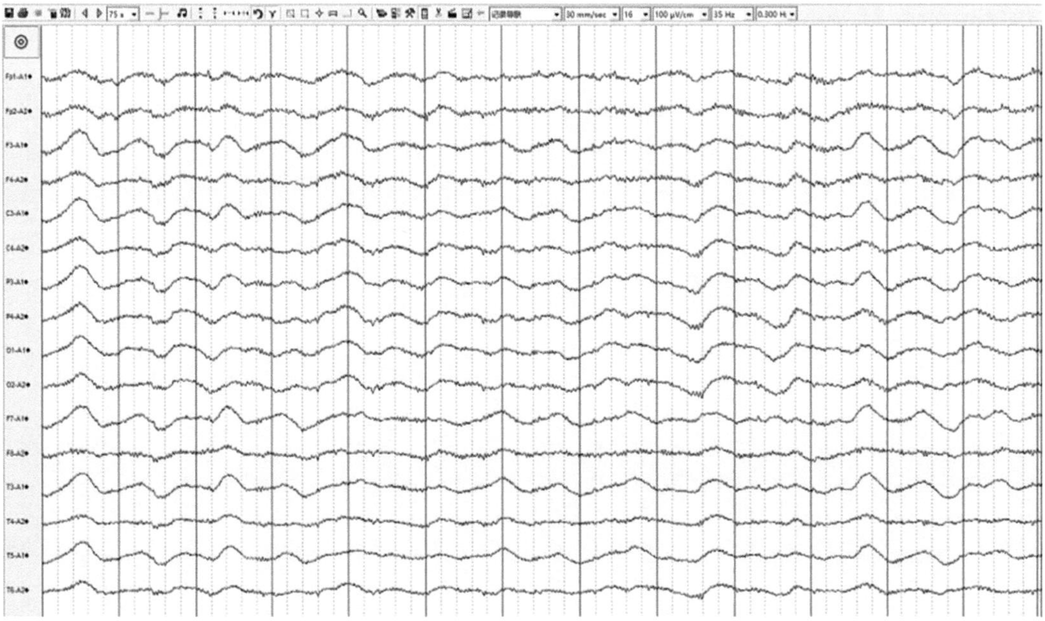

**Fig. 11.1** Female, 58 years old, anti-NMDAR encephalitis. EEG background activity showed diffuse low amplitude δ activity of 1.0 Hz

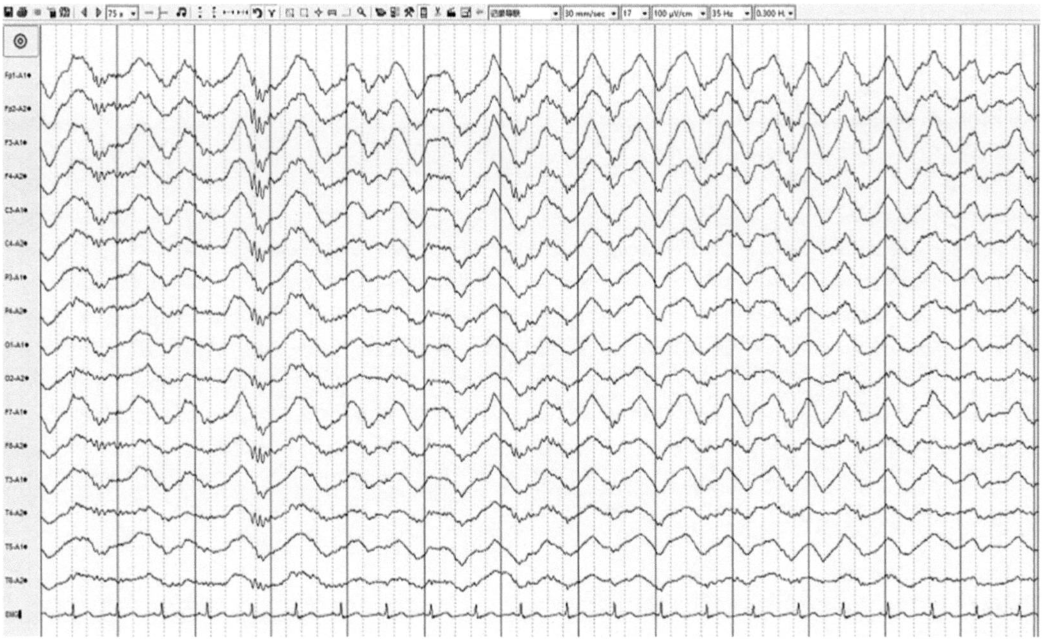

**Fig. 11.2** GRDA is different from background activity. EEG can be seen in diffuse, synchronous or nonsynchronous, continuous RDA

pattern of SE [23]. However, studies on critically ill or comatose patients have found that because GRDA lacks a clear evolution in frequency, location, and morphology, it does not indicate the origin of epilepsy [24]. In addition, GRDA does not respond to AEDs, so there is no correlation between it and seizures. The latest study found that GRDA is related to abnormal

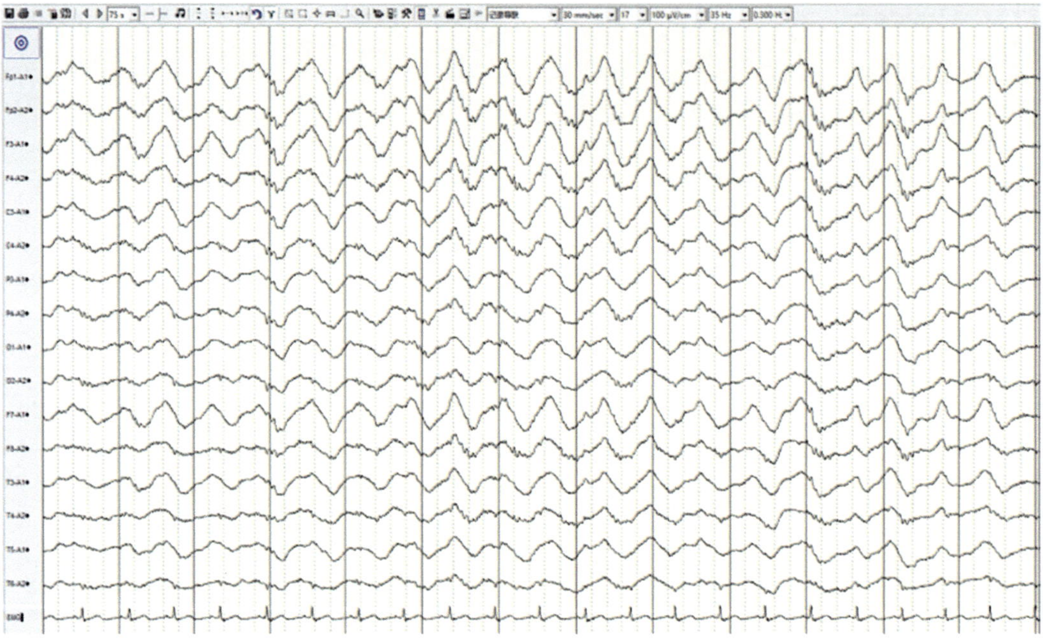

**Fig. 11.3** This kind of waveform is relatively single, without acceleration or recruitment, lasting from several minutes to several hours

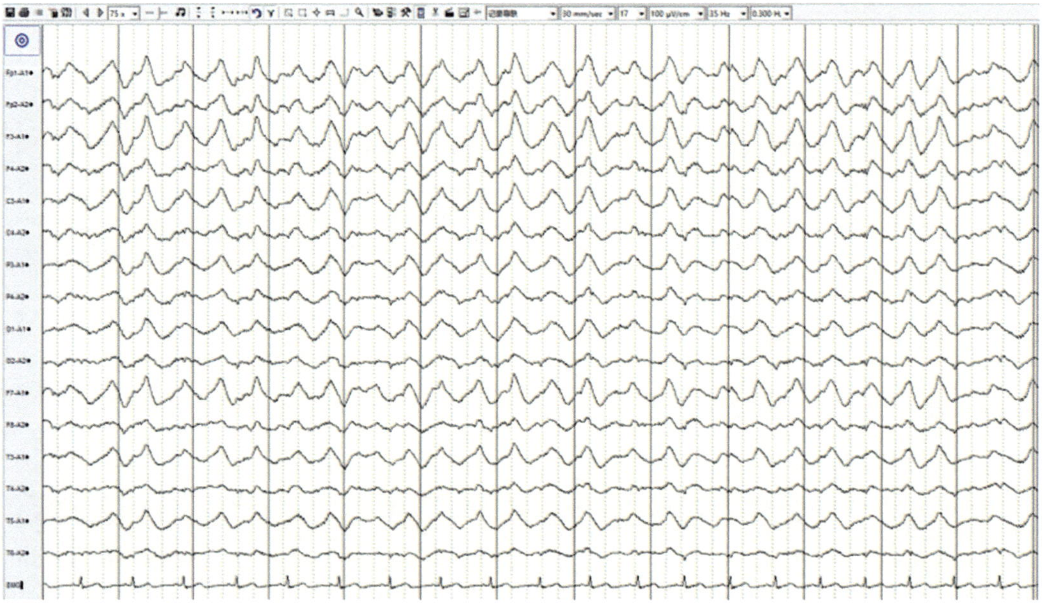

**Fig. 11.4** The waveform did not disappear after intravenous injection of diazepam

movements, suggesting that this EEG pattern originated from the basal ganglia. At the same time, MRI and FDG-PET examinations also confirmed the significance of the basal ganglia in anti-NMDAR encephalitis [22]. In addition, GRDA also appears in other diseases of basal ganglia nerve dysfunction, such as Creutzfeldt-Jakob disease, diffuse Lewy body disease, subcortical disease, and deep midline disease that affects thalamic-cortical projection [25, 26].

### 11.3.2 Epilepsy Waves

Acute symptomatic epilepsy is a common symptom of AE, and some scholars believe that AE is the most common cause of new-onset RSE [26]. EEG is of great significance in the diagnosis and evaluation of epileptic seizures or SE. Patients with AE with epileptic seizures should be routinely tested by video EEG to determine the type of seizures and guide the clinical application of AEDs. In anti-NMDAR encephalitis [27], the incidence of epileptic seizures is approximately 80%, and the seizures occur in various forms, including generalized epileptic seizures such as GTCSs, focal or mixed epileptic seizures, and SE (convulsive or nonconvulsive). Epileptic seizures in patients with LGI1 antibody-related encephalitis are common in various forms of temporal lobe epilepsy. The aura is more common with vertical hair seizures ("goose bumps"). Faciobrachial dystonic seizures (FBDSs) are the characteristic symptom of the disease, manifesting as frequent and short-lived dystonia-like involuntary unilateral movements of the arms, face, and even lower extremities. The onset time is short, usually only a few seconds. Frequent attacks can reach dozens of times a day accompanied by bilateral dystonia-like episodes, paresthesia aura, daze, and changes in consciousness. EEGs can manifest mild diffuse slow waves or bilateral frontotemporal slow waves, or they can be completely normal [15]. Anti-GABA (B) receptor encephalitis is usually dominated by GTCSs, and patients can quickly progress to SE. The EEGs of patients with anti-GABA receptor encephalitis show epileptic discharges originating from the temporal lobe and diffuse or scattered slow waves.

Related studies have reported that some patients with AE have clinically obvious epileptic seizures, but only a small number of patients have EEG records with clear epileptic discharges. For example, the detection rate of abnormal EEGs during FBDS episodes is low (only 21–30%). The possible reason is that some epileptic seizures and SE are easily controlled by drugs, so they are not found during EEG monitoring, or the clinically observed seizures are actually involuntary movements, resulting in a lower detection rate of EEG epileptic discharges [28, 29]. In anti-NMDAR encephalitis, the symptoms of NCSE are not specific. The clinical diagnosis mainly depends on EEG monitoring. Existing study [27] describes NCSE EEG activity in anti-NMDAR encephalitis as follows: extensive persistence of a 2–3 Hz rhythmic δ slow wave, which is more pronounced in the frontotemporal lobe, has a spatiotemporal evolution form, it is not affected by AEDs, it is incompletely inhibited by anesthetic drugs (propofol, midazolam), and gradually disappears after immunosuppressive therapy or felbamate therapy. However, some scholars [30] believe that this type of brain electrical activity does not reflect the NCSE of anti-NMDAR encephalitis, so there is still no unified definition of its typical brain electrical activity.

### 11.3.3 EBA

EBA is β activity with a frequency of 14–20 Hz, which is similar to the large amount of β activity caused by barbiturates, benzodiazepines, and other sedative hypnotic drugs under normal conditions, but compared to drug-induced β activity, the amplitude of EBA is higher, the frequency is slower, and the occurrence has nothing to do with the use of sedative drugs. EBA is more common in the early stages of anti-NMDAR encephalitis. Therefore, when the disease is highly suspected and changes are seen in EEGs, EBA can provide a basis for the early diagnosis of the disease. At the same time, the overlapping β-wave activities of EBA and EDB are similar, and the two have time correlations. EBA can be seen in patients with dysplasia of the cortex [22]. This EEG pattern may originate in the cerebral cortex.

### 11.3.4 EDB Wave

EDB refers to extensive and continuous 0.3–1.0 Hz δ-wave complex β-wave activity in both cerebral hemispheres during waking and sleeping periods, and the activity is more prominent in the front head. EDB can appear in newborns, with EEGs showing a transient δ rhythm compounded with an 8.0–20 Hz fast wave, which is usually symmetrical but not synchronous, and it can appear in various brain regions but is rare in the frontal lobe [13] (Figs. 11.5 and 11.6). EDB is a specific EEG manifestation of anti-NMDAR encephalitis, with an incidence of 16–41% [21, 31]. EDB appears in the early stage of anti-NMDAR encephalitis, mainly in the peak period, and gradually disappears during the recovery period [13]. Studies have found that EDB is not an artifact caused by involuntary movement, nor it is a drug-related fast wave caused by AEDs or

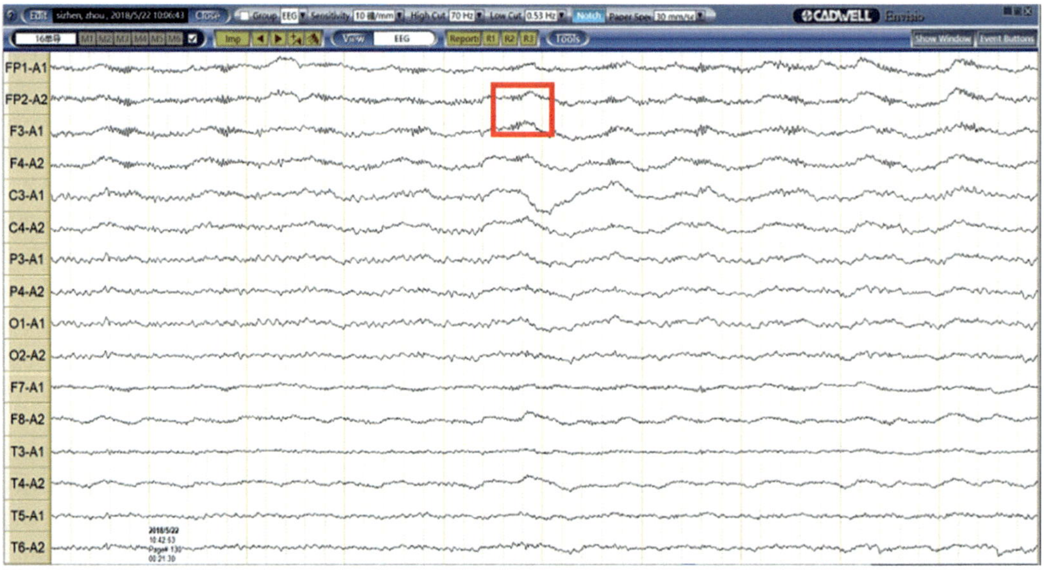


**Fig. 11.5** A 16-year-old female presented with a 12-day history of mental and behavioral abnormalities, aggravation, and limb rigidity for 3 days and was subsequently diagnosed with anti-NMDA encephalitis. The EEG showed EDB

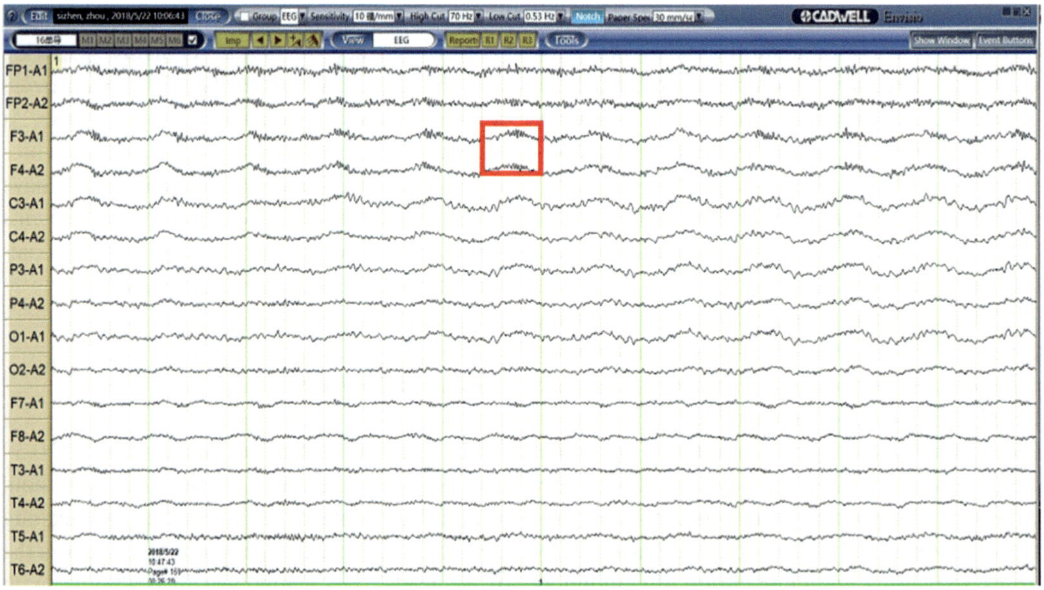


**Fig. 11.6** The EEG showed EDB characterized by a diffuse, full-lead, medium-amplitude δ slow wave superimposed with a 15–20 Hz β wave

sedative drugs, and it has nothing to do with the sleep cycle; therefore, EDB is a type of brain electrical activity that is specific to anti-NMDAR encephalitis. If EDB is found in clinical practice, anti-NMDAR encephalitis should be highly suspected. The origin of EDB is still unclear [22], but in newborns, δ brush is described as an endogenous cortical EEG pattern that is triggered by sensory input and seems to play an important role in brain development, so EDB may be produced by the cortex in patients with anti-NMDAR encephalitis.

Studies [22] have found that in patients with anti-NMDAR encephalitis, the three patterns, EDA, EBA, and GRDA, have a significant time correlation. EDA appears in the early stage, followed by EBA, and GRDA appears last. This time correlation provides electrophysiological support for the time progression of anti-NMDAR encephalitis from the initial damage of the main cortex to the subcortex, especially basal ganglia dysfunction.

## 11.4 The Clinical Value of EEG in AE

### 11.4.1 Role in Early Diagnosis

According to the different parts of the brain tissue involved, AE can manifest different clinical symptoms, such as damage to the frontal and temporal lobes. Patients often present with abnormal mental behavior, seizures, and cognitive dysfunction. Mental symptoms are one of the common clinical symptoms of AE. Almost eighty-one percent of AE patients have psychotic symptoms as the first onset; young and middle-aged patients with acute or subacute onset are often misdiagnosed with "functional mental illness", leading to delays in the optimal treatment time and adverse consequences [32]. The probability of poor prognosis of AE reaches 29.38%, and it is positively correlated with the degree of brain damage, indicating that early diagnosis and treatment can improve the prognosis [17]. At present, CBF examination and head imaging examination, as common auxiliary examination methods, can provide certain clues for disease diagnosis, but the positive rate is not high. In anti-NMDAR encephalitis, more than 90% of patients have abnormal EEGs, and the positive rate of imaging is less than 50% [33]. With the increase in related research, specific EEG patterns are gradually recognized by clinicians; therefore, EEG is more sensitive than imaging in the diagnosis of anti-NMDAR encephalitis, and it has important significance in early diagnosis.

### 11.4.2 Effect on Epilepsy and SE

Studies have shown that most (nearly 80%) AE patients have limb twitches, but only a small proportion of patients have epileptic waves on EEGs [17]. The possible reasons are as follows: (a) Many patients have epileptic seizures or even SE at the early stage of onset, but some patients have seizures that are easier to control, and epileptic waves cannot be recorded during EEG detection; (b) Epilepsy and involuntary movements coexist, or clinical epileptiform seizures are actually involuntary movements; therefore, the detection rate of EEG epileptic waves is low. It is sometimes difficult to distinguish anti-NMDAR encephalitis epilepsy and involuntary movements based on clinical manifestations alone, especially in patients with impaired consciousness. Clinically, AEDs are overadministered, which are likely to cause many adverse consequences [32].

SE is a common symptom of anti-NMDAR encephalitis [24]. If a patient shows CSE, it is often easy for doctors to determine and provide timely treatment. However, when a patient has manifestations that are inconsistent with the anti-NMDAR encephalitis itself, such as changes in cognition, behavior, and consciousness, accompanied by slight twitching of limbs or face but no obvious convulsion-like symptoms, then NCSE should be suspected, and it is necessary for the patient to undergo EEG or qEEG monitoring in a timely manner to avoid a delay in treatment. Therefore, EEG is essential for the diagnosis, differential diagnosis, and medication guidance of epilepsy in AE.

### 11.4.3 Role in Prognostic Evaluation

The use of EEG to determine the prognosis of AE has been a hot research topic in recent years. There are many related studies on the effect of EDB on the prognosis of anti-NMDAR encephalitis, and there is much controversy. It has been reported in the literature [33] that EDB is related to the length of the patient's disease. Patients with EDB in their EEGs have a longer hospital stay and a worse prognosis. However, another study [34] found that the median mRS score of patients with anti-NMDAR encephalitis who developed EDB was 0 point (0–3 points) during the recovery period, suggesting a better prognosis. Some scholars [35] have proposed that patients with β waves superimposed between the peaks of the δ waves rather than on the peaks have a better prognosis than patient with EDB. The latest study [31] of a long-term follow-up of patients with anti-NMDAR encephalitis found that there was no significant difference in prognosis between the two groups with or without EDB, indicating that EDB has no specificity in predicting poor prognosis. The possible reason for this difference in results is that the sample size was too small and the test power was too low. In addition to EDB, other EEG patterns have also been reported to affect the prognosis of anti-NMDAR encephalitis. Studies have found that persistent unilateral or focal abnormal EEG activity with normal background activity in at least one cerebral hemisphere suggests a better prognosis, while diffuse abnormal EEG activity lacking physiological background activity is associated with severe neurological function injury and is associated with a poor prognosis [36]; some scholars have suggested that patients with normal background activity, epileptiform discharges, pleomorphic δ rhythm, and diffuse β activity at the peak of the disease have a good prognosis after 6–54 months [31].

In recent years, qEEGs (Fig. 11.7) have attracted the attention of medical workers as an important tool for evaluating the prognosis of patients with AE, and the clinical value of qEEGs has attracted the attention of medical workers. Jiang et al. [37] included 26 patients with anti-NMDA encephalitis. In this study, these patients were divided into a critical group and a

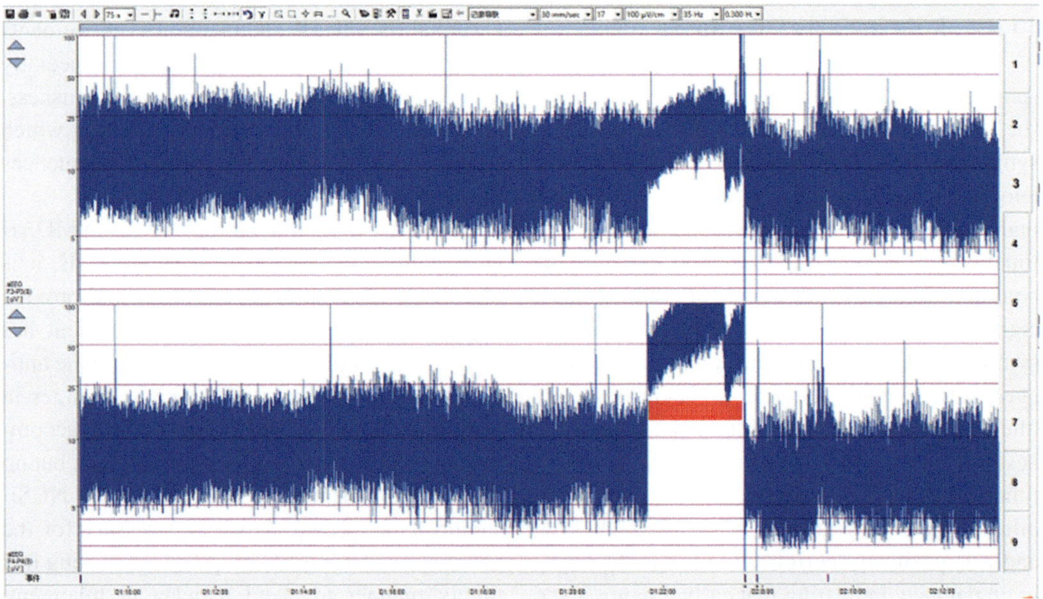

**Fig. 11.7** A 31-year-old female presented with sleep disorder for 1 month and abnormal mental behavior for 7 days and was diagnosed with LGI1 encephalitis. The patient had frequent NCSE episodes, and the aEEG showed elevated upper and lower boundaries

noncritical group, and their short-term and long-term prognoses were compared. The results showed that most qEEG parameters, including aEEG background, total power, 95% SEF, and the power of different brainwave frequency bands, cannot reflect the severity of anti-NMDA encephalitis. However, studies have found that parietal aEEG bandwidth is related to prognosis. Logistic regression analysis shows that expanded parietal aEEG bandwidth can be used as an objective indicator to predict poor long-term results. A narrower parietal aEEG bandwidth is associated with good long-term prognosis. The corresponding sensitivity and specificity are 90.00% and 56.25%, respectively [37]. This is a new discovery, and its mechanism has not been explained yet. Therefore, the use of aEEGs may have value in predicting the prognosis of patients with anti-NMDAR encephalitis, but further research is needed. EEGs and qEEGs are controversial in judging the prognosis of anti-NMDAR encephalitis, but with the gradual increase in related research, EEGs will become more reliable in judging the prognosis.

## References


1. Iizuka T, Sakai F. [Anti-nMDA receptor encephalitis—clinical manifestations and pathophysiology]. Brain Nerve. 2008;60(9):1047–60.
2. Dalmau J, Bataller L. [Limbic encephalitis: the new cell membrane antigens and a proposal of clinical-immunological classification with therapeutic implications]. Neurologia. 2007;22(8):526–37.
3. Bien CG, Vincent A, Barnett MH, et al. Immunopathology of autoantibody-associated encephalitides: clues for pathogenesis. Brain. 2012;135(Pt 5):1622–38.
4. Wang Y, Yu Y, Hu Y, et al. Clinical and electroencephalographic features of the seizures in neuronal surface antibody-associated autoimmune encephalitis. Front Neurol. 2020;11:280.
5. Gu Y, Zhong M, He L, et al. Epidemiology of antibody-positive autoimmune encephalitis in Southwest China: a multicenter study. Front Immunol. 2019;10:2611.
6. Venkatesan A. Immune-mediated encephalitis for the infectious disease specialist. Curr Opin Infect Dis. 2019;32(3):251–8.
7. Liu B, Xie Z, Liu G, et al. Elevated neuron-specific enolase and S100 calcium-binding protein B concentrations in cerebrospinal fluid of patients with anti-N-methyl-d-aspartate receptor encephalitis. Clin Chim Acta. 2018;480:79–83.
8. Bacchi S, Franke K, Wewegama D, et al. Magnetic resonance imaging and positron emission tomography in anti-NMDA receptor encephalitis: a systematic review. J Clin Neurosci. 2018;52:54–9.
9. Neo S, Yeo T, Chen Z, et al. Acute radiological features facilitate diagnosis and prognosis of anti-N-methyl-d-aspartate receptor (NMDAR) and anti-voltage-gated potassium channel (VGKC) encephalitis in adults. J Neurol Sci. 2020;419:117216.
10. Freund B, Ritzl EK. A review of EEG in anti-NMDA receptor encephalitis. J Neuroimmunol. 2019;332:64–8.
11. Kirkpatrick MP, Clarke CD, Sonmezturk HH, et al. Rhythmic delta activity represents a form of nonconvulsive status epilepticus in anti-NMDA receptor antibody encephalitis. Epilepsy Behav. 2011;20(2):392–4.
12. Johnson N, Henry C, Fessler AJ, et al. Anti-NMDA receptor encephalitis causing prolonged nonconvulsive status epilepticus. Neurology. 2010;75(16):1480–2.
13. Schmitt SE, Pargeon K, Frechette ES, et al. Extreme delta brush: a unique EEG pattern in adults with anti-NMDA receptor encephalitis. Neurology. 2012;79(11):1094–100.
14. Nosadini M, Boniver C, Zuliani L, et al. Longitudinal electroencephalographic (EEG) findings in pediatric anti-N-methyl-D-aspartate (anti-NMDA) receptor encephalitis: the Padua experience. J Child Neurol. 2015;30(2):238–45.
15. Irani SR, Michell AW, Lang B, et al. Faciobrachial dystonic seizures precede Lgi1 antibody limbic encephalitis. Ann Neurol. 2011;69(5):892–900.
16. Carvajal FJ, Mattison HA, Cerpa W. Role of NMDA receptor-mediated glutamatergic signaling in chronic and acute neuropathologies. Neural Plast. 2016;2016:2701526.
17. Gable M, Glaser C. Anti-N-methyl-d-aspartate receptor encephalitis appearing as a new-onset psychosis: disease course in children and adolescents within the California encephalitis project. Pediatr Neurol. 2017;72:25–30.
18. Shi Y, Serial EEG. Monitoring in a patient with anti-NMDA receptor encephalitis. Clin EEG Neurosci. 2017;48(4):301–3.
19. Gresa-Arribas N, Titulaer MJ, Torrents A, et al. Antibody titres at diagnosis and during follow-up of anti-NMDA receptor encephalitis: a retrospective study. Lancet Neurol. 2014;13(2):167–77.
20. Sutter R, Kaplan PW, Cervenka MC, et al. Electroencephalography for diagnosis and prognosis of acute encephalitis. Clin Neurophysiol. 2015;126(8):1524–31.
21. Veciana M, Becerra JL, Fossas P, et al. EEG extreme delta brush: an ictal pattern in patients with anti-NMDA receptor encephalitis. Epilepsy Behav. 2015;49:280–5.
22. Jeannin-Mayer S, Andre-Obadia N, Rosenberg S, et al. EEG analysis in anti-NMDA receptor encephali-

tis: description of typical patterns. Clin Neurophysiol. 2019;130(2):289–96.
23. Gataullina S, Plouin P, Vincent A, et al. Paroxysmal EEG pattern in a child with N-methyl-D-aspartate receptor antibody encephalitis. Dev Med Child Neurol. 2011;53(8):764–7.
24. Chanson E, Bicilli E, Lauxerois M, et al. Anti-NMDA-R encephalitis: should we consider extreme delta brush as electrical status epilepticus? Neurophysiol Clin. 2016;46(1):17–25.
25. Trinka E, Leitinger M. Which EEG patterns in coma are nonconvulsive status epilepticus? Epilepsy Behav. 2015;49:203–22.
26. Rodriguez RA, Vlachy J, Lee JW, et al. Association of periodic and rhythmic electroencephalographic patterns with seizures in critically ill patients. JAMA Neurol. 2017;74(2):181–8.
27. Kadoya M, Onoue H, Kadoya A, et al. Refractory status epilepticus caused by anti-NMDA receptor encephalitis that markedly improved following combination therapy with rituximab and cyclophosphamide. Intern Med. 2015;54(2):209–13.
28. Song L, Liu AH. [Anti-N-methyl-D-aspartic acid receptor encephalitis: clinical analysis of 7 cases]. Zhonghua Yi Xue Za Zhi. 2013;93(31):2508–10.
29. Liu X, Guo L, Liang C. [Research progress on electroencephalogram characteristics of anti-N-methyl-D-aspartate receptor encephalitis]. Zhejiang Da Xue Xue Bao Yi Xue Ban. 2020;49(1):118–23.
30. Da SF, Castro LH, Andrade JQ, et al. Serial and prolonged EEG monitoring in anti-N-methyl-d-aspartate receptor encephalitis. Clin Neurophysiol. 2014;125(8):1541–4.
31. Zhang Y, Liu G, Jiang MD, et al. Analysis of electroencephalogram characteristics of anti-NMDA receptor encephalitis patients in China. Clin Neurophysiol. 2017;128(7):1227–33.
32. Yildirim M, Konuskan B, Yalnizoglu D, et al. Electroencephalographic findings in anti-N-methyl-d-aspartate receptor encephalitis in children: a series of 12 patients. Epilepsy Behav. 2018;78:118–23.
33. VanHaerents S, Stillman A, Inoa V, et al. Early and persistent 'extreme delta brush' in a patient with anti-NMDA receptor encephalitis. Epilepsy Behav Case Rep. 2014;2:67–70.
34. Li H, Wang XH, Fang F, et al. [Clinical and electroencephalographic analysis of anti-N-methyl-D-aspartate receptor encephalitis in children]. Zhonghua Er Ke Za Zhi. 2016;54(7):510–14.
35. Wang J, Wang K, Wu D, et al. Extreme delta brush guides to the diagnosis of anti-NMDAR encephalitis. J Neurol Sci. 2015;353(1–2):81–3.
36. Gitiaux C, Simonnet H, Eisermann M, et al. Early electro-clinical features may contribute to diagnosis of the anti-NMDA receptor encephalitis in children. Clin Neurophysiol. 2013;124(12):2354–61.
37. Jiang N, Guan H, Lu Q, et al. Features and prognostic value of quantitative electroencephalogram changes in critically ill and non-critically ill anti-NMDAR encephalitis patients: a pilot study. Front Neurol. 2018;9:833.

# Application of Multimodal EEG in ICP Monitoring

12

Wei Dan and Weina Chai

## Contents



**Abstract**

Increased ICP is a common clinicopathological syndrome in neurology that can cause a cerebral herniation crisis and lead to respiratory and circulatory failure and death in patients. The prevention and treatment of ICP are keys to the treatment of acute intracranial trauma, stroke, intracranial tumors, and hydrocephalus. Monitoring intracranial pressure plays a crucial role in improving the treatment effect. With the development of science and technology, the monitoring of ICP has gradually expanded from the initial lumbar puncture to more noninvasive and invasive measurement methods, among which the continuous monitoring of EEG is also one of them. In this chapter, we introduce many methods of ICP monitoring, enumerate possible EEG changes that may occur with increased ICP, and summarize the effects of multimodal monitoring on ICP to help readers understand increased ICP and the application of related multimodal monitoring.

**Keywords**

ICP monitoring · Increased ICP · Ischemia-reperfusion injury · Hydrocephalus · Multimodal monitoring · EEG · BIS

W. Dan (✉) · W. Chai
Department of Neurosurgery, The First Affiliated Hospital of Chongqing Medical University, Chongqing, China
e-mail: weinachai@hospital.cqmu.edu.cn





X. Wang et al. (eds.), *Multi-Modal EEG Monitoring of Severely Neurologically Ill Patients*,
https://doi.org/10.1007/978-981-16-4493-1_12

## 12.1 Common Methods and Importance of ICP Monitoring

The technique of lumbar puncture created in the late nineteenth century to measure ICP is still in use today and has become a traditional measurement method. However, for patients with acute TBI and intracranial hypertension, lumbar puncture has the risk of inducing cerebral hernia and is not recommended as a clinical method for ICP monitoring.

At present, ICP measurement methods can be divided into two categories: noninvasive and invasive. Noninvasive methods of measuring and evaluating ICP have been developed, but they are not reliable enough to be used routinely. Noninvasive methods are classified into five categories. These methods include analyses of fluid dynamics, ophthalmology, eye movement, electrophysiology, MRI, transcranial Doppler ultrasonography (TCD), CBF velocity analysis, near-infrared spectroscopy (NIRS), transcranial time-of-flight technology, spontaneous venous pulsation measurement, venous ophthalmodynamometry, optical coherence tomography (OCT) of the retina, optic nerve sheath diameter (ONSD) assessment, pupillometry, tympanic membrane displacement (TMD) measurement, otoacoustic emission (OAE)/acoustic measurement analysis, estimations based on transcranial acoustic (TCA) signals, VEPs, EEG, skull vibration analysis, brain tissue resonance analysis, estimations based on jugular vein blood flow, etc. Currently, none of the noninvasive methods have demonstrated sufficient accuracy and ease of use while allowing continuous monitoring in routine clinical applications. However, these methods allow ICP measurement in patients when invasive monitoring is contraindicated or unavailable [1].

At present, ICP measurement methods used in clinical practice belong to the invasive category. According to whether pressure sensors are directly placed in the intracranial space, invasive ICP measurement methods can be divided into the following two categories: (a) implantation methods, in which pressure sensors are directly implanted inside the skull by drilling or craniotomy; (b) catheterization methods, in which a catheter is inserted into the ventricles, cistern or subarachnoid space. The sensor is located outside the skull but in contact with the fluid or CSF that fills the catheter for pressure measurement. Different pressure sensors convert ICP into electrical and digital signals, which can be amplified to display and record ICP.

The various ICP monitoring devices have been compared in terms of their accuracy, stability, and ability to drain CSF and were ranked in order of their performance as follows: (a) intraventricular devices, such as a pressure sensor with probe tip or a fluid conduction catheter with an external pressure sensor; (b) intraparenchymal probes; (c) subdural probes; and (d) extradural probes. Intraventricular catheters are considered the preferred clinical device. The method of placing intraventricular catheters is simple and accurate, and the catheter can be used to release CBF to reduce ICP. However, this method cannot be used in patients with a loss of ventricular compression. Then, the second choice is to use one of the methods of placing the ICP probe in the extradural, subdural or intraparenchymal region. The invasive ICP probe can be placed in multiple intracranial areas, with little resulting injury and stable performance [2].

## 12.2 Effects of Increased ICP on EEGs

Studies have shown that increased ICP can manifest as disordered pleomorphic slow waves at the lesion side, and with a further increase in ICP, BS, and even ECS may occur [3].

A study found that bursts of electrical activity were more common in patients with high ICP due to obstructive hydrocephalus than in patients with benign intracranial hypertension. However, there was no significant correlation between the amplitude and number of the bursts and the numerical changes in ICP or the duration of symptoms of increased ICP [4]. A study [5] reported the EEG manifestation of three cases of adult hydrocephalus and pointed out that the EEGs of hydrocephalus patients were characterized by low voltage. In one patient, some fast electrical activity was observed. Zuidema, Cohen [6] and Bradshaw [7] reported no EEG findings and no slow activity in patients with intracranial hypertension due to intracranial tumors; associated with some results of CBF examination, patients with intracranial hypertension, and normal EEGs may be found because CBF is not significantly affected. An in vivo study of rhesus monkeys showed that when ICP reached 160 mmHg, CBF dropped to 12 ml/min, and arterial pressure was 140/90 mmHg, there was no significant change in EEGs compared with the control group [8]. An 8-year-old boy with increased ICP caused by a malfunction of a cerebrospinal diverter pump showed symptoms including GTCSs that lasted for a few minutes, intermittent headaches, gaze, no response to voice command, increased bilateral muscle tone, and incontinence. The EEG showed a sudden decay of electrical activity, and the background activity was replaced by low-voltage single-rhythm wide-ranging β activity. The above symptoms disappeared after the diverter pump was repaired [9].

## 12.3 Common EEG Changes Due to Intracranial Hypertension

As mentioned above, the EEGs of patients with intracranial hypertension can be characterized by pleomorphic slow waves (Figs. 12.1, 12.2, 12.3, and 12.4) and even BS and ECS (Fig. 12.5).

## 12.4 EEG Manifestations of Ischemia-Reperfusion Injury

Patients with cardiac arrest often die from brain injury mediated by hypoxia and ischemia-reperfusion. Even if these patients survive, most show varying degrees of neurological sequelae of language, perception, and motor dysfunction, and these patients may even enter VS. EEG can show the real-time characteristics of the functional state of the brain, and EEGs have become an important indicator of the progression of HIE [10].

When the cerebral blood supply is stopped due to cardiac arrest, the BIS value of an EEG decreases [11]. Goodman observed that the BIS values dropped to zero after cardiac arrest in two patients undergoing cardiothoracic surgery. Although CPR was successful, the BIS value was still low. Both patients had severe brain damage after surgery [12].

BS is a common mode of brain function that is severely degraded due to hypoxic-ischemic brain injury, and BS can be detected under general anesthesia. The BS rate is a parameter that quantifies the degree of suppression of EEG activity. Borges et al. [13] conducted a prospective study in which, based on the main results of emergency EEGs, patients' 3-month (or longer) survival rates were determined. They found that for coma patients who showed BS, diffuse suppression,

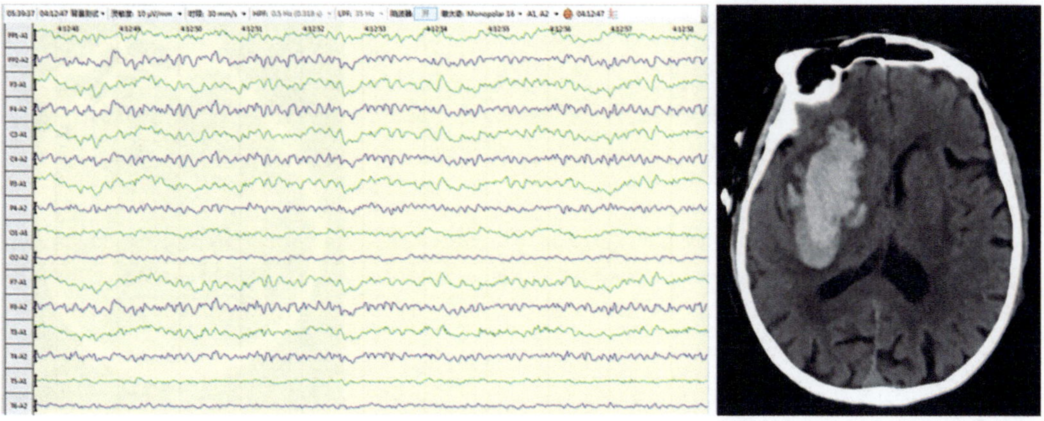

**Fig. 12.1** EEG from an 87-year-old male with cerebral hemorrhage in the right basal ganglia region, showing increased slow-wave activity in each lead group, most prominently on the right

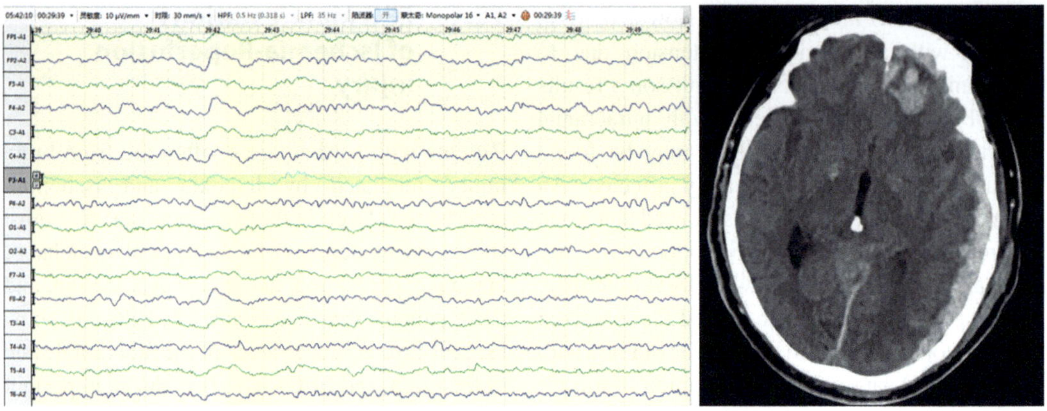

**Fig. 12.2** EEG from a 74-year-old male with severe TBI, showing increased slow-wave activity in each lead group

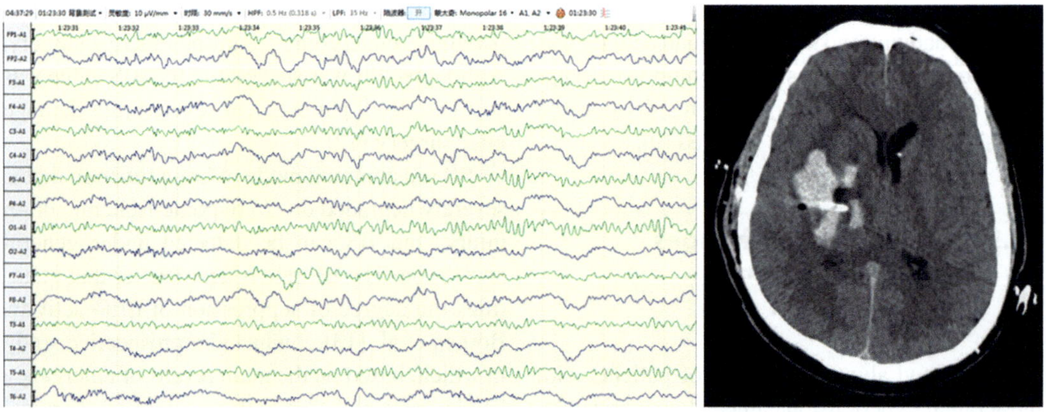

**Fig. 12.3** EEG from a 32-year-old male with cerebral hemorrhage in the right basal ganglia region, showing increased slow-wave activity on one side

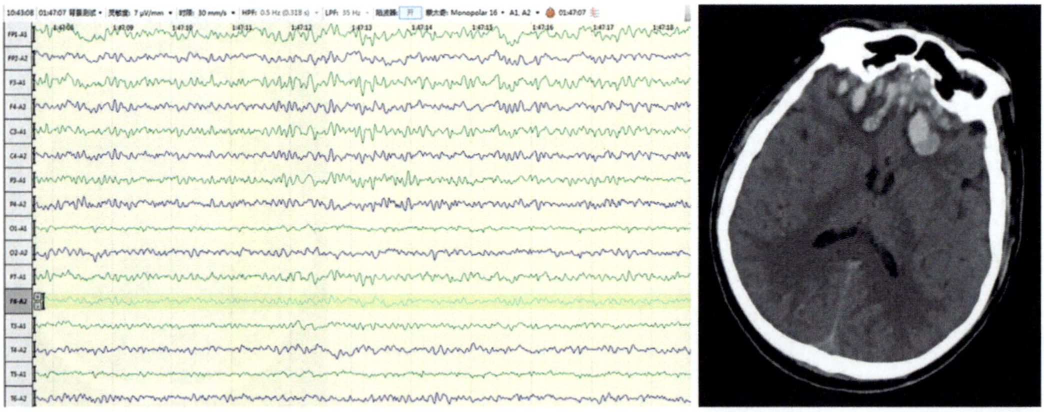

**Fig. 12.4** EEG from a 54-year-old male with bilateral cerebral contusions in the frontal lobes, showing scattered increased slow-wave activity

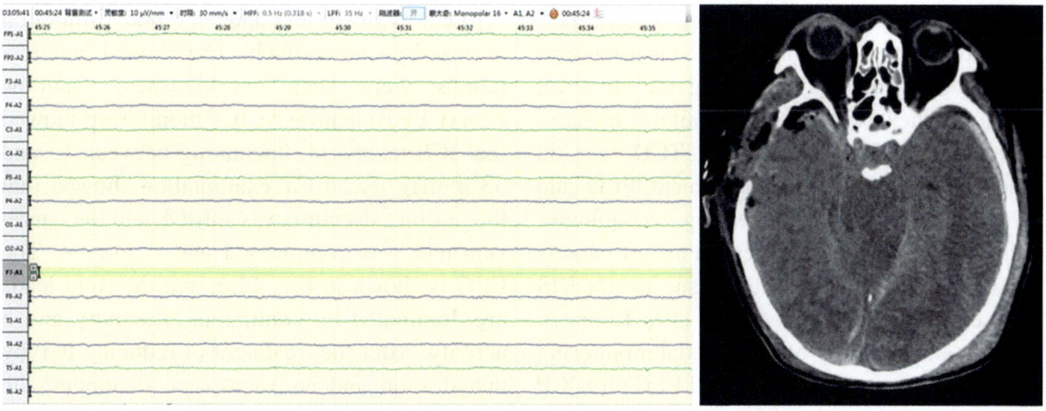

**Fig. 12.5** EEG from a 69-year-old male with extremely severe TBI, showing low voltage in each lead

and α/θ patterns, the 3-month (or longer) survival rate was 25% whereas good EEG patterns RDA was associated with a better prognosis. In 21 clinical trials, they found that abnormal EEG background activity (nonreactive EEG, abnormal background activity, periodic firing, low voltage or BS) was associated with increased mortality. Another prospective study included 681 patients who underwent emergency EEG examinations to determine predictors of the 3-month survival rate, and the Kaplan-Meier curve was used to estimate survival probability. This study found that for those who showed continuous δ activity and extensive epileptiform discharge, the survival rate was 50% [14].

EEG, SEP, and BAEP results were recorded in 161 patients with severe ischemic brain injuries (GCS score ≤ 8) and 77 patients with hypoxic-ischemic brain damage after CPR. The GCS was used for scoring the outcome 6 months after the onset of the disease, and it was found that a lack of EEG responsiveness and the presence of pathological N20 (short-latency somatosensory evoked potential, SLSEP) and pathological wave V (BAEP) showed good sensitivity for predicting prognosis, and the prognosis of patients with nonhypothermic treatment and nonresponsive EEGs was poor [15].

SIRPIDs are defined as periodic, rhythmic or repetitive discharges. Alvarez et al. [16] conducted a prospective cohort study to observe the prevalence of SIRPIDs in cardiac arrest survivors in a coma and examine the potential association of SIRPIDs with the results. A total of 105 coma patients underwent EEG monitoring after cardiac arrest and were studied during hypothermic or nonhypothermic treatment. It was found that patients with both SIRPIDs and noncontinuous or nonreactive EEGs showed stronger neurological dysfunction than patients with SIRPIDs alone. Therefore, these researchers speculated that SIRPIDs were related to adverse outcomes during the low-temperature period, and SIRPIDs in the normal-temperature period after being awake may indicate a good prognosis.

After hypothermia treatment in patients with hypoxic-ischemic brain damage, the background activity of EEGs may manifest as isoelectric or low-pressure activity, epileptiform discharges, BS, and diffuse slow waves or normal rhythm [17]. After CPR, EEGs show generalized inhibition, BS, GEDs, or unresponsiveness, often suggesting hypoxic-ischemic brain damage and poor prognosis [18].

## 12.5 The Clinical Application Value of Multimodal Monitoring in Patients with Intracranial Hypertension

Clinical examination is the gold standard for monitoring the function of the CNS; however, it is usually unavailable when vital signs are unstable. In such cases, bedside monitoring of CNS function should include measuring cerebral perfusion pressure, estimating CBF, evaluating cerebral oxygenation, and evaluating the electrical activity of the CNS. Currently available technologies include ICP monitoring, TCD, carotid blood oxygen saturation measurement, EEG, and EP monitoring. Newly emerging technologies include NIRS and PbtO2 measurement to assess the oxygenation status of brain tissue and the BIS to assess the depth of anesthesia [19]. Research supports the necessity of multimodal monitoring (ICP, CBF, brain metabolism, and EEG) for ICP measurement and emphasizes the potential advantages of EEG in children [3].

**Case**

A 50-year-old woman was diagnosed with a right middle cerebral artery aneurysm (unruptured).

The patient underwent right middle cerebral artery aneurysmal neck clipping, and severe cerebral vasospasm and cerebral infarction occurred postoperatively. The clinical manifestations were deep consciousness (shallow coma). Bedside invasive ICP monitoring showed that ICP increased, fluctuating between 15 and 33 mmHg. Head CT examination showed that the midline structure was shifted, and the lateral ventricle was compressed and deformed. The EEG is shown in Fig. 12.6, and the right leads are dominated by continuous θ activity and δ activity. After the treatment of reducing ICP by dehydration and antivasospasm treatment, the level of consciousness gradually improved (drowsiness). Head CT reexamination showed that the midline structure shift and lateral ventricle compression were improved. The EEG reexamination is shown in Fig. 12.7. The abovementioned θ activity and δ activity were slightly reduced and replaced by a low-amplitude β rhythm.

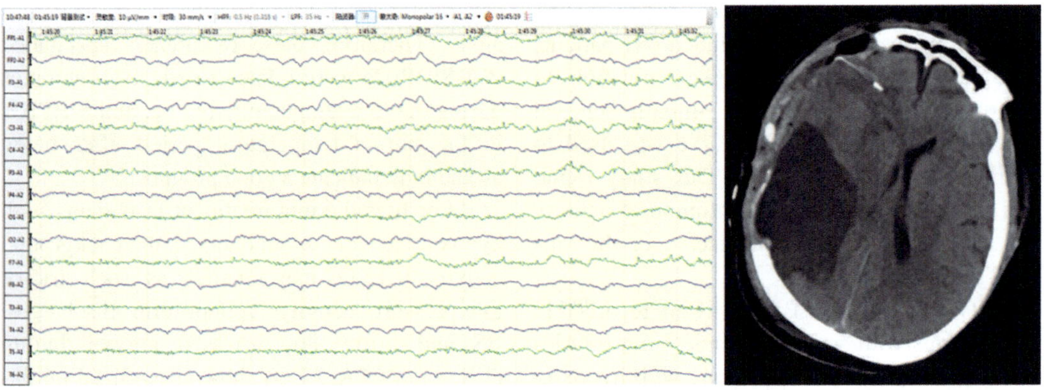

**Fig. 12.6** EEG from Yu X, a 50-year-old female, showing a continued increase in slow activity in the right EEG leads

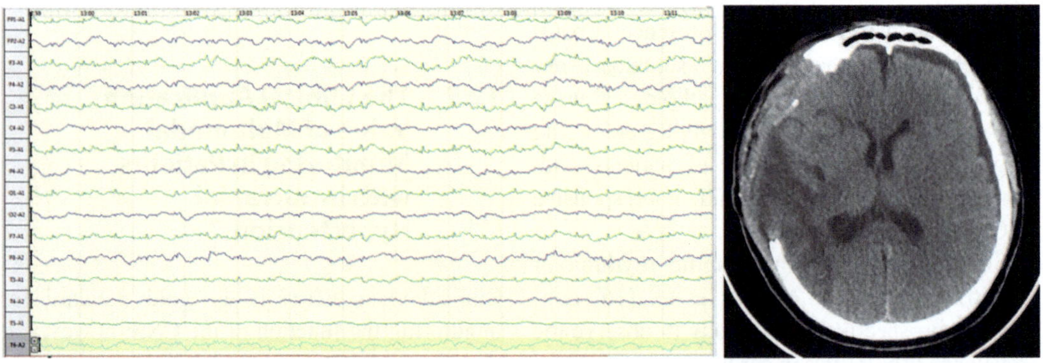

**Fig. 12.7** EEG from Yu X, a 50-year-old female, showing improvement in the slow activity in the right leads

The common EEG changes in intracranial hypertension are mainly slow-wave activity, which may be related to the decrease in cerebral perfusion pressure and cerebral ischemia and hypoxia caused by intracranial hypertension.

## References


1. Zhang X, Medow JE, Iskandar BJ, et al. Reply to Comment on 'Invasive and noninvasive means of measuring intracranial pressure: a review'. Physiol Meas. 2018;39(5):58002.
2. Evensen KB, Eide PK. Measuring intracranial pressure by invasive, less invasive or non-invasive means: limitations and avenues for improvement. Fluids Barriers CNS. 2020;17(1):34.
3. Kane NM, Germon TJ, Nelson RJ. Effect of sudden episodic intracranial hypertension on the electroencephalogram in a child with head injury. J Neurol Neurosurg Psychiatry. 1994;57(10):1277–8.
4. Mani KS, Townsend HR, The EEG. In benign intracranial hypertension. Electroencephalogr Clin Neurophysiol. 1964;16:604–10.
5. Bodensteiner J, Matsuo F. EEG in benign intracranial hypertension. Dis Nerv Syst. 1977;38(12):1007–10.
6. Zuidema GD, Cohen SJ. Pseudotumor cerebri. J Neurosurg. 1954;11(5):433–41.
7. Bradshaw P. Benign intracranial hypertension. J Neurol Neurosurg Psychiatry. 1956;19(1):28–41.
8. Lucas S, Solomon G, Labar D, et al. Episodic brainstem compression masquerading as electrodecremental seizures. J Child Neurol. 1994;9(2):167–9.
9. Kochs E. Monitoring of the central nervous system[J]. Acta Anaesthesiol Scand Suppl. 1996;109:60–1.
10. Feng G, Jiang G, Li Z, et al. Prognostic value of electroencephalography (EEG) for brain injury after cardiopulmonary resuscitation. Neurol Sci. 2016;37(6):843–9.
11. Chawla LS, Akst S, Junker C, et al. Surges of electroencephalogram activity at the time of death: a case series. J Palliat Med. 2009;12(12):1095–100.
12. Goodman PG, Mehta AR, Castresana MR. Predicting ischemic brain injury after intraoperative cardiac arrest during cardiac surgery using the BIS monitor. J Clin Anesth. 2009;21(8):609–12.
13. Borges MA, Botos HJ, Bastos RF, et al. Emergency EEG: study of survival. Arq Neuropsiquiatr. 2010;68(2):174–8.
14. Soholm H, Kjaer TW, Kjaergaard J, et al. Prognostic value of electroencephalography (EEG) after out-of-hospital cardiac arrest in successfully resuscitated patients used in daily clinical practice. Resuscitation. 2014;85(11):1580–5.
15. Zhang Y, Su YY, Haupt WF, et al. Application of electrophysiologic techniques in poor outcome prediction among patients with severe focal and diffuse ischemic brain injury. J Clin Neurophysiol. 2011;28(5):497–503.
16. Alvarez V, Oddo M, Rossetti AO. Stimulus-induced rhythmic, periodic or ictal discharges (SIRPIDs) in comatose survivors of cardiac arrest: characteristics and prognostic value[J]. Clin Neurophysiol. 2013;124(1):204–8.
17. Tjepkema-Cloostermans MC, van Meulen FB, Meinsma G, et al. A Cerebral Recovery Index (CRI) for early prognosis in patients after cardiac arrest[J]. Crit Care. 2013;17(5):R252.
18. Fugate JE, Wijdicks EF, Mandrekar J, et al. Predictors of neurologic outcome in hypothermia after cardiac arrest. Ann Neurol. 2010;68(6):907–14.
19. Langfitt TW, Tannanbaum HM, Kassell NF, et al. Acute intracranial hypertension, cerebral blood flow, and the EEG. Electroencephalogr Clin Neurophysiol. 1966;20(2):139–48.

# Application of Multimodal EEG in Sedation and Analgesia

# 13

Suyue Pan and Yao Wang

## Contents



**Abstract**

Sedation and analgesia in the ICU are particularly important for patients. They can reduce human–machine confrontation and reduce patients' stress response. Accurate evaluation of sedation is the basis for sedation. At present, subjective evaluation of sedation effects is not ideal, and more objective brain function indicators, such as EEG and EP, need to be adopted. However, the original EEG waveform is complicated, and various artifacts are generated in the ICU due to clinical treatment and surgery. Professional EEG interpretation training is required, which is time-consuming. Multimodal EEG includes BIS, aEEG, 95% SEF, entropy index, and RBP, which are primarily displayed in digital form and can continuously and objectively assess the level of sedation. This chapter primarily introduces the effects of sedative drugs on EEG, focusing on the evaluation and application of multimodal EEG on the effect of sedation and anal-

S. Pan (✉) · Y. Wang
Department of Neurology, Nanfang Hospital of Southern Medical University, Guangzhou, Guangdong, China
e-mail: pansuyue@smu.edu.cn



X. Wang et al. (eds.), *Multi-Modal EEG Monitoring of Severely Neurologically Ill Patients*,
https://doi.org/10.1007/978-981-16-4493-1_13

gesia, and discusses the performance of multimodal EEG of different drugs and excessive sedation, hoping to provide a valuable reference for improving the clinical management of critically ill patients under sedation.

**Keywords**

Sedation · Analgesia · Benzodiazepines · Propofol · Ketamine · Dexmedetomidine · EEG · Multimodal EEG · Excessive sedation

In the ICU, mechanical ventilation is a commonly used treatment for critically ill patients, but body stimulation through tracheal intubation, invasive operation, instrument noise, and the unfamiliar environment can cause the patient to experience irritability, which is where human–machine confrontation comes into being. Human–machine confrontation has a very adverse effect on the treatment and prognosis of patients. Therefore, sedation is particularly necessary for mechanical ventilation. In clinical practice, the use of sedatives is often adjusted to maintain the depth of sedation. However, it is difficult to control the depth of clinical sedation. Insufficient sedation can lead to increased oxygen consumption, human–machine confrontation, and accidental decoupling; excessive sedation can lead to ventilator-related pneumonia, delayed weaning, gastrointestinal bleeding, and bacteremia. The ideal sedative effect should be that the patient is relatively quiet, easily awakened, and maintains a sleep–wake cycle, but it is difficult to achieve this goal. Therefore, accurate sedation evaluation is an important basis for the implementation of sedation. According to the results of sedation evaluation, the dosage of the drug can be adjusted in a timely manner to achieve an effective sedation effect.

Parameters of sedation include consciousness, amnesia, arousal, and analgesia. Sedation is difficult to express with a single parameter. The clinical evaluation of sedation depends on the patient's response to external stimuli. However, stimulation through evaluation itself changes the patient's level of sedation. According to the guidelines for the management of pain, restlessness/sedation, delirium, immobility, and sleep interruption in adult patients in the ICU issued by the American Academy of Critical Care Medicine in 2018 [1], for most critically ill patients, ensuring their comfort and maintaining mild sedation can improve clinical outcomes. The guidelines state that the most commonly used clinical evaluation systems currently include subjective evaluations such as the Richmond Agitation and Sedation Scale (RASS) and the Riker Sedation–Agitation Scale (SAS). However, for patients with neurological impairment, subjective scoring alone is not enough. The clinical evaluation score depends on the patient's movement and response; therefore, the depth of sedation cannot be measured accurately. In addition, due to the influence of social, personal, and professional factors on sedation monitoring, subjective evaluation of sedation effects is not ideal. Objective evaluation indicators of brain function can be used, such as BAEPs and the BIS.

## 13.1 The Effect of Sedative Drugs on EEG

### 13.1.1 Benzodiazepines

The effect of benzodiazepines on EEGs is related to the plasma concentration and the pharmacokinetics of the drug. The most commonly used are valium and midazolam, both of which are highly lipophilic and have a wide tissue distribution. Only 1–2% of plasma proteins do not bind to diazepam, and 3–4% do not bind to midazolam, but the clearance rates of the two are inconsistent. Diazepam has a very long half-life and low clearance rate; in contrast, midazolam has a short half-life and high metabolic clearance rate. Both have a rapid effect on EEGs. Diazepam reaches its maximum effect 1 min after intravenous injection, and the proportion of 13–30 Hz EEG activity is significantly increased; then, it drops rapidly until 5 h after the injection, but the frequency of EEG activity is still significantly faster than at baseline. After 6–8 h, the change in EEGs is not particularly obvious. Midazolam had the greatest effect on EEGs 5–10 min, on average, after administration. The background activity is replaced by a low-amplitude fast wave. The increase in frequency (13 ~ 30 Hz) is similar to that observed with diazepam. All these changes occur 5–10 min after drug administration. From 5–10 min to 2.5 h after administration, the effect of midazolam on the basic rhythm is not obvious [2, 3], and the background activity returns to baseline in the next 3–4 h.

In the research of Kurowskj et al. [2], subjects received 1, 2, and 3 mg of clonazepam, and soon the amplitude of the α wave decreased, followed by regular β activity. When 1 mg clonazepam was given, EEG activity took 3–4 h to return to the level observed with placebo administration. When 2 mg clonazepam was given, the total power decreased, the average frequency and the frequency with the highest power were reduced, δ (1.5–3.5 Hz) and θ (3.5–7.5 Hz) activity increased, and α power decreased; all parameters returned to predose levels after 3–5 h. When 3 mg clonazepam was administered, the changes in the frequency of δ (1.5–3.5 Hz), α2 (9–13 Hz), and β1 (13–20 Hz) waves slowly decreased and returned to predose levels approximately 7 h later.

### 13.1.2 Propofol

Propofol is a fat-soluble inhibitor of synapses that binds to the postsynaptic membrane of GABA (A) receptors; widely acts on the cortex, thalamus, brainstem, and spinal cord; and can produce anesthesia and sedation through multiple sites. Propofol produces slow δ activity on EEGs by reducing the output of the thalamus and brainstem to the cortex and by strengthening the hyperpolarization of cortical pyramidal cells. In most cases of anesthesia records, only a few electrodes on the forehead are used. The EEG of a conscious patient with closed eyes shows the alpha activity of the occipital lobe. With the loss of consciousness, slow activity appears, and α activity is activated (α and β are transferred from the occipital lobe to the forehead in the EEG). Some studies have shown that the amount of propofol is related to EEG changes during the induction of anesthesia [4]. For example, in a PICU study, researchers randomly divided children (21, 7–8 years old) into a 3 mg/kg propofol group, a 5 mg/kg propofol group, or a 5–7 mg/kg sodium thiopental group. The baseline EEG activity of all children was normal, and the induced EEG patterns of the three groups were similar: After the 12-s average incubation period, EEGs showed that the frequency changed from 9 to 10 Hz (α activity) to 14 Hz (β activity), and this change lasted up to 2 s, followed by δ activity (2–3 Hz) that lasted approximately 1–2 min, and finally, β activity reappeared, but it did not completely replace the δ activity in the next 5 min [5]. δ activity was most obvious in the orbitofrontal area [6].

### 13.1.3 Ketamine

As an anesthetic adjuvant and analgesic, ketamine mainly binds to NMDARs in the brain and spinal cord. Ketamine is a channel receptor blocker. The suppression induced by ketamine at low to moderate doses results in increased brain metabolism, CBF, and hallucinations. When a small dose of ketamine was given for 2 min, the EEG showed fast β waves or low-frequency γ waves (25–32 Hz). Although β/γ activity lasted for only 27 min, the patient anesthetic effect of an inability to respond to oral instructions will continue for several minutes after β/γ activity disappears [7].

### 13.1.4 Dexmedetomidine

Dexmedetomidine is an α2 receptor agonist that mainly acts on the locus coeruleus under the cerebral cortex and the midline nucleus of the thalamus. Compared with patients who are administered propofol, those who are administered dexmedetomidine are more likely to be awakened, the dosage is smaller, and there is no respiratory depression. Dexmedetomidine is the most commonly used drug for shallow sedation in the ICU.

The level of sedation produced when a small dose of dexmedetomidine is given is a weak patient response to auditory and tactile stimuli, and the EEGs of these patients show slow δ activity and spindle (9–15 Hz) activity, lasting approximately 1–2 s. Spindles are represented by α and slow β activities, with a frequency range of 9–15 Hz. Compared with the spindles induced by propofol, the frequencies of spindles induced by dexmedetomidine are lower. The spindles are similar to those that appear in stage II NREM sleep [8].

## 13.2 The Role of Multimodal EEG Monitoring to Evaluate the Sedative Effect

### 13.2.1 The Role of BIS Monitoring in Evaluating Sedation and Analgesia

In BIS monitoring, the original EEG signal is collected through a sensor placed on the forehead. A series of signals, such as spectrum, amplitude, and rhythm signals, are analyzed through energy spectrum analysis, dual-spectrum technology analysis, and time-domain analysis. After processing, this signal is fitted into a value from 0 to 100: 0 means resting-state EEG activity, and 100 means wide-awake EEG activity. BIS monitoring is mainly designed for anesthesia monitoring during various operations and can reduce the amount of anesthesia, monitor the depth of anesthesia, reduce intraoperative awareness, and monitor the degree of sedation. The BIS sedation range is generally 80–60 for mild sedation, 60–40 for moderate sedation, below 40 for deep sedation, 20 for close to inhibition, and 0 for resting-state electrical activity [9, 10].

BIS monitoring was officially approved by the U.S. Food and Drug Administration in 1996, and the BIS was used clinically as an anesthesia depth monitoring indicator. BIS monitoring was initially used for intraoperative anesthesia monitoring, and later, it was extended to ICU sedation monitoring [11]. There are five subparameters that affect the BIS value: the singal quality index (SQI), EMG, suppression ratio, SEF, and total power. When recording BIS data, if SQI ≥ 80% and EMG < 40, data recording can be started. At this time, the data are less affected, the signal quality is the best, and the reliability is high. The BIS can quickly reflect the functional status of the cerebral cortex; therefore, it is considered to be the most sensitive and accurate objective indicator to assess the state of consciousness, including the depth of sedation.

BIS monitoring in the ICU can continuously and objectively assess the level of sedation. Using BIS monitoring, sedatives can be titrated to the target BIS value, BIS < 60, so that the smallest dose of sedatives can be used to achieve the least awakening (awareness <5%) [12]. BIS monitoring can reduce excessive sedation in nonparalyzed patients. Appropriate sedation treatment for ICU patients is conducive to the recovery of their body's physiological and psychological state, and reasonable sedation can also shorten patient mechanical ventilation time.

Although there is still controversy about whether the BIS can accurately reflect the depth of sedation, a large number of studies have confirmed that BIS monitoring of sedation is practical and effective [13–17]. There is a good correlation between BIS values and Ramsay scores and SAS scores. Among them, the BIS is significantly positively correlated with the SAS score and significantly negatively correlated with the Ramsay score. The BIS can better reflect the depth of sedation [13]. Yamashita et al. [14] found that the BIS value decreases with the depth of sedation, and there is a significant correlation between the BIS value and the Ramsay score. In deep sedation (defined as a Ramsay score of 5–6 points), the BIS value in the high-age group (over 65 years old) was significantly lower than that in the low-age group (18–65 years old). Qadeer et al. [15] defined deep sedation as 1 ~ 2 points according to the Observer's Assessment of Alertness/Sedation Scale (OAA/S) score, and they found that when the BIS was ≤75 points, the BIS predicted deep sedation with low sensitivity and high specificity. In addition to monitoring the degree of sedation in ICU patients, BIS monitoring can also guide the sedation of severely ill patients in the ICU. Olson et al. [16] found that the amount of propofol in patients with increased BIS monitoring was significantly reduced, and the infusion rate was lower. Patients who are evaluated with BIS monitoring and Ramsay score assessment wake up much faster than those who are evaluated with Ramsay score alone. Therefore, it is believed that BIS monitoring, as a sedation assessment tool, is a useful means for improving the care of critically ill patients under sedation. Mahmood et al. [17] found that the use of BIS monitoring for trauma ICU patient management was associated with a better prognosis. BIS monitoring can guide the adjustment of the dosage of sedatives, which can minimize restlessness, extubation failure rate, and time in the ICU.

### 13.2.2 The Role of aEEG in Evaluating Sedation and Analgesia

aEEGs are different from standard EEGs. aEEGs are the records of the signal of only one channel. The signal usually comes from a pair of electrodes placed in bilateral parietal leads (equivalent to the 10/20 international electrode placement method, P3 and P4). aEEGs express the various and complex EEG data recorded intuitively in the form of output parameters through amplitude integration and semilogarithmic compression based on the real-time background EEG signal recording, and the output signal represents the change in the voltage of all EEG background activity. The interpretation of aEEGs mainly depends on their upper and lower boundaries, spectrum shape and other indicators, and the upper and lower boundaries are quantitative parameters that are more objective and accurate and can reduce the influence of human interpretation on the research results.

Giordano et al. [18] defined aEEG activity based on the amplitude and background rhythm as continuous normal-voltage activity (the lower boundary is 7–10 μV, and the upper boundary is 10–25 μV), DNV activity (the lower boundary is variable but always lower than 5 μV and the upper boundary is above 10 μV), BS (discontinuous background with a lower boundary of 0–2 μV and a burst amplitude >25 μV), and ECI/FT (0 potential). They found that the use of both aEEGs and Neonatal Pain, Agitation, and Sedation Scale (N-PASS) scores can more accurately distinguish light sedation and deep sedation to effectively adjust the drug dose. Compared with the use of the Burdjalov score, the use of aEEG parameters could better distinguish between nonsedation and mild sedation and nonsedation and deep sedation but could not distinguish between light sedation and deep sedation. However, a decrease in aEEG parameters was related to an increase in the use of sedative drugs. In a small number of children who were deeply sedated, BS activities could be observed. At the same time, the study found that the discontinuity of aEEG activity increased with the patient's sedation level, which was also confirmed by the effects of sufentanil, morphine, and pethidine on the brain electrical activity of premature infants. At the same time, Giordano et al. [18] found that there were fewer sleep cycles but longer intervals in deeply sedated patients. However, Olischar et al. [19] found that the sleep–wake cycle did not increase significantly with the increase in narcotic sedative drugs.

### 13.2.3 95% SEF

The 95% SEF is a simple quantitative indicator for monitoring brain function, and it is the frequency of the highest edge at 95% of the total power spectrum [20]. The 95% SEF is the frequency index of the power spectrum analysis, which means that 95% of the brain electrical energy exists at this frequency, which can be considered the highest frequency of the brain electrical signal. The 95% SEF combines the power spectrum and frequency to obtain a value. Simplifying the EEG power spectrum into a single parameter and making it an indicator can be observed separately and can quickly and clearly show the shift in EEG frequency and power. In EEG monitoring, the higher the proportion of slow activity, such as δ and θ wave activity, the lower the 95% SEF. When awake, the cerebral cortex is active, with more fast-wave components, the power value of fast waves is higher, and the 95% SEF value is higher. In contrast, when cerebral cortex function is inhibited, the 95% SEF shifts to a lower frequency.

A number of studies have shown that the 95% SEF has a good correlation with the depth of sedation and has a linear relationship with the concentration of sedatives [21, 22]. The results of the study of Itamoto et al. [23] on dogs showed that after the use of dexmedetomidine, the δ-band power of the EEG increased, prompting the 95% SEF to shift to the low-frequency region. When studying the effect of sedative drugs on rats, researchers found that the 95% SEF decreased with the increase in the amount of anesthetic sedative drugs such as halothane but did not change with the amount of isoflurane [24]. Sleigh et al. [20] studied patients under general anesthesia and showed that the 95% SEF has a good correlation with the depth of anesthesia and sedation.

BIS and 95% SEF monitoring can accurately assess the depth of sedation of propofol; however, it has only slight ability to assess the depth of midazolam sedation, and it cannot assess the depth of ketamine sedation. The accuracy of BIS monitoring in evaluating the depth of sedation of anesthetics is higher than that of 95% SEF monitoring.

### 13.2.4 Entropy Index

Entropy index monitoring is a new method in which the original EEG and frontal muscle EMG signals are collected and converted into numerical values through entropy calculation formulas and spectral entropy applications. As a physical concept, entropy was first used in information theory and later used in the power spectrum of information processing to express the irregularity of information: The more irregular the signal is, the higher the entropy value; the more regular the signal is, the lower the entropy value is; and the entropy value is 0 when the signal is completely regular [25]. In the awake state, the brain electrical activity is very irregular, and its entropy is high. When most anesthetics induce deep anesthesia, they first cause BS, and then suppression appears on the EEG. If the EEG signal is completely suppressed, its entropy value is 0. Entropy is divided into state entropy and reaction entropy. State entropy is calculated based on EEG signals, and response entropy is based on the integrated calculation of EEG and frontal muscle electromyography signals. Currently, Kolmogorov entropy, approximate entropy, spectral entropy, and Hilbert yellow entropy are commonly used in anesthesia sedation monitoring research. A large number of comparative studies on entropy and the BIS have shown that there is a good correlation between the two, which can effectively monitor the depth of sedation. The entropy index due to the difference in the signal source and the operation component of its algorithm, entropy, and BIS also reflect their own characteristics [26].

Iannuzzi et al. [27] found that when propofol was used for sedation, 90% of people had a BIS value of 70.2 (70.2–90.2) and a state entropy value of 60.3 (60.3–75.5) when they were unable to speak and a BIS value of 38.2 (38.2–70.4) and a state entropy value of 42.2 (42.2–60.4) when they lost consciousness. In the discovery of the loss of speech and loss of consciousness, state entropy had a smaller range than BIS and an obvious correlation.

### 13.2.5 RBP

The RBP is an indicator used to quantify the changes in the frequency of response of EEG parameters. The EEG power of different frequency bands is presented as a percentage, indicating the proportion of energy in different frequency bands of brain electrical activity. Changes in EEG frequency can be caused by sedative drugs, and the frequency changes are also different under different sedation depths.

The β wave induced by small doses of propofol is related to abnormal excitation of neurons [28]. Akeju et al. [29] found that dexmedetomidine and propofol induced different states of brain function in patients. Propofol induces large-scale slow-wave activity by producing a long-term neuronal resting state so that the patient is in a deeper unconscious state. When dexmedetomidine induces the patient to be in an unconscious state, their EEG activity is more similar to that of a sleep state. The lower spindle wave has an energy frequency band of 13 Hz, and its amplitude is significantly lower than that of propofol-induced unconscious brainwaves. Scheinin et al. [30] randomly divided 47 patients into a propofol group and a dexmedetomidine group and found that as the depth of sedation increased, both groups showed an increase in slow-wave band energy and state-dependent α generalization, especially the propofol group. Maksimow et al. [31] reported that the energy of the δ and θ bands increased compared to baseline after the use of high concentrations of dexmedetomidine in humans.

## 13.3 Multimodal EEG and Different Sedative Drugs

Dexmedetomidine and propofol cause an increase in low-frequency, high-amplitude brain electrical activity (δ waves at 0.5–4 Hz and θ waves at 4.1–8 Hz). As the drug concentration increases, consciousness gradually changes from wakefulness to a loss of consciousness. Propofol will cause an increase in power from α to slow β (8.1–15 Hz) activity. In the unconscious state, EEG responsiveness to commands is still observed with propofol administration. BIS and spectrum entropy monitoring are poor in evaluating different states of consciousness to unconsciousness [32].

Maksimow et al. [31] conducted a study on 11 healthy volunteers and administered different doses of dexmedetomidine. The plasma concentrations of the low-dose group and the high-dose group were 0.5 ng/ml and 5 ng/ml, respectively. The spectral entropy decreased from 84 ± 5 to 66 ± 16, and the spectral entropy of the high-dose group decreased from 84 ± 5 to 20 ± 12. Analyzing the loss of consciousness and regaining consciousness separately, the spectrum entropy decreased from 76 ± 8 to 43 ± 10 before the loss of consciousness occurred and increased from 14 ± 4 to 63 ± 13 once consciousness was regained. These changes were consistent in all subjects.

## 13.4 Multimodal EEG Manifestations of Excessive Sedation

The results of a study showed that, as the dosages of propofol and dexmedetomidine were increased, the frontal-head α activity and the whole-head slow-wave activity increased, while the β activity was inhibited. As the dose of dexmedetomidine was increased, spindles disappeared, and the amplitude of slow δ activity increased. At this time, EEG activity was similar to that of stage III of NREM sleep and REM sleep, and the slow-wave energy at high doses increased compared with that at lower doses [33]. When high doses of sedatives, including propofol, barbiturates, and some inhaled anesthetics, are administered, BS occurs. If the EEG of a patient shows BS, then as the dose of sedatives is increased, the length of suppression between bursts will increase, and the dosage can be increased until the EEG is equipotent.

**Cases**

1. A 48-year-old man, with a diagnosis of cerebral infarction after the removal of a thrombus from the left middle cerebral artery (Fig. 13.1a, b).
2. A 47-year-old man, was admitted to the hospital with "left limb weakness for 18 days, with aggravation and a disturbance of consciousness for 7 days." He had a history of hypertension and was admitted to the hospital with a shallow coma. Head CT showed a large-area cerebral infarction on the right side encompassing the frontal, temporal–parietal, and occipital lobes. Bilateral BIS monitoring was performed (Fig. 13.2).

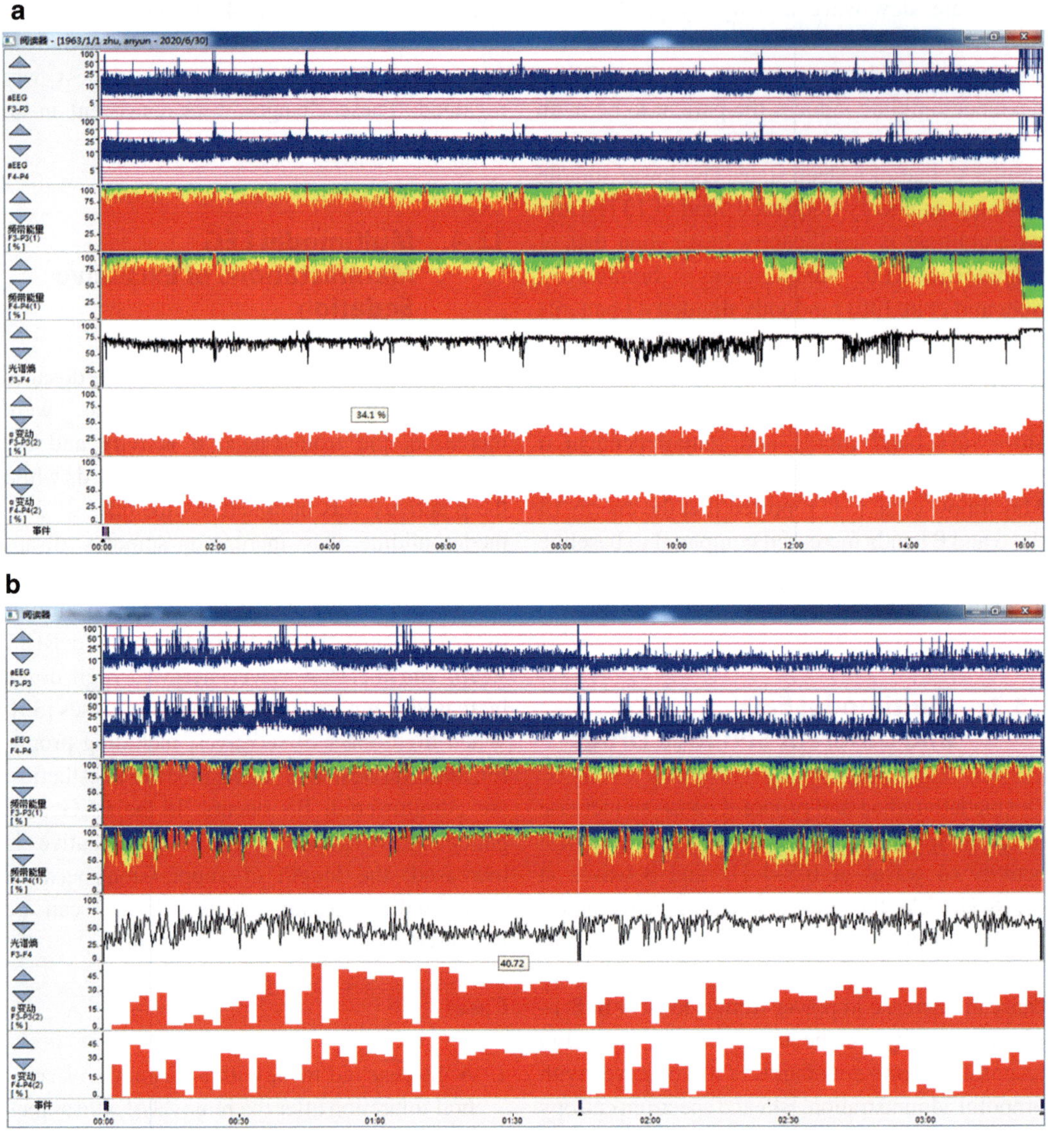

**Fig. 13.1** (**a**) Dexmedetomidine was continuously pumped for sedation. aEEG activity shows 5 μV < lower boundary < 10 μV, 10 μV < upper boundary < 25 μV, continuous background activity, spectral entropy of 50–75, and the RBP mainly of δ activity was higher in the left hemisphere. (**b**) After dexmedetomidine was stopped in the patient in (**a**), the upper boundary of aEEG activity increased, and the RBP of δ activity in both hemispheres was lower than before

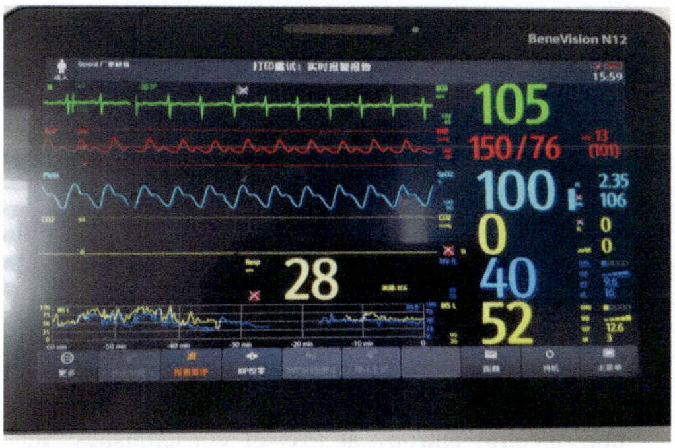


**Fig. 13.2** BIS on the left was 52, and the BIS on the right was 40

## References

1. Devlin JW, Skrobik Y, Gélinas C, et al. Clinical practice guidelines for the prevention and Management of Pain, agitation/sedation, delirium, immobility, and sleep disruption in adult patients in the ICU. Crit Care Med. 2018;46(9):e825–73.
2. Kurowski M, Ott H, Herrmann WM. Relationship between EEG dynamics and pharmacokinetics of the benzodiazepine lormetazepam. Pharmacopsychiatria. 1982;15(3):77–83.
3. Greenblatt DJ, Ehrenberg BL, Gunderman J, et al. Pharmacokinetic and electroencephalographic study of intravenous diazepam, midazolam, and placebo. Clin Pharmacol Ther. 1989;45(4):356–65.
4. San-juan D, Chiappa KH, Cole AJ. Propofol and the electroencephalogram. Clin Neurophysiol. 2010;121(7):998–1006.
5. Borgeat A, Wilder-Smith OH, Despland PA, et al. Spontaneous excitatory movements during recovery from propofol anaesthesia in an infant: EEG evaluation. Br J Anaesth. 1993;70(4):459–61.
6. Johnson BW, Sleigh JW, Kirk IJ, et al. High-density EEG mapping during general anaesthesia with xenon and propofol: a pilot study. Anaesth Intensive Care. 2003;31(2):155–63.
7. McMillan R, Muthukumaraswamy SD. The neurophysiology of ketamine: an integrative review. Rev Neurosci. 2020;31(5):457–503.
8. Kallionpaa RE, Valli K, Scheinin A, et al. Alpha band frontal connectivity is a state-specific electroencephalographic correlate of unresponsiveness during exposure to dexmedetomidine and propofol. Br J Anaesth. 2020;125(4):518–28.
9. Rampil IJ. A primer for EEG signal processing in anesthesia. Anesthesiology. 1998;89(4):980–1002.
10. Blackburn P, Vissers R. Pharmacology of emergency department pain management and conscious sedation. Emerg Med Clin North Am. 2000;18(4):803–27.
11. De Deyne C, Struys M, Decruyenaere J, et al. Use of continuous bispectral EEG monitoring to assess depth of sedation in ICU patients. Intensive Care Med. 1998;24(12):1294–8.
12. Shetty RM, Bellini A, Wijayatilake DS, et al. BIS monitoring versus clinical assessment for sedation in mechanically ventilated adults in the intensive care unit and its impact on clinical outcomes and resource utilization. Cochrane Database Syst Rev. 2018;2:D11240.
13. Karamchandani K, Rewari V, Trikha A, et al. Bispectral index correlates well with Richmond agitation sedation scale in mechanically ventilated critically ill patients. J Anesth. 2010;24(3):394–8.
14. Yamashita K, Terao Y, Inadomi C, et al. Age-dependent relationship between bispectral index and sedation level. J Clin Anesth. 2008;20(7):492–5.
15. Qadeer MA, Vargo JJ, Patel S, et al. Bispectral index monitoring of conscious sedation with the combination of meperidine and midazolam during endoscopy[J]. Clin Gastroenterol Hepatol. 2008;6(1):102–8.
16. Olson DM, Zomorodi MG, James ML, et al. Exploring the impact of augmenting sedation assessment with physiologic monitors. Aust Crit Care. 2014;27(3):145–50.
17. Mahmood S, Parchani A, El-Menyar A, et al. Utility of bispectral index in the management of multiple trauma patients. Surg Neurol Int. 2014;5:141.
18. Giordano V, Deindl P, Goeral K, et al. The power of N-PASS, aEEG, and BIS in detecting different levels of sedation in neonates: a preliminary study. Paediatr Anaesth. 2018;28(12):1096–104.
19. Olischar M, Davidson AJ, Lee KJ, et al. Effects of morphine and midazolam on sleep-wake cycling in amplitude-integrated electroencephalography in post-surgical neonates >/= 32 weeks of gestational age. Neonatology. 2012;101(4):293–300.
20. Sleigh JW, Donovan J. Comparison of bispectral index, 95% spectral edge frequency and approximate entropy of the EEG, with changes in heart rate variability during induction of general anaesthesia. Br J Anaesth. 1999;82(5):666–71.
21. Roustan JP, Valette S, Aubas P, et al. Can electroencephalographic analysis be used to determine sedation levels in critically ill patients? Anesth Analg. 2005;101(4):1141–51.
22. Bruhn J, Bouillon TW, Radulescu L, et al. Correlation of approximate entropy, bispectral index, and spectral edge frequency 95 (SEF95) with clinical signs of "anesthetic depth" during coadministration of propofol and remifentanil. Anesthesiology. 2003;98(3):621–7.
23. Itamoto K, Taura Y, Wada N, et al. Effect of medetomidine on electroencephalography and use of a quantitative electroencephalograph for evaluating sedation levels in dogs. J Vet Med A Physiol Pathol Clin Med. 2001;48(9):525–35.
24. Antunes LM, Golledge HD, Roughan JV, et al. Comparison of electroencephalogram activity and auditory evoked responses during isoflurane and halothane anaesthesia in the rat. Vet Anaesth Analg. 2003;30(1):15–23.

25. Schwilden H. Concepts of EEG processing: from power spectrum to bispectrum, fractals, entropies and all that. Best Pract Res Clin Anaesthesiol. 2006;20(1):31–48.
26. Muller JN, Kreuzer M, Garcia PS, et al. Monitoring depth of sedation: evaluating the agreement between the Bispectral Index, qCON and the Entropy Module's State Entropy during flexible bronchoscopy. Minerva Anestesiol. 2017;83(6):563–73.
27. Iannuzzi M, Iannuzzi E, Rossi F, et al. Relationship between bispectral index, electroencephalographic state entropy and effect-site EC50 for propofol at different clinical endpoints. Br J Anaesth. 2005;94(5):613–6.
28. McCarthy MM, Brown EN, Kopell N. Potential network mechanisms mediating electroencephalographic beta rhythm changes during propofol-induced paradoxical excitation. J Neurosci. 2008;28(50):13488–504.
29. Akeju O, Pavone KJ, Westover MB, et al. A comparison of propofol- and dexmedetomidine-induced electroencephalogram dynamics using spectral and coherence analysis. Anesthesiology. 2014;121(5):978–89.
30. Scheinin A, Kallionpaa RE, Li D, et al. Differentiating drug-related and state-related effects of Dexmedetomidine and propofol on the electroencephalogram. Anesthesiology. 2018;129(1):22–36.
31. Maksimow A, Snapir A, Sarkela M, et al. Assessing the depth of dexmedetomidine-induced sedation with electroencephalogram (EEG)-based spectral entropy. Acta Anaesthesiol Scand. 2007;51(1):22–30.
32. Kaskinoro K, Maksimow A, Langsjo J, et al. Wide inter-individual variability of bispectral index and spectral entropy at loss of consciousness during increasing concentrations of dexmedetomidine, propofol, and sevoflurane. Br J Anaesth. 2011;107(4):573–80.
33. Kasuya Y, Govinda R, Rauch S, et al. The correlation between bispectral index and observational sedation scale in volunteers sedated with dexmedetomidine and propofol. Anesth Analg. 2009;109(6):1811–5.

# Application of Multimodal EEG in Predicting the Risk of Suicide

# 14

Xiaojiang Jiang and Li Kuang

## Contents



**Abstract**

Suicide has become a serious social and public health problem in the world, and it has conveyed a heavy burden to society and families. Effective research to identify suicide risk warning indicators using evidence-based medical technology to promote suicide prevention has become a top priority in the global

X. Jiang (✉)
Department of Neurology, The Third Affiliated Hospital of Army Medical University, Chongqing, China

L. Kuang
Department of Psychiatry, The First Affiliated Hospital of Chongqing Medical University, Chongqing, China



X. Wang et al. (eds.), *Multi-Modal EEG Monitoring of Severely Neurologically Ill Patients*,
https://doi.org/10.1007/978-981-16-4493-1_14

medical research field. Although mental health awareness and global suicide prevention strategies have made unprecedented progress, the suicide rate has been worryingly increasing for a long time. Therefore, exploring the neurobiological mechanism underlying suicidal behavior and suicide risk warning indicators is very important to systematically prevent suicide. This chapter introduces the more typical EEG biological markers and analyzes their possible neurophysiological mechanisms. It focuses on the role of PSG in predicting the risk of suicide in patients, proposes to strengthen the observation of sleep indicators for people at high risk of suicide, and guides the clinical development of targeted sleep disorder treatment, which may reduce the risk of suicidal ideation and behavior implementation in patients. At the same time, it further summarizes the common manifestations of multimodal EEG in suicide patients and the relevant research progress of multimodal EEG for predicting suicide in patients, which is significant for further exploring suicide risk warning indicators and treatment targets.

**Keywords**

Suicide · Suicide prediction · Depression · qEEG · EEG · EEG power spectrum · Event-related potential (ERP) · Machine learning

## 14.1 The Neurophysiological Mechanism of EEG Changes in Suicidal Patients

Depression is one of the main causes of social burdens worldwide. Depression is characterized by a lack of motivation and difficulty in experiencing happiness. Depression affects activities of daily living and can lead to suicide in extreme cases. Suicide not only brings huge medical costs and job losses to society but also brings a heavy emotional burden to loved ones. Therefore, the exploration of the neurobiological mechanisms underlying suicidal behavior is essential for systematic suicide prevention. The diagnosis of neuropsychiatric disorders, including depression, mostly relies on questionnaires, which lack objective quantitative indicators and are easily affected by the subjectivity of physicians and patients. With the development of EEG technology, it is possible to conduct noninvasive research on neuropsychiatric disorders, including depression. qEEG is a digital computer processing method that converts the digital format of EEG data for statistics and analysis. For example, the power or frequency of a specific waveform is a useful biomarker for evaluating neurophysiological changes and predicting mental state. Using this technology can help researchers achieve a better understanding of the mechanism behind depression and identify the corresponding biological markers. These characteristics can be accurately measured and become a tool to identify or diagnose suicide attempts in patients with depression.

de Aguiar et al. [1] systematically summarized multiple studies using qEEG to detect biomarkers of depression. Their article mentions that brainwaves can reflect the neurophysiological state. Among brainwaves, $\alpha$ waves reflect the inactivity and relaxation of the brain, $\beta$ waves are related to anxiety and introversion, $\theta$ waves are related to emotional processing, $\gamma$ waves are related to attention and cognition and may also be related to mood swings (a large number of $\gamma$ waves provides emotional balance), and $\delta$ waves are related to deep sleep. Fernando summarized some biological signs of depression and suicidal ideation. Subjects with suicidal ideation had increased $\alpha$ activity during a whole night of sleep; their $\alpha$ activity was asymmetrical, and their $\alpha$ activity in the left hemisphere was increased. To obtain a deeper understanding, we have specifically analyzed several previous studies. Graae et al. [2] studied the changes in resting qEEGs of individuals who attempted suicide and healthy controls in Spanish female teenagers. The EEGs of 16 suicide attempters and 22 healthy controls during eyes-opened and eyes-closed periods were recorded. After calculation, it was found that the individuals who attempted suicide were different from the healthy control group in terms of α wave asymmetry. The right brain of the healthy control group had a larger α power spectrum than the left brain, and the asymmetry of the suicide attempt group was not as significant as that of the healthy control group. This is because the α power spectrum of the left brain in the suicide attempt group increased; therefore, the asymmetry gap decreased. The suicide attempt group had abnormal alpha-wave asymmetry, especially in the posterior cerebrum, which was related to the severity of the suicide attempt but not to the severity of depression. Consistent with the results of Fernando's study, Lee et al. [3] used a mood scale to divide subjects into depression and healthy control groups for routine EEG recordings. The depression group had a higher α power spectrum in the left central cortex (C3). The α wave is derived from the depolarization of the membrane potential of thalamic–cortical neurons, and the generated potential is recruited to the cortex and recorded. It is one of the basic waveforms of brainwaves. The frequency range of α waves is 8–13 Hz, which can be further divided into slow α waves (8–9 Hz), intermediate α waves (9–12 Hz), and fast α waves (12–13 Hz). The amplitude is 20–100 μV. When the eyes are closed, the most obvious recording is in the occipital lobe and the posterior parietal lobe. When the eyes are open, the incoming visual stimulus increases the activity of the occipital cortex, and the α rhythm is blocked and replaced by desynchronized low-amplitude fast waves. qEEG calculates the power spectrum of each band, which is directly proportional to the number and voltage of the band. Given this information, the increase in the α-band power spectrum of the left hemisphere (the dominant hemisphere) of the depression group and suicide attempt group means that the number or amplitude of α waves was increased. This is probably because of the transition of the wave band from α waves to β waves as α waves became fast α waves, reflecting a state of high alertness or anxiety. This may also be due to the increase in the amplitude of waves, indicating that the dominant hemisphere had recruited more α waves. Because the α wave reflects the state of relaxation and nonfunctioning, this phenomenon may reflect the weakened activity of the dominant hemisphere. Therefore, depressed patients, especially those with suicidal ideation, have higher α band power on the left side of the brain and abnormal α asymmetry, which can be used as biomarkers of depression and suicidal ideation.

Bruderet et al. [4] studied depression patients receiving fluoxetine treatment and found that fluoxetine treatment responders had greater alpha power than nonresponders and healthy controls, especially in the occipital region, which can be understood as the relaxation ability of patients who responded to fluoxetine being restored. The study also found that the alpha asymmetry of responders and nonresponders was different. The right hemisphere of the responders showed greater alpha power than the left hemisphere.

This finding is consistent with the results of previous studies showing that the right brain of a healthy control group had a larger α power spectrum than the left brain. This shows that the performance of patients with curative effects tends to have normal α asymmetry, which is a manifestation of effective treatment. Gerard E's research also mentioned that serotonergic activity was closely related to wakefulness. Serotonergic cells in the raphe nucleus exhibit a constant discharge pattern. When patient changes from arousal to sleep, the discharge rate decreases. Based on this theory, it is hypothesized that the increase in α power in depressed patients who respond to selective serotonin reuptake inhibitors (SSRIs) reflects that low arousal before treatment is related to low serotonergic activity [4]. Glenn et al. [5] also mentioned that previous studies have compared the levels of serotonin receptors in depressed patients with suicidal behaviors and nondepressed patients. It was found that depressed patients who attempted suicide or died of suicide had increased expression of serotonin 1A receptors in certain areas of the cerebral cortex than the control group. This receptor inhibits the further release of serotonin into the synapse, causing a loss of serotonin transduction signals and resulting in an impaired ability to use serotonin in suicidal people. Therefore, SSRIs are more effective than other antidepressants in suppressing suicidal tendencies and suicidal behaviors [5]. This serotonergic mechanism may be the common basis for depression and abnormal EEG activity.

Benschop Lars et al. [6] used qEEG to study the characteristics of EEG power spectra at rest in female patients with major depression disorder (MDD). Compared with depressed patients without suicidal tendency, individuals who attempted suicide and depressed patients with suicidal ideation both showed low γ activity in the frontal region and high β and low γ activity in the left occipital area. Compared with depressed patients with suicidal ideation, people who attempted suicide had reduced β and γ activities in the right temporal region. As mentioned earlier, β waves are related to anxiety, γ waves may be related to mood swings, and a large amount of γ power provides emotional balance. Therefore, low γ activity in the frontal area reflects the disorder of emotional balance, and high β activity in the left occipital region reflects an increase in anxiety. The study also examined whether these suicide-based frequency features appeared in the relevant brain regions previously reported in the neuroimaging literature. The results of this analysis showed that the activities were reduced in depressed patients who attempted suicidal and suicidal ideation in the orbitofrontal, medial, middle, upper, and lower frontal regions and the anterior cingulate cortex (ACC). In patients who attempted suicide, the reduction in the activity of the right temporal lobe was limited to the right inferior temporal lobe, middle temporal lobe, epithelial layer of the temporal lobe, and fusiform gyrus. Ding et al. [7] used MRI to comprehensively evaluate the cortical volume, surface area, and thickness of depression patients who attempted suicide, patients with mood disorders but no suicidal behaviors, and healthy people. This study included evaluations of the orbitofrontal cortex (OFC), ventrolateral prefrontal cortex (VLPFC), dorsal prefrontal cortex (DPFC), and medial prefrontal cortex (MPFC, including the ACC). Compared with the other two groups, the volume of the left VLPFC was decreased in depressed patients who had attempted suicide. In addition, the study found that, compared with the healthy control group, depressed patients who had attempted suicide had reduced OFC and DFPC volumes, but the volume of the MFPC was not decreased. For patients with a history of mood disorders, the volume of the left VLPFC had certain specificity in identifying patients who had attempted suicide. When combining the results of the above two studies, it can be concluded that the brainwave abnormality of depressed patients who have attempted suicide may be related to the changes in the cortical volume of the corresponding area. In particular, the frontal lobe is mainly responsible for the regulation of emotions; therefore, the γ rhythm changes in this area are more significant. The amount of brain-derived neurotrophic factor (BDNF) secreted in this part is abnormal and may also be involved in the abnormal regulation of EEGs. Neural network dysfunction or impaired neuroplasticity of the brain may be an important factor in inducing suicidal behavior. BDNF exists in various parts of the brain. Increased levels of BDNF can enhance neuronal activity and increase intersynaptic connections. After an autopsy of patients who committed suicide, it was found that the levels of BDNF in the brains of depressed and nondepressed patients were significantly reduced, which was particularly noticeable in the prefrontal lobe and hippocampus [8]. Liu et al. [9] summarized the high expression of several inflammatory cytokines (such as IL-6) found in the prefrontal cortex of deceased individuals with depression who committed suicide. Abnormalities in neuroinflammation increase the risk of suicide by impairing the executive control of the frontal lobe, which is consistent with the inflammatory response caused by sleep interruption. That is, sleep disorders participate in the stress process, which leads to impaired brain prefrontal function by stimulating neuroinflammatory processes, thereby impairing executive control ability and leading to an increased risk of suicide.

Fitzgerald et al. [10] reviewed the related content of γ power as a biomarker of MDD. In one study, when depressed patients performed spatial and arithmetic tasks, the resting γ power in the prefrontal and temporal lobes increased, while the resting γ power in the ACC decreased. When subjects with MDD performed emotion-related tasks, the γ power of the prefrontal cortex also decreased. These changes all reflect the abnormalities of emotional regulation and cognition in the corresponding brain regions of patients with depression. Arikan et al. [11] used qEEG to investigate the neurophysiological changes in depressed patients with suicidal ideation and suicide attempts. In participants sitting calmly with their eyes closed, 7 min of qEEG data were recorded in a quiet, dimly lit room. The results showed that the high γ power of F4, Fz, F8, C4, Cz, O2, T5, and T6 in the suicide attempt group was greater than that in the nonsuicide attempt group. In addition, there were significant differences in the high γ power of Fz, Cz, and F8 between the suicide attempt group and the suicidal ideation group. In the high waveband of each electrode, the γ power of the suicide attempt group was higher than that of the suicidal ideation group. The γ rhythm is mainly the high-frequency brain electrical activity of approximately 30–140 Hz that occurs when healthy people are highly concentrated or performing working memory activities. The γ rhythm can be divided into the slow γ rhythm (25–50 Hz) and the fast γ rhythm (80–145 Hz). The fast γ rhythm plays an important role in spatial attention and memory coding. The slow γ rhythm is often related to the successful distribution of attention, information perception, integrated processing, and working memory. Abnormalities in neurotransmitters or receptors may cause abnormal γ rhythms, including abnormal levels of serotonin or the dysfunction of receptors, NMDAR-mediated glutamate transmission dysfunction, abnormal dopaminergic pathway signaling, and GABA system abnormalities, such as structural changes in the GABA receptor that can lead to abnormal γ rhythms [12, 13].

These previous conclusions have certain differences. The heterogeneity may be due to the different conditions used in different studies, and different experimental operations may reflect different underlying physiological mechanisms. However, there is no doubt that the γ rhythm has obvious changes in different brain regions in patients with depression and suicidal ideation. The alteration mechanism involves the disorder of multiple neural circuits and transmitter regulation, and further research is needed.

Lee et al. [14] studied the qEEG changes in the frontal lobe area associated with suicidal ideation in young healthy subjects. The subject sat quietly and relaxed on a chair with their eyes closed, and brainwaves were recorded from 10:00 am to 5:00 pm. It was found that subjects with high scores on the suicidal ideation scale had higher θ-band power in the frontal lobe and median area, and there was a positive correlation. The results indicate that cerebral electrical activity in the central prefrontal region of young healthy subjects may be related to suicidal ideation. Therefore, brain electrical activity in the θ-wave band in this area has clinical application value as a biomarker for suicide prevention. The θ rhythm usually occurs during brain work, rest, and sleep. The frequency of the theta wave is 4–7 Hz, and the amplitude is 100–150 μV. The θ wave appears when drowsiness occurs, which generally indicates that the CNS has entered a state of depression. The θ wave appears only in the frontal lobe when the eyes are closed and individuals are quiet. It also appears in other parts of the cortex when individuals' eyes are open or when they hear sudden noises or think about problems. θ waves appear when healthy people are sleeping, and if they have the same amplitude as the α waves during awakening, it is an abnormal phenomenon. Hunter et al. [15] used qEEG to analyze whether suicidal ideation related to antidepressant treatment in patients with MDD was related to neurophysiological changes. It was found that after 48 h of medication, the power of the midline and right frontal (MRF) dropped sharply instantly, and there was no clear correlation with the type of medication. The instantaneous θ-wave reduction associated with suicidal ideation induced by antidepressants and the θ-wave performance of suicidal ideation at rest may be affected by different neural mechanisms.

Suicidal behavior is divided into three types: suicidal ideation, suicide attempt, and suicide completion. Suicidal ideation precedes suicide attempts and is an important predictor of suicide attempts and suicide completion. Therefore, the identification of suicidal ideation is the primary task of suicide prevention. At present, there are many studies using qEEG to detect individuals with depression and suicidal ideation or suicide attempts. Although there are some differences in the research results, the conclusions of most studies are consistent, suggesting that some of the characteristics of EEG changes can be used as biological markers of depression and suicidal ideation. However, there are few in-depth explanations of the specific mechanisms of EEG changes in such patients. The generation mechanism of EEG changes is intricate and involves multiple neurophysiological systems. Patients with depression and suicidal ideation have complex changes in a variety of neurotransmitters, neural circuits, and the structure of the cerebral cortex, which jointly participate in the physiological mechanism of EEG changes. We summarized some of the more typical biological markers monitored by qEEG and analyzed their possible neurophysiological mechanisms as some enlightenment for further in-depth research.

## 14.2 The Role of PSG in Predicting the Risk of Suicide in Patients

Suicide causes nearly one million deaths every year worldwide, which greatly increases the global burden of disease [16]. The global annual suicide rate after age standardization is 11.4 per 100,000 (15.0 per 100,000 for men and 8.0 per 100,000 for women), and suicide is also the second leading cause of death among people aged 15–29. Suicide is a serious social and public health problem worldwide. The prevention of suicide has been listed as a top priority for national medical research by the medical departments of many countries. They also called for effective research to obtain early warning indicators of suicide risk factors based on evidence-based medicine to promote the prevention of suicide. Although mental health consciousness and global suicide prevention strategies have made unprecedented progress, the suicide rate has been growing at an alarming rate for a long time [17]. In 2013, the WHO proposed the first mental health action plan, and the suicide prevention plan is part of the whole plan, striving to achieve the goal of reducing suicide rates by 10% in all countries in the world by 2020 [18, 19]. In recent years, many studies have shown that problems related to sleep disorders are closely associated with suicidal behavior and suicidal ideation [20, 21]. However, the description of sleep-related issues, especially the quantitative indicators obtained through objective sleep monitoring (PSG, actigraphy, etc.) to warn of suicide risk, is still in the preliminary research stage. Sleep disorder as a potentially significant risk factor for suicide has received increasing attention. Studies have shown that reducing sleep duration by only 1 h may also significantly increase the risk of suicide [22].

### 14.2.1 The Neurobiological Mechanism of Suicide

The mechanism of suicide is currently unclear. Most views believe that it is a result of the interaction of multiple complex factors such as genetics, social environment, and psychology. However, there is currently no animal model that can stimulate a certain nucleus in the cerebral cortex and absolutely lead to suicide attempts or behaviors. There are few studies from China on brain imaging of patients who attempted suicide, but more reports from abroad. Brain structure imaging has become the most commonly used method. Through research in recent years, it has been found that the abnormal brain structure characteristics of suicide are mainly changes in the volume and density of white matter and gray matter, white matter hyperintensities, and damaged nerve fibers of white matter [23–25].

Although existing studies have found a series of predictors in interdisciplinary fields, the related neurobiological mechanisms of suicide risk have not been determined. However, among many mechanisms, sleep disorders have become an important link between suicide and the primary mental disorders leading to suicide; that is, sleep disorders are the triggering factors for suicidal ideation and behavior implementation in many mental illnesses including MDD and treatment-resistant depression.

### 14.2.2 Progress in Research on Suicide Risk and Objective Sleep Monitoring

Previous evidence has shown that subjective sleep disorders are closely related to suicidal ideation and behavior (including suicide death) [26]. Sleep EEG has been identified as a monitoring method, and sleep EEGs have been identified as a potential biomarker for diseases closely related to suicide, such as MDD. Previous studies have shown that subjective complaints about sleep problems may be related to the risk of suicidal behavior. This complaint is not affected by affective episodes or depression, and in some cases, the risk of suicide is greater than that of depression-related symptoms [21].

Preliminary studies support the possible biomarker utility of sleep disorders as suicide risk and treatment targets. However, to date, most studies investigating the link between sleep and suicide have evaluated only subjective sleep disorders, such as prolonged subjective sleep latency, nightmares and poor sleep quality [27]. Subjective and objective sleep assessments have not been performed simultaneously, which has led to inconsistent results in studies on the correlation between sleep disorders and increased suicide risk. Therefore, objective sleep measurements, such as PSG parameters, should be actively used to systematically assess the relationship between sleep and suicidal symptoms and increased behavioral risk, especially for patients with bipolar depression or MDD.

#### 14.2.2.1 Suicide Risk and Changes in Macroscopic Sleep Structure

Previous evidence has reported that increased suicide risk is related to prolonged sleep latency, increased REM, less sleep in stage 4 of NREM, lower sleep efficiency, and an increased number of awakenings during sleep. Existing studies on abnormal sleep EEG activity and suicide provide important evidence for the relationship between changes in the macroscopic structure of sleep or the overall pattern of sleep stages and the risk of suicide [28].

**Prolonged Sleep Latency**

Suicidal patients have more rumination during the onset of sleep; that is, they repeatedly recall the unpleasant and even traumatic events they experienced during the day and in the past. The risk of acute suicide often occurs during relatively brief periods of high arousal or exaltation. When a suicidal patient's sleep latency is prolonged, it will inevitably lead to excessive wakefulness (including excessive cognitive and cortical wakefulness) before falling asleep, which creates more opportunities for suicidal thoughts and behaviors to occur, thereby increasing the risk of suicide. Therefore, by improving sleep disorders with prolonged sleep latency, it is of great significance to correct the bad behaviors and excessive wakefulness that are highly concerned with the ability to fall asleep and block the vicious cycle of suicide risk due to prolonged sleep latency [28, 29].

**Increased REM Sleep**

An increase in REM sleep indicates an increase in the number of dreams in an individual's night of sleep, including nightmares and night terrors, which often aggravates a suicidal patient's bad mood, especially when they wake up from a nightmare; they are more likely to have suicidal ideation and even commit suicidal behavior [28, 30].

**Sleep Reduction in Stage 4 of NREM**

It is a sign of deep sleep. Therefore, a decrease in NREM indicates that an individual is easily awakened at night, fragmenting sleep, and increasing the number of awakenings. When the individual wakes up the next morning, they will not feel the recovery of the brain after sleep. In suicidal patients, accumulated ideas of suicide and/or bad memories of severe traumatic events cannot be erased due to the lack of good sleep. In addition, due to the lack of deep sleep at night, the loss of executive control in the following morning and day is also one of the important reasons leading to the implementation of suicidal behavior [28].

**Lower Sleep Efficiency**

Sleep efficiency is calculated by an individual's bedtime and sleep time as reflected by PSG and indicates an individual's total sleep quality. When sleep efficiency decreases, it ineffectively prompts a suicidal patient to sleep too long in bed, and the fixed thinking pattern when tossing and turning in bed without sleep may strengthen previous suicidal ideation and lead to the implementation of suicidal behavior, similar to repeated awakenings at night [28].

#### 14.2.2.2 Suicide Risk and Changes in Microscopic Sleep Structure

Although the analysis of sleep macrostructure is necessary for the study of the relationship between suicide risk and sleep disorders, some people criticize that simple sleep macrostructure analysis will result in the loss of records of microscopic sleep-related events of REM and NREM during sleep monitoring. Therefore, when studying the relationship between suicide risk and sleep EEG monitoring, supplementing quantitative sleep EEG (or sleep microstructure) may be a more complete method because it also describes the different EEGs of brain activity during sleep frequency changes.

The cyclic alternating pattern reflects microstructural changes during sleep [31]. An increase in frequency of the cyclic alternating pattern indicates an increase in light sleep in NREM, which leads to patients often misunderstanding the stage 2 sleep distributed between arousals as an awakened state, which leads to the delusion of being "up all night." Conventional treatment has difficulty correcting this delusion, which causes patients to lose confidence in the treatment of insomnia and ultimately increases the risk of suicidal ideation and suicidal behavior.

#### 14.2.2.3 The Correlation Between Suicide Risk and OSAS

The apnea–hypopnea index (AHI) indicates the severity of OSAS during sleep. The risk of suicide in patients with MDD combined with OSAS is higher than that in patients without OSAS. The reason is that most patients with OSAS suffer from awakening due to nocturnal hypoxia and increased nocturia during PSG, which causes poor sleep continuity and a significant increase in nights with awakenings and leads to an increase in suicidal attempts and behaviors in patients with suicidal tendencies, which is similar to the increase in the risk of suicide in individuals with changes in macroscopic sleep structure. A long period of uncorrected OSAS leads to impaired daytime cognitive function and decreased work efficiency, which will further aggravate the patient's anxiety and depression, leading to an increased risk of suicide [32].

### 14.2.3 The Role of Objective Sleep Monitoring Indicators in Determining the Early Warning Signs of and Guiding Interventions for Suicide Risk

When implementing objective sleep monitoring for people at risk of suicide, significantly prolonged night sleep latency, increased number of sleep awakenings, shortened sleep time of stage III and IV, increased REM, decreased sleep efficiency, and increased number of cyclic alternating patterns in the sleep microstructure may indicate an increased risk of suicide [9]. Therefore, strengthening the observation of these relevant sleep monitoring indicators for people at high risk of suicide to guide clinical treatment programs of targeted sleep disorder may reduce the risk of suicidal ideation and behavior implementation.

The potential importance of sleep as a neurobiological factor may provide new insights into the pathogenesis of suicide risk. In addition, because sleep disorders can be monitored in the weeks and months before suicide, this sleep disorder is completely treatable. Therefore, it is of great significance to carry out long-term and further research on sleep disorders as a hypothetical biomarker and therapeutic target for suicide prevention.

In short, the long-term comprehensive dynamic tracking of the big data (including shopping history, chat history, medical treatment, facial expression changes, wearable sleep monitors, and machine learning) [33] of individuals at high risk of suicide in the future may be the most effective suicide risk warning indicator.

Comparing suicidal ideation, suicide attempts, and death by suicide in clinical research is helpful to discover the pathophysiological mechanism of suicide. At the same time, studies before and after suicide treatment are also crucial to find effective treatment methods to control suicide. In conclusion, research on the early warning signs, prevention, and control of suicide risk should include a comprehensive collection of various information to extract the most valuable susceptibility factors. It is never possible to accurately predict the risk of suicide through a single medical indicator. Only by tracing and observing long-term comprehensive big data and finding relevant risk indicators that have significantly changed recently (especially changes that cannot be explained by normal reasons), it can be possible to achieve short-term early warning of suicide risk.

## 14.3 Common Multimodal EEG Manifestations in Suicide Patients

### 14.3.1 Background

Suicide refers to a dangerous behavior in which individuals deliberately or voluntarily take various means to end their lives under the influence of complex psychological activities. Suicide has become a serious social and public health problem worldwide and has brought a heavy burden to society and families. According to a report by the WHO in 2019, more than 800,000 people die by suicide every year, and one person dies every 40 s globally [16]. Severe depression or epilepsy can lead to suicide. The lifetime prevalence of mental disorders in patients with epilepsy is usually approximately 50–60%. In particular, the prevalence of mental disorders in temporal lobe epilepsy is relatively high. Mental disorders of patients with epilepsy mostly manifest as mood disorders of anxiety or depression. Compared with the general population, the risk of suicide in patients with epilepsy is greatly increased. In addition, AEDs can also increase the risk of suicidal ideation and suicidal behavior [34]. EEG is the most important examination tool in the diagnosis and treatment of neuropsychiatric diseases. It is a method of using electrophysiological indicators to record brain activity. Although high-resolution anatomy and functional imaging are constantly developing, EEG is irreplaceable by other detection methods in the diagnosis and treatment of neuropsychiatric disorders. Therefore, it is of great significance to explore the electrophysiological characteristics of suicide patients, including their EEGs.

### 14.3.2 EEG Manifestations

The human brain is composed of tens of thousands of neurons. Brainwaves are electrical signals generated by the activities between neurons and are the overall reflection of the electrophysiological activities of brain nerve cells on the cerebral cortex or scalp surface. In EEG research, there are at least four important wavebands, the frequency range of which is between 1 and 30 Hz, namely the δ wave (1–3 Hz), θ wave (4–7 Hz), α wave (8–13 Hz), and β wave (14–30 Hz). The range of the wave amplitudes is uncertain, and other normal brainwaves with special waveforms may appear during sleep, such as the hump wave, K-complex wave, μ wave, λ wave, and σ wave. Normal EEG activity is mainly an α rhythm waveform, usually in the occipital area. The EEG activities of the two sides are basically synchronized and symmetrical, and the amplitude difference is less than 20%; if these conditions are not met, the EEG activity is considered abnormal. The dominant frequency characteristics of the α wave represent the order and unity of brain electrical activity. If brain function is disordered, the characteristics of the α wave will change.

The common EEG waveform abnormalities in patients with depression are α-wave asymmetry, α-wave generalization or forward shift, a low-amplitude α wave, a low-amplitude β wave, a low-amplitude δ wave, a low-amplitude θ wave, increased β-wave activity, and widely low voltage. The EEGs of suicide patients can show nonspecific abnormalities in a wide range of brain areas and a variety of frequency domains. The more severe the disease, the higher the degree of abnormality.

Van der Vinne et al. [35] proposed that α wave asymmetry may be an important biomarker for the evaluation of depression, and it is also related to the treatment response of patients. α-wave asymmetry measures the relative α-wave activity between the two hemispheres of the brain, especially on the frontal lobe electrodes. α-wave asymmetry is associated with suicidal behavior. Greater α-wave activity in the left cerebral hemisphere than in the right cerebral hemisphere is observed in depressed suicidal adolescents. Lee et al. [3] showed that, compared with emotionally stable subjects, patients with depression have a higher α-wave level in the left cerebral hemisphere, which means that left cerebral hemisphere activity is reduced. Dolsen et al. [36] found that, compared with depression patients with lower suicidal ideation, depression patients with suicidal ideation had increased α-wave activity during a whole night of sleep.

In addition, Liu et al. [37] used working memory task assessment to find that the amplitude of slow waves (θ waves and δ waves) in the central region, parietal lobe, and lateral electrode was greater in patients with depression after treatment than in the control group, and the β wave in the center of the left cerebral hemisphere decreased in the depression patients.

### 14.3.3 EEG Power Spectrum Manifestations

The EEG power spectrum is based on ordinary EEG and processed by a computer to quantify and objectify EEG activity. It can accurately quantify and locate the functional status of each brain area. Each band of brainwaves is related to specific mechanisms in the brain. For example, the α wave reflects inactivity and relaxation in the brain; the β wave is related to expectation, anxiety, and introversion; the θ wave is related to emotional processing; the γ wave is related to attention; and the δ wave is related to deep sleep [1].

According to the different frequencies of the α band, researchers such as Park et al. [38] further divided the α wave into two sub-bands, the low α wave (8–10 Hz) and the high α wave (10–12 Hz), and discussed the relationship between the asymmetry of the α wave and the risk of suicide. It is generally believed that the low α band is related to attention and may be more related to suicidal behavior. The α-band index, especially the frontal low α-band index, is associated with increased suicidal behavior. The possible reason is that suicide patients have a certain degree of cognitive rigidity and attention bias, and they often pay attention to the relevant clues of suicide.

Previous studies have shown that in patients with major depression, the β band ranging from 12 to 30 Hz has a significant negative correlation with the correlation scale for measuring inattention [39]. Koshiyama et al. [40] followed up patients with depression for 3 years and recorded the quality of life as well as the β band and power spectrum of resting-state EEG and found that the high resting-state power of the β band may be a potentially useful biomarker. It helps predict the development of treatment for patients with depression. Lars Benschop et al. [6] used qEEG technology to evaluate the EEG power characteristics of patients with depression at rest. Compared with depression patients without suicidal tendencies, suicide attempters and individuals with suicidal ideations showed high β-band activity in the left occipital area and decreased β-band activity in the right temporal area, which may be related to the anxiety response of depressed patients.

Researchers such as Lee et al. [14] explored the changes in the frontal θ-wave qEEGs related to suicidal ideation in young healthy subjects. The results showed that brain electrical activity in the frontal–central area may be related to differences in suicidal ideation in young healthy subjects. θ-band brain electrical activity has clinical potential as a biomarker for suicide prevention. The θ-band activity of the frontal lobe on the right side of the midline is related to changes in suicidal ideation.

Researchers such as Lee et al. [14] studied the neurophysiological biomarkers of suicidal ideation in healthy people using qEEGs to detect the frontal lobe (FP1, FP2, F7, F3, Fz, F4, and F8) and central midline electrodes (FCz and Cz) θ band. It was found that people with high scores on the Baker Suicidal Ideation Scale had higher relative powers of θ waves at F3, Fz, FCz, and Cz than those with low scores on the Baker Suicidal Ideation Scale. In addition, the relative power of θ waves in the frontal–central area of the group with high scores on the Baker Suicidal Ideation Scale was significantly higher than that of the group with low scores on the Baker Suicidal Ideation Scale. These findings suggest that electrical activity in the central area of the frontal lobe may be related to suicidal ideation in young healthy individuals. In addition, a study based on the hypothesis that depression patients with suicidal ideation and those who had attempted suicide had a higher γ-rhythm, using qEEG analysis, found that suicidal ideation patients had significantly higher γ-wave power in areas F4, Fz, C4, Cz, O2, F8, T5, and T6 than the control group. Therefore, it is believed that high γ waves may be used as a biomarker for suicide screening [11].

In addition, a study evaluating suicidal ideation in teenage female patients showed that, compared with patients with low suicidal ideation, patients with high suicidal ideation had relatively lower δ power overnight [36].

### 14.3.4 ERP Manifestations

ERPs are based on attention and are related to mental activities such as recognition, comparison, judgment, memory, and decision. They reflect different aspects of the cognitive process and are a window to understand the cognitive function of the brain. The classic ERP components include P1, N1, P2, N2, and P3 (P300), among which P1, N1, and P2 are the exogenous (physiological) components of the ERP, which are affected by the physical characteristics of the stimulus, and N2 and P3 are the endogenous (psychological) components of the ERP, which are not affected by the physical characteristics of the stimulus and are related to the mental state and attention of the subjects. However, there are few studies about using ERPs to predict suicide. ERP research may improve the understanding of suicidal thoughts and suicidal behaviors in a large number of complex processes.

Tsypes et al. [41] used EEG and ERP research to explore the Research Domain Criteria (RdoC) substructure and the initial response to rewards for adult suicide attempters compared with non-suicide attempters. The subjects completed clinical interviews and self-report questionnaires, computer-based monetary incentive delay tasks (MIDTs), and Doors tasks, and their cEEGs were recorded. Time–space principal component analysis was used to separate each ERP of interest and its components that overlap with other times or spaces. Exploratory time–frequency analysis is used to supplement ERP analysis. The results show that suicide attempters, compared with nonattempters, have specific defects in reward expectation (the ERP component of clue P3 becomes dull during MIDTs) and the initial response to reward (a decrease in δ power under the condition of Doors task gain).

### 14.3.5 Summary

Suicidal behavior has a major impact on both individuals and society, and early recognition of suicidal ideation can help prevent suicidal behavior. As an important inspection tool for neuropsychiatric disorders, EEG and other neuroelectrophysiological techniques are of great significance for the recognition and prediction of suicidal ideation and can be regarded as important biomarkers of suicidal behavior. However, there are certain differences in the results of various studies. Further study should explore the EEG and neurophysiological manifestations of suicidal behavior.

## 14.4 Research Progress on the Use of Multimodal EEG in Predicting Suicide

### 14.4.1 Background

According to a report by the WHO in 2019, more than 800,000 people die by suicide every year, and one person dies every 40 s around the world [16]. The number of suicide deaths exceeds the sum of war and homicide victims. Suicide can be prevented, and timely intervention is the key to reducing tragedies. Psychological counseling and medication can dispel this idea to a certain extent. However, assessing the risk of suicide is a major challenge faced by clinicians [5]. First, suicidal behavior is an extremely strong personal behavior. Patients with suicidal thoughts often cover up their own intentions. Nearly 80% of people who successfully committed suicide denied suicidal thoughts in their last clinical interview [42]. Second, due to the subjectivity of self-reports, the effect of investigating suicidal tendencies in the form of questionnaires is not ideal. Meta-analysis suggests the limitations of current suicide prediction methods. Matthew et al. [43] included a group of individuals from a longitudinal cohort study who had previous suicide attempts, divided them into high-risk and low-risk groups, and observed the actual circumstances due to suicide death of the two groups. The results showed that the suicide mortality rate of the high-risk group was indeed higher than that of the low-risk group, approximately half of suicide deaths occurred in the low-risk group, and 95% of individuals in the high-risk group did not die from suicide. In another systematic review, Chan et al. [44] summarized individuals with a history of self-harm in a prospective study and found that a history of self-harm, suicidal intentions, poor physical condition, and male sex were significantly associated with suicide risk, but these factors are very common in the population, and the clinical value is weak, which means limitations of the scale and existing evaluation models. And recent article stated that the role of mental health services is to prevent death and relieve the suffering of patients and their families, rather than wasting energy and resources on risk evaluation [45].

Therefore, finding an objective method and indicator to detect suicidal tendency in advance and intervene in time has become an urgent need for clinicians.

### 14.4.2 Multiple Cognitive Deficits Are Associated with Suicide

Previous studies have partially revealed possible cognitive deficits in people with suicide-related problems, such as cognitive rigidity, deficits in executive function, decreased problem-solving ability, decreased decision-making ability, ruminative thinking, decreased ability to control attention and impulses, and attention to information bias [46–48].

#### 14.4.2.1 Defects in Decision-Making Functions

Individuals who have recently attempted suicide may have obstacles in decision-making functions, and their behavior is reflected in the attention to the best results at hand, not the adverse consequences in the future, and they cannot learn or reflect on the consequences of previous decisions [46]. Studies on veterans with posttraumatic stress disorder (PTSD) have shown that the higher the degree of self-reported impulse, the greater the likelihood of suicidal ideation and self-harm, and the lower the ability to inhibit behavior, the more likely they are to attempt suicide [49]. Another study using the Cambridge Automated Neuropsychological Test Battery (CANTB) showed that suicidal ideation was associated with a higher overall proportion of betting and risk-taking in the Cambridge gambling test task [50], implying abnormal impulse control and decision-making ability. Moreover, individuals who attempted suicides may have selective attention to negative information [51].

#### 14.4.2.2 Insufficient Anti-interference Ability

Continuous insufficiency of anti-interference ability and deficits in learning or memory may lead to an increased risk of suicidal behavior. Keilp et al. [52] revealed the neuropsychological defects of suicide attempts at different levels of depression. The results showed that suicide attempters performed poorly in attention and working memory and had lower intelligence before being ill. Individuals who attempted suicides also performed poorly in the computerized Stroop task and the Buschke Selective Reminder Test. These defects may be characteristic markers independent of current symptomology.

#### 14.4.2.3 Deficits in Cognitive Control

In the case of emotional stimulation, general deficits in cognitive control may be a sign of adolescent suicide risk. Stewart et al. [53] included 99 young people with recent suicidal thoughts or suicidal behaviors and asked them to complete the Suicide Stroop Task, presenting negative or positive suicide-related words in the task. The results showed that, compared with adolescents who stayed at the level of suicide conception, individuals who attempted suicides were more disturbed by suicide and positive stimuli. Individuals who attempted suicides showed greater interference with emotional stimulation, which means individuals who attempted suicides have significant cognitive control defects in the face of emotional stimuli. However, the specificity of the Suicide Stroop Task as a suicide screening tool and whether cognitive control deficits are related to stimulus valence remain unclear.

#### 14.4.2.4 Abnormality in the Expectation and Initial Reaction to Rewards

A study of the RdoC substructure and the initial response to rewards of adult individuals who attempted suicides compared with nonindividuals who attempted suicides used EEG and ERP. The subjects completed the self-report questionnaire and the computer MIDT and Doors task. Researchers recorded cEEGs in these two tasks using time–space principal component analysis to separate each ERP component of interest from other components that overlap in time or space. Exploratory time–frequency analysis is also used to supplement ERP analysis. The results showed that, compared with nonindividuals who attempted suicides, individuals who attempted suicides have specific defects in reward expectations (the ERP component of clue P3 becomes dull during MIDT) and the initial response to rewards (the feedback-related $\delta$ power decreases under the condition of Doors task gain). These results are at least partially independent of current symptoms or diagnoses of depression and anxiety [41].

The measurement of ERPs is a stable and direct neurophysiological method. It can be used as a test for clinical changes and a predictor of clinical changes. Unfortunately, the literature on neurocognitive testing combined with EEG, ERP measurement, and other brain imaging techniques for suicide prediction is still rare. Multimodal cognitive assessment of impulsivity, cognitive flexibility, decision-making ability, response to rewards, etc., may be helpful for suicide screening of susceptible and high-risk populations, and it is more predictive if combined with EEG and imaging techniques.

### 14.4.3 EEG Abnormalities Related to Suicide

EEG signals are special and complex bioelectrical signals that reflect the functional state of the brain. Alpha waves in EEGs are the main wave bands of the brain when an individual is in a quiet state with closed eyes. In this state, significant alpha-wave activity indicates the order and unity of brain electrical activity and that the body is calm and tranquil. In contrast, beta-wave activity when an individual is in a quiet state with closed eyes may mean that the body is in a state of tension and stress. This pathological change may indicate a disorder of mood and brain function. If the brain is dysfunctional and the individual is under negative stress for a long time, brain electricity may transition from alpha waves to beta waves. Other specific EEG changes that may exist are as follows.

#### 14.4.3.1 Changes in EEG Power Spectra

EEG power spectra quantify and objectify brain electrical activity through computer processing on the basis of ordinary EEGs. EEG power spectra can accurately quantify and locate the brain function status of each brain area.

Suicidal ideation and attempts are common phenomena of depression spectrum disorder. Previous studies have found that patients with depression and suicide have changes in the spatial distribution of their EEG power spectra [11]. However, the specific relationship between its changes and suicide is still uncertain. A study on suicide attempts in depression patients showed that the average high $\gamma$ power of the right central electrode in the suicide attempt group was significantly higher than that of the nonsuicide attempt group; the high $\gamma$ power of the right lateral prefrontal electrode in the suicide attempt group was significantly higher than that of the nonsuicide attempt group and suicidal ideation group [11]. The average high $\gamma$ power in the posterior temporal lobe of the suicide attempt group was significantly higher than that of the nonsuicide attempt group ($p = 0.05$). In addition, Benschop et al. [6] also found a phenomenon of low activation of the frontal lobe in the orbitofrontal area, the medial frontal area, the middle frontal area, the upper and lower frontal areas, and the ACC in a suicide attempt group. This low activation of the right temporal lobe of the attempter group was confined to the right inferior, middle, and superior cortexes and fusiform gyrus.

#### 14.4.3.2 Abnormal Spatial Distribution of EEG Frequency

A study of female adolescents who had attempted suicide [2] showed that there was no significant difference in overall alpha power between individuals who attempted suicides and a healthy control group, and alpha block (indicating no deviation in occipital lobe function) existed in the two groups. In the overall power of other frequency bands, there was no significant difference between the groups. There were significant differences in the $\alpha$ asymmetry of EEGs between the two groups. The healthy control group had higher $\alpha$ power in the right hemisphere as a whole, while individuals who attempted suicides had no obvious asymmetry. 68% of the control group had greater alpha power in the right hemisphere than in the left hemisphere, while only 44% of individuals who attempted suicides showed this asymmetry. Repeated-measures analysis of variance was performed on the attempters grouped by intention, and the results showed that intention, area, and hemisphere had significant interactions. Among them, only the suicidal intention group showed abnormal posterior asymmetry. In another study of night EEGs [36], compared with participants with low suicidal ideation, the absolute alpha power of people with high suicidal ideation increased throughout the night. The relative $\delta$ power of participants with low suicidal ideation decreased overnight compared with that of participants with high suicidal ideation. Compared with participants with low suicidal ideation, participants with high suicidal ideation had a higher percentage of $\alpha$-$\delta$ sleep throughout the night.

In addition, another study [6] showed that the bilateral $\beta$ (15–30 Hz) and low-$\gamma$ (31–60 Hz) activities of an attempt group and an ideation group were reduced compared with those of a control group. The suicidal ideation group also showed bilateral $\alpha$ hyperactivity in the posterior occipital zone and high-$\beta$ (25–30 Hz) and low-$\gamma$ hyperactivity in the left occipital lobe. When the attempt group was compared with the ideation group, the attempt group's high $\beta$ and low-$\gamma$ activity in the right temporal lobe was decreased.

### 14.4.4 Suicide-Related Brain Structural and Functional Changes

#### 14.4.4.1 Various Brain Structural and Functional Abnormalities

Despite the small sample sizes of studies and the heterogeneity of the neuroimaging techniques and analysis methods used, there is increasing evidence that specific brain regions and circuits play an important role in suicidal thoughts and behavior. This is especially true for the cortex–striatal system that supports emotion and impulse regulation, including the prefrontal lobe, cingulate and insular cortex, amygdala, hippocampus, thalamus, and striatal regions. Since the ventral prefrontal cortex (VPFC), DPFC, ACC, insula, proximal temporal lobe, basal ganglia, thalamus, and posterior regions are the most frequently studied regarding the relationship between suicidal thoughts and behavior, and because there is the most consistent evidence for the participation of these regions, special attention should be paid to these regions and the connection between them [54].

Lianne et al. [54] also summarized the relevant literature on brain imaging manifestations of suicide patients in the past 20 years and believed that the cortex–striatal system, including the prefrontal lobe, cingulate and insular cortex, amygdala, hippocampus, thalamus, and striatum, is subject to emotion and impulse regulation. The serotonergic changes in the amygdala and hippocampus are related to suicide attempts and suicidal ideation across mental disorders. The changes in the function of these areas are related to the increased autobiographical recall of mental pain, the inactivation of immediate reward processing, and the impaired prospects of individuals who made suicide attempts. In the process of emotional processing and suppression, the activation rate of the thalamus is higher, and it is related to adult suicide attempts and suicidal ideation in major depressive disorder. The VPFC (ACC, OFC, and right prefrontal cortex (RPFC)), insula, amygdala, hippocampus, medial temporal area, posterior midline structure (posterior cingulate cortex and anterior cuneiform), dorsal ACC, ventral striatum, thalamus, and cerebellum contribute to the generation of suicidal ideation through their roles in overly negative and inactive positive inner states, negative self-suggestion, obstacles to future thinking, and contemplation. Diffusion tensor imaging studies [55] have shown that the depressed suicidal brain may be a result of defective connectivity, which subsequently leads to reduced brain volumes and neural inhibition of suicidal thoughts. Mark et al. [56] believe that previous studies on the neural mechanisms of suicide have different results, which may be due to the different susceptibilities of different people to suicide. Due to differences in the brain regions, neurotransmitter systems, population age, and white matter fiber bundles involved in suicide, a variety of neural mechanisms may be involved.

#### 14.4.4.2 Machine Learning-Assisted Imaging Diagnosis of Suicide

Previous studies have shown that young people are likely to post online statements about suicidal thoughts and suicide risk factors. Posts, instant messages, text messages, and emails on social networking sites to express pain may be becoming more common [57]. In addition, pain and suicidal thoughts expressed online may not be disclosed to doctors. It is not clear to what extent this online expression represents real suicidal ideation and risk, but a study has shown that suicidal thoughts expressed online are correlated with psychologically assessed suicide risk [57].

Researchers have developed a "Suicide Artificial Intelligence Prediction Heuristic" [58], which can predict the risk of users' suicidal thoughts in the future by analyzing publicly available Twitter data. They used Twitter data to inquire about suicide-related psychological structures (including burden, stress, loneliness, hopelessness, insomnia, depression, and anxiety) and trained a series of neural networks based on the model to evaluate the probability of user suicide in the near future.

### 14.4.5 Summary and Outlook

In the past, suicide assessment and prediction relied more on doctors' interviews with patients. At present, examinations based on EEG and fMRI partially reveal the neural mechanisms related to suicide. With the gradual application of machine learning in brain imaging data analysis, we will be able to better interpret the thoughts of each scanned person, including suicide-related ideas. However, the quality and sample size of current EEG and imaging studies are limited. At the same time, these techniques are used only to examine superficial phenomena or secondary changes related to suicide. Scientists have tried to skip the appearances related to suicide and search for the cause of suicide from the perspective of genes and heredity, but disappointingly, some meta-analyses have reported inconsistent relationships between specific genes and suicidal behavior [59–61].

In the future, a multimodal algorithm that integrates data from EEG, brain structural and function imaging, well-designed neurocognitive experiments, genetic and epigenetic marker analyses, demographics, and machine learning, as well as personal data from social networks, self-report scales, clinical interviews, and other tools, is expected to build a more efficient suicide risk assessment and prediction model.

## References


1. de Aguiar NF, Rosa J. Depression biomarkers using non-invasive EEG: a review. Neurosci Biobehav Rev. 2019;105:83–93.
2. Graae F, Tenke C, Bruder G, et al. Abnormality of EEG alpha asymmetry in female adolescent suicide attempters. Biol Psychiatry. 1996;40(8):706–13.
3. Lee PF, Kan D, Croarkin P, et al. Neurophysiological correlates of depressive symptoms in young adults: a quantitative EEG study. J Clin Neurosci. 2018;47:315–22.
4. Bruder GE, Sedoruk JP, Stewart JW, et al. Electroencephalographic alpha measures predict therapeutic response to a selective serotonin reuptake inhibitor antidepressant: pre- and post-treatment findings. Biol Psychiatry. 2008;63(12):1171–7.
5. Glenn CR, Nock MK. Improving the short-term prediction of suicidal behavior. Am J Prev Med. 2014;47(3 Suppl 2):S176–80.
6. Benschop L, Baeken C, Vanderhasselt MA, et al. Electroencephalogram resting state frequency power characteristics of suicidal behavior in female patients with major depressive disorder. J Clin Psychiatry. 2019;80(6):18m12661.
7. Ding Y, Lawrence N, Olie E, et al. Prefrontal cortex markers of suicidal vulnerability in mood disorders: a model-based structural neuroimaging study with a translational perspective. Transl Psychiatry. 2015;5:e516.
8. Banerjee R, Ghosh AK, Ghosh B, et al. Decreased mRNA and protein expression of BDNF, NGF, and their receptors in the hippocampus from suicide: an analysis in human postmortem brain. Clin Med Insights Pathol. 2013;6:1–11.
9. Liu RT, Steele SJ, Hamilton JL, et al. Sleep and suicide: a systematic review and meta-analysis of longitudinal studies. Clin Psychol Rev. 2020;81:101895.
10. Fitzgerald PJ, Watson BO. Gamma oscillations as a biomarker for major depression: an emerging topic. Transl Psychiatry. 2018;8(1):177.
11. Arikan MK, Gunver MG, Tarhan N, et al. High-gamma: a biological marker for suicide attempt in patients with depression. J Affect Disord. 2019;254:1–6.
12. Puig MV, Watakabe A, Ushimaru M, et al. Serotonin modulates fast-spiking interneuron and synchronous activity in the rat prefrontal cortex through 5-HT1A and 5-HT2A receptors. J Neurosci. 2010;30(6):2211–22.
13. Ferando I, Mody I. Altered gamma oscillations during pregnancy through loss of delta subunit-containing GABA(a) receptors on parvalbumin interneurons. Front Neural Circuits. 2013;7:144.
14. Lee SM, Jang KI, Chae JH. Electroencephalographic correlates of suicidal ideation in the Theta band. Clin EEG Neurosci. 2017;48(5):316–21.
15. Hunter AM, Leuchter AF, Cook IA, et al. Brain functional changes (QEEG cordance) and worsening suicidal ideation and mood symptoms during antidepressant treatment. Acta Psychiatr Scand. 2010;122(6):461–9.
16. Fleischmann A, De Leo D. The World Health Organization's report on suicide: a fundamental step in worldwide suicide prevention. Crisis. 2014;35(5):289–91.
17. Cratsley K, Mackey TK. Health policy brief: global mental health and the United Nations' sustainable development goals. Fam Syst Health. 2018;36(2):225–9.
18. Rodrigues CD, de Souza DS, Rodrigues HM, et al. Trends in suicide rates in Brazil from 1997 to 2015. Braz J Psychiatry. 2019;41(5):380–8.
19. Thomas SP. World health assembly adopts comprehensive mental health action plan for 2013–2020. Issues Ment Health Nurs. 2013;34(10):723–4.
20. Lopez-Castroman J, Jaussent I. Sleep disturbances and suicidal behavior. Curr Top Behav Neurosci. 2020;46:211–28.
21. Drapeau CW, Nadorff MR. Suicidality in sleep disorders: prevalence, impact, and management strategies. Nat Sci Sleep. 2017;9:213–26.
22. Winsler A, Deutsch A, Vorona RD, et al. Sleepless in Fairfax: the difference one more hour of sleep can make for teen hopelessness, suicidal ideation, and substance use. J Youth Adolesc. 2015;44(2):362–78.
23. Alexopoulos GS, Meyers BS, Young RC, et al. 'Vascular depression' hypothesis. Arch Gen Psychiatry. 1997;54(10):915–22.
24. Pompili M, Innamorati M, Mann JJ, et al. Periventricular white matter hyperintensities as predictors of suicide attempts in bipolar disorders and

unipolar depression. Prog Neuro-Psychopharmacol Biol Psychiatry. 2008;32(6):1501–7.
25. Cyprien F, Courtet P, Malafosse A, et al. Suicidal behavior is associated with reduced corpus callosum area. Biol Psychiatry. 2011;70(4):320–6.
26. Bernert RA, Kim JS, Iwata NG, et al. Sleep disturbances as an evidence-based suicide risk factor. Curr Psychiatry Rep. 2015;17(3):554.
27. Goldschmied JR, Cheng P, Armitage R, et al. Examining the effects of sleep delay on depressed males and females and healthy controls. J Sleep Res. 2014;23(6):664–72.
28. Bernert RA, Luckenbaugh DA, Duncan WC, et al. Sleep architecture parameters as a putative biomarker of suicidal ideation in treatment-resistant depression. J Affect Disord. 2017;208:309–15.
29. Sabo E, Reynolds CR, Kupfer DJ, et al. Sleep, depression, and suicide. Psychiatry Res. 1991;36(3):265–77.
30. Boafo A, Armitage R, Greenham S, et al. Sleep architecture in adolescents hospitalized during a suicidal crisis. Sleep Med. 2019;56:41–6.
31. Terzano MG, Parrino L, Spaggiari MC, et al. CAP variables and arousals as sleep electroencephalogram markers for primary insomnia. Clin Neurophysiol. 2003;114(9):1715–23.
32. McCall WV, Benca RM, Rumble ME, et al. Prevalence of obstructive sleep apnea in suicidal patients with major depressive disorder. J Psychiatr Res. 2019;116:147–50.
33. Mellem MS, Liu Y, Gonzalez H, et al. Machine learning models identify multimodal measurements highly predictive of Transdiagnostic symptom severity for mood, anhedonia, and anxiety. Biol Psychiatry Cogn Neurosci Neuroimaging. 2020;5(1):56–67.
34. Kaufman KR, Struck PJ. Psychogenic nonepileptic seizures and suicidal behavior on a video/EEG telemetry unit: the need for psychiatric assessment and screening for suicide risk. Epilepsy Behav. 2010;19(4):656–9.
35. van der Vinne N, Vollebregt MA, van Putten M, et al. Frontal alpha asymmetry as a diagnostic marker in depression: fact or fiction? A meta-analysis. Neuroimage Clin. 2017;16:79–87.
36. Dolsen MR, Cheng P, Arnedt JT, et al. Neurophysiological correlates of suicidal ideation in major depressive disorder: hyperarousal during sleep. J Affect Disord. 2017;212:160–6.
37. Liu M, Zhou L, Wang X, et al. Deficient manipulation of working memory in remitted depressed individuals: behavioral and electrophysiological evidence. Clin Neurophysiol. 2017;128(7):1206–13.
38. Park Y, Jung W, Kim S, et al. Frontal alpha asymmetry correlates with suicidal behavior in major depressive disorder. Clin Psychopharmacol Neurosci. 2019;17(3):377–87.
39. Dominguez-Rodriguez A, Chavez-Valdez SM, Avitia GC, et al. Unified protocol for anxiety disorders in two cities of Mexico measuring gamma activity: study protocol for a randomized controlled trial. Contemp Clin Trials Commun. 2020;18:100556.
40. Koshiyama D, Kirihara K, Usui K, et al. Resting-state EEG beta band power predicts quality of life outcomes in patients with depressive disorders: a longitudinal investigation. J Affect Disord. 2020;265:416–22.
41. Tsypes A, Owens M, Gibb BE. Reward responsiveness in suicide attempters: an electroencephalography/event-related potential study. Biol Psychiatry Cogn Neurosci Neuroimaging. 2020;6(1):99–106.
42. Busch KA, Fawcett J, Jacobs DG. Clinical correlates of inpatient suicide. J Clin Psychiatry. 2003;64(1):14–9.
43. Matthew L, Muthusamy K, Nicholas M, et al. Meta-analysis of longitudinal cohort studies of suicide risk assessment among psychiatric patients: heterogeneity in results and lack of improvement over time. PLoS One. 2016;11(6):e0156322.
44. Chan MKY, Bhatti H, Meader N, et al. Predicting suicide following self-harm: systematic review of risk factors and risk scales. Br J Psychiatry. 2016;209(4):277–83.
45. Graney J, Hunt IM, Quinlivan L, et al. Suicide risk assessment in UK mental health services: a national mixed-methods study. Lancet Psychiatry. 2020;7(12):1046–53.
46. Hegedus KM, Szkaliczki A, Gal BI, et al. Decision-making performance of depressed patients within 72 h following a suicide attempt. J Affect Disord. 2018;235:583–8.
47. Ponsoni A, Branco LD, Cotrena C, et al. Self-reported inhibition predicts history of suicide attempts in bipolar disorder and major depression. Compr Psychiatry. 2018;82:89–94.
48. Pustilnik A, Elkana O, Vatine JJ, et al. Neuropsychological markers of suicidal risk in the context of medical rehabilitation. Arch Suicide Res. 2017;21(2):293–306.
49. Hausman C, Meffert BN, Mosich MK, et al. Impulsivity and cognitive flexibility as neuropsychological markers for suicidality: a multi-modal investigation among military veterans with alcohol use disorder and PTSD. Arch Suicide Res. 2020;24(3):313–26.
50. Vilma L, Naomi AF, Aurelija P, et al. Neurocognitive markers of suicidal ideation in patients with anxiety and mood disorders. Int J Psychiatry Clin Pract. 2020;24(2):116–9.
51. Richard-Devantoy S, Ding Y, Turecki G, et al. Attentional bias toward suicide-relevant information in suicide attempters: a cross-sectional study and a meta-analysis. J Affect Disord. 2016;196:101–8.
52. Keilp JG, Beers SR, Burke AK, et al. Neuropsychological deficits in past suicide attempters with varying levels of depression severity. Psychol Med. 2014;44(14):2965–74.
53. Stewart JG, Glenn CR, Esposito EC, et al. Cognitive control deficits differentiate adolescent suicide Ideators from attempters. J Clin Psychiatry. 2017;78(6):e614–21.
54. Lianne S, Anne-Laura VH, Vasiliki C, et al. Imaging suicidal thoughts and behaviors: a comprehensive

review of 2 decades of neuroimaging studies. Mol Psychiatry. 2020;25(2):1–20.
55. Bijttebier S, Caeyenberghs K, van den Ameele H, et al. The vulnerability to suicidal behavior is associated with reduced connectivity strength. Front Hum Neurosci. 2015;9:632.
56. Mark DU, Victoria A. Evidence for neurodegeneration and neuroplasticity as part of the neurobiology of suicide. Biol Psychiatry. 2011;70(4):306–7.
57. Zheng W, Guang Y, Xianyun T. Exploring behavior of people with suicidal ideation in a Chinese Online Suicidal Community. Int J Environ Res Public Health. 2018;16(1):54.
58. Roy A, Nikolitch K, McGinn R, et al. A machine learning approach predicts future risk to suicidal ideation from social media data. NPJ Digit Med. 2020;3:78.
59. Zhang J, Shen Y, He G, et al. Lack of association between three serotonin genes and suicidal behavior in Chinese psychiatric patients. Prog Neuro-Psychopharmacol Biol Psychiatry. 2008;32(2):467.
60. Hung CF, Lung FW, Hung TH, et al. Monoamine oxidase A gene polymorphism and suicide: an association study and meta-analysis. J Affect Disord. 2012;136(3):643–9.
61. Clayden RC, Zaruk A, Meyre D, et al. The association of attempted suicide with genetic variants in the SLC6A4 and TPH genes depends on the definition of suicidal behavior: a systematic review and meta-analysis. Transl Psychiatry. 2012;2:e166.

# Application of Multimodal EEG in the Determination of Brain Death

# 15

Feng Li

## Contents



**Abstract**

Clinically, if a brain dead patient uses a life support system, the patient can typically be maintained for a few days or even a few months until the heart stops naturally. However, this consumes considerable manpower and material resources, causing serious economic and psychological burdens on the patient's family and simultaneously wasting social resources. However, if you consider removing the support system, the key issue to be solved is still ensuring that the diagnosis of brain death is accurate. Accurately determining whether a patient has experienced brain death at an early stage is a thorny issue in clinical work. The determination of brain death is a serious process, and its legislation involves many fields, such as morality, ethics, religion, and law. Reliable diagnostic criteria for brain death are not only conducive to scientifically determining the death of a person, maintain-

F. Li (✉)
Department of Neurology, The First Affiliated Hospital of Chongqing Medical University, Chongqing, China



X. Wang et al. (eds.), *Multi-Modal EEG Monitoring of Severely Neurologically Ill Patients*,
https://doi.org/10.1007/978-981-16-4493-1_15

ing the dignity of the deceased, saving health and medical resources, and reducing the burden on the family, but also for providing better donors for organ transplantation and bringing the hope of survival to more patients to save the lives and health of more people. This chapter briefly describes the concept and related history of brain death, combined with legends, and elaborates on the Chinese brain death criteria and specific steps, including the specific content and determination methods of clinical determination, confirmation test, and spontaneous breathing provocation test, as well as the relevant content determination steps. Frequency is described to help medical workers understand brain death determination and provide guarantee for their clinical decision-making and the successful implementation of organ transplantation.

**Keywords**

Brain death · Spontaneous breathing challenge test · Brainstem reflex · EEG SLSEP · TCD

Neurologically severe patients often experience severe brain damage due to cerebrovascular disease, craniocerebral injury, intracranial infection, SE, and cardiac arrest. After brain injury, due to the combination of various mechanisms, such as neuroinflammation, oxidative stress, and the toxic effect of glutamate excitatory transmitters, blood–brain barrier damage, microvascular failure, and brain edema can be aggravated, which directly leads to neuronal cell death, thereby leading to secondary brain damage. This secondary brain damage is an important mechanism for the deterioration of the condition of neurologically severe patients and even brain death in the late stage [1, 2].

The concept of "brain death" first came into being in France. In 1959, French scholars Mollaret and Goulon first proposed the concept of "irreversible coma" at the 23rd International Congress of Neurology and at the same time reported 23 cases of this pathological state and used the term "CNS death." Their report suggests that all patients who are diagnosed with "irreversible coma" have almost zero chance of waking up. The medical profession accepted and approved this formulation. On this basis, the concept of brain death began to sprout, and clinicians began to doubt the traditional death standards. In 1966, the USA proposed that brain death is a sign of clinical death. In 1968, at the 22nd World Medical Congress, the Special Committee for the Review of the Definition of Brain Death at Harvard Medical School proposed the concept of an "irreversible loss of brain function" as a new death standard and formulated the world's first brain death standard [3, 4]. Recent standards [5] indicate that brain death refers to the irreversible loss of whole brain function, including brainstem function. With the accumulation of global brain death diagnostic practice experience and further research, China drafted the "Brain Death Judgment Criteria and Technical Specifications" (adult quality control version) in 2015. In 2019, this version was revised, and the judgment criteria and processes are outlined here [6].

## 15.1 Prerequisites for Judgment

### 15.1.1 The Cause of the Coma Is Clear

Primary brain injuries that lead to coma include craniocerebral trauma and cerebrovascular disease. Secondary brain injuries that lead to coma are mainly hypoxic encephalopathy caused by cardiac arrest, anesthesia accidents, drowning, and suffocation. If the cause of the coma is not clear, brain death judgment cannot be implemented [7].

### 15.1.2 The Exclusion of Various Causes of Reversible Coma

Cause of reversible coma includes acute poisoning, such as carbon monoxide poisoning, alcohol poisoning, sedative and hypnotic poisoning, narcotic poisoning, antipsychotic poisoning, and muscle relaxant poisoning; low temperature (bladder temperature or rectal temperature ≤32 °C); severe electrolyte and acid–base balance disorder; and severe metabolic and endocrine dysfunction, such as hepatic encephalopathy, uremic encephalopathy, hypoglycemia, or hyperglycemia encephalopathy [8].

## 15.2 Clinical Judgment

### 15.2.1 Deep Coma

**Inspection Method and Result Judgment** In patients in a deep coma, when the thumbs are strongly pressed against the supraorbital notch on both sides of the subject or the face is needled, there is no facial muscle activity. In addition, the GCS score is 2T points (exercise = 1 point, eyes open = 1 point, language = T). The inspection results need to be confirmed repeatedly.

**Notes** (a) Any stimulation must be limited to the head and face; (b) in cases of neuropathy of the trigeminal nerve or facial nerve, the judgment of deep coma should be made with caution; and (c) spinal reflexes can be caused by stimulation below the neck. The spinal cord may survive brain death; therefore, there may still be spinal reflexes and/or spinal autoreflexes. No spontaneous movement of the limbs will be observed in patients with brain death; (d) no decerebrated rigidity, decorticated rigidity, or spasticity will be observed in patients with brain death [7].

### 15.2.2 All Brainstem Reflexes Disappeared [8]

(a) Pupil reflex; (b) corneal reflex; (c) head–eye reflex; (d) vestibular reflex; and (e) cough reflex.

If all the above five brainstem reflexes disappear, brainstem function can be considered to have disappeared, but this needs to be checked repeatedly. If one or more of the five brainstem reflexes cannot be determined, examinations for those that can be determined should be repeated at least 2 times (with an interval of 5 min), and confirmation test items should be added.

### 15.2.3 No Spontaneous Breathing

In patients with no spontaneous breathing, the patient does not breathe spontaneously and must rely on a ventilator to maintain breathing. This also needs to be verified by the spontaneous breathing provocation test, and the following steps and methods should be strictly followed to determine that there is no spontaneous breathing [7, 8].

**Prerequisites for the Test** (a) Core body temperature ≥36.5 °C; if lower than this standard, the body can be healed physically; (b) systolic blood pressure (SBP) ≥90 mmHg (1 mmHg = 0.133 kPa) or mean arterial pressure (MAP) ≥60 mmHg; if lower than this standard, hypertensive drugs can be given; (c) arterial partial pressure of oxygen (PaO2) ≥200 mmHg; if lower than this standard, 100% oxygen can be provided for 10–15 min to achieve PaO2 ≥ 200 mmHg; and (d) PaCO2 35–45 mmHg; if lower than this standard, the ventilation per minute can be reduced. For patients with chronic carbon dioxide retention, PaCO2 should be >45 mmHg. Before the spontaneous breathing provocation test is implemented, life support and organ function support should be strengthened.

**Test Methods and Procedures** (a) Draw arterial blood to detect PaCO2; (b) remove the ventilator; (c) immediately place the oxygen catheter through the artificial airway at the carina level, and input 100% oxygen at 6 L/min; (d) closely observe the patient to see whether there is breathing movement in the chest and/or abdomen; (e) 8–10 min after the ventilator is removed, draw arterial blood again to test PaCO2; and (f) resume mechanical ventilation.

**Test Result Judgment** If the prerequisite PaCO2 is 35–45 mmHg, the test result shows that

$PaCO_2 \geq 60$ mmHg or $PaCO_2$ exceeds the original level of 20 mmHg, and there is no breathing movement, and it can be judged that there is no spontaneous breathing. If the prerequisite $PaCO_2$ is >45 mmHg, the test results show that $PaCO_2$ exceeds the original level by 20 mmHg and there is no breathing movement, it can be judged that there is no spontaneous breathing.

**Notes** (a) During the spontaneous breathing provocation test, if there is a significant drop in blood oxygen saturation or blood pressure, heart rate slows, or arrhythmia is observed, the test should be terminated immediately. At this time, if $PaCO_2$ rises to meet the judgment requirements, the result judgment can still be made. If the increase in $PaCO_2$ does not meet the criteria, the test should be declared a failure. To avoid the spontaneous breathing provocation test influencing the confirmation test, it can be placed in the final step of brain death judgment. (b) At least 2 doctors (one doctor is responsible for monitoring breathing, heart rate, blood pressure, and oxygen saturation, and the other doctor is responsible for observing whether there is breathing movement in the chest and/or abdomen) and one doctor or nurse (responsible for managing the breathing machine, oxygen catheterization, and drawing arterial blood) are needed.

All the above three clinical criteria must be met.

## 15.3 Confirmation Tests

### 15.3.1 EEG

In patients with brain death, the EEG shows electrical resting activity at the standard parameter setting requirements (such as impedance <5 kΩ and sensitivity 2 μV/mm) in all leads (at least 8) for 30 min, with an average amplitude ≤2 μV and no response to stimulation (Fig. 15.1). EEG is relatively safe for monitoring the electrophysiology of the cerebral cortex in patients with deep coma. With the development of science and technology, various portable EEG instruments provide conditions for the monitoring of brain death. In the observation of patients with brain death by Vicenzini et al. [9] compared with CBF assessment, cerebrovascular angiography, or even TCD monitoring, EEG can confirm brain death by first monitoring equipotential EEGs, which shortens the diagnosis time.

### 15.3.2 SLSEP Monitoring

SLSEPs refer to the electrical responses of the somatosensory system (peripheral nerve containing sensory fibers or sensory nerve conduction pathway) that can be detected in a short period of time when receiving appropriate stimulation. Obtained by computer technology superposition and extraction, SEP waveforms have a time-dependent relationship with stimuli. The waveform is stable if the stimulus type and intensity remain unchanged, and SEP monitoring has the advantages of objective, sensitive, safe, noninvasive, repeatable, and bedside operation, making it especially suitable for assessing the brain function of critically ill patients. SLSEP monitoring began to be used in the determination of brain death in 1980 [10]. To date, many studies have confirmed the existence of bilateral SLSEPs N9 and/or N13 in the median nerve and the disappearance of P14, N18, and N20 [11–13] (Fig. 15.2a–c). The sensitivity of SLSEP monitoring for judging brain death is as high as 100%, the specificity is 78–100% [11, 14], and the results are not affected by anesthetics.

### 15.3.3 TCD Monitoring

TCD monitoring directly determines whether there is cerebral circulatory arrest, and TCD monitoring has high sensitivity and specificity for the determination of brain death. Because of its advantages, such as being noninvasive, economical, rapid, reproducible, and unaffected by drugs, and because it can be carried out at the bedside, TCD monitoring has been used in con-

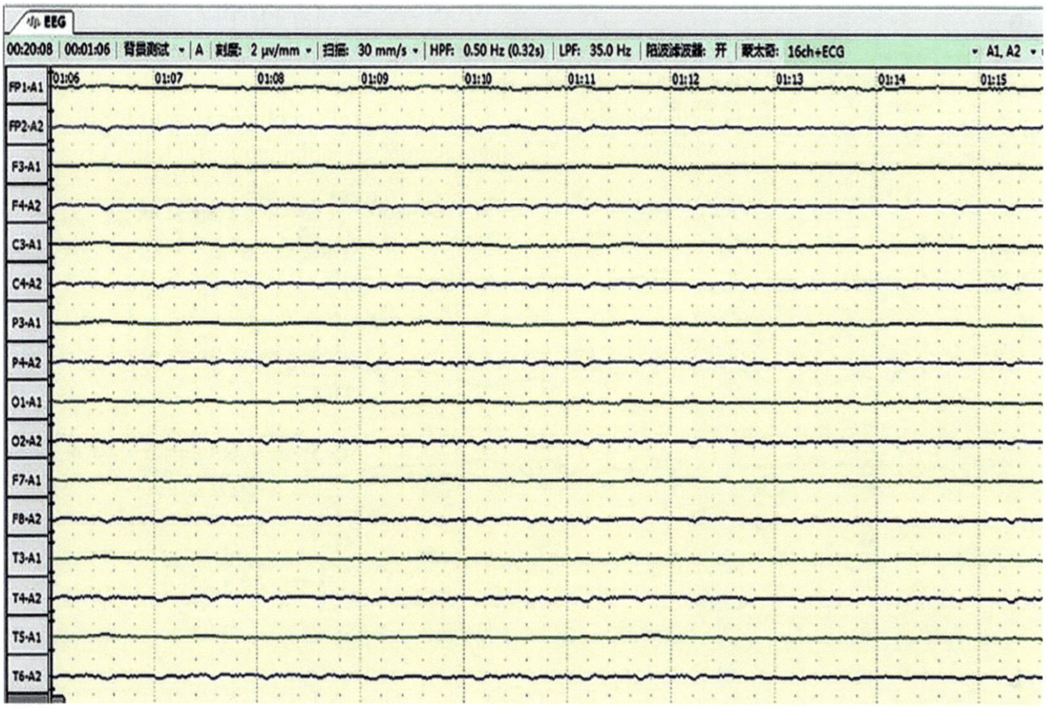


**Fig. 15.1** EEG, showing that electrical activity at all leads is at rest (brainwave activity ≤2 μV), which meets the criteria for determining brain death by EEG

firmation tests for brain death judgment in various countries around the world. TCD monitoring of patients with brain death shows oscillating waves for the blood flow in the anterior and posterior circulation of the brain, sharp systolic waves, or the disappearance of blood flow signals (Fig. 15.3a–c). Brunser et al. [15] showed that the sensitivity, specificity, and positive and negative rates of TCD monitoring in the diagnosis of brain death reached 100%, 96%, 96.1%, and 100%, respectively, confirming the role of TCD monitoring in the diagnosis of brain death.

### 15.3.4 Order of Confirmation Tests

The preferred order for confirmation test items is EEG, SLSEP monitoring, and TCD monitoring. The results of at least two confirmation tests must meet the criteria for brain death. If EEG or SLSEP monitoring is combined with TCD monitoring, the false-positive rate of judgment can be reduced, and the consistency of judgment can be improved. If TCD monitoring is not possible, clinicians can refer to the results of computed tomography angiography (CTA) or digital subtraction angiography (DSA).

## 15.4 Judgment Steps

The judgment of brain death is divided into the following 3 steps: *Step 1* is the clinical judgment of brain death. If the criteria of clinical judgment are met (deep coma, a loss of brainstem reflexes, no spontaneous breathing), the clinician can proceed with the next judgment step. *Step 2* is to carry out the brain death confirmation tests, and when the brain death criteria are met in at least two of the items, the clinician can proceed with the next judgment step. In *step 3*, the spontaneous breathing provocation test is performed to verify that there is no spontaneous breathing.

a

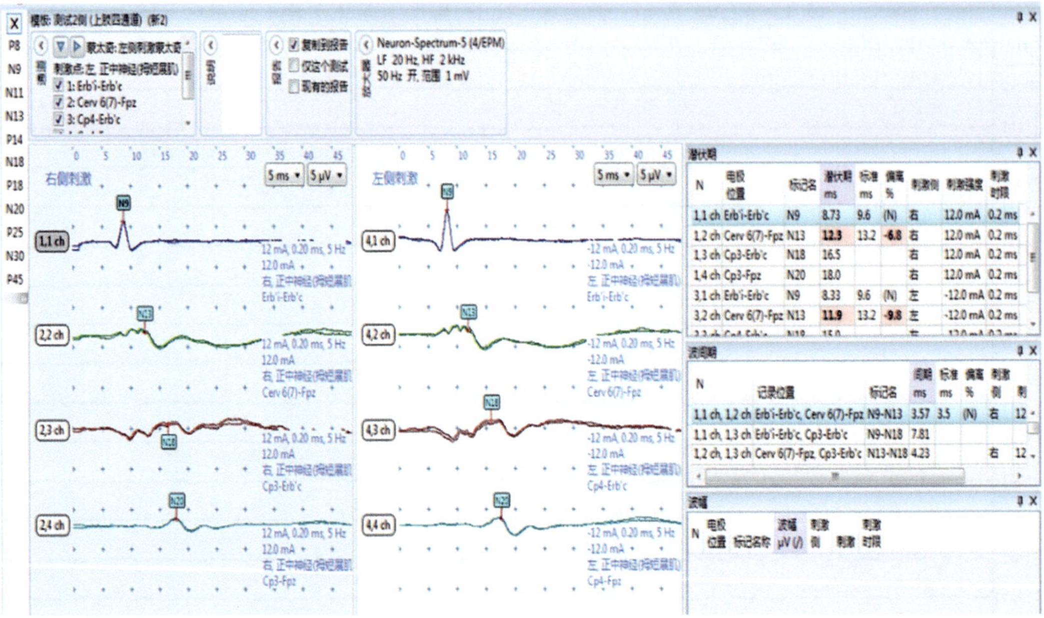

b

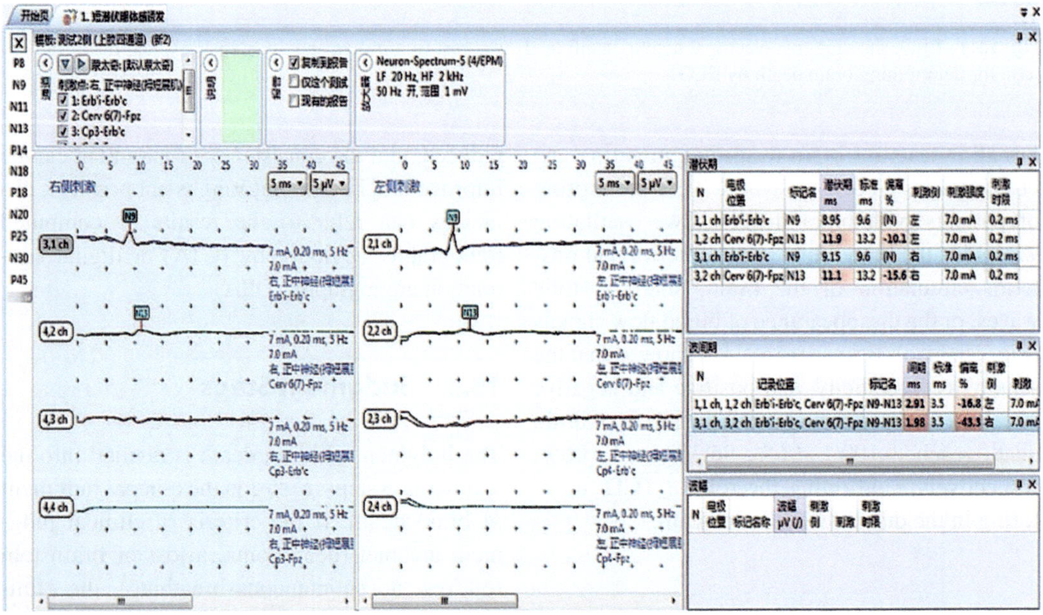

**Fig. 15.2** (**a–c**) The SLSEPs of the median nerve. (**a**) Normal SLSEP; (**b** and **c**) N9 and N13 are present on both sides, and P14, N18, and N20 are absent on both sides, which meets the criteria for SLSEP-determined brain death

c

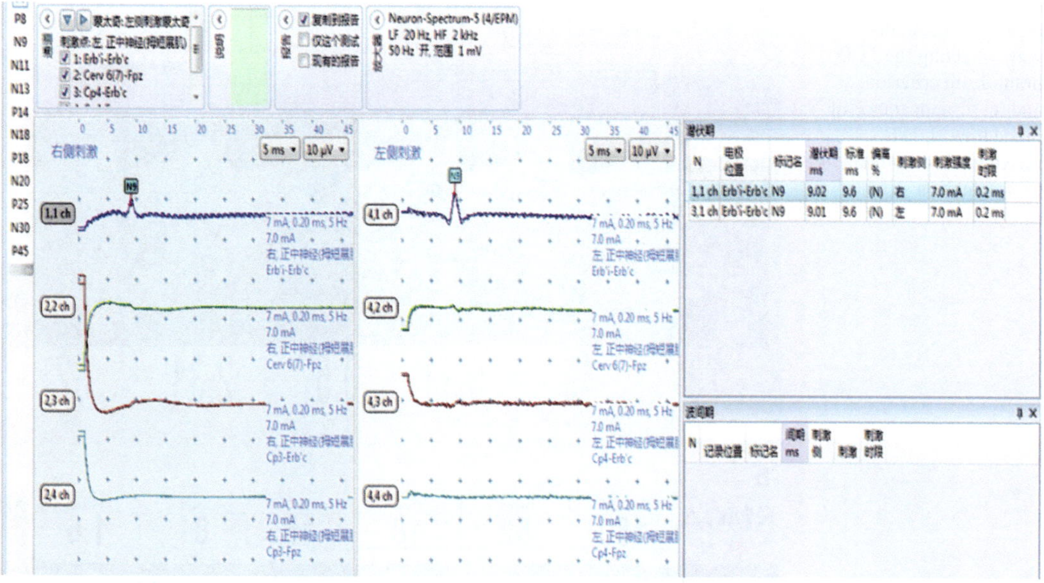

**Fig. 15.2** (continued)

## 15.5 Judgment Times

Brain death can be judged on the premise that the prerequisites for the determination of brain death are met, the three clinical judgments and two confirmation tests are complete and the results are unequivocal, and all brain death judgment standards are met. If a clinical judgment step cannot be performed or a result is in doubt, another confirmation test item can be added (three items in total), and brain death can be judged again 6 h after the first judgment (at least one spontaneous breathing provocation test should be conducted and the results should confirm there is no spontaneous breathing). If the results of the re-judgment meet the criteria for brain death, then brain death can be confirmed (Fig. 15.4).

### Case

The patient was admitted to the hospital on 2018.03.01, because of "headache for 1 month, lack of speech for 5 h, and a disturbance of consciousness for 2+ h". She was diagnosed with "miliaris phthisis" 3+ months prior and was hospitalized with isoniazid, rifampicin, ethambutol, and pyrazinamide (HREZ) quadruple anti-tuberculosis treatment in the Department of Pulmonary and Infectious Diseases of our hospital. 1+ month prior, labor was induced at 16 weeks of pregnancy. Admission diagnosis was tuberculous meningoencephalitis. The patient was resistant to multiple tuberculosis drugs, and the treatment effect was poor. She had been hospitalized for 3+ months and had complained of headaches. Lumbar puncture and CBF examination did not indicate improvement. Because of the worsening of headaches, she had transient consciousness disturbance and was transferred to the ICU twice.

At 13:54 on 2018.08.27, the patient responded suddenly and did not breathe spontaneously. The patient was given airbag-assisted breathing, prepared for intubation, and given mannitol and furosemide for dehydration to lower ICP. At 13:59, the patient's heartbeat slowed to a stop, his pupils dilated, and the light reflex disappeared. CPR was immediately followed by atropine and epinephrine intravenous injections. The heart rate recovered at 14:00. The blood pressure dropped to 68/40 mmHg at 14:02. Dopamine was pushed.

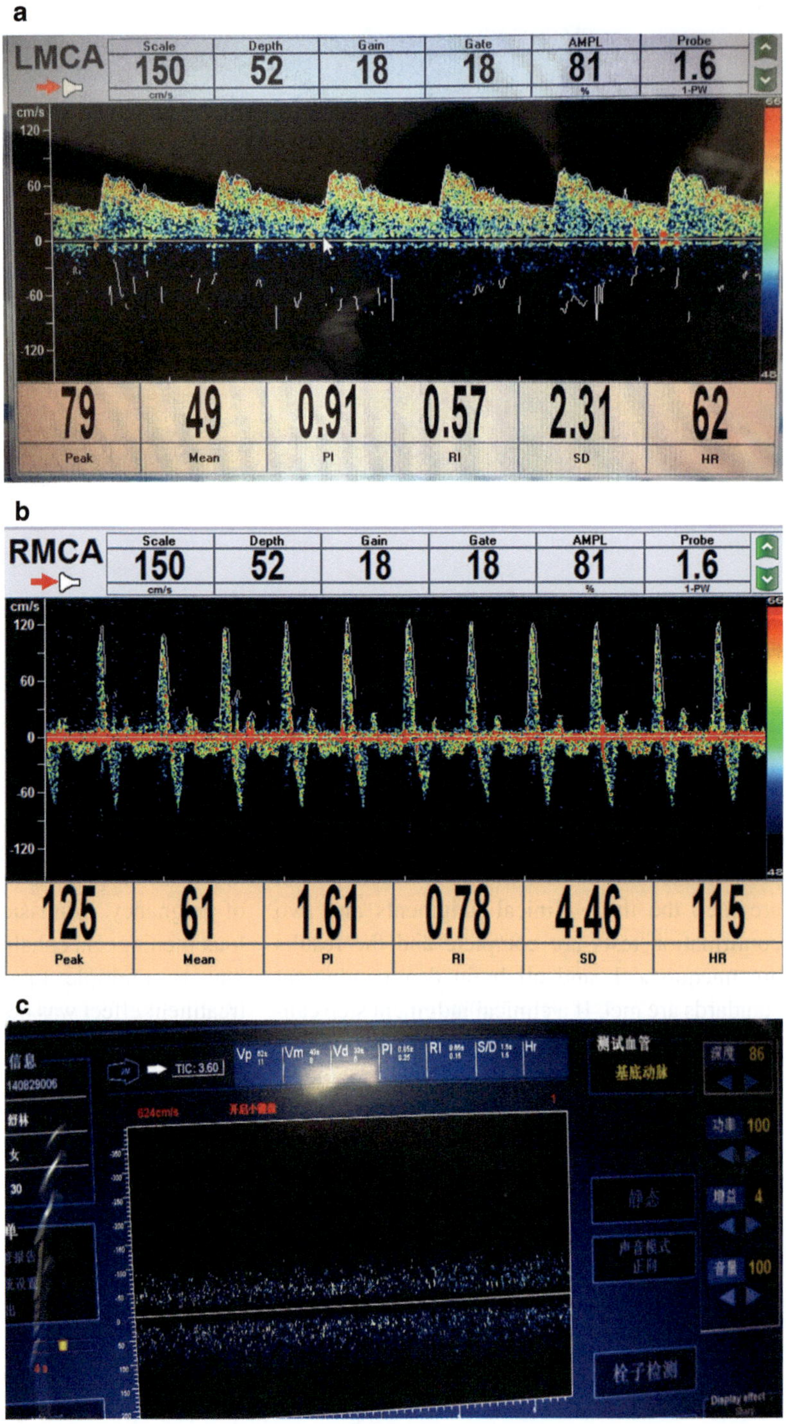


**Fig. 15.3** (**a**–**c**) TCD. (**a**) Normal blood flow signal; (**b**) oscillatory wave, meeting the TCD brain-death criterion; and (**c**) disappearance of blood flow signals, meeting the TCD brain death criterion

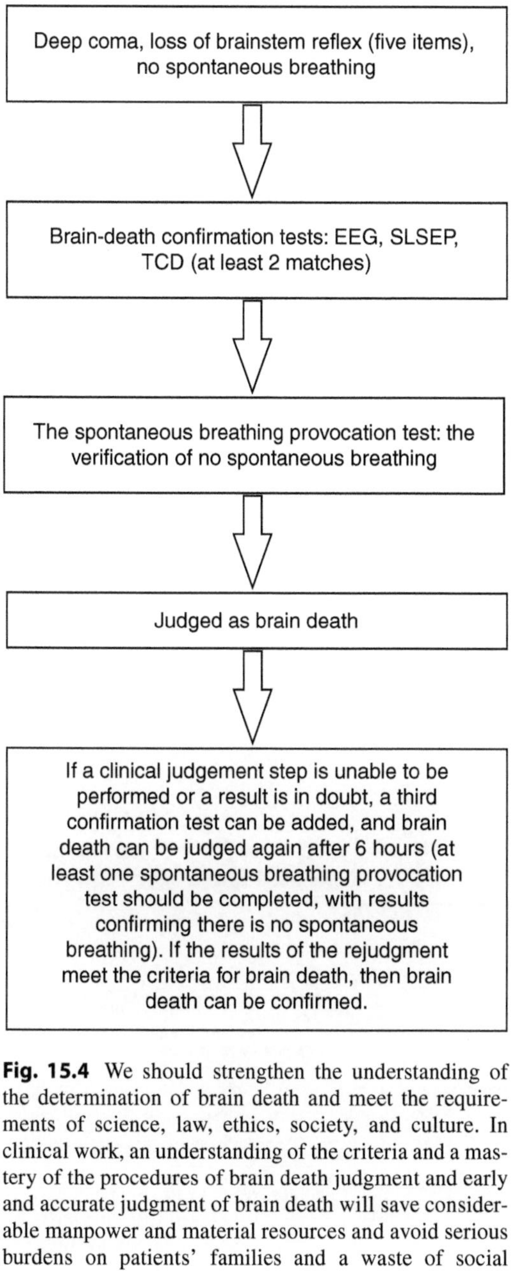


**Fig. 15.4** We should strengthen the understanding of the determination of brain death and meet the requirements of science, law, ethics, society, and culture. In clinical work, an understanding of the criteria and a mastery of the procedures of brain death judgment and early and accurate judgment of brain death will save considerable manpower and material resources and avoid serious burdens on patients' families and a waste of social resources

Tracheal intubation was performed at 14:05, the heartbeat stopped at 14:10, and atropine static push was administered. Heart rate recovered at 14:12, and the patient was transferred to the ICU at 14:15. After the transfer, the patient was in a deep coma, his pupils were dilated by 6 mm, and the light reflex had disappeared. Active dehydration was given to lower ICP, ventilator-assisted ventilation was provided, and dopamine was administered to maintain blood pressure.

The patient was diagnosed with brain death through assessment, and the judgment process was as follows:

1. *Clinical assessment*: (a) Deep coma GCS: 2T points; (b) brainstem reflexes: Both pupils were 6 mm in diameter, and the pupils' light reflex, corneal reflex, head–eye reflex, vestibular reflex, and cough reflex had disappeared.
2. *Confirmation tests*: (a) EEG: In continuous recording for more than 30 min, the EEG was in an electrical resting state at 2 μV/mm, and there was no obvious response to sound, light, or pain stimulation in the EEG (Fig. 15.5); (b) EP: N9 is seen in the bilateral median nerve SEP, and N13, P14, N18 and N20 are absent on both sides (Fig. 15.6).
3. *Spontaneous breathing confirmation test*: The preliminary PaCO2 was 41 mmHg. Eight to ten minutes after the ventilator was removed, the PaCO2 was ≥60 mmHg, and no breathing movement was observed. Therefore, the patient was determined to have no spontaneous breathing. Blood gas analysis before ventilator removal was as follow: pH: 7.36, PaCO2: 41 mmHg, and PaO2: 503 mmHg. Blood gas analysis 8–10 min after ventilator removal was as follow: pH: 7.07, PaCO2: 87 mmHg, and PaO2: 316 mmHg.

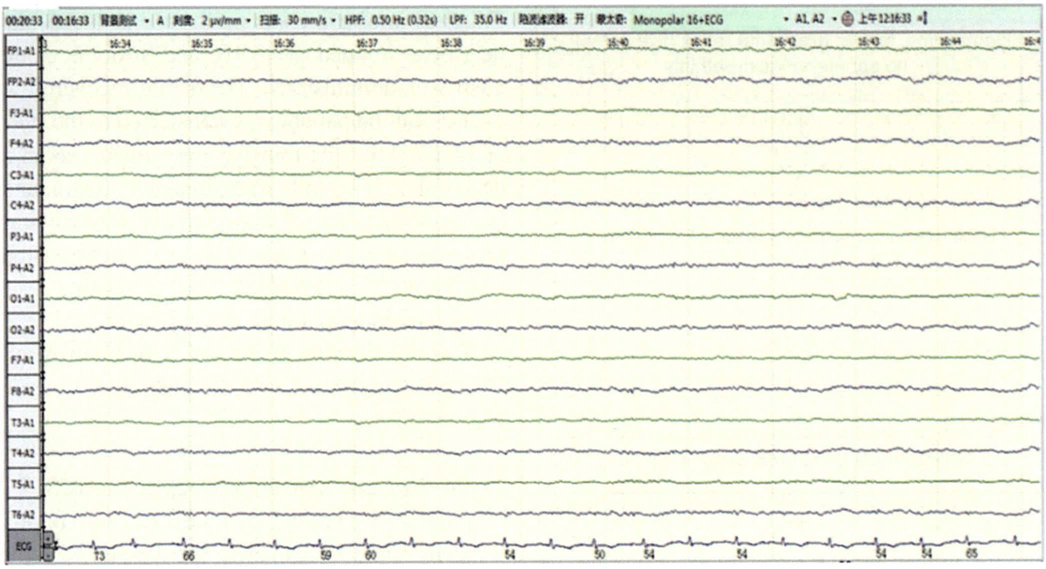


**Fig. 15.5** EEG showed an electrical resting state

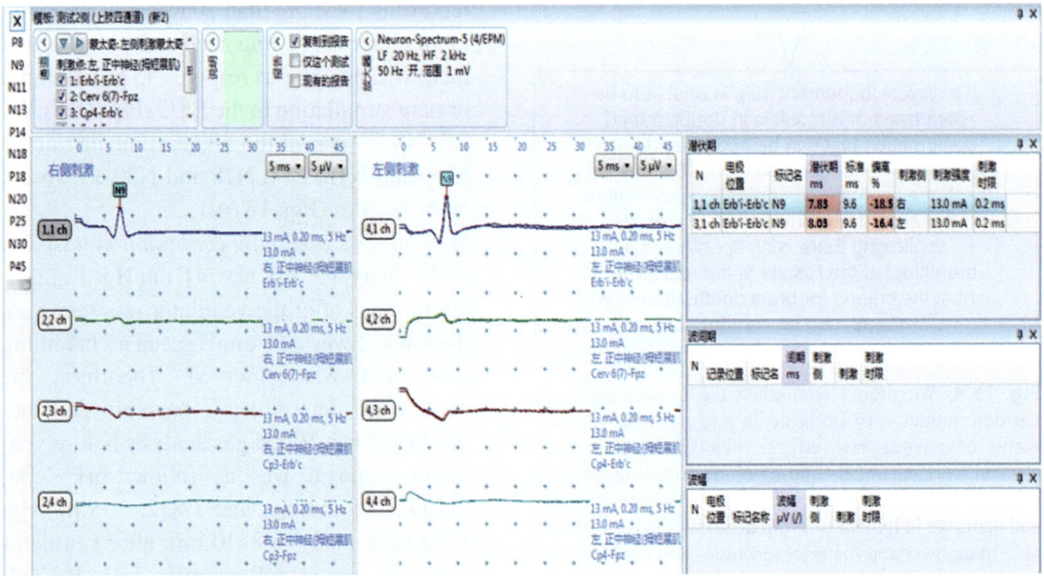


**Fig. 15.6** EP: N9 is seen in the bilateral median nerve SEP, and N13, P14, N18, and N20 are absent on both sides

## References


1. Lauritzen M, Dreier JP, Fabricius M, et al. Clinical relevance of cortical spreading depression in neurological disorders: migraine, malignant stroke, subarachnoid and intracranial hemorrhage, and traumatic brain injury. J Cereb Blood Flow Metab. 2011;31(1):17–35.
2. Reithmeier T, Isaak R, Sanchez-Porres R. [Multimodal Neuromonitoring and its impact on therapeutic and diagnostic decisions in critical ill patients]. Anasthesiol Intensivmed Notfallmed Schmerzther. 2018;53(10):682–95.
3. Paqueron A. A definition of irreversible coma. Report of the Ad Hoc Committee of the Harvard Medical School to Examine the Definition of Brain Death. JAMA. 1968;205(6):337–40.

4. Citerio G, Murphy PG. Brain death: the European perspective. Semin Neurol. 2015;35(2):139–44.
5. Aboubakr M, Alameda G. Brain death criteria. 2021.
6. Brain Injury Evaluation Quality Control Center of National Health Commission. Criteria and practical guidance for determination of brain death in adults (2nd edition). Chin Med J (Engl). 2019;132(3):329–35.
7. Su Y, Yang Q, Liu G, et al. Diagnosis of brain death: confirmatory tests after clinical test. Chin Med J. 2014;127(7):1272–7.
8. Su YY, Zhao H, Zhang Y, et al. [Studies on evaluation of brain death]. Zhonghua Nei Ke Za Zhi. 2004;43(4):250–3.
9. Vicenzini E, Pro S, Pulitano P, et al. Current practice of brain death determination and use of confirmatory tests in an Italian university hospital: a report of 66 cases. Minerva Anestesiol. 2013;79(5):485–91.
10. Anziska BJ, Cracco RQ. Short latency somatosensory evoked potentials in brain dead patients. Arch Neurol. 1980;37(4):222–5.
11. Facco E, Munari M, Gallo F, et al. Role of short latency evoked potentials in the diagnosis of brain death. Clin Neurophysiol. 2002;113(11):1855–66.
12. Sonoo M, Tsai-Shozawa Y, Aoki M, et al. N18 in median somatosensory evoked potentials: a new indicator of medullary function useful for the diagnosis of brain death. J Neurol Neurosurg Psychiatry. 1999;67(3):374–8.
13. Wagner W. Scalp, earlobe and nasopharyngeal recordings of the median nerve somatosensory evoked P14 potential in coma and brain death. Detailed latency and amplitude analysis in 181 patients. Brain. 1996;119(Pt 5):1507–21.
14. Machado C, Valdes P, Garcia O, et al. Short latency somatosensory evoked potentials in brain-dead patients using restricted low cut filter setting. J Neurosurg Sci. 1993;37(3):133–40.
15. Brunser A, Hoppe A, Carcamo DA, et al. [Validation of transcranial Doppler in the diagnosis of brain death]. Rev Med Chil. 2010;138(4):406–12.

# Application of the BIS in the ICU

# 16

Suyue Pan and Yongming Wu

## Contents



**Abstract**

With the continuous development of modern medical technology and the increasing demand of patients, most critically ill patients need anesthesia, sedation, and analgesia due to disease or treatment. At the same time, issues such as medical ethics and disease treatment costs have become increasingly prominent. Accurate and effective monitoring of patient awareness can provide important information for clinical intervention and prognostic judgment, assisting ICU clinicians in optimizing clinical intervention strategies. This not only helps to improve the patient's medical treatment experience but also reduces unnecessary medical burden and economic costs. The BIS index is a quantitative value obtained after data processing and analysis of the original EEG signal. Because more original EEG information is integrated, its changes are related to the degree of oxygen consumption of cerebral cortex cells and the degree of brain cell damage. It can reflect the function of the cerebral cortex to further evaluate the degree of brain injury and its prognosis. It has the advantages of objectiveness, accuracy, noninvasiveness, and convenience and has good application prospects in the ICU. This chapter briefly describes the principle of BIS and related influencing factors, further introduces the correlation between BIS value and

S. Pan (✉) · Y. Wu
Department of Neurology, Nanfang Hospital of Southern Medical University, Guangzhou, Guangdong, China
e-mail: pansuyue@smu.edu.cn



X. Wang et al. (eds.), *Multi-Modal EEG Monitoring of Severely Neurologically Ill Patients*,
https://doi.org/10.1007/978-981-16-4493-1_16

clinical anesthetics, and focuses on the clinical application of BIS in the depth of sedation and analgesia monitoring in ICU patients to provide a new monitoring tool for critically ill patients. At the same time, we summarize the correlation between BIS and the degree of brain damage and prognosis in critically ill patients, which can provide new ideas for the early observation and prognostic judgment in critically ill patients.

**Keywords**

BIS · ICU · State of consciousness · Sedation · Analgesia · Anesthesia · Clinical application · Prognostic evaluation

In BIS monitoring, raw EEG signals are collected through a sensor placed on the forehead, and the spectrum, amplitude, rhythm, and other signals of the original EEG, including the energy spectrum and time domain, are analyzed. After processing, this information is fitted into a numerical value, from 0 to 100: 0 means the brain electrical activity in a resting state, and 100 means the brain is awake. BIS monitoring is mainly designed for anesthesia during various operations, reducing the amount of anesthesia, monitoring the depth of anesthesia, and reducing intraoperative awareness, and the BIS can be used to monitor the degree of sedation. The sedation range is generally 80–60 for light anesthesia, 60–40 for moderate anesthesia, 40 or less for deep anesthesia, approximately 20 for inhibition of brain electrical activity, and 0 for the resting state of brain electrical activity [1, 2] (Fig. 16.1).

## 16.1 Principle of BIS Monitoring

BIS monitoring was initially used for intraoperative anesthesia monitoring. Later, it was extended to ICU sedation monitoring. BIS monitoring means that a computer uses a bispectral analysis method (a statistical technique for studying nonlinear indicators) to convert the time and amplitude relationship of the original EEG signal into a frequency and power relationship. The dimensionless index is obtained by quantitative analysis and the calculation of the degree of coupling between phase and power. Because the BIS integrates the characteristics of frequency, power, phase, and harmonics in the EEG, it contains more original EEG information. There are 5 subparameters that affect the BIS value: the SQI, EMG, suppression ratio, SEF, and total power. When recording BIS data, data recording starts when SQI is ≥80% and EMG is <40. At this time, the data are less affected, and the signal quality is the best, which can improve reliability. The BIS can quickly reflect the functional status of the cerebral cortex, so it is considered to be the most sensitive and accurate objective indicator to assess the state of consciousness, including the depth of sedation [3, 4]. At present, there have been reports of BIS monitoring of the depth of anesthesia, ICU sedation evaluation, etc., as well as evaluation reports of brain function recovery in patients with acute brain injury and CPCR. This monitoring result has been confirmed by a large number of clinical studies to be the only clinically proven safe and effective monitoring index for the depth of consciousness [3].

## 16.2 Factors Influencing the BIS

The main factors affecting the BIS are as follows: (a) The most common is the EMG signal from the forehead. The EMG frequency (30–300 Hz) often overlaps with the EEG frequency. If a patient's EMG signal is 30–50 Hz, the BIS value will increase. The patient's activity, turning over, sputum suction, and physical therapy can increase myoelectric interference. In addition, as the depth of anesthesia increases, the myoelectric activity will decrease (Fig. 16.2); (b) the inhibition ratio mainly quantifies the percentage of time that the EEG of the last 1960s has equal potential, and the value is also between 0 and 100. The inhibition ratio is the most effective in monitoring neurological patients when the target is barbiturate coma. The inhibition ratio is also effective in

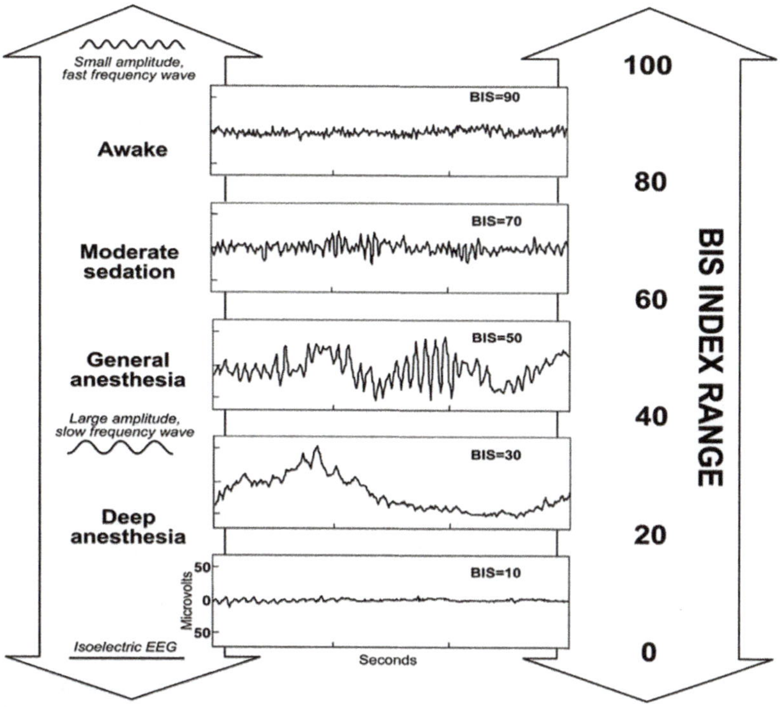


**Fig. 16.1** BIS classification standard

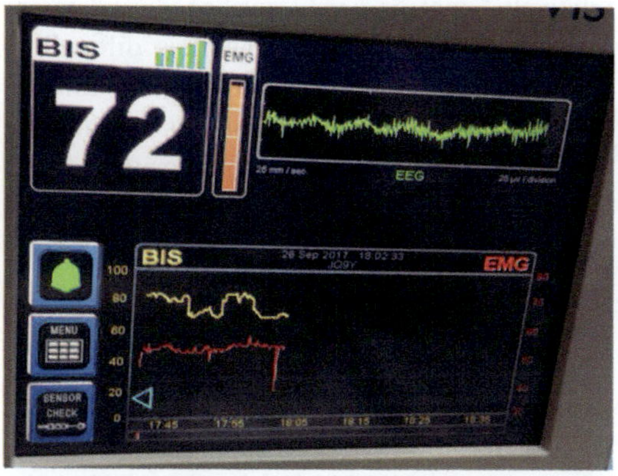


**Fig. 16.2** Increased frontal muscle myoelectricity leads to an increased BIS value

patients who are not deeply anesthetized. When the inhibition ratio decreases close to 0 until the BIS value drops below 20, as the BIS value decreases in the later stage, the suppression ratio increases rapidly; (c) hypoglycemia can lower the BIS; (d) low body temperature can reduce the BIS; (e) when sound is greater than 80 dB, it can increase the BIS. The sound range of ICUs is generally between 50 dB and 70 dB; therefore, sound has no significant effect on the BIS in ICUs; (f) a reduction in the BIS can be seen during sleep, except for during REM sleep when the BIS is increased; (g) CNS disease, severe TBI, cerebrovascular accidents, etc., can result in a reduction in the BIS on the affected side [3].

## 16.3 Correlation Between the BIS and Clinical Anesthetics

Since the emergence of BIS monitoring, it has been widely proven to be effective in monitoring the depth of general anesthesia during surgery. The BIS value is also related to the sleep phase and is also closely related to the metabolic activity of the whole brain. Compared with multiple anesthesia scoring systems, BIS monitoring has also proven to be effective in ICU patients [5].

A study found that in general anesthesia, the BIS is not affected by age, but the use of some anesthetic drugs, such as ketamine and xenon, will affect the BIS [6]. The BIS can reflect the concentration of anesthetics. For example, when BIS analysis is used for monitoring, the use of propofol, pentobarbital, and volatile drugs shows lower induced consciousness; the use of low doses of opioids will result in a higher BIS value. Relevant studies [7, 8] have confirmed that the BIS and propofol have a good correlation. Anesthesiologists can rely on the BIS value to more accurately determine the depth of sedation in patients during surgery. The reason is that propofol mainly acts on the cerebral cortex to inhibit it. However, the analgesic effect of opioids mainly acts on the subcortical center (including the spinal cord), and opioids have no inhibitory effect on the cerebral cortex. At least 5 times the analgesic dose is needed to induce obvious EEG suppression. The use of remifentanil and propofol has a synergistic effect. A study has shown that when propofol is combined with remifentanil, it can increase the sedative effect of the former without changing the BIS value [9]. Yang Gu et al. [10] found that dexmedetomidine reduced the dosage of propofol required during sedation, and dexmedetomidine increased the BIS value produced by propofol. If the sensitivity is reduced during deep sedation, some drugs (ketamine, such as opioids) will affect the BIS assessment of sedation. The BIS is lower when using propofol and pentobarbital for deep sedation than when using midazolam and chloral hydrate [11].

## 16.4 Clinical Application of the BIS

In the initial stage, BIS monitoring was mainly used for intraoperative monitoring of the depth of anesthesia. Later, this concern for consciousness gradually expanded to the ICU and emergency room with more anesthesia and mechanical ventilation. Using BIS monitoring in the ICU can continuously and objectively assess the level of anesthesia. Using BIS monitoring, the anesthetic can be titrated to the target BIS value, BIS < 60, so that the smallest dose of anesthetic to achieve awakening is the least possible (awareness < 5%) [12]. BIS monitoring can reduce excessive anesthesia for nonparalyzed patients. The anesthesiologists implement individualized administration based on the intraoperative BIS value and the patient's vital signs, to avoid anesthesia that is too shallow or deep to improve the quality of anesthesia and accurately predict the anesthesia effect to ensure patient safety during the perioperative period.

Appropriate sedation treatment for ICU patients is conducive to the recovery of their body's physiological functions and psychological state, and reasonable sedation can also shorten the time of mechanical ventilation for patients. The application of BIS monitoring in the ICU provides a new method for clinically solving the problem of excessive sedation that easily occurs during sedation treatment.

### 16.4.1 Monitoring the Depth of Sedation

The most important application area of BIS monitoring in the ICU is the depth monitoring of sedation in critically ill patients. Ideally, the sedative effect in the ICU should be that the patient is relatively quiet, is easily awakened, and maintains a sleep–wake cycle, but it is difficult to achieve this ideal goal. Sedation is a multimodal concept, including consciousness, amnesia, arousal, analgesia, and other parameters; therefore, it is difficult to express with a single parameter. The clinical evaluation of sedation depends on the patient's response to external stimuli; however, stimulation itself changes the patient's level of sedation. In the course of the disease, patients have different needs for sedation and analgesia. For most critically ill patients, ensuring patient comfort while maintaining mild sedation can improve clinical outcomes. The Clinical Practice Guidelines for the Management of Pain, Agitation, and Delirium in American adult ICU patients [13] recommend subjective evaluations such as the RASS, SAS, and Ramsay scores, which are currently the most commonly used clinical evaluation systems. When subjective sedation assessment is not possible, objective evaluation indicators of brain function can be used, such as BAEPs, the BIS, and the patient status index. For patients with neurological impairment, subjective scoring alone is not enough. The clinical evaluation score depends on the patient's movement and response; therefore, the depth of sedation cannot be accurately measured. In addition, due to the influence of social, personal, and professional factors on sedation monitoring, subjective evaluation of sedation effects is not ideal.

Mechanical ventilation is a commonly used treatment for critically ill patients. However, the stimulation of tracheal intubation, invasive operation, instrument noise, and unfamiliar environment during the treatment process can cause the patient to experience irritability and other emotions, forming a human–machine confrontation. This confrontation has a very adverse effect on the treatment and prognosis of patients. Therefore, sedation is particularly necessary for mechanical ventilation therapy. Clinically, the patient's depth of sedation is often maintained by adjusting the dose of sedatives. However, clinically, it is difficult to control the depth of sedation for patients. Insufficient sedation can lead to increased oxygen consumption, human–machine confrontation, accidental decoupling, etc. Excessive sedation can lead to ventilator-related pneumonia, delayed weaning, gastrointestinal bleeding, and bacteremia. The evaluation of sedation is an important basis for the implementation of sedation. According to the results of the evaluation of sedation, the dosage of the drug can be adjusted in time to achieve an effective sedation effect.

Although there is still controversy as to whether the BIS can accurately reflect the depth of sedation, adult ICU studies suggest that BIS monitoring of sedation is practical and effective. The BIS has a good correlation with the Ramsay score and SAS score. Among them, the BIS has a significant positive correlation with SAS scores and a significant negative correlation with Ramsay scores. The BIS can better reflect the depth of sedation [14, 15]. For example, Yamashita et al. [16] found that the BIS value decreased with the depth of sedation, and there was a significant correlation between the BIS value and the Ramsay score. In deep sedation (defined as a Ramsay score of 5–6 points), the BIS value in the older group (over 65 years) was significantly lower than that in the younger group (18–65 years). Qadeer et al. [17] defined deep sedation as the OAA/S scale. When the OAA/S scale score is 1–2 points and BIS $\leq$ 75 points, BIS predicts deep sedation with low sensitivity and high specificity. In the PICU, John et al. [18] found that RASS score, SAS score, and the BIS have a good correlation in the evaluation of sedation in children on mechanical ventilation. Within the range of sedation goals that PICU mechanically ventilated patients need to achieve, that is, SAS is 2–4 points, BIS monitoring as a continuous real-time objective method may more accurately and objectively reflect the degree of sedation in children. However, some studies have contrasting results. Vazquez [15] conducted a meta-analysis on the effects of BIS monitoring and subjective scoring scale assessment in ICU mechanical ventilation, providing a reference for choosing better sedation assessment tools in clinical practice. The results indicated that there is no sufficient evidence to show that the application of BIS monitoring in mechanically ventilated ICU patients is better than subjective scoring scale assessment. However, in some patients who cannot be assessed by subjective scoring scales, such as those with neurological paralysis, the use of BIS monitoring will not overestimate the patient's sedation due to the lack of muscle activity.

In addition to monitoring the degree of sedation in ICU patients, the BIS can also guide the sedation of critically ill patients in the ICU. A study by Olson et al. [19] found that the dosage of propofol in patients with additional BIS monitoring was significantly reduced, and the infusion rate was lower. The patients in the group with additional BIS monitoring woke up much faster than those in the group assessed by the Ramsay score alone. It is believed that the sedation assessment tool of BIS monitoring can provide a useful means for improving the care of critically ill patients with sedation. Mahmood et al. [20] found that BIS monitoring in the management of multiple trauma patients in the trauma ICU was associated with a better prognosis. BIS monitoring is a guide to adjust the dosage of sedatives, and it can also minimize restlessness, extubation failure, and ICU residence time.

With the in-depth research and the use of BIS monitoring, the development of individualized and precise sedation has been promoted, such as goal-directed sedation and BIS monitoring combined with closed-loop target-controlled infusion. The 2018 Adult ICU Analgesia and Sedation Treatment Guidelines [13] recommend that the choice of the depth of sedation in ICU patients is based on the state of organ function and the implementation of target-guided sedation strategies. Goal-directed shallow sedation is the mainstream sedation. Early goal-directed sedation (EGDS) was first proposed by Shehabi [21] in 2013 and recognized at home and abroad. EGDS is a more individualized and titrated sedation strategy. Compared with standard traditional-directed sedation (STDS), EGDS can significantly increase the rate of reaching the standard for shallow sedation and reduce the cumulative dose of sedative drugs. Yang et al. [22] reported that there was no statistically significant difference in mechanical ventilation time between an EGDS group and a STDS group. The time spent in the ICU in the EGDS group was longer than that in the STDS group ($P < 0.05$). The 90-day mortality rate in the EGDS group was higher than that in the STDS group ($P < 0.05$). The BIS has a good correlation with the RASS score and can be used for sedation assessment of patients in the ICU; a large-sample study comparing EGDS and STDS on the basis of the BIS is still needed.

The BIS combined with closed-loop target-controlled infusion has been used to guide the level of anesthesia in surgical patients. The BIS can be used to monitor brain function status indicators in real time and is a more reliable signal source for closed-loop target-controlled infusion. A study has shown that in the closed-loop target control group during anesthesia, the amount of anesthetic propofol was lower, and the BIS value and MAP were more stable [23]. The comparison of BIS monitoring combined with closed-loop target-controlled infusion and manual target-controlled intravenous infusion of propofol after surgery showed that the sedation of patients receiving BIS-guided closed-loop target-controlled infusion was more stable. This principle can also be applied to guide the sedation of critically ill patients: The actual BIS value of the patient is automatically fed back to the target-controlled pump as a control variable, and the target-controlled pump automatically adjusts the drug dose for sedation therapy according to the patient's BIS value. BIS monitoring combined with a closed-loop target-controlled infusion system enables clinicians to achieve the best depth of sedation through real-time monitoring of patient sedation levels and drug–dosage adjustments.

### 16.4.2 Analgesia

Pain is a common symptom of ICU patients. Many patients experience varying degrees of pain during ICU admission. The primary diseases, medical care operations, passive immobilization, sleep deprivation, etc., make it very common for ICU patients to feel pain, physical discomfort, and anxiety. Most patients are unable to actively express their pain through language due to coma, mechanical ventilation, sedation, etc. Pain is one of the important reasons why patients remember the bad experience of critical illness. To address the pain of critically ill patients, we must first obtain an accurate pain assessment. The pain assessment of ICU patients unable to communicate verbally remains a major challenge for clinicians. Using objective and effective measures to detect and even quantify pain behavior will help adjust the level of analgesia in critically ill patients and will help to obtain pain relief. Tracheal tube aspiration is a bad stimulus for patients and causes physiological reactions, including changes in heart rate, respiration, and blood oxygen saturation. However, in the study of Grap et al. [24], it was shown that the physiological response may not be a good or consistent pain marker, and changes in the physiological response did not change the level of sedation. Coleman et al. [25] monitored the BIS while stimulating the forearms of 30 subjects after general induction of anesthesia and found that the BIS was significantly increased with moderately harmful stimuli (from 35.00 increased to 40.00, $P = 0.003$) and severe noxious stimuli (from 37.67 to 40.00, $P = 0.007$). When the BIS value was >45, the ROC curve showed a sensitivity of 40.0% and a specificity of 73.3% for predicting pain. The analysis of participants with a baseline BIS > 40 showed a higher increase in the BIS value following painful stimulation, indicating that the increase in the BIS value for harmful procedures is likely to be higher when the level of sedation in ICU patients is lower. Faritous et al. [26] used the Critical Care Pain Observation Tool (CPOT) and BIS as pain assessment tools in 70 patients with tracheal intubation after coronary artery bypass graft and valve operation and found that the CPOT and the baseline BIS, BIS during pain stimulation, and BIS during recovery were positively correlated. BIS monitoring and the CPOT can be used to evaluate pain in patients with tracheal intubation. BIS monitoring is more sensitive than hemodynamic indicators, and it can play a more effective role in monitoring pain in intubated patients with deep anesthesia in the ICU. Arbour et al. [27] found that only the right BIS in the case of left-brain trauma is closely related to the frequency of painful behaviors. Research supports that the bilateral BIS is useful for pain monitoring in patients with only left-brain trauma who cannot speak.

### 16.4.3 The Use of BIS Monitoring to Evaluate the Degree and Prognosis of Brain Injury

Because changes in the BIS are related to the degree of oxygen consumption and brain damage of cells in the cerebral cortex, the BIS can be monitored to reflect the level of function of the cerebral cortex and then to evaluate whether brain resuscitation has been successful in the early treatment of patients with acute brain injury and cardiopulmonary arrest.

The BIS is related to the state of consciousness and can be used to assess the level of consciousness of patients and to predict the prognosis of brain damage. Gilbert et al. [28] were the first to apply BIS monitoring outside of sedation anesthesia. They studied the use of the BIS to assess the neurological function of 31 patients with unsedated consciousness in the ICU. They found that the BIS was significantly correlated with a variety of neurological function scores, including the GCS score. The higher the BIS is, the better the neurological function is. A later study supported the positive correlation between the BIS and GCS scores [29]. Fabregas et al. [30] suggested that the BIS is not only related to the level of consciousness of patients during sedation in the operating room but can also be used to predict the neurological prognosis of patients with brain trauma. Dunham et al. [31] studied 18 patients with severe brain injury caused by various etiologies (such as cerebral hemorrhage, epidural and subdural hemorrhage, brain contusion, SAH), including the patients' cranial artery pressure (CAP) indexes (CAP index = ICP/MAP − ICP) and BIS and the relationship between $StcO_2$ and prognosis. Most patients who survived and had good prognoses had higher BIS and higher levels of StcO2, while their ICPs, and CAP indexes were lower (BIS > 60, $StcO_2 > 70$, low ICP and CAP index), whereas most patients who died and had poor prognoses had lower BIS and lower levels of $StcO_2$ but increased ICPs and CAP indexes (BIS < 60, $StcO_2 < 70$, high ICP and CAP index). Schnakers et al. [32] studied 43 patients with brain injury due to various causes (such as brain trauma, HIE, ischemic or hemorrhagic stroke, SAH caused by aneurysm, metabolic encephalopathy, SE, encephalitis). In patients with severe brain damage, the BIS was used to distinguish the level of consciousness, such as a VS and MCS, and the BIS was used to predict the recovery of consciousness in patients with severe brain damage and coma 1 year later. The follow-up results after 1 year showed that the BIS in the good prognosis group was significantly higher than that in the poor prognosis group and that there was no significant difference in the BIS values of patients with brain injury due to different etiologies. Myles et al. [33] studied 25 patients with severe hypoxic–ischemic brain injury after emergency surgery. They obtained that compared with other indicators, such as injury duration, clinical evaluation, laboratory tests, and pupil reflex, the BIS was more useful than the other indicators in predicting the prognosis of severe hypoxic–ischemic brain injury. An abnormal BIS indicated a 6.6-fold increase in the possibility of poor neurological prognosis, while a normal BIS suggested a fivefold increase in the possibility of good neurological prognosis, and a low BIS accompanied by a high inhibition ratio was highly suggestive of brain injury. Regarding patients with craniocerebral injury in whom sedative drugs are used, Deogaonkar et al. [34] studied the relationship between the BIS and various sedation scores, such as RASS, SAS, and GCS scores, of 30 patients with craniocerebral injury in the NICU. The BIS was significantly correlated with various sedation scores.

However, some researchers hold the opposite view. Gill et al. [35] studied the relationship between the BIS and the GCS scores of 38 patients with changes in consciousness in the emergency department. The results showed that although there was statistical significance, the correlation coefficient between the BIS and the GCS score was only 0.387, and the fluctuation between the two was relatively large. Therefore, the authors believed that there was no reliable correlation between the BIS and the GCS score, and there was no accurate assessment of the role of consciousness impairment in emergency room patients. Nasraway et al. [36] studied the relationship between the sedation score (SAS score) and the BIS of 20 critically ill patients and found that there was no clear relationship between the BIS and the sedation score. At the same time, they believed that BIS software and hardware are unreliable or unconsistent in monitoring the consciousness level of intensive care patients. However, a previous study by Deogaonkar et al. [34] simultaneously compared the two BIS software versions and found that the correlation coefficients between the new version, BIS-XP, and RASS, SAS, and GCS scores were significantly higher than those between BIS 2.1.1 and these scores. Therefore, considering that the BIS software version used in the above two articles was not the new version, the inference ability of the studies is poor, which may lead to bias in their research results.

There are many studies on the BIS in patients with HIE after CPR following cardiopulmonary arrest. The main research aim of these studies was to judge patient prognosis and present different views. Stammet et al. [37] studied 47 patients who entered the ICU after CPR for treatment with mild hypothermia (two of them were excluded due to the inconsistent use of sedative drugs). BIS monitoring was used as one of the tools to predict the prognosis of these patients. The result was that when the BIS was 0, none of the patients had recovered their neurological function during ICU stay. A follow-up of 6 months after discharge found that in the ICU, when the BIS value was 0, the positive predictive value of poor prognosis was 100%, and when the BIS was not 0, the negative predictive value of good prognosis was 55%. Dumans-Nizard et al. [38] reported two cases of double lung transplantation. During the operation, hypotension and cardiac arrest occurred. Rescue measures such as cardiopulmonary bypass were successful. The intermediate BIS monitoring indicated that the BIS value increased from 0 to approximately 40. However, one patient died 6 days after surgery, and the other patient recovered after hypothermia treatment without any symptoms of neurological deficit. Therefore, the author believed that the BIS after CPR was not a reliable indicator for predicting prognosis. Myles and Cairo [39] reported a case of a patient with pulmonary hypertension who underwent double lung transplantation. Sudden pulmonary embolism caused cardiac arrest. The patient was given CPR and thrombectomy. The patient's BIS was continuously monitored during this process. The BIS fluctuated between 2 and 10 when muscle relaxants were not used, the BIS fluctuated from 0 to 5 after the use of muscle relaxants, the BIS rose to 38 after surgery, the SQI was between 90 and 100%, and suppression ratio was 0–2%. However, brain death was determined on the basis of the patient's clinical manifestations and EEGs. After being identified, the BIS changes were considered to be due to pulse interference. The author finally suggested that BIS monitoring was not designed to monitor ischemic brain damage, and there was no basis for the use of BIS monitoring in patients with ischemic brain damage.

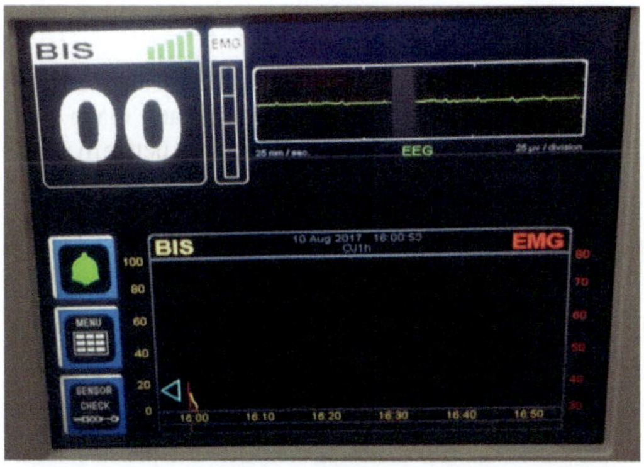


**Fig. 16.3** Male, 22 years old, HIE, deep coma, and brain death. The EEG showed ECS, and the BIS value was 0

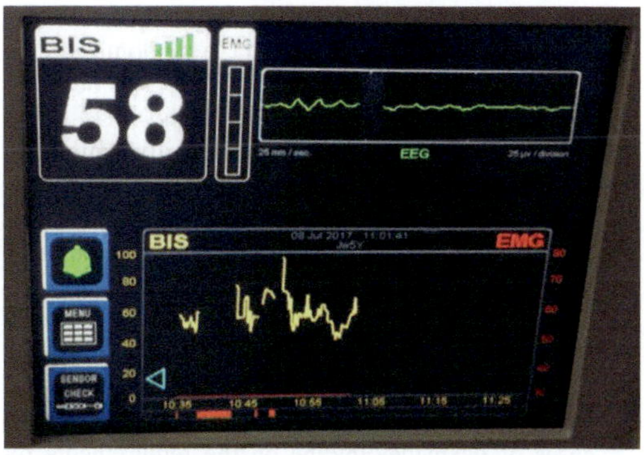


**Fig. 16.4** BIS on the left was 58

Previous studies [32, 40] observed the BIS values and prognoses of 56 patients with severe coma and found that BIS monitoring can be used to assess the occurrence of brain death in patients with severe coma (Fig. 16.3).

BIS monitoring still has a shortcoming; that is, it monitors only the unilateral EEG information of the forehead and then integrates it. Therefore, when a unilateral brain injury occurs, the bilateral data may be asymmetric, and is the use of the BIS reliable? This is worth considering. Fudickar et al. [41] studied 20 patients with unilateral supratentorial brain injury and compared their bilateral cranial BIS and mid-latency BAEPs and found that, compared with mid-latency BAEPs, the BIS was associated with unilateral brain injury. There are obvious differences between the injured side of the brain and the healthy side; therefore, the author suggests that in the process of monitoring the BIS, the BIS of the opposite side of the lesion should be monitored. However, mid-latency BAEP is more reliable in patients with unilateral head injury without significant bilateral differences.

As a tool for objective evaluation of sedation and analgesia, BIS monitoring can overcome the human error of subjective scoring. BIS monitoring is intuitive and digital and can avoid repeated stimulation of patients. Its advantages are its quantitative nature, noninvasiveness, bedside implementation, and dynamic monitoring. BIS monitoring is used to monitor and evaluate ICU sedation and analgesia and to assess the level of consciousness.

**Case**

A 47-year-old man was admitted to the hospital with "left limb weakness for 18 days, with aggravation and a disturbance of consciousness for 7 days." He had a history of hypertension, was admitted to the hospital with superficial coma, and had a GCS score of E2VTM3. Head CT showed a massive cerebral infarction on the right frontotemporal–occipital side. Bilateral BIS monitoring was performed (Fig. 16.4).

## References


1. Rampil IJ. A primer for EEG signal processing in anesthesia. Anesthesiology. 1998;89(4):980–1002.
2. Sandler NA. Additional clinical observations utilizing bispectral analysis. Anesth Prog. 2000;47(3):84–6.
3. Shetty RM, Bellini A, Wijayatilake DS, et al. BIS monitoring versus clinical assessment for sedation in mechanically ventilated adults in the intensive care unit and its impact on clinical outcomes and resource utilization. Cochrane Database Syst Rev. 2018;2:D11240.
4. Paul B, Robert V. Pharmacology of emergency department pain management and conscious sedation. Emerg Med Clin North Am. 2000;18(4):803–27.
5. Yaman F, Ozcan N, Ozcan A, et al. Assessment of correlation between bispectral index and four common sedation scales used in mechanically ventilated patients in ICU. Eur Rev Med Pharmacol Sci. 2012;16(5):660–6.
6. Johansen JW. Update on bispectral index monitoring. Best Pract Res Clin Anaesthesiol. 2006;20(1):81–99.

7. Rusch D, Arndt C, Eberhart L, et al. Bispectral index to guide induction of anesthesia: a randomized controlled study. BMC Anesthesiol. 2018;18(1):66.
8. Araujo AM, Machado H, de Pinho PG, et al. Population pharmacokinetic-pharmacodynamic modeling for propofol anesthesia guided by the bispectral index (BIS). J Clin Pharmacol. 2019;60:617–28.
9. Tukenmez B, Memis D, Pamukcu Z. The addition of haloperidol, propofol, or midazolam to sufentanil for intravenous sedation in the intensive care unit using bispectral index. J Opioid Manag. 2008;4(1):34–40.
10. Gu Y, Yang F, Zhang Y, et al. The effects of different doses of dexmedetomidine on the requirements for propofol for loss of consciousness in patients monitored via the bispectral index: a double-blind, placebo-controlled trial. BMC Anesthesiol. 2020;20(1):96.
11. Finger RG, Mallmann C, Nedel WL. BIS monitoring in sedated, mechanically ventilated patients: right tool in the wrong patients? A meta-analysis. Intensive Care Med. 2016;42(6):1086–7.
12. Kelley SD, Manberg PJ, Sigl JC. Anesthesia awareness and the bispectral index. N Engl J Med. 2008;359(4):427–8, 430–1.
13. Devlin JW, Skrobik Y, Gélinas C, et al. Clinical practice guidelines for the prevention and management of pain, agitation/sedation, delirium, immobility, and sleep disruption in adult patients in the ICU. Crit Care Med. 2018;46(9):e825–73.
14. Karamchandani K, Rewari V, Trikha A, et al. Bispectral index correlates well with Richmond agitation sedation scale in mechanically ventilated critically ill patients. J Anesth. 2010;24(3):394–8.
15. Vazquez MJ. Assessing sedation in PICU: clinical scales or BIS analysis? Minerva Anestesiol. 2012;78(3):286–7.
16. Yamashita K, Terao Y, Inadomi C, et al. Age-dependent relationship between bispectral index and sedation level. J Clin Anesth. 2008;20(7):492–5.
17. Qadeer MA, Vargo JJ, Patel S, et al. Bispectral index monitoring of conscious sedation with the combination of meperidine and midazolam during endoscopy. Clin Gastroenterol Hepatol. 2008;6(1):102–8.
18. John WB, Christopher RF, Joseph DT. The correlation of the bispectral index monitor with clinical sedation scores during mechanical ventilation in the pediatric intensive care unit. Anesth Analg. 2002;94(3):506–11.
19. Olson DM, Zomorodi MG, James ML, et al. Exploring the impact of augmenting sedation assessment with physiologic monitors. Aust Crit Care. 2014;27(3):145–50.
20. Mahmood S, Parchani A, El-Menyar A, et al. Utility of bispectral index in the management of multiple trauma patients. Surg Neurol Int. 2014;5:141.
21. Shehabi Y. Early goal directed sedation, a bridge to better clinical outcomes. Chin Med J. 2014;127(10):1969–72.
22. Yang G, Guo X, Mao G, et al. [Clinical research of early goal directed sedation applying in acute brain injury]. Zhonghua Wei Zhong Bing Ji Jiu Yi Xue. 2020;32(3):345–9.
23. Hemmerling TM, Charabati S, Zaouter C, et al. A randomized controlled trial demonstrates that a novel closed-loop propofol system performs better hypnosis control than manual administration. Can J Anaesth. 2010;57(8):725–35.
24. Grap MJ, Munro CL, Wetzel PA, et al. Responses to noxious stimuli in sedated mechanically ventilated adults. Heart Lung. 2014;43(1):6–12.
25. Coleman RM, Tousignant-Laflamme Y, Gelinas C, et al. Changes in the bispectral index in response to experimental noxious stimuli in adults under general anesthesia. ISRN Pain. 2013;2013:583920.
26. Faritous Z, Barzanji A, Azarfarin R, et al. Comparison of bispectral index monitoring with the critical-care pain observation tool in the pain assessment of intubated adult patients after cardiac surgery. Anesth Pain Med. 2016;6(4):e38334.
27. Arbour C, Gelinas C, Loiselle CG, et al. An exploratory study of the bilateral bispectral index for pain detection in traumatic-brain-injured patients with altered level of consciousness. J Neurosci Nurs. 2015;47(3):166–77.
28. Gilbert TT, Wagner MR, Halukurike V, et al. Use of bispectral electroencephalogram monitoring to assess neurologic status in unsedated, critically ill patients. Crit Care Med. 2001;29(10):1996–2000.
29. Haug E, Miner J, Dannehy M, et al. Bispectral electroencephalographic analysis of head-injured patients in the emergency department. Acad Emerg Med. 2004;11(4):349–52.
30. Fabregas N, Gambus PL, Valero R, et al. Can bispectral index monitoring predict recovery of consciousness in patients with severe brain injury? Anesthesiology. 2004;101(1):43–51.
31. Dunham CM, Ransom KJ, McAuley CE, et al. Severe brain injury ICU outcomes are associated with Cranial-Arterial Pressure Index and noninvasive Bispectral Index and transcranial oxygen saturation: a prospective, preliminary study. Crit Care. 2006;10(6):R159.
32. Schnakers C, Ledoux D, Majerus S, et al. Diagnostic and prognostic use of bispectral index in coma, vegetative state and related disorders. Brain Inj. 2008;22(12):926–31.
33. Myles PS, Daly D, Silvers A, et al. Prediction of neurological outcome using bispectral index monitoring in patients with severe ischemic-hypoxic brain injury undergoing emergency surgery. Anesthesiology. 2009;110(5):1106–15.
34. Deogaonkar A, Gupta R, DeGeorgia M, et al. Bispectral Index monitoring correlates with sedation scales in brain-injured patients. Crit Care Med. 2004;32(12):2403–6.
35. Gill M, Green SM, Krauss B. Can the bispectral index monitor quantify altered level of consciousness in emergency department patients? Acad Emerg Med. 2003;10(2):175–9.

36. Nasraway SSJ, Wu EC, Kelleher RM, et al. How reliable is the Bispectral Index in critically ill patients? A prospective, comparative, single-blinded observer study. Crit Care Med. 2002;30(7):1483–7.
37. Stammet P, Werer C, Mertens L, et al. Bispectral index (BIS) helps predicting bad neurological outcome in comatose survivors after cardiac arrest and induced therapeutic hypothermia. Resuscitation. 2009;80(4):437–42.
38. Dumans-Nizard V, Hamada S, Fischler M. Bispectral index during cardiopulmonary resuscitation: a poor indicator of recovery. Two very different cases. Anaesthesia. 2010;65(2):196–8.
39. Myles PS, Cairo S. Artifact in the bispectral index in a patient with severe ischemic brain injury. Anesth Analg. 2004;98(3):706–7.
40. Shehabi Y, Bellomo R, Kadiman S, et al. Sedation intensity in the first 48 hours of mechanical ventilation and 180-day mortality: a multinational prospective longitudinal cohort study. Crit Care Med. 2018;46(6):850–9.
41. Fudickar A, Jacobsen JH, Weiler N, et al. Bilateral measurement of bispectral index and mid-latency auditory evoked potentials in patients with unilateral brain lesions. J Crit Care. 2009;24(4):545–50.

# Application of aEEG in Severely Ill Patients

# 17

Yuanfeng Zhou and Feng Li

## Contents



**Abstract**

Critically ill patients are characterized by rapid onset and development of severity. Damage to the nervous system and other organs and metabolic abnormalities will eventually lead to brain dysfunction and even brain death. However, clinically, it is difficult for ICU doctors to judge the degree of brain damage based on clinical symptoms alone, and it is difficult to identify epileptic seizures with atypical clinical manifestations and clinical electrical seizures. Therefore, in critically ill patients, it is necessary to monitor changes in brain function and seizures in real time to allow timely and corresponding treatment to correct the occurrence of reversible brain

Y. Zhou (✉)
Department of Neurology, Children's Hospital of Fudan University, Shanghai, China
e-mail: yuanfengzhou@fudan.edu.cn

F. Li
Department of Neurology, The First Affiliated Hospital of Chongqing Medical University, Chongqing, China



X. Wang et al. (eds.), *Multi-Modal EEG Monitoring of Severely Neurologically Ill Patients*,
https://doi.org/10.1007/978-981-16-4493-1_17

damage. Early detection and correction of reversible brain injury, accurate and objective evaluation of brain function status, guidance of clinicians to formulate and adjust treatment plans, and minimization of the occurrence of complications are of great significance for improving the prognosis and quality of life in patients. As a supplement to conventional EEG, compared to traditional EEG, aEEG is being gradually applied in the NICU due to its more intuitive results, easy interpretation, simple operation, convenience, long range, and high-quality monitoring at the bedside. aEEG can simply and effectively monitor neuroelectrophysiological changes in neurocritically ill patients, dynamically reflecting the state of brain function and detecting brain function changes and convulsions or seizures in an early stage to guide treatment and predict prognosis in real time. This chapter briefly describes aEEG principles, parameter indicators, and monitoring requirements. At the same time, it introduces aEEG result analysis indicators, pattern classification, and diagnostic criteria to help readers quickly understand the basic knowledge of aEEG. This chapter focuses on the application of aEEG in the intensive care of children and adults in combination with the legend and provides a reference for the clinical evaluation of brain function and the prognosis of critically ill patients.

**Keywords**

ICU · aEEG · Children · Brain function · Brain damage · Neonatal convulsion · HIE · Epilepsy · Prognosis

## 17.1 Overview

At present, methods for monitoring brain function in critical patients are still very limited. Head imaging, TCD monitoring, and ICP and cerebral oxygen monitoring can indirectly reflect changes in brain structure, blood flow, ICP, and oxygenation metabolism but cannot fully reflect changes in brain function.

EEG activity is very sensitive to pathophysiological changes in the cerebral cortex, especially ischemia and hypoxia. EEG activity has a good correlation with changes in CBF, and EEG can also be used to judge whether seizures are convulsive or nonconvulsive. Due to the limitations of conventional EEG, cEEG or continuous video EEG, which can conveniently, dynamically, and noninvasively evaluate the function of brain neurons and monitor epileptic seizures, is more suitable for monitoring brain function in critically ill patients. According to the existing EEG grading standards, cEEGs can be used to locate initial brain injury in severe patients, reflect the degree of brain injury and monitor convulsion, and judge the short-term and long-term prognosis of children according to the dynamic changes in EEG and the response to external stimuli. However, the following problems still exist in the practical application of cEEG: (a) The amount of cEEG monitoring data is large, which requires considerable time and professional neuroelectrophysiologists to play back and analyze the changes in amplitude and frequency, which often delays the timely diagnosis and treatment of the disease; and (b) cEEGs can reflect EEG activity at that time, but they cannot reflect the continuous change and trend in brain function in real time. Therefore, it is impossible to judge the prognosis of and treat critically ill children on the basis of whether brain injury is reversible.

Therefore, simple, real-time, and reliable EEG monitoring methods are needed to solve the above problems in ICUs, and the continuous brain function monitoring trend chart is an effective auxiliary means to solve these problems [1]. The trend chart of continuous brain function monitoring is simple in clinical operation. It is more intuitive and simple, and it analyzes in real-time changes in the trends of the amplitude and frequency of brainwaves in the unit of "hours." The trend charts of brain function monitoring are mainly divided into two categories: One is based on amplitude analysis, such as aEEGs and ET charts; the other is based on frequency analysis, such as the energy power spectrum and spectrum trend chart. At present, aEEG can meet the requirements of bedside EEG monitoring for critically ill patients to a certain extent.

## 17.2 aEEG

aEEG is not a new technology. In the 1960s, Maynard and Priors [2] developed the earliest brain function monitor and introduced aEEG into clinical practice. It was used as a means of monitoring brain function in adults undergoing cardiac bypass surgery and after CPR [3]. aEEG has the ability of time compression output, which can simulate the traditional EEG system. The application of aEEG does not require professional EEG technicians or neuroelectrophysiologists. Timely analysis by ICU clinicians and nurses provides a simpler means for monitoring the changing trends of brain function in ICUs and operating rooms.

### 17.2.1 Signal Processing of aEEG

aEEG is not a specific EEG instrument, and in essence, it is a simplified form of conventional EEG monitoring in which the trend graph of brain function is formed after the conventional EEG signals are reprocessed. aEEG signals are obtained from conventional EEG amplifiers. With a frequency range of 2–15 Hz, EEG signals are amplified and filtered by asymmetric bandpass filters, followed by semilogarithmic amplitude compression, correction, smoothing, integration, and finally time compression, followed by output on the computer screen at a slow paper feeding speed (6 cm/h). The output signals are no longer the original EEG signals but signals representing the change in the background brain electrical activity voltage of the whole EEG; that is, they are integrated trend graphs of the change in the amplitude of brain electrical activity and indirectly reflect the range of the change in the EEG amplitude; thus, they are aEEGs.

### 17.2.2 Monitoring Channels of aEEG

Early aEEG was mostly single channel. According to the international standard for the placement of electrodes in the 10–20 lead system, dual-top recording electrodes (P3–P4) are generally recommended as recording electrodes for traditional single-channel aEEG. Priors et al. [3] suggested the selection of dual-top recording electrodes because the area near the parietal bone is in the marginal zone of the middleand posterior cerebral arteries, which is sensitive to ischemia and hypoxia, and the top area was less susceptible to the interference of muscle activity and eye movements. However, due to limited monitoring electrodes for single-channel aEEG, aEEGs can reflect the changes in brain electrical activity and brain function in only local brain regions; the connection mode using P3–P4 electrodes cannot be used to judge whether brain electrical activity is different between hemispheres. Therefore, it is recommended to add F3/F4 recording electrodes for dual-channel (F3–P3 and F4–P4) aEEG monitoring. Dual-channel monitoring can detect and reflect the trend in unilateral brain electrical activity and/or the asymmetry of epilepsy, better reflect the electrical activity of various brain regions, increase the positive rate of seizure detection, and provide accurate evidence for clinical diagnosis and treatment [4].

### 17.2.3 Analysis Indexes of aEEGs, the Classification of aEEG Patterns, and Criteria for the Classification of aEEGs

#### 17.2.3.1 Analysis Indexes of aEEGs

Analysis indexes of aEEGs mainly include (a) background amplitude morphology and upper and lower boundaries of the EEG amplitude; (b) periodic changes in sleep–wake background activity; and (c) convulsions or seizures. The amplitude trend band of aEEGs fluctuates up and down around the baseline average value to form an amplitude band with sine wave-like changes, which is presented in two dimensions (the horizontal axis represents the time and the vertical axis represents the amplitude value) on the coordinate axis, with the upper boundary (≤100 μV) and lower boundary (>0 μV) of amplitude. The numerical values and average values of the upper and lower boundaries of the amplitude can be quantitatively analyzed with the software. The aEEG sleep–wake cycle is characterized by smooth periodic changes, mainly in the lower boundary. The wide-band phase of aEEGs in neonates represents discontinuous background activity during quiet sleep (an alternating pattern in full-term infants), and the narrow-band phase represents continuous background activity during wake or active sleep (Fig. 17.1). The wide-band phase of aEEGs in infants and children represents medium- and high-amplitude slow-wave background activity in NREM sleep (stages I, II, and III), and the narrow-band phase represents background activity of awakening or low- and medium-amplitude activity in REM sleep (Fig. 17.2). aEEGs during convulsions or seizures are primarily characterized by transient increases in the upper and lower boundaries of the amplitude band (Fig. 17.3), sometimes only in the lower boundary, and in rare cases by transient decreases in the upper and lower boundaries of the amplitude band.

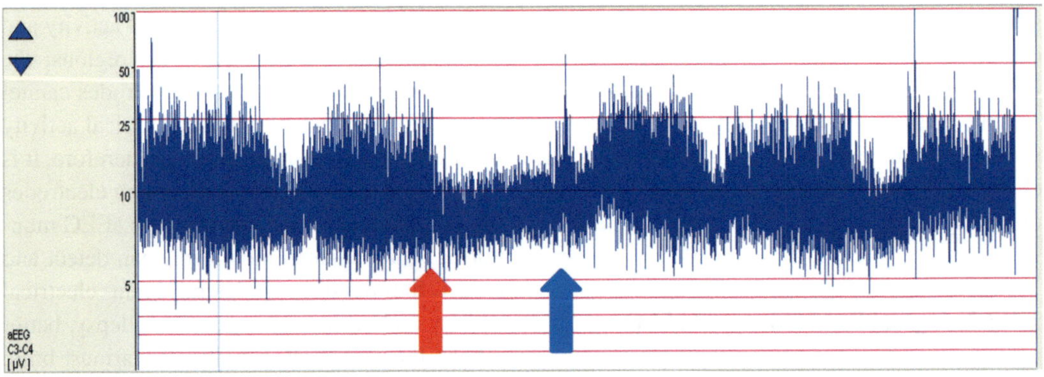


**Fig. 17.1** Neonatal aEEG: The wide-band period (red arrow) represents discontinuous background activity in quiet sleep (alternating pattern in full-term infants), while the narrow-band period (blue arrow) represents continuous background activity in awake periods or periods of active sleep

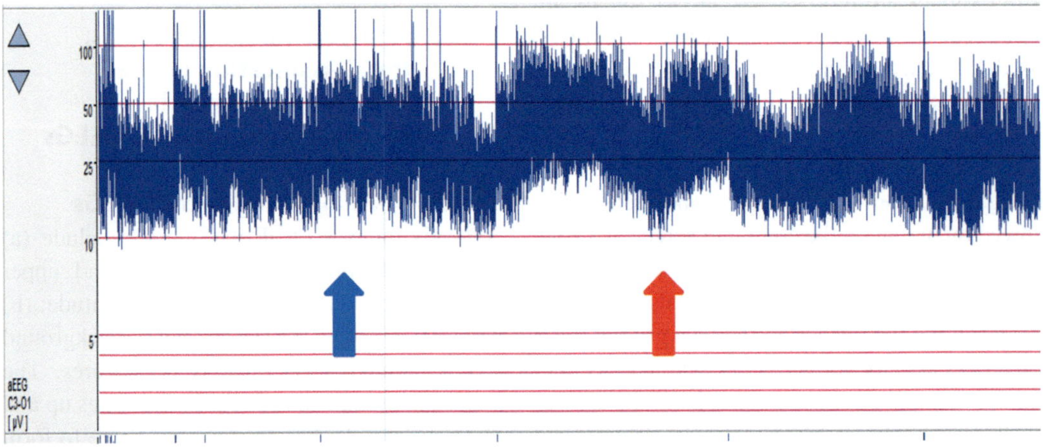


**Fig. 17.2** Wide-band phase (red arrow) of aEEGs in infants and children represents the background activities of moderate- to high-amplitude slow waves in NREM sleep (I, II, and III), while the narrow-band phase (blue arrow) represents the low- to medium-amplitude background activities in awakening or REM sleep

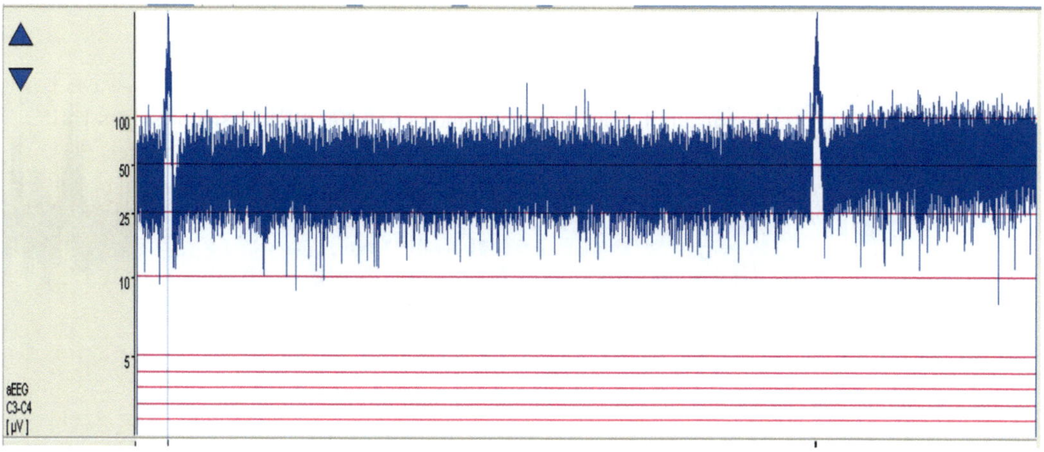


**Fig. 17.3** Seizures on aEEG are characterized by sudden rise in short upper and lower boundaries

#### 17.2.3.2 Classification of aEEG Patterns

As early as the 1980s, some authors described aEEG patterns in relation to the development process of normal-term and premature infants [5]. To date, several aEEG patterns have been classified, mainly on the basis of amplitude. Naqeeb et al. [6] proposed three types of normal-term infant aEEG amplitudes: (a) normal amplitude, the upper boundary of the amplitude of electrical activity is >10 μV and the lower boundary is >5 μV; (b) mildly abnormal amplitude, the upper boundary is >10 μV and the lower boundary is ≤5 μV; and (c) severely abnormal amplitude, the upper boundary is <10 μV and the lower boundary is <5 μV. The disadvantage of this classification is that it does not define the BS pattern or the type of sleep–wake cycle.

Hellström-Westas [7] proposed another definition of background activity based on EEG terms, which was applicable to the classification of sleep–wake cycles of all neonates, and this classification method is currently commonly used in clinical practice.

1. Classification of background activity patterns.
   (a) Continuous activity is defined as the lower boundary (minimum amplitude) at (5) 7–10 μV and the upper boundary (maximum amplitude) at 10–25 (~50) μV, which is often referred to as CNV (Fig. 17.4).
   (b) DNV is defined as an upper boundary at >10 μV and a variable lower boundary at <5 μV (Fig. 17.5).
   (c) CLV, also known as continuous extremely low-amplitude activity, is approximately or < 5 μV (Fig. 17.6).
   (d) BS is defined as the lower boundary being constant within 0–1 (2) μV and the burst amplitude being >25 μV (Fig. 17.7). BS+ refers to the background activity of BS with more than one burst (≥100/h). BS means BS background activity with few bursts (<100/h).
   (e) ECS or FT is defined as a background activity amplitude <5 μV (Fig. 17.8).
2. Sleep–wake cycle classification.
   (a) Absence of sleep–wake cycle: no sinusoidal change in aEEG background activity.
   (b) Immature sleep–wake cycle: The lower boundary has some periodic changes but is not fully developed compared with the normal boundary.
   (c) Mature sleep–wake cycle: There is a clearly identifiable sinusoidal change in the aEEG between discrete and continuous background activities that last for at least 20 min.
3. Classification of convulsions or seizures
   (a) Seizure only once.
   (b) Repeated convulsion: discharges ≥3 times within 30 min.

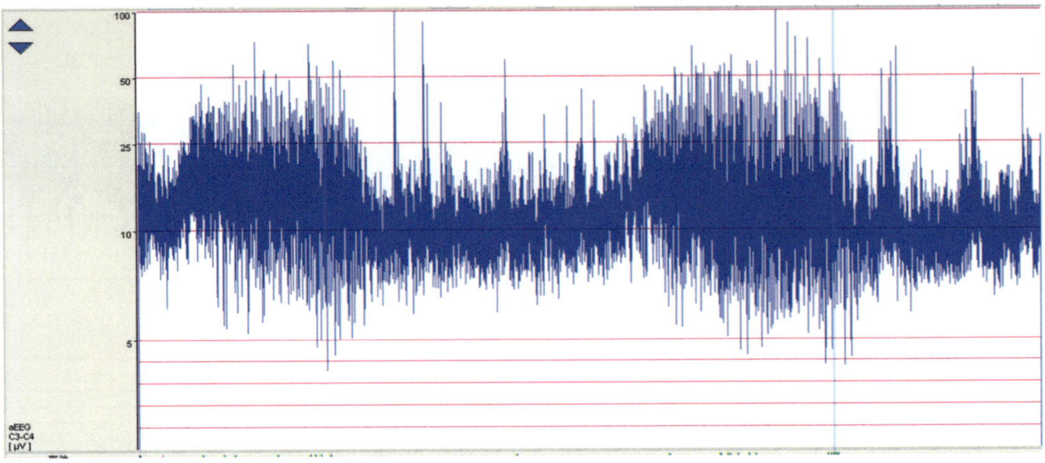


**Fig. 17.4** Continuous activity, with the lower boundary (minimum amplitude) at (5) 7–10 μV and the upper boundary (maximum amplitude) at 10–25 (~50) μV

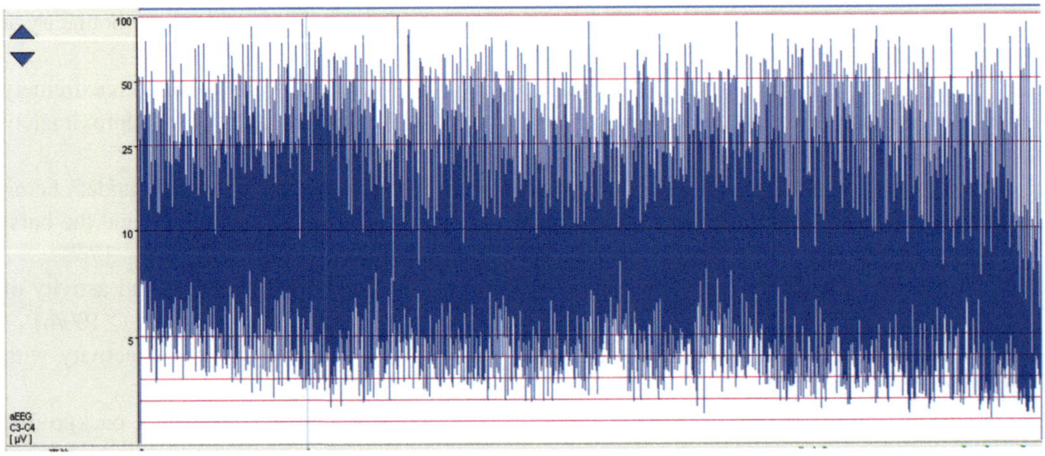


**Fig. 17.5** DNV is defined as an upper boundary >10 μV and a variable lower boundary <5 μV

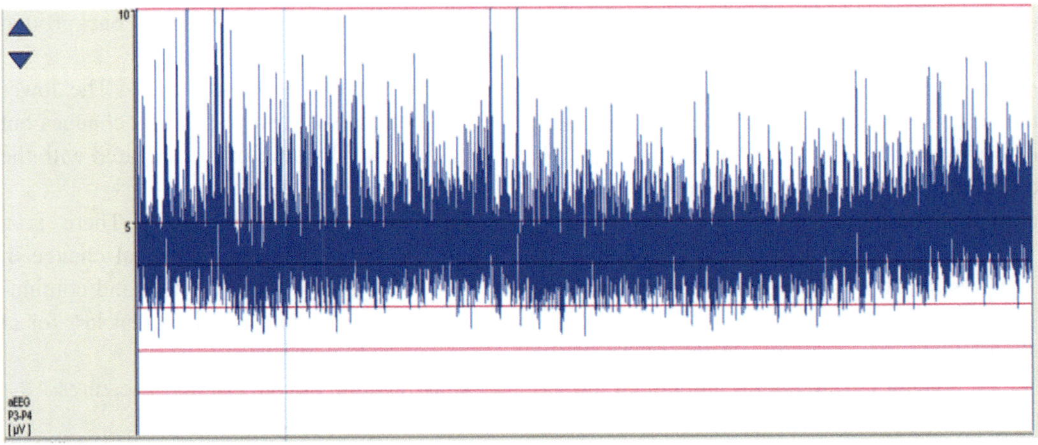


**Fig. 17.6** CLV, also known as continuous extremely low-amplitude activity, is approximately or <5 μV

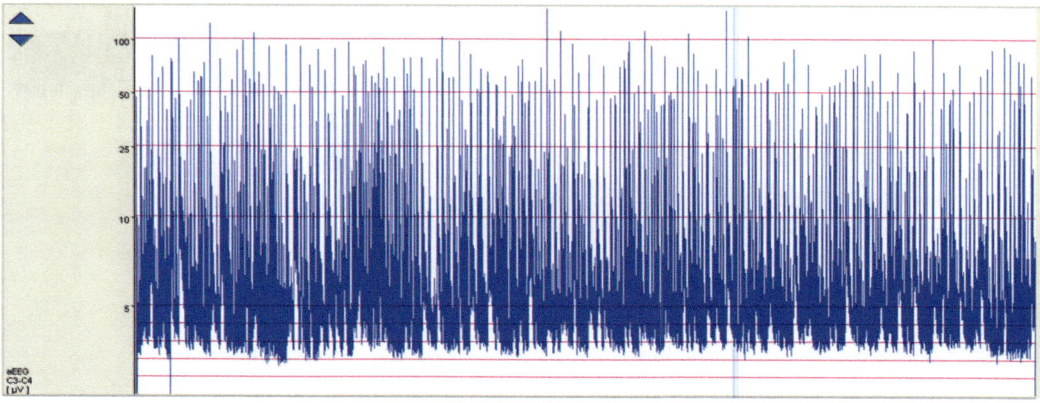


**Fig. 17.7** BS is defined as the lower boundary being constant within 0–1 (2) μV and the burst amplitude being >25 μV

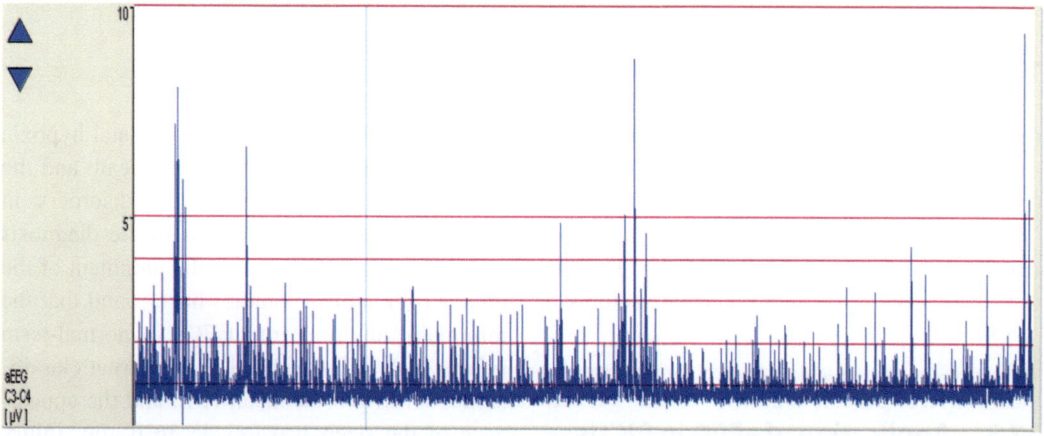


**Fig. 17.8** Inactive or FT: The background activity is mainly ECS, <5 μV

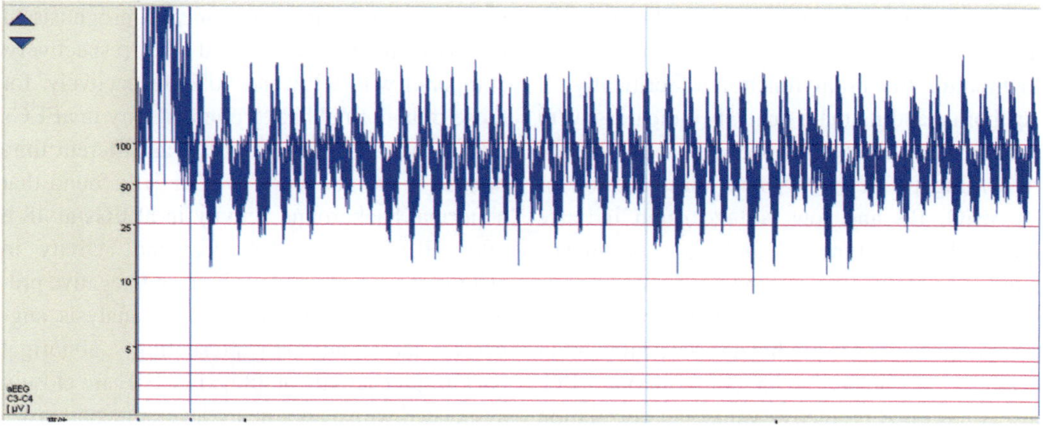


**Fig. 17.9** SE: discharge lasting more than 30 min, characterized by a "sawtooth pattern"

(c) SE: discharge lasting more than 30 min characterized by either a "sawtooth pattern" (Fig. 17.9) or a continuous increase in the amplitude of the peaks and valleys (Fig. 17.10).

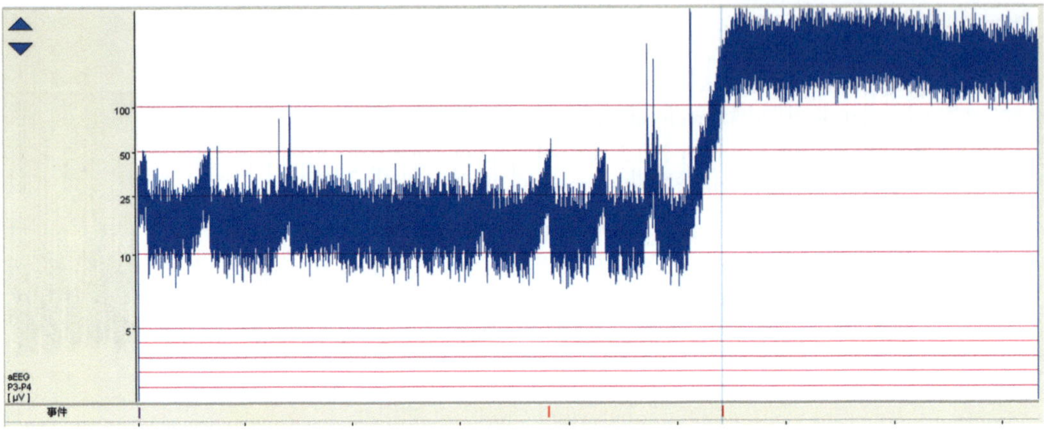


**Fig. 17.10** SE: discharge ≥30 min, the amplitude of the wave crest and trough increased continuously

#### 17.2.3.3 Criteria for the Classification of aEEGs [6]

(a) Normal aEEG: continuous activity and a mature sleep–wake cycle.
(b) Mildly abnormal aEEG: DNV, an immature sleep–wake cycle, and only one seizure.
(c) Severely abnormal aEEG: CLV, BS, ECS, no sleep–wake cycle, and recurrent seizures or SE.

## 17.3 Application of aEEG in PICUs

At present, aEEG has become a routine method for monitoring brain function in PICUs. In pediatrics, aEEG was first used in the neonatal ICU to monitor the brain function of critically ill newborns, and its main analysis indicators were background activity, sleep cycle, and seizures. According to the background classification of the EEG, BS and low voltage often indicate impaired brain function and poor prognosis, requiring timely intervention to improve prognosis. The isoelectric point is equivalent to ECS, which can be used to predict and determine brain death [8]. Compared with conventional EEG, aEEG has good predictive value and correlation in the prognosis of HIE, premature brain injury, neonatal seizures, epilepsy diagnosis, and monitoring.

### 17.3.1 HIE

In neonates, HIE is caused by perinatal hypoxia and is the main cause of neonatal death and the development of nervous system disorders in infants. EEG is of great value in the diagnosis and prognosis of HIE and in the judgment of the effects of treatment. Studies have found that the minimum amplitude of aEEGs in normal-term infants with HIE is related to the Sarnat classification severity of neonatal HIE, and the appearance of the sleep–wake cycle 36 h after injury with HIE suggests a good prognosis [9]. The sensitivity and specificity of conventional EEG in predicting the neurodevelopmental prognosis of infants with HIE are 92% and 83%, respectively, compared with 93% and 90%, respectively, for those of abnormal background activity in aEEGs [10]. A meta-analysis of aEEG at different time points (6, 24, 48, or 72 h) after HIE found that abnormal background activity in aEEGs at 48 h after HIE or normal background activity in aEEGs at 6 h had good positive and negative predictive values, respectively. This analysis suggests that aEEGs presenting abnormal background activity at 48 h after HIE are closely associated with a poor neurodevelopmental prognosis and that those presenting normal background activity at 6 h after HIE are closely associated with a good neurodevelopmental prognosis [11]. Another meta-analysis of neonatal HIE after mild hypothermia treatment evaluated the accuracy of different examination methods in predicting neural development, and the same conclusion was reached that aEEG at 24 h after HIE showed that the positive predictive value of abnormal background activity in patients with dysplasia was reliable [12]. A pattern of recurrent seizures in aEEGs was strongly associated with early lethality and the severity of brain injury on head MRI in a prospective study of HIE in normal-term infants [13].

Among the critically ill children admitted to PICUs, 2 ~ 6% had cardiac arrest, which may lead to severe neurological sequelae. Therefore, early brain function monitoring and early intervention and prognosis judgment of brain function in children with cardiac arrest are of great value. A retrospective study of 30 children using dual-channel aEEG monitoring early after cardiac arrest found that continuous background activity and spontaneous appearance of the sleep cycle within 24 h after cardiac arrest were indicators of a good prognosis [14]. It is suggested that early aEEG monitoring after cardiac arrest in children can be used to predict their prognosis.

### 17.3.2 Brain Injury in Premature Infants

Brain injury is a common complication seen in premature infants. The common types of brain injury in premature infants are periventricular–intraventricular hemorrhages and periventricular leukomalacia. Survivors often have severe neurodevelopmental disorders. As premature infants usually need respiratory support, head MRI is difficult to perform early. Therefore, the value of EEG in the early diagnosis and prediction of the prognosis of brain injury in premature infants are very important. In a double-blind prospective cohort study, the aEEGs of 23 premature infants less than 31 gestational weeks were continuously monitored for 4 h each day for 3 days. Severe abnormal background activity, discontinuous low-voltage background activity, and the absence of the sleep–wake cycle were aEEG changes associated with poor early prognosis, including death or severe paraventricular/internal bleeding or leukomalacia on MRI [13]. A retrospective study included 95 premature infants with a gestational age of less than 30 weeks, and aEEG monitoring was used to evaluate the correlation between seizures and periventricular–intraventricular hemorrhage, periventricular leukomalacia, and death within 3 days after birth. The study found that the incidence of seizures reached 48% within 3 days after brain injury in premature infants. Recurrent seizures 1, 2, and 3 days after birth were related to periventricular–intraventricular hemorrhage, periventricular–intraventricular hemorrhage, periventricular leukomalacia, death and severe periventricular–intraventricular hemorrhage, and language development delay at the age of 2 years [15]. A systemic review, including seven conventional EEGs and six aEEGs, evaluated the accuracy of background EEG activity in predicting late neurological development in premature infants. The results showed that abnormal background activity in aEEGs could be used as a predictor of late adverse prognosis, which is death, intelligence quotient less than 70, and cerebral palsy, with the sensitivity and specificity reaching 83% and 83%, respectively [16].

### 17.3.3 Neonatal Convulsions

Neonatal convulsions occur with high incidence in high-risk neonates and are a risk factor for death or disability in the neonatal period. Neonatal convulsions have mild and atypical clinical manifestations, but they also can appear only subclinically (i.e., in EEGs). The early diagnosis and treatment of neonatal convulsions are still of great significance and challenge for pediatricians [17]. The diagnosis of neonatal convulsions based on clinical observation or empirical diagnosis is not reliable. Therefore, a reliable detection method in neonates with clinically suspected convulsions is cEEG monitoring. Despite increasing attention to the role of aEEG at the bedside, real-time monitoring, and timely detection by neonatal healthcare personnel in the diagnosis and treatment of neonatal convulsions, multichannel cEEG monitoring remains the gold standard for the diagnosis of neonatal convulsions. A systematic review including and comparing ten studies concerning the diagnosis of neonatal convulsions with aEEG revealed that for the diagnosis of neonatal convulsions, the average sensitivity and specificity of aEEG (with conventional EEG) were 76% and 85%, respectively, while those of aEEG (without conventional EEG) were 39% and 95%, respectively. This study suggested that aEEG combined with multichannel raw EEG synchronous display can significantly improve the sensitivity and specificity of neonatal seizure diagnosis [18]. As a supplement to multichannel conventional EEG monitoring, aEEG can detect neonatal seizures in a timely manner and can be used as a good bedside screening method for neonatal seizures. In addition, trained and experienced neonatal healthcare personnel can better explain aEEG results and detect seizures in a timely manner [19].

### 17.3.4 Epilepsy

Similar to neonatal convulsions, due to the particularity and sensitivity of children's brain development, diseases of the CNS and diseases of various organs involving the CNS in children will lead to epileptic seizures and SE, including convulsive and nonconvulsive seizures. Common causes of epilepsy include CNS infection, cerebrovascular disease, and metabolic disorders. Repeated seizures or SE can lead to secondary epilepsy, cognitive impairment, behavioral abnormalities, focal neurological damage and other neurological sequelae, and even death. Therefore, the timely detection, diagnosis, and treatment of seizures and SE are particularly important in PICUs. At present, there is still a lack of meta-analyses and systematic reviews on the value of aEEG in the diagnosis of epileptic seizures in PICUs. A prospective observational study analyzed the ability of trained PICU clinicians to identify seizures via dual-channel aEEG and found that PICU clinicians had 100% sensitivity and 88% specificity for bedside recognition of seizures using aEEG. The average time from the onset of an epileptic seizure to recognition was 25 min, suggesting that PICU clinicians can identify an epileptic seizure well through aEEG. Standardized training plans and regular examinations can reduce the misdiagnosis rate and shorten the recognition time [20]. Other retrospective studies have found that the sensitivity of aEEG for seizure recognition in PICUs is 46–73.7%; therefore, more prospective studies and meta-analyses are needed to further confirm the value of aEEG for seizure recognition in PICUs [21, 22].

### 17.3.5 Others

In addition to the application of aEEG in monitoring the brain function of patients with HIE, premature brain injury, neonatal convulsions, epilepsy, and other diseases, the clinical application of aEEG in the perioperative intensive care of neonates with CHD has also been reported [23]. A study found that the rate of abnormal aEEG activity in children with CHD and persistent pulmonary hypertension was as high as 50%, which often indicates poor neurological function prognosis.

## 17.4 Application of aEEG in Adult ICUs

The adult brain is well developed, and there are some differences in brain electrical activity between neonates and adults; the electrical activity level of each part of the brain is not consistent. Therefore, the number of electrodes in monitoring the electrical activity of adults should be as large as possible to reflect whole-brain function. Currently, aEEG is mainly used for the diagnosis and monitoring of coma after cardiac arrest and epilepsy, and related research in adult ICUs is rare.

### 17.4.1 Prognosis Assessment of Coma Patients After Cardiac Arrest

Therapeutic hypothermia is an effective method recommended by the current guidelines for the treatment of coma patients after CPR that can improve the survival rate at discharge and the neurological prognosis [24]. Predicting the prognosis of patients with cardiac arrest during TTM remains a challenge. Conventional evaluation methods mainly focus on GCS scores combined with neuroimaging and biochemical tests, but these methods have limitations when used as bedside tools in the NICU. During therapeutic hypothermia, patients need mechanical ventilation, sedation, and intermittent administration of muscle relaxants, which can also prolong drug metabolism due to hypothermia [25]. Patients receiving therapeutic hypothermia will not be able to undergo clinical neurological testing in the first few days after cardiac arrest, and subsequent neurological examinations may be unreliable [26, 27]. Although conventional EEG has been reported as a useful examination method in the early prediction of neurological prognosis [28], it is difficult to identify by critical care physicians and emergency physicians. aEEG solves this issue and is applied to the assessment of neurological prognosis in comatose patients after cardiac arrest in ICUs.

aEEG can better evaluate the prognosis of coma patients after cardiac arrest under the condition of hypothermia. Rundgren et al. [29] used continuous aEEG to monitor the EEG activity of patients with cardiac arrest after mild hypothermia treatment, and a total of 34 comatose patients after cardiac arrest were included. Within 4 h after the initiation of hypothermia treatment, all patients with continuous normal EEG monitoring recovered consciousness. Most of the patients with flat aEEG activity recovered normal aEEG activity and consciousness after rewarming. However, patients with BS did not recover consciousness and died. It is suggested that continuous normal aEEG activity in the early stage of hypothermia therapy is a useful predictor of good prognosis. However, flat aEEG activity in the early stage cannot predict poor prognosis, and the effect of sedatives on aEEG activity in the early stage of disease needs to be considered. Another study [30] included 95 comatose patients after cardiac arrest, and the aEEG monitoring time was extended to 120 h. A similar conclusion was drawn: Continuous normal aEEG activity in the early stage of hypothermia treatment or continuous normal aEEG activity after the return to normal body temperature was related to the recovery of consciousness, while initial flat aEEG activity was not related to the prognosis. Therefore, early continuous normal aEEG activity is a prognostic factor for coma patients after cardiac arrest.

Further study showed that the dynamic changes in aEEG activity had good prediction ability. Sangho et al. [31] included 130 comatose patients after cardiac arrest. After hypothermia treatment, when abnormal aEEG activity evolved into normal aEEG activity within 24 h, the overall prognosis was good; however, taking 36 h as the cutoff point, patients in whom aEEG activity did not return to normal had a poor neurological prognosis (specificity 100%, sensitivity 78.7%, positive predictive value 100%, and negative predictive value 77.5%). Another study [32] found that patients with abnormal aEEG activity not returning to normal within 72 h may have a poor neurological prognosis (specificity 100%, sensitivity 77.8%, positive predictive value 100%, and negative predictive value 82.4%). Sugiyama et al. [33] showed that patients in whom aEEG activity did not return to normal within 23 h had a poor neurological prognosis (specificity 100%, sensitivity 89%, positive predictive value 100%, and negative predictive value 86%). Another study [34] also found that patients with abnormal aEEG developing into normal CNV within 12 h after the restoration of spontaneous circulation after hypothermia treatment have a good prognosis. However, patients without CNV or BS within 36 h in aEEGs have poor prognosis and a low survival rate. In conclusion, aEEGs showing BS or SE at any time indicated a poor prognosis.

In addition, aEEG may also be helpful to evaluate the prognosis of other brain injury patients.

You et al. [35] analyzed the aEEGs of 128 comatose patients after acute brain injury to understand the prognostic value of aEEG in comatose patients with acute brain injury, and the causes of coma included not only cardiac arrest but also brain injury, stroke, SAH, etc. The results showed that most of the patients (44/56, 78.6%) with continuous normal voltage aEEG activity had a good follow-up outcome after 6 months, while the majority (62/81, 76.5%) with continuous extremely low voltage, BS, and a FT had poor neurological outcome after 6 months of follow-up.

### 17.4.2 Application in Epilepsy Patients

Epilepsy or subclinical seizures occur in 16–48% of patients with severe brain injury in NICUs and seriously affect their prognosis [36, 37]. Conventional EEG monitoring should be performed when seizures are clinically suspected, as timely and appropriate treatment can reduce damage to the brain. Subclinical seizures require cEEG monitoring to be detected promptly and reliably. aEEG can be used to detect epilepsy because of its advantages of long-term detection/easy bedside application. In comatose patients after cardiac arrest, SE in EEGs is very common and can be divided into two types: one evolves from BS and the other evolves from CNV. Most patients with SE in EEGs do not recover consciousness and die, suggesting that SE in EEGs is associated with adverse prognosis [30]. Consistent with the results in previous studies, the presentation of SE in aEEGs at any time in comatose patients after cardiac arrest is predictive of poor prognosis, which indicated that aEEG could be used to monitor SE after brain injury and evaluate the prognosis of the disease [31, 33]. In a randomized controlled trial, after short-term (3 h) training, three neurophysiologists compared aEEGs with the original EEGs in patients with suspected epilepsy. The results showed that aEEG had high sensitivity and a low false-positive rate in the recognition of adult epilepsy in the NICU [38].

### 17.4.3 Prognosis Assessment of Anti-NMDAR Encephalitis

Anti-NMDAR encephalitis is an AE, and it accounts for 1% of all ICU admissions of young adults [39]. The presence of the "δ brush" in EEGs is an important marker of anti-NMDAR encephalitis in some but not all patients. Similarly, the presence of the "δ brush" in EEGs does not necessarily indicate anti-NMDAR encephalitis [40, 41]. Therefore, it is necessary to explore additional EEG markers to determine the severity and predict the outcome of anti-NMDAR encephalitis, and aEEG may have predictive value for the prognosis of NMDAR encephalitis. To understand the prognostic value of qEEG in patients with anti-NMDAR encephalitis, Jiang et al. [42] included 26 patients with anti-NMDAR encephalitis and divided them into a critical group and a noncritical group. The short-term and long-term prognoses of these patients were compared. The results showed that most qEEG parameters, including aEEG background activity, total power, 95% SEF, and the power of different brainwave bands, could not reflect the severity of anti-NMDAR encephalitis. However, the study also found that parietal aEEG bandwidth was related to prognosis. Logistic regression analysis showed that the expansion of apical aEEG bandwidth could be used as an objective index to predict poor long-term results. Narrower apical aEEG bandwidth was associated with good long-term prognosis, and the corresponding sensitivity and specificity were 90.00% and 56.25%, respectively. This is a new discovery, and its mechanism cannot be explained. Thus, the role that aEEG may play in predicting the prognosis of NMDAR encephalitis needs further investigation.

At present, aEEG is widely used in PICUs and increasingly used in adult ICUs. In PICUs, aEEG can be used to better evaluate brain maturity and predict the prognosis of encephalopathy, HIE, or SE in newborns. In adult ICUs, aEEG can be used to predict the prognosis of coma patients after CPR and recognize SE. There is a lack of research on the application of aEEG in adult ICUs, and the standards for newborn aEEG interpretation are used to interpret adult aEEGs.

Therefore, more studies are needed to confirm the role of aEEG in predicting the prognosis of brain injury and identifying epileptic discharge in children and adults.

## References


1. Grocott HP, Davie S, Fedorow C. Monitoring of brain function in anesthesia and intensive care. Curr Opin Anaesthesiol. 2010;23(6):759–64.
2. Maynard D, Prior PF, Scott DF. Device for continuous monitoring of cerebral activity in resuscitated patients. Br Med J. 1969;4(5682):545–6.
3. Prior PF, Maynard DE, Sheaff PC, et al. Monitoring cerebral function: clinical experience with new device for continuous recording of electrical activity of brain. Br Med J. 1971;2(5764):736–8.
4. Arnaez J, Sanchez-Acosta CG, Fasce J, et al. Usefulness of two-channel amplitude-integrated EEG recording in a neonatal setting. J Matern Fetal Neonatal Med. 2019;34:1–11.
5. Viniker DA, Maynard DE, Scott DF. Cerebral function monitor studies in neonates. Clin Electroencephalogr. 1984;15(4):185–92.
6. Al NN, Edwards AD, Cowan FM, et al. Assessment of neonatal encephalopathy by amplitude-integrated electroencephalography. Pediatrics. 1999;103(6 Pt 1):1263–71.
7. Hellstrom-Westas L, Rosen I. Continuous brain-function monitoring: state of the art in clinical practice. Semin Fetal Neonatal Med. 2006;11(6):503–11.
8. Awal MA, Lai MM, Azemi G, et al. EEG background features that predict outcome in term neonates with hypoxic ischaemic encephalopathy: a structured review. Clin Neurophysiol. 2016;127(1):285–96.
9. Thoresen M, Hellstrom-Westas L, Liu X, et al. Effect of hypothermia on amplitude-integrated electroencephalogram in infants with asphyxia. Pediatrics. 2010;126(1):e131–9.
10. van Laerhoven H, de Haan TR, Offringa M, et al. Prognostic tests in term neonates with hypoxic-ischemic encephalopathy: a systematic review. Pediatrics. 2013;131(1):88–98.
11. Chandrasekaran M, Chaban B, Montaldo P, et al. Predictive value of amplitude-integrated EEG (aEEG) after rescue hypothermic neuroprotection for hypoxic ischemic encephalopathy: a meta-analysis. J Perinatol. 2017;37(6):684–9.
12. Ouwehand S, Smidt L, Dudink J, et al. Predictors of outcomes in hypoxic-ischemic encephalopathy following hypothermia: a meta-analysis. Neonatology. 2020;117:1–17.
13. Variane G, Magalhaes M, Gasperine R, et al. Early amplitude-integrated electroencephalography for monitoring neonates at high risk for brain injury. J Pediatr. 2017;93(5):460–6.
14. Bourgoin P, Barrault V, Joram N, et al. The prognostic value of early amplitude-integrated electroencephalography monitoring after pediatric cardiac arrest. Pediatr Crit Care Med. 2020;21(3):248–55.
15. Vesoulis ZA, Inder TE, Woodward LJ, et al. Early electrographic seizures, brain injury, and neurodevelopmental risk in the very preterm infant. Pediatr Res. 2014;75(4):564–9.
16. Fogtmann EP, Plomgaard AM, Greisen G, et al. Prognostic accuracy of electroencephalograms in preterm infants: a systematic review. Pediatrics. 2017;139(2):e20161951.
17. Cristina U, Neil M, Janet MR. Outcome following neonatal seizures. Semin Fetal Neonatal Med. 2013;18(4):224–32.
18. Rakshasbhuvankar A, Paul S, Nagarajan L, et al. Amplitude-integrated EEG for detection of neonatal seizures: a systematic review. Seizure. 2015;33:90–8.
19. Kadivar M, Moghadam EM, Shervin BR, et al. A comparison of conventional electroencephalography with amplitude-integrated EEG in detection of neonatal seizures. Med Devices (Auckl). 2019;12:489–96.
20. Rowberry T, Kanthimathinathan HK, George F, et al. Implementation and early evaluation of a quantitative electroencephalography program for seizure detection in the PICU. Pediatr Crit Care Med. 2020;21(6):543–9.
21. Din F, Lalgudi GS, Akiyama T, et al. Seizure detection algorithms in critically ill children: a comparative evaluation. Crit Care Med. 2020;48(4):545–52.
22. Bruns N, Sanchez-Albisua I, Weiss C, et al. Amplitude-integrated EEG for neurological assessment and seizure detection in a German pediatric intensive care unit. Front Pediatr. 2019;7:358.
23. El-Dib M, Chang T, Tsuchida TN, et al. Amplitude-integrated electroencephalography in neonates. Pediatr Neurol. 2009;41(5):315–26.
24. Nolan JP, Deakin CD, Soar J, et al. European Resuscitation Council guidelines for resuscitation 2005. Section 4. Adult advanced life support. Resuscitation. 2005;67(Suppl 1):S39–86.
25. Tortorici MA, Kochanek PM, Poloyac SM. Effects of hypothermia on drug disposition, metabolism, and response: a focus of hypothermia-mediated alterations on the cytochrome P450 enzyme system. Crit Care Med. 2007;35(9):2196–204.
26. Rossetti AO, Oddo M, Logroscino G, et al. Prognostication after cardiac arrest and hypothermia: a prospective study. Ann Neurol. 2010;67(3):301–7.
27. Al TE, Savard M, Sharpe M, et al. Predictors of poor neurologic outcome after induced mild hypothermia following cardiac arrest. Neurology. 2008;71(19):1535–7.
28. Chen R, Bolton CF, Young B. Prediction of outcome in patients with anoxic coma: a clinical and electrophysiologic study. Crit Care Med. 1996;24(4):672–8.
29. Rundgren M, Westhall E, Cronberg T, et al. Continuous amplitude-integrated electroencephalogram predicts outcome in hypothermia-treated cardiac arrest patients. Crit Care Med. 2010;38(9):1838–44.

30. Rundgren M, Rosen I, Friberg H. Amplitude-integrated EEG (aEEG) predicts outcome after cardiac arrest and induced hypothermia. Intensive Care Med. 2006;32(6):836–42.
31. Oh SH, Park KN, Shon YM, et al. Continuous amplitude-integrated electroencephalographic monitoring is a useful prognostic tool for hypothermia-treated cardiac arrest patients. Circulation. 2015;132(12):1094–103.
32. Oh SH, Park KN, Kim YM, et al. The prognostic value of continuous amplitude-integrated electroencephalogram applied immediately after return of spontaneous circulation in therapeutic hypothermia-treated cardiac arrest patients. Resuscitation. 2013;84(2):200–5.
33. Sugiyama K, Kashiura M, Akashi A, et al. Prognostic value of the recovery time of continuous normal voltage in amplitude-integrated electroencephalography in out-of-hospital cardiac arrest patients treated with therapeutic hypothermia: a retrospective study. J Intensive Care. 2016;4:25.
34. Sugiyama K, Miyazaki K, Ishida T, et al. Categorization of post-cardiac arrest patients according to the pattern of amplitude-integrated electroencephalography after return of spontaneous circulation. Crit Care. 2018;22(1):226.
35. You W, Tang Q, Wu X, et al. Amplitude-integrated electroencephalography predicts outcome in patients with coma after acute brain injury. Neurosci Bull. 2018;34(4):639–46.
36. Friedman D, Claassen J, Hirsch LJ. Continuous electroencephalogram monitoring in the intensive care unit. Anesth Analg. 2009;109(2):506–23.
37. DeLorenzo RJ, Waterhouse EJ, Towne AR, et al. Persistent nonconvulsive status epilepticus after the control of convulsive status epilepticus. Epilepsia. 1998;39(8):833–40.
38. Sun J, Ma D, Lv Y. Detection of seizure patterns with multichannel amplitude-integrated EEG and the color density spectral array in the adult neurology intensive care unit. Medicine (Baltimore). 2018;97(38):e12514.
39. Gable MS, Sheriff H, Dalmau J, et al. The frequency of autoimmune N-methyl-D-aspartate receptor encephalitis surpasses that of individual viral etiologies in young individuals enrolled in the California Encephalitis Project. Clin Infect Dis. 2012;54(7):899–904.
40. Zhang Y, Liu G, Jiang MD, et al. Analysis of electroencephalogram characteristics of anti-NMDA receptor encephalitis patients in China. Clin Neurophysiol. 2017;128(7):1227–33.
41. Limotai C, Denlertchaikul C, Saraya AW, et al. Predictive values and specificity of electroencephalographic findings in autoimmune encephalitis diagnosis. Epilepsy Behav. 2018;84:29–36.
42. Jiang N, Guan H, Lu Q, et al. Features and prognostic value of quantitative electroencephalogram changes in critically ill and non-critically ill anti-NMDAR encephalitis patients: a pilot study. Front Neurol. 2018;9:833.

GPSR Compliance

*The European Union's (EU) General Product Safety Regulation (GPSR) is a set of rules that requires consumer products to be safe and our obligations to ensure this.*

*If you have any concerns about our products, you can contact us on ProductSafety@springernature.com*

In case Publisher is established outside the EU, the EU authorized representative is:

Springer Nature Customer Service Center GmbH
Europaplatz 3
69115 Heidelberg, Germany

**Batch number: 10731383**

Printed by Printforce, the Netherlands